a LANGE medical book

Katzung & Trevor's Pharmacology

Examination & Board Review

sixth edition

Anthony J. Trevor, PhD
Professor of Pharmacology and Toxicology
Department of Cellular & Molecular Pharmacology
University of California, San Francisco

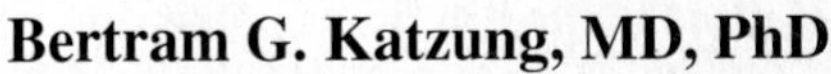
Bertram G. Katzung, MD, PhD
Professor of Pharmacology
Department of Cellular & Molecular Pharmacology
University of California, San Francisco

Susan B. Masters, PhD
Associate Professor of Pharmacology
Department of Cellular & Molecular Pharmacology
University of California, San Francisco

Lange Medical Books/McGraw-Hill
Medical Publishing Division

New York Chicago San Francisco Lisbon London Madrid Mexico City
Milan New Delhi San Juan Seoul Singapore Sydney Toronto

McGraw-Hill

*A Division of The **McGraw-Hill** Companies*

Katzung & Trevor's Pharmacology: Examination & Board Review, Sixth Edition

3 4 5 6 7 8 9 0 DOWDOW 0 9 8 7 6 5 4 3

ISBN: 0-8385-8147-1
ISSN: 1063-8636

Notice

Medicine is an ever-changing science. As new research and clinical experience broaden our knowledge, changes in treatment and drug therapy are required. The authors and the publisher of this work have checked with sources believed to be reliable in their efforts to provide information that is complete and generally in accord with the standards accepted at the time of publication. However, in view of the possibility of human error or changes in medical sciences, neither the authors nor the publisher nor any other party who has been involved in the preparation or publication of this work warrants that the information contained herein is in every respect accurate or complete, and they disclaim all responsibility for any errors or omissions or for the results obtained from use of the information contained in this work. Readers are encouraged to confirm the information contained herein with other sources. For example and in particular, readers are advised to check the product information sheet included in the package of each drug they plan to administer to be certain that the information contained in this work is accurate and that changes have not been made in the recommended dose or in the contraindications for administration. This recommendation is of particular importance in connection with new or infrequently used drugs.

This book was set in Times Roman by Rainbow Graphics.
The editors were Janet Foltin, Harriet Lebowitz, and Peter J. Boyle.
The production supervisor was Catherine Saggese.
The art manager was Charissa Baker.
The index was prepared by Katherine Pitcoff.
RR Donnelley was printer and binder.

This book was printed on acid-free paper.

INTERNATIONAL EDITION ISBN: 0-07-112463-2

Contents

VIII. CHEMOTHERAPEUTIC DRUGS

IX. TOXICOLOGY

X. SPECIAL TOPICS

Preface

This book is designed to help students review pharmacology and to prepare for both regular course examinations and board examinations. The sixth edition has been extensively revised to make such preparation as efficient as possible. As with earlier editions, rigorous standards of accuracy and currency have been maintained, in keeping with the book's status as companion to the textbook *Basic & Clinical Pharmacology*. Several strategies are employed to make reviewing more effective.

First, the book divides pharmacology into the topics used in most courses and textbooks. Major introductory chapters (eg, autonomic pharmacology and CNS pharmacology) are included for integration with relevant physiology and biochemistry. The chapter-based approach facilitates use of this review book in conjunction with course notes or a larger text.

Second, each chapter explicitly lists a set of objectives, providing students with a checklist against which they can challenge themselves as they progress through the book.

Third, each chapter provides a concise review of the core subject matter. Core content is based on careful analysis of the content of current board examinations as well as of major medical school courses. Tables of definitions and diagrams illustrating the major subdivisions within each drug group are provided.

Fourth, tables of important drug names are provided in each chapter dealing with specific drug groups. Recognition of drug names is important for both board and course examinations. Learning the names is made more efficient by distinguishing between drugs important as prototypes, those recognized as major variants, and those that should simply be recognized as belonging to a particular drug group.

Fifth, each chapter ends with practice questions followed by a list of answers and explanations. Questions that require analysis of graphic or tabular data are included. Most of the questions are of the "A" (single best answer) type in keeping with the format adopted by the United States Medical Licensure Examination (USMLE); many are set in the "clinical vignette" format currently favored. Case histories are included in 20 chapters, with questions and answers, providing additional review and testing of the student's preparation for questions about clinical pharmacology. A small proportion of questions are of the "R" (matching and extended matching) type. Appendices II and III present two complete examinations, each covering the entire field of pharmacology. More than 1150 questions (with answers) are provided in this book.

Sixth, Appendix I is an updated list of key drugs that appear frequently in board and course examination questions with concise key word descriptions of their characteristics. This learning aid serves also as an efficient flash-card list of the drugs and those drug properties most likely to appear on an examination.

When studying a discipline, it is important to continually review the basic principles and key information learned previously. To help students do this, most chapters now include a new Skill Keeper feature that consists of questions linking material in the chapter to information presented in previous chapters. Skill Keepers are intended to remind students of important principles discussed in earlier chapters and to facilitate the integration of drug information.

A short appendix on test strategies, which summarizes time-saving devices for approaching specific types of questions used on most objective examinations, is also included.

We recommend that this book be used with a regular text. *Basic & Clinical Pharmacology,* 8th edition (McGraw-Hill, 2001), follows the chapter sequence used here. However, this review book is designed to complement any standard medical pharmacology text. The student who completes and understands *Pharmacology: Examination and Board Review* will greatly improve his or her performance on examinations and will have an excellent command of pharmacology.

Because it was developed in parallel with the textbook *Basic & Clinical Pharmacology,* this review book represents the authors' interpretations of chapters written by contributors to that text. We are very grateful to these contributors, to our other faculty colleagues, and to our students—who have taught us most of what we know about teaching.

Suggestions and criticisms regarding this study guide should be sent to us at the following address: Department of Cellular and Molecular Pharmacology, Box 0450, University of California School of Medicine, San Francisco, CA 94143-0450, USA.

San Francisco
August 2001

Anthony J. Trevor, PhD
Bertram G. Katzung, MD, PhD
Susan B. Masters, PhD

Part I: Basic Principles

Introduction 1

OBJECTIVES

You should be able to:

- Predict the relative ease of permeation of a weak acid or base from a knowledge of its pK_a and the pH of the medium.
- List and discuss the common routes of drug administration and excretion.
- Draw graphs of the blood level versus time for drugs subject to zero-order elimination and for drugs subject to first-order elimination.

Learn the definitions that follow.

Table 1–1. Definitions.

Term	Definition
Pharmacology	The study of the interaction of chemicals with living systems
Drugs	Substances that act on living systems at the chemical (molecular) level
Drug receptors	The molecular components of the body with which a drug interacts to bring about its effects
Medical pharmacology	The study of drugs used for the diagnosis, prevention, and treatment of disease
Toxicology	The study of the undesirable effects of chemical agents on living systems; considered an area of pharmacology. In addition to the adverse effects of therapeutic agents on individuals, toxicology deals with the actions of industrial pollutants, natural organic and inorganic poisons, and other chemicals on species and ecosystems as well
Pharmacodynamics	The actions of a drug on the body, including receptor interactions, dose-response phenomena, and mechanisms of therapeutic and toxic action
Pharmacokinetics	The actions of the body on the drug, including absorption, distribution, metabolism, and excretion. Elimination of a drug may be achieved by metabolism or by excretion. Biodisposition is a term sometimes used to describe the processes of metabolism and excretion

CONCEPTS

A. The Nature of Drugs:

1. **Size and molecular weight (MW):** Drugs in common use vary in size from MW 7 (lithium) to over MW 50,000 (thrombolytic enzymes). The majority of drugs, however, have molecular weights between 100 and 1000.
2. **Drug-receptor bonds:** Drugs bind to receptors with a variety of chemical bonds. These include very strong covalent bonds (which usually result in irreversible action), somewhat weaker electrostatic bonds (eg, between a cation and an anion), and much weaker interactions (eg, hydrogen, van der Waals, and hydrophobic bonds).

B. The Movement of Drugs in the Body: In order to reach its receptors and bring about a biologic effect, a drug molecule (eg, a benzodiazepine sedative) must travel from the site of administration (eg, the gastrointestinal tract) to the site of action (eg, the brain).

1. **Permeation:** Permeation is the movement of drug molecules into and within the biologic environment. It involves several processes, of which the following are the most important:
   a. **Aqueous diffusion:** Aqueous diffusion is the movement of molecules through the watery extracellular and intracellular spaces. The membranes of most capillaries have small water-filled pores that permit the aqueous diffusion of molecules up to the size of small proteins between the blood and the extravascular space. This is a passive process governed by Fick's law (see below).
   b. **Lipid diffusion:** Lipid diffusion is the movement of molecules through membranes and other lipid structures. Like aqueous diffusion, this is a passive process governed by Fick's law (see below).
   c. **Transport by special carriers:** Drugs may be transported across barriers by mechanisms that carry similar endogenous substances, eg, the amino acid carriers in the blood-brain barrier and the weak acid carriers in the renal tubule. Unlike aqueous and lipid diffusion, carrier transport is not governed by Fick's law and is capacity-limited. Selective inhibitors for these carriers may have clinical value; eg, probenecid, which inhibits transport of uric acid, penicillin, and other weak acids, is used to increase the excretion of uric acid in gout. The family of P-glycoprotein transport molecules, previously identified as one cause of cancer drug resistance, has recently been identified in the epithelium of the gastrointestinal tract and appears to be responsible for expulsion of certain drugs into the intestinal lumen.
   d. **Endocytosis, pinocytosis:** Endocytosis occurs through binding to specialized components (receptors) on cell membranes, with subsequent internalization by infolding of that area of the membrane. The contents of the resulting vesicle are subsequently released into the cytoplasm of the cell. Endocytosis permits very large or very lipid-insoluble chemicals to enter cells. For example, large molecules such as peptides may enter cells by this mechanism. Smaller, polar substances such as vitamin B_{12} and iron combine with special proteins (B_{12} with intrinsic factor and iron with transferrin), and the complexes enter cells by this mechanism. Exocytosis is the reverse process, ie, the expulsion of membrane-encapsulated material from cells.
2. **Fick's law of diffusion:** Fick's law predicts the rate of movement of molecules across a barrier; the concentration gradient ($C_1 - C_2$) and permeability coefficient for the drug and the area and thickness of the barrier membrane are used to compute the rate, as follows:

$$\textbf{Rate} = (C_1 - C_2) \times \frac{\textbf{Permeability coefficient}}{\textbf{Thickness}} \times \textbf{Area} \qquad (1)$$

   This relationship quantifies the observations that drug absorption is faster from organs with large surface areas, eg, the small intestine, than from organs with small absorbing areas, eg, the stomach. Furthermore, drug absorption is faster from organs with thin membrane barriers, eg, the lung, than from those with thick barriers, eg, the skin.
3. **Water and lipid solubility of drugs:**
   a. **Aqueous diffusion:** The aqueous solubility of a drug is often a function of the electrostatic charge (degree of ionization, polarity) of the molecule, because water molecules behave as dipoles and are attracted to charged drug molecules, forming an aqueous shell around them. Conversely, the lipid solubility of a molecule is inversely proportionate to its charge.
   b. **Lipid diffusion:** Many drugs are weak bases or weak acids. For such molecules, the *pH of the medium* determines the fraction of molecules charged (ionized) versus uncharged (nonionized). If the pK_a of the drug and the pH of the medium are known, the fraction of molecules in the ionized state can be predicted by means of the Henderson-Hasselbalch equation:

$$\log\left(\frac{\textbf{Protonated form}}{\textbf{Unprotonated form}}\right) = \textbf{pK}_a - \textbf{pH} \qquad (2)$$

"Protonated" means *associated with a proton* (a hydrogen ion); this form of the equation applies to both acids and bases.

c. **Ionization of weak acids and bases:** Weak bases are ionized—and therefore more polar and more water-soluble—when they are protonated; weak acids are not ionized—and so are less water-soluble—when they are protonated.

The following equations summarize these points:

$RNH_3^+ \rightleftharpoons$	RNH_2 +	H^+	
protonated weak base (charged, more water-soluble)	**unprotonated weak base (uncharged, more lipid-soluble)**	**proton**	**(3)**

$RCOOH \rightleftharpoons$	$RCOO^-$ +	H^+	
protonated weak acid (uncharged, more lipid-soluble)	**unprotonated weak acid (charged, more water-soluble)**	**proton**	**(4)**

The Henderson-Hasselbalch relationship is clinically important when it is necessary to accelerate the excretion of drugs by the kidney, eg, in the case of an overdose. Most drugs are freely filtered at the glomerulus, but lipid-soluble drugs can be rapidly reabsorbed from the tubular urine. When a patient takes an overdose of a weak acid drug, its excretion may be accelerated by alkalinizing the urine, eg, by giving bicarbonate. This is because a drug that is a weak acid dissociates to its charged, polar form in alkaline solution and this form cannot readily diffuse from the renal tubule back into the blood. Conversely, excretion of a weak base may be accelerated by acidifying the urine, eg, by administering ammonium chloride (Figure 1–1).

C. Absorption of Drugs:

1. **Routes of administration:** Drugs usually enter the body at sites remote from the target tissue or organ and thus require transport by the circulation to the intended site of action. To enter the bloodstream, a drug must be absorbed from its site of administration (unless the drug has been injected directly into the bloodstream). The rate and efficiency of absorption differ depending on a drug's route of administration. In fact, for some drugs, the amount absorbed into the circulation may be only a small fraction of the dose administered

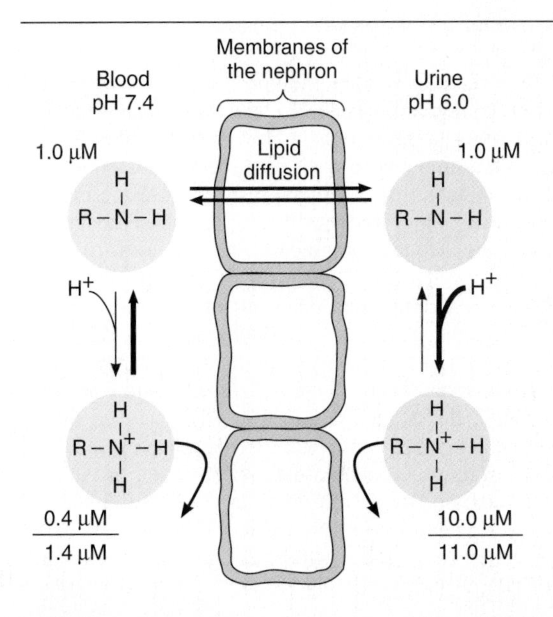

Figure 1–1. "Trapping" is a method for accelerating excretion of drugs. Because the nonionized form diffuses readily across the lipid barriers of the nephron, this form will equilibrate and may reach equal concentrations in the blood and urine; the ionized form will not. Protonation will occur within the blood and the urine according to the Henderson-Hasselbalch equation. Pyrimethamine, a weak base of pK_a 7.0, is used in this example. At blood pH, only 0.4 μmol of the protonated species will be present for each 1.0 μmol of the unprotonated form. The total concentration in the blood will thus be 1.4 μmol/L if the concentration of the unprotonated form is 1.0 μmol/L. In the urine at pH 6.0, 10 μmol of the nondiffusible ionized form will be present for each 1.0 μmol of the unprotonated, diffusible, form. Therefore, the total urine concentration (11 μmol/L) may be almost eight times higher than the blood concentration.

when given by certain routes. The amount absorbed divided by the amount administered constitutes its **bioavailability.** Common routes of administration and some of their features include the following:

a. **Oral (swallowed):** The oral route offers maximum convenience, but absorption may be slower and less complete than when parenteral routes are used. Ingested drugs are subject to the **first-pass effect,** in which a significant amount of the agent is metabolized in the gut wall and the liver before it reaches the systemic circulation. Thus, some drugs have low bioavailability when given orally.

b. **Intravenous:** The intravenous route offers instantaneous and complete absorption (by definition, bioavailability is 100%). This route is potentially more dangerous, however, because of the high blood levels that are produced if administration is too rapid.

c. **Intramuscular:** Absorption from an intramuscular injection site is often (not always) faster and more complete (higher bioavailability) than with oral administration. Large volumes (eg, > 5 mL into each buttock) may be given. First-pass metabolism is avoided.

d. **Subcutaneous:** The subcutaneous route offers slower absorption than the intramuscular route. Large volume bolus doses are less feasible. First-pass metabolism is avoided.

e. **Buccal and sublingual:** The buccal route (in the pouch between gums and cheek) permits direct absorption into the systemic venous circulation, bypassing the hepatic portal circuit and first-pass metabolism. This process may be fast or slow depending on the physical formulation of the product. The sublingual route (under the tongue) offers the same features as the buccal route.

f. **Rectal (suppository):** The rectal route offers partial avoidance from the first-pass effect (though not as completely as the sublingual route). Larger amounts of drug and drugs with unpleasant taste are better administered rectally than by the buccal or sublingual routes. Some drugs administered rectally may cause significant irritation.

g. **Inhalation:** In the case of respiratory diseases, the inhalation route offers delivery closest to the target tissue. This route often provides rapid absorption because of the large alveolar surface area available.

h. **Topical:** The topical route includes application to the skin or to the mucous membrane of the eye, nose, throat, airway, or vagina for *local* effect. The rate of absorption varies with the area of application and the drug formulation, but is usually slower than any of the routes listed above.

i. **Transdermal:** The transdermal route involves application to the skin for *systemic* effect. Absorption usually occurs very slowly, but the first-pass effect is avoided.

D. Distribution of Drugs:

1. **Determinants of distribution:** The distribution of drugs to the tissues depends upon the following:

a. **Size of the organ:** The size of the organ determines the concentration gradient between blood and the organ. For example, skeletal muscle can take up a large amount of drug because the concentration in the muscle tissue remains low (and the blood-tissue gradient high) even after relatively large amounts of drug have been transferred; this occurs because skeletal muscle is a very large organ. In contrast, because the brain is smaller, distribution of a smaller amount of drug into it will raise the tissue concentration and reduce to zero the blood-tissue concentration gradient, preventing further uptake of drug.

b. **Blood flow:** Blood flow to the tissue is an important determinant of the *rate* of uptake, although blood flow may not affect the steady state amount of drug in the tissue. As a result, well-perfused tissues (eg, brain, heart, kidneys, splanchnic organs) will often achieve high tissue concentrations sooner than poorly perfused tissues (eg, fat, bone). If the drug is rapidly eliminated, the concentration in poorly perfused tissues may never rise significantly.

c. **Solubility:** The solubility of a drug in tissue influences the concentration of the drug in the extracellular fluid surrounding the blood vessels. If the drug is very soluble in the cells, the concentration in the perivascular extracellular space will be lower and diffusion from the vessel into the extravascular tissue space will be facilitated. For example, some organs (including the brain) have a high lipid content and thus dissolve a high concentration of lipid-soluble agents. As a result, a very lipid-soluble anesthetic will transfer out of the blood and into the brain tissue to a greater extent than a drug with low lipid solubility.

d. **Binding:** Binding of a drug to macromolecules in the blood or a tissue compartment will tend to increase the drug's concentration in that compartment. For example, warfarin is strongly bound to plasma albumin, which restricts warfarin's diffusion out of the vascular compartment. Conversely, chloroquine is strongly bound to tissue proteins, which results in a marked reduction in the plasma concentration of chloroquine.

2. **Apparent volume of distribution:** The apparent volume of distribution (V_d) is an important pharmacokinetic parameter that reflects the above determinants of drug distribution in the body. V_d relates the amount of drug in the body to the concentration in the plasma. (See Chapter 3 and Table 1–2.)

E. **Metabolism of Drugs:** Metabolism of a drug sometimes terminates its action, but other effects of drug metabolism are also important. Some drugs, when given orally, are metabolized before they enter the systemic circulation. This **first-pass metabolism** was referred to above as one cause of low bioavailability. Other drugs are administered as inactive **prodrugs** and must be metabolized to active agents. Some drugs are not metabolized at all—their action must be terminated by excretion.

1. **Drug metabolism as a mechanism of termination of drug action:** The action of many drugs (eg, phenothiazines) is terminated before they are excreted because they are metabolized to biologically inactive derivatives.
2. **Drug metabolism as a mechanism of drug activation: Prodrugs** (eg, levodopa, methyldopa, parathion) are inactive as administered and must be metabolized in the body to become active. Many drugs are active as administered and have active metabolites as well, eg, many benzodiazepines.
3. **Drug elimination without metabolism:** Some drugs (eg, lithium) are not modified by the body; they continue to act until they are excreted.

F. **Elimination of Drugs:** Along with the dosage, the rate of elimination (disappearance of the active molecule from the bloodstream or body) determines the duration of action for most drugs. Therefore, knowledge of the time course of concentration in plasma is important in predicting the intensity and duration of effect for most drugs. ***Note:*** Drug *elimination* is not the same as drug *excretion:* a drug may be eliminated by metabolism long before the modified molecules are excreted from the body. Furthermore, for drugs with active metabolites (eg, diazepam), elimination of the parent molecule by metabolism is not synonymous with termination of action. For drugs that are not metabolized, excretion is the mode of elimination. A small number of drugs combine irreversibly with their receptors, so that disappearance from the bloodstream is not equivalent to cessation of drug action: these drugs may have a very prolonged action. For example, phenoxybenzamine, an irreversible inhibitor of alpha adrenoceptors, is eliminated from the bloodstream in an hour or less after administration. The drug's action, however, lasts for 48 hours.

1. **First-order elimination:** The term *first-order elimination* implies that the rate of elimination is proportionate to the concentration, ie, the higher the concentration, the greater the amount of drug eliminated per unit time. The result is that the drug's concentration in plasma decreases exponentially with time (Figure 1–2, left). Drugs with first-order elimination have a characteristic **half-life of elimination** that is constant regardless of the amount

Table 1–2. Average values for some physical volumes within the adult human body.

Compartment	Volume (L/kg Body Weight)
Plasma	0.04
Blood	0.08
Extracellular water	0.2
Total body water	0.6
Fat	0.2–0.35

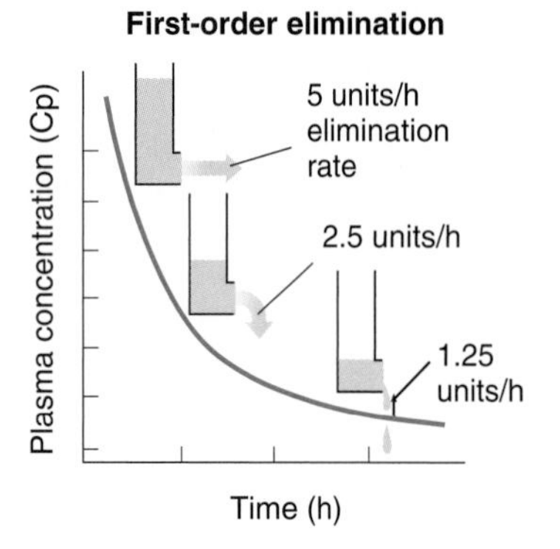

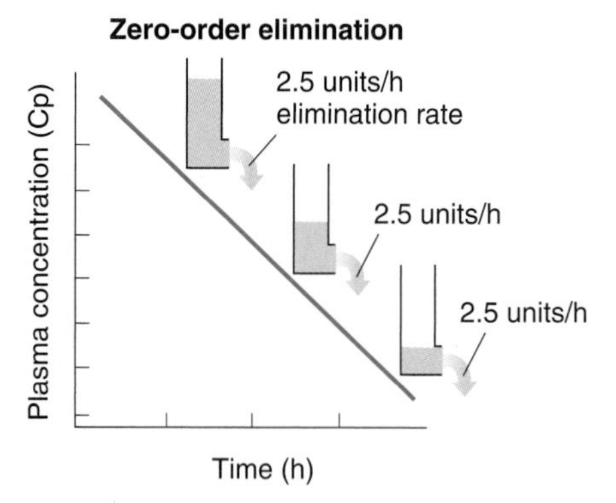

Figure 1–2. Comparison of first-order and zero-order elimination. For drugs with first-order kinetics (left panel), rate of elimination is proportionate to concentration; in the case of zero-order elimination (right panel), the rate is constant and independent of concentration.

of drug in the body. The concentration of such a drug in the blood will decrease by 50% for every half-life. Most drugs in clinical use demonstrate first-order kinetics.

2. **Zero-order elimination:** The term *zero-order elimination* implies that the rate of elimination is constant regardless of concentration (Figure 1–2, right panel). A few drugs saturate their elimination mechanisms even at low concentrations. As a result, the drug's concentration in plasma decreases in a linear fashion over time. This is typical of ethanol (over most of its plasma concentration range) and of phenytoin and aspirin at high therapeutic or toxic concentrations.

G. Pharmacokinetic Models:

1. **Multicompartment distribution:** After absorption, many drugs undergo an early distribution phase followed by a slower elimination phase. Mathematically, this behavior can be modeled by means of a "two-compartment model" as shown in Figure 1–3. (Note that each phase is associated with a characteristic half-life: $t_{1/2\alpha}$ for the first phase, $t_{1/2\beta}$ for the second phase.)
2. **Single-compartment distribution:** A few drugs may behave as if they are distributed to only one compartment (eg, if they are restricted to the vascular compartment). Others have more complex distributions that require more than two compartments for construction of accurate mathematical models.

QUESTIONS

DIRECTIONS: Each of the numbered items or incomplete statements in this section is followed by answers or by completions of the statement. Select the ONE lettered answer or completion that is BEST in each case.

1. A 3-year-old child is brought to the emergency department having just ingested a large overdose of promethazine, an antihistaminic drug. Promethazine is a weak base with a pK_a of 9.1. It is capable of entering most tissues, including the brain. On physical examination, the heart rate is 100/min, blood pressure 110/60 mm Hg, and respiratory rate 20/min. In this case of promethazine overdose,
   (A) Urinary excretion would be accelerated by administration of NH_4Cl
   (B) Urinary excretion would be accelerated by giving $NaHCO_3$
   (C) More of the drug would be ionized at blood pH than at stomach pH
   (D) Absorption of the drug would be faster from the stomach than from the small intestine
   (E) Hemodialysis is the only effective therapy
2. All of the following are general mechanisms of drug permeation EXCEPT
   (A) Aqueous diffusion
   (B) Aqueous hydrolysis
   (C) Lipid diffusion
   (D) Pinocytosis or endocytosis
   (E) Special carrier transport

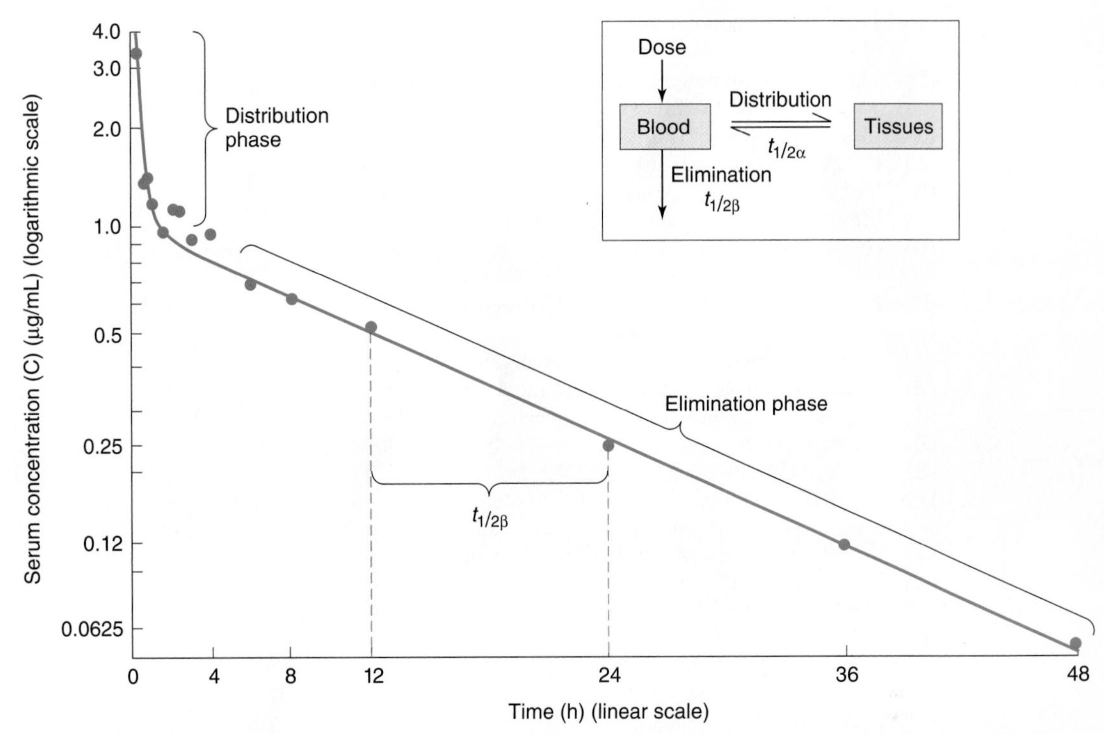

Figure 1–3. Serum concentration-time curve after administration of chlordiazepoxide as an intravenous bolus. The experimental data are plotted on a semilogarithmic scale as filled circles. This drug follows first-order kinetics and appears to occupy two compartments. The initial curvilinear portion of the data represents the distribution phase, with drug equilibrating between the blood compartment and the tissue compartment. The linear portion of the curve represents drug elimination. The elimination half-life ($t_{1/2\beta}$) can be extracted graphically as shown by measuring the time between any two plasma concentration points that differ by twofold. (See Chapter 3 for additional details.) (Modified and reproduced, with permission, from Greenblatt DJ, Koch-Weser J: Drug therapy: Clinical pharmacokinetics. N Engl J Med 1975;293:702.)

3. A patient with a history of episodic attacks of coughing, wheezing, and shortness of breath is being evaluated in the asthma clinic. Several drug treatments with different routes of administration are under consideration. Which of the following statements about routes of administration is MOST correct?
- **(A)** Blood levels often rise more slowly after intramuscular injection than after oral dosing
- **(B)** The "first-pass" effect is the result of metabolism of a drug after administration and before it enters the systemic circulation
- **(C)** Administration of antiasthmatic drugs by inhaled aerosol is usually associated with more adverse effects than is administration of these drugs by mouth
- **(D)** Bioavailability of most drugs is greater with rectal (suppository) administration than with sublingual administration
- **(E)** Administration of a drug by transdermal patch is often faster but is associated with more first-pass metabolism than oral administration

4. Aspirin is a weak organic acid with a pK_a of 3.5. What percentage of a given dose will be in the lipid-soluble form at a stomach pH of 2.5?
- **(A)** About 1%
- **(B)** About 10%
- **(C)** About 50%
- **(D)** About 90%
- **(E)** About 99%

5. If the plasma concentration of a drug declines with "first-order kinetics," this means that
- **(A)** There is only one metabolic path for drug disposition
- **(B)** The half-life is the same regardless of the plasma concentration

(C) The drug is largely metabolized in the liver after oral administration and has low bioavailability
(D) The rate of elimination is proportionate to the rate of administration at all times
(E) The drug is not distributed outside the vascular system

6. Regarding termination of drug action,
(A) Drugs must be excreted from the body to terminate their action
(B) Metabolism of drugs always increases their water solubility
(C) Metabolism of drugs always abolishes their pharmacologic activity
(D) Hepatic metabolism and renal excretion are the two most important mechanisms involved
(E) Distribution of a drug out of the bloodstream terminates the drug's effects

7. Distribution of drugs to specific tissues
(A) Is independent of blood flow to the organ
(B) Is independent of the solubility of the drug in that tissue
(C) Depends on the unbound drug concentration gradient between blood and the tissue
(D) Is increased for drugs that are strongly bound to plasma proteins
(E) Has no effect on the half-life of the drug

8. Pilocarpine is being considered for the treatment of glaucoma in a 58-year-old patient. Except for elevated intraocular pressure, the patient's history and physical exam are unremarkable. Pilocarpine is a weak base of pK_a 6.9. Which of the following statements is FALSE?
(A) After parenteral administration, the concentration of pilocarpine in the aqueous humor (pH 7.8) will be lower than the concentration in the duodenum (pH 5.5)
(B) When administered as eye drops, absorption into the eye will be faster if the drops are alkaline (pH 8.0) than if they are acidic (pH 5.0)
(C) Excretion in the urine will be faster if urine pH is alkaline (pH 8.0) than if the urine pH is acidic (pH 5.8)
(D) The proportion of pilocarpine in the protonated form will be approximately 90% at pH 5.9
(E) The proportion of pilocarpine in the more lipid soluble form will be approximately 99% at pH 8.9

9. For which of the following drugs will excretion be most significantly accelerated by acidification of the urine?
(A) Weak acid with pK_a of 5.5
(B) Weak base with pK_a of 3.5
(C) Weak acid with pK_a of 7.5
(D) Weak base with pK_a of 6.5

10. A physical process by which a weak acid becomes less water-soluble and more lipid-soluble at low pH is:
(A) Distribution
(B) Elimination
(C) First-pass effect
(D) Permeation
(E) Protonation

DIRECTIONS (Items 11–15): Each set of matching questions in this section consists of a list of lettered options followed by several numbered items. For each numbered item, select the ONE lettered option that is most closely associated with it. Each lettered option may be selected once, more than once, or not at all.

Items 11–15:
(A) Distribution
(B) Elimination
(C) Endocytosis
(D) First-pass effect
(E) First-order kinetics
(F) Lipid solubility
(G) Permeation
(H) Pharmacodynamics
(I) Pharmacokinetics

(J) Protonation
(K) Volume of distribution
(L) Zero-order kinetics

11. Properties that characterize the effects of a drug on the body
12. Properties that describe the effects of the body on a drug
13. Process by which the amount of active drug in the body is reduced after absorption into the systemic circulation
14. Process by which drug in the body is reduced after administration but before entering the systemic circulation
15. Kinetics that are characteristic of the excretion of ethanol and high doses of phenytoin and aspirin

ANSWERS

1. Questions that deal with acid-base (Henderson-Hasselbalch) manipulations are common. Since absorption involves permeation across lipid membranes, we can treat an overdose by decreasing absorption from the gut and reabsorption from the tubular urine by making the drug *less lipid-soluble*. Ionization attracts water molecules and decreases lipid solubility. Promethazine is a weak base—which means that it will be more ionized (protonated) at acid pH than at basic pH. Choice **(C)** suggests that the drug would be more ionized at pH 7.4 than at pH 2.0: clearly wrong. **(D)** says (in effect) that the more ionized form will be absorbed faster, and that is wrong. **(A)** and **(B)** are opposites, since NH_4Cl is an acidifying salt and sodium bicarbonate an alkalinizing one. From the point of view of test strategy, opposites always deserve careful attention and, in this case, encourage us to exclude **(E),** a distracter. Since an acid environment favors ionization of a weak base, we should give NH_4Cl. The answer is **(A).**

2. Hydrolysis has nothing to do with the mechanisms of permeation; rather, hydrolysis is one mechanism of drug metabolism. The answer is **(B).**

3. Blood levels usually rise more *rapidly* after intramuscular injection than after oral administration. **(C)** is wrong: delivering the drug directly to the target organ usually *reduces* adverse effects, because the required total dose is smaller and the concentration reaching other organs is lower. Bioavailability is usually greater after sublingual than after rectal administration. This is because suppositories tend to migrate upward in the rectum and absorption from this location is partially into the portal circulation. Onset of effect is usually slower with transdermal administration than with any other route; but it does permit absorption directly into the systemic venous circulation. The answer is **(B).**

4. Aspirin is an acid, so it will be more ionized at alkaline pH and less ionized at acidic pH. The Henderson-Hasselbalch equation predicts that the ratio will change from 50/50 at the pH equal to the pK_a to 10/1 (protonated/unprotonated) at 1 pH unit more acidic than the pK_a. For acids, the protonated form is the nonionized, more lipid-soluble form. The answer is **(D).**

5. See pages 5–6 of this unit. First-order means that the elimination rate is proportionate to the concentration perfusing the organ of elimination. One result of this proportionality is that a plot of the logarithm of the plasma concentration on the vertical axis versus time on the horizontal axis is a straight line. The half-life is a constant. The rate of elimination is proportionate to the rate of administration only at steady state. Zero-order elimination means that a constant number of moles or grams are eliminated per unit time regardless of the plasma concentration. The half-life will then be concentration-dependent and is not a useful variable. Ethanol is the most common drug with zero-order elimination. The answer is **(B).**

6. Note the "trigger" words ("must," "always") in choices **(A), (B),** and **(C).** All drugs that affect tissues other than the blood or vascular endothelium act outside of the "bloodstream." The answer is **(D).**

7. This is a straightforward question of distribution concepts. There are no trigger words to give the answer away, but it can be deduced without much trouble. From the list of determinants of drug distribution given previously, choice **(C)** is correct.

8. More Henderson-Hasselbalch concepts. Weak bases are more protonated in an acidic environment because more protons (hydrogen ions) are available. In the protonated state, weak bases are ionized, polar, and less lipid soluble. Therefore, less pilocarpine is lipid-soluble and able to diffuse through the duodenum (pH 5.5) than is able to diffuse through the surface of the eye (pH 7.8). By the same reasoning, the drug diffuses faster if the eye drops are alkaline than if they are acidic. Less drug diffuses back into the body from the urine if the urine pH is acidic than if it is alkaline, so excretion will be faster in acidic urine. The answer is **(C).**

9. The excretion of weak bases is accelerated by acidification of the urine. Which of the weak bases listed would be more responsive to acidification? Consider that urine pH can be modified over the range of 5.5 to 8.0. The weak base of pK_a 6.5 would shift from 90% nonionized at pH 7.5 to 90% ionized at pH 5.5. A major increase in excretion might be expected. On the other hand, the weak base of pK_a 3.5 would be 99.99% ionized at pH 7.5 and still 99% ionized at pH 5.5. This would not result in a major change in excretion. The answer is **(D).**
10. Protonation (combination with a proton, H^+) causes a weak acid to lose its negative electrical charge and become less polar and more lipid soluble. The answer is **(E).**
11. More definitions. Pharmacodynamics is the term given to the properties of drug action on the body. The answer is **(H).**
12. Pharmacokinetics is the general term that describes all of the body's actions on the drug. The answer is **(I).**
13. The amount of active drug is reduced by excretion and metabolism, processes that are included in the term "elimination." The answer is **(B).**
14. "First-pass effect" is the term given to elimination of a drug before it enters the systemic circulation, ie, on its first pass through the liver. The answer is **(D).**
15. The excretion of most drugs is determined by first-order kinetics. However, ethanol—and, in higher doses, aspirin and phenytoin—follow zero-order kinetics, ie, their elimination rates are constant regardless of blood concentration. The answer is **(L).**

2 Pharmacodynamics

OBJECTIVES

You should be able to:

- Compare the efficacy and the potency of two drugs on the basis of their dose-response curves.
- Predict the effect of a partial agonist in a patient in the presence and in the absence of a full agonist.
- Name two proteins in blood that have important inert drug binding sites.
- Predict the effect of adding drug B when a barely subtoxic dose of drug A is present, if drug A and drug B both bind to the same inert binding sites.
- Specify whether an antagonist is competitive or irreversible based on its effect on the dose-response curve of an agonist.
- Give examples of competitive and irreversible pharmacologic antagonists, and physiologic and chemical antagonists.
- Name the coupling and effector proteins activated by muscarinic (M_1, M_2, M_3), alpha, and beta receptors.
- Name five transmembrane signaling methods by which drug-receptor interactions exert their effects.

Learn the definitions that follow.

Table 2–1. Definitions.

Term	Definition
Receptor	Component of the biologic system to which a drug binds to bring about a change in function of the system
Inert binding site	Component of the biologic system to which a drug binds without changing any function
Receptor site	Specific region of the receptor molecule at which the drug binds
Agonist	A drug that activates its receptor upon binding
Effector	Component of the biologic system that accomplishes the biologic effect after being activated by the receptor; often a channel or enzyme
Pharmacologic antagonist	A drug that binds to its receptor without activating it
Competitive antagonist	A pharmacologic antagonist that can be overcome by increasing the dose of agonist
Irreversible antagonist	A pharmacologic antagonist that cannot be overcome by increasing the dose of agonist
Physiologic antagonist	A drug that counters the effects of another by binding to a different receptor and causing opposing effects
Chemical antagonist	A drug that counters the effects of another by binding the drug and preventing its action
Partial agonist	A drug that binds to its receptor but produces a smaller effect at full dosage than a full agonist
Graded dose-response curve	A graph of the increasing responses to increasing doses of a drug
Quantal dose-response curve	A graph of the fraction of a population that shows a specified response to increasing doses of a drug
EC_{50}	In graded dose-response curves, the concentration or dose that produces 50% of the maximum possible response; in quantal dose-response curves, the dose that causes the specified response in 50% of the population
K_d	The concentration of drug that results in binding to 50% of the receptors
Efficacy	The maximum effect a drug can bring about, regardless of dose
Potency	The dose or concentration required to bring about 50% of a drug's maximal effect
Spare receptors	Receptors that do not have to bind drug in order for the maximum effect to be produced; ie, K_d greater than the EC_{50}

PHARMACODYNAMIC CONCEPTS

Pharmacodynamics (this chapter) deals with the effects of drugs on biologic systems, while pharmacokinetics (Chapter 3) deals with actions of the biologic system on the drug. The principles of pharmacodynamics apply to all biologic systems, from isolated receptors in the test tube to patients with specific diseases. The most important principles are discussed below.

A. **Receptors:** Receptors are the specific molecules in a biologic system with which drugs interact to produce changes in the function of the system. Receptors must be selective in their ligand-binding characteristics (so as to respond to the proper chemical signal and not to meaningless ones). Receptors also must be modified as a result of binding an agonist molecule (so as to bring about the functional change). Many receptors have been identified, purified, chemically characterized, and cloned. The majority of the receptors characterized to date are proteins; a few are other macromolecules such as DNA. The **receptor site** or **recognition site** for a drug is the specific binding region of the macromolecule and has a high and selective affinity for the drug molecule. The interaction of a drug with its receptor is the fundamental event that initiates the action of the drug.

B. **Effectors:** Effectors are molecules that translate the drug-receptor interaction into a change in cellular activity. The best examples of effectors are enzymes such as adenylyl cyclase. Some receptors are also effectors in that a single molecule may incorporate both the drug binding site and the effector mechanism, eg, the tyrosine kinase effector of the insulin receptor, or the sodium-potassium channel of the nicotinic acetylcholine receptor.

C. Graded Dose-Response Relationships: When the response of a particular receptor-effector system is measured against increasing concentrations of a drug, the graph of the response versus the drug concentration or dose is called a graded dose-response curve (Figure 2–1, panel A). Plotting the same data on semilogarithmic axes usually results in a sigmoid curve, which simplifies the mathematical manipulation of the dose-response data (Figure 2–1, panel B). The efficacy (**E_{max}**) and potency (**EC_{50}**) parameters are derived from these data. The *smaller* the EC_{50}, the *greater* the potency of the drug.

D. Graded Dose-Drug Binding Relationship and Binding Affinity: It is possible to measure the fraction of receptors bound by drug and by plotting this fraction against the log of the concentration of drug, a graph similar to the dose-response curve is obtained (Figure 2–1, panel C). The concentration of drug required to bind 50% of the receptor sites is denoted the **K_d** and is a useful measure of the affinity of a drug molecule for its binding site on the receptor molecule. The smaller the K_d, the greater the affinity of the drug for its receptor. If the number of binding sites on each receptor molecule is known, it is possible to determine the total number of receptors in the system from the **B_{max}**.

E. Quantal Dose-Response Relationships: When the minimum dose required to produce a specified response is determined in each member of a population, the quantal dose-response relationship is defined (Figure 2–2). When plotted as the fraction of the population that responds at each dose versus the log of the dose administered, a cumulative quantal dose-response curve, usually sigmoid in shape, is obtained. The **median effective (ED_{50}), median toxic (TD_{50}),** and **median lethal doses (LD_{50})** are extracted from experiments carried out in this manner.

F. Efficacy: Efficacy, often called maximal efficacy, is the maximal effect (E_{max}) an agonist can produce if the dose is taken to very high levels. Efficacy is determined mainly by the nature of the receptor and its associated effector system. It can be measured with a graded dose-response curve (Figure 2–1) but not with a quantal dose-response curve. By definition, partial agonists have lower maximal efficacy than full agonists (see below).

G. Potency: Potency denotes the amount of a drug needed to produce a given effect. In graded dose-response measurements, the effect usually chosen is 50% of the maximal effect and the dose causing this effect is called the **EC_{50}** (Figure 2–1, panels A and B). Potency is determined mainly by the affinity of the receptor for the drug. In quantal dose-response measurements **ED_{50}, TD_{50},** and **LD_{50}** are typical potency variables (median effective, toxic, and lethal doses, respectively, in 50% of the population studied). Thus, potency can be determined from either graded or quantal dose-response curves (eg, Figures 2–1 and 2–2), but the numbers obtained are not identical.

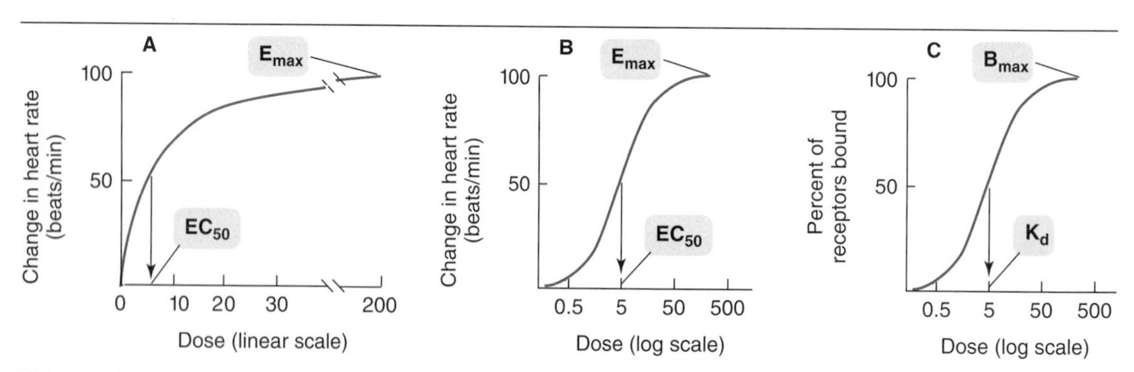

Figure 2–1. Graded dose-response and dose-binding graphs. ***A.*** Relation between drug dose or concentration and drug effect. When the dose axis is linear, a hyperbolic curve is commonly obtained. ***B.*** Same data, logarithmic dose axis. The dose or concentration at which effect is half-maximal is denoted EC_{50}, while the maximal effect is E_{max}. ***C.*** If the percentage of receptors that bind drug is plotted against drug concentration, a similar curve is obtained, and the concentration at which 50% of the receptors are bound is denoted K_d and the maximal number of receptors bound is termed B_{max}.

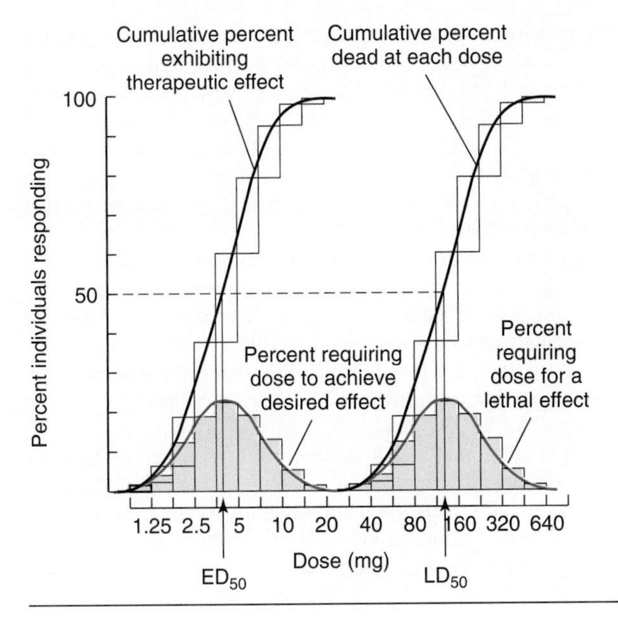

Figure 2–2. Quantal dose-response plots from a study of the therapeutic and lethal effects of a new drug in mice. Shaded boxes (and the accompanying curves) indicate the frequency distribution of doses of drug required to produce a specified effect, ie, the percentage of animals that required a particular dose to exhibit the effect. The open boxes (and corresponding curves) indicate the cumulative frequency distribution of responses, which are lognormally distributed. (Reproduced, with permission, from Katzung BG [editor]: *Basic & Clinical Pharmacology,* 8th ed. McGraw-Hill, 2001.)

H. Spare Receptors: Spare receptors are said to exist if the maximal drug response is obtained at less than maximal occupation of the receptors. In practice, the determination is usually made by comparing the concentration for 50% of maximal effect (EC_{50}) with the concentration for 50% of maximal binding (K_d). If the EC_{50} is less than the K_d, spare receptors are said to exist (Figure 2–3). This might result from one of several mechanisms. First, the effect of the drug-receptor interaction may persist for a much longer time than the interaction itself. Second, the actual number of receptors may exceed the number of effector molecules available. The presence of spare receptors increases sensitivity to the agonist because the likelihood of a drug-receptor interaction increases in proportion to the number of receptors available. (For contrast, the system depicted in Figure 2–1, panels B and C, does not have spare receptors, since the EC_{50} and the K_d are equal.)

I. Inert Binding Sites: Inert binding sites are components of endogenous molecules that bind a drug without initiating events leading to any of the drug's effects. In some compartments of the body (eg, the plasma), inert binding sites play an important role in buffering the concentration of a drug because bound drug does not contribute directly to the concentration gradient that drives diffusion. The two most important plasma proteins with significant binding capacity are **albumin** and **orosomucoid (α_1-acid glycoprotein).**

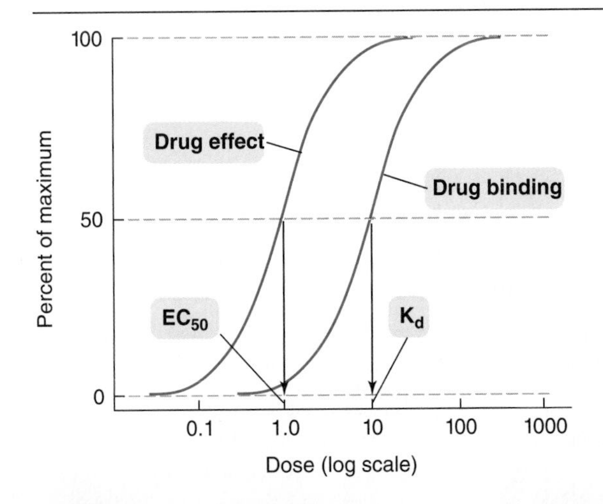

Figure 2–3. In a system with spare receptors, the EC_{50} is lower than the K_d, indicating that to achieve 50% of maximal effect, fewer than 50% of the receptors must be activated. Explanations for this phenomenon are discussed in the text.

J. Agonists and Partial Agonists: An agonist is a drug capable of fully activating the effector system when it binds to the receptor. A partial agonist produces less than the full effect, even when it has saturated the receptors (Figure 2–4). In the presence of a full agonist, a partial agonist acts as an inhibitor.

K. Competitive and Irreversible Pharmacologic Antagonists: Competitive antagonists are drugs that bind to the receptor in a reversible way without activating the effector system for that receptor. In the presence of a competitive antagonist, the log dose-response curve is shifted to higher doses (ie, horizontally to the right on the dose axis) but the same maximal effect is reached (Figure 2–5A). In contrast, an irreversible antagonist causes a downward shift of the maximum, with no shift of the curve on the dose axis unless spare receptors are present (Figure 2–5B). The effects of competitive antagonists can be overcome by adding more agonist. Irreversible antagonists cannot be overcome by adding more agonist. Competitive antagonists increase the ED_{50}; irreversible antagonists do not (unless spare receptors are present).

L. Physiologic Antagonists: A physiologic antagonist is a drug that binds to a different receptor, producing an effect opposite to that produced by the drug it is antagonizing. Thus it differs from a pharmacologic antagonist, which interacts with the same receptor as the drug it is inhibiting. A common example is the antagonism of the bronchoconstrictor action of histamine (mediated at histamine receptors) by epinephrine's bronchodilator action (mediated at beta adrenoceptors).

M. Chemical Antagonists: A chemical antagonist is a drug that interacts directly with the drug being antagonized to remove it or to prevent it from reaching its target. A chemical antagonist does not depend on interaction with the agonist's receptor (although such interaction may occur). A common example of a chemical antagonist is dimercaprol, a chelator of lead and some other toxic metals. Pralidoxime, which combines avidly with the phosphorus in organophosphate cholinesterase inhibitors, is another type of chemical antagonist.

N. Therapeutic Index, Therapeutic Window: The therapeutic index is the ratio of the TD_{50} (or LD_{50}) to the ED_{50}, determined from quantal dose-response curves. The therapeutic index represents an estimate of the safety of a drug, since a very safe drug might be expected to have a very large toxic dose and a small effective dose. For example, in Figure 2–2, the ED_{50} is approximately 3 mg and the LD_{50} is approximately 150 mg. The therapeutic index is therefore approximately 50 (150/3). Unfortunately, factors such as the varying slopes of dose-response curves make this estimate a poor safety index. The therapeutic window, a more clinically relevant index of safety, describes the dosage range between the minimum effective therapeutic concentration or dose, and the minimum toxic concentration or dose. For example, if the average minimum therapeutic plasma concentration of theophylline is 8 mg/L and toxic effects are observed at 18 mg/L, the therapeutic window is 8–18 mg/L.

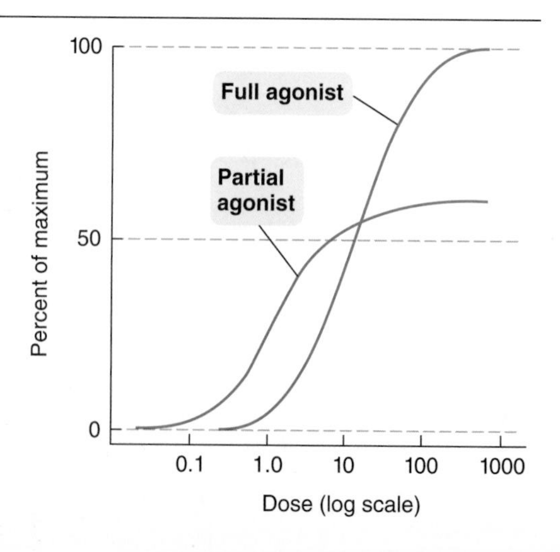

Figure 2–4. Comparison of dose-response curves for a full agonist and a partial agonist. The partial agonist acts on the same receptor system as the full agonist but cannot produce as large an effect (it has lower maximal efficacy), no matter how much the dose is increased. A partial agonist may be more potent (as in the figure), less potent, or equally potent; potency is an independent factor.

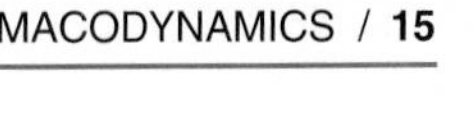

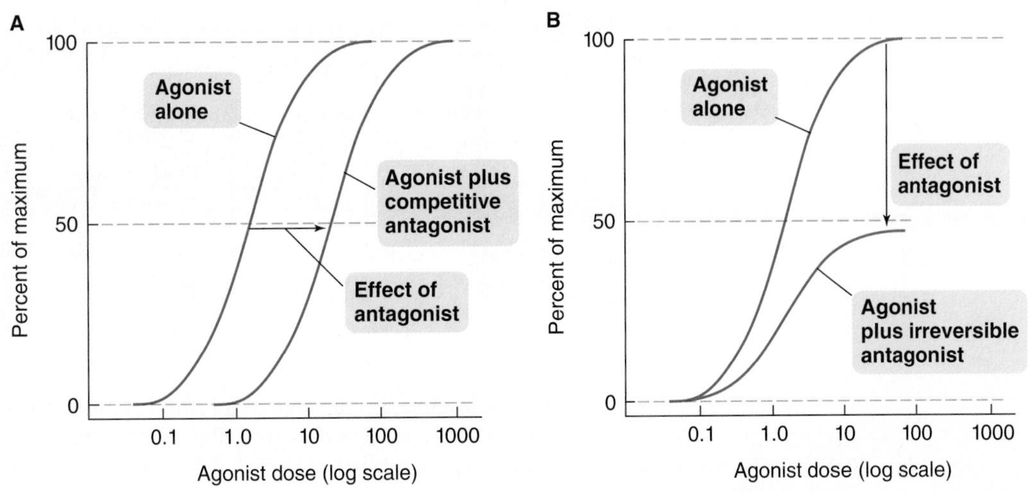

Figure 2–5. Agonist dose-response curves in the presence of competitive and irreversible antagonists. Note the use of a logarithmic scale for drug concentration. ***A.*** A competitive antagonist has an effect illustrated by the shift of the agonist curve to the right. ***B.*** A noncompetitive antagonist shifts the agonist curve downward.

O. Signaling Mechanisms: Once an agonist drug has bound to its receptor, some effector mechanism is activated. For most drug-receptor interactions, the drug is present in the extracellular space while the effector mechanism resides inside the cell and modifies some intracellular process. Thus, signaling across the membrane must occur. Five major types of transmembrane signaling mechanisms for receptor-effector systems have been defined (Figure 2–6):

1. **Receptors that are intracellular:** Some drugs, especially more lipid-soluble or diffusible agents (eg, steroid hormones, nitric oxide) may cross the membrane and combine with an intracellular receptor that affects an intracellular effector molecule. No specialized transmembrane signaling device is required.
2. **Receptors located on membrane-spanning enzymes:** Drugs that affect membrane-spanning enzymes combine with a receptor on the extracellular portion of enzymes and

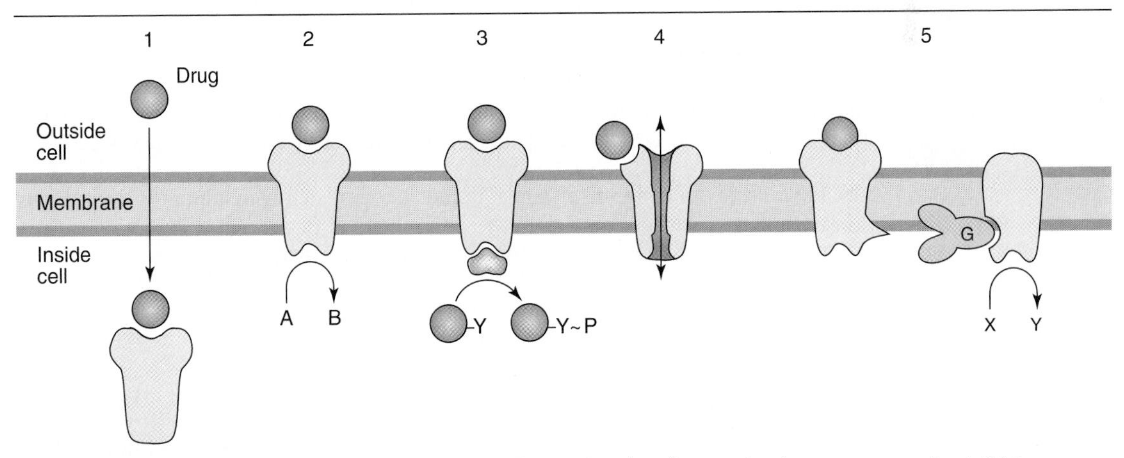

Figure 2–6. Signaling mechanisms for drug effects. Five major signaling mechanisms are recognized: (1) transmembrane diffusion of the drug to bind to an intracellular receptor; (2) transmembrane enzyme receptors, whose outer domain provides the receptor function and inner domain provides the effector mechanism; (3) transmembrane receptors that, after activation by an appropriate ligand, activate separate mobile protein tyrosine kinase molecules (JAKs), which phosphorylate STAT molecules that regulate transcription; (4) transmembrane channels that are gated open or closed by the binding of a drug to the receptor site; and (5) G protein-coupled receptors, which utilize a coupling protein to activate a separate effector molecule. (Reproduced, with permission, from Katzung BG [editor]: *Basic & Clinical Pharmacology,* 8th ed. McGraw-Hill, 2001.)

Table 2–2. Examples of receptors that are coupled to their effectors by G proteins.

Receptor Types	Coupling Protein	Effector	Effector Substrate	Second Messenger Response	Result
M_1, M_3, α	G_q	Phospholipase C	Membrane lipids	↑ IP_3 ↑ DAG	↑ Ca^{2+} ↑ Protein kinase
β, D_1	G_s	Adenylyl cyclase	ATP	↑ cAMP	↑ Ca^{2+} influx ↑ Enzyme activity
α_2, M_2	G_i	Adenylyl cyclase	ATP	↓ cAMP	↓ in Ca^{2+} influx and enzyme activity

modify their intracellular activity. For example, insulin acts on a tyrosine kinase that is located in the membrane. The insulin receptor site faces the extracellular environment and the enzyme catalytic site is on the cytoplasmic side. When activated, the receptors dimerize and phosphorylate specific protein substrates.

3. **Receptors located on membrane-spanning molecules that bind separate intracellular tyrosine kinase molecules:** Like receptor tyrosine kinases, these receptors have extracellular and intracellular domains and form dimers. However, after receptor activation by an appropriate drug, the tyrosine kinase molecules (Janus kinases; JAKs) are activated, resulting in phosphorylation of "STAT" molecules (signal transducers and activators of transcription). STAT dimers then travel to the nucleus, where they regulate transcription.
4. **Receptors located on membrane ion channels:** Receptors that regulate membrane ion channels may directly cause the opening of an ion channel (eg, acetylcholine at the nicotinic receptor) or modify the ion channel's response to other agents (eg, benzodiazepines at the GABA channel). The result is a change in transmembrane electrical potential.
5. **Receptors linked to effectors via G proteins:** A very large number of drugs bind to receptors that are linked by coupling proteins to intracellular or membrane effectors. The best defined examples of this group are the sympathomimetic drugs, which activate or inhibit adenylyl cyclase (formerly called adenylate cyclase) by a multistep process: activation of the receptor by the drug results in activation of G proteins that either stimulate or inhibit the cyclase. More than 20 types of G proteins have been identified; three of the most important are listed in Table 2–2.

QUESTIONS

DIRECTIONS: Each of the numbered items or incomplete statements in this section is followed by answers or by completions of the statement. Select the ONE lettered answer or completion that is BEST in each case.

1. A 55-year-old woman with congestive heart failure is to be treated with a diuretic drug. Drugs X and Y have the same mechanism of diuretic action. Drug X in a dose of 5 mg produces the same magnitude of diuresis as 500 mg of drug Y. This suggests that

(A) Drug Y is less efficacious than drug X
(B) Drug X is about 100 times more potent than drug Y
(C) Toxicity of drug X is less than that of drug Y
(D) Drug X is a safer drug than drug Y
(E) Drug X will have a shorter duration of action than drug Y because less of drug X is present for a given effect

2. Dose-response curves are used for drug evaluation in the animal laboratory and in the clinic. *Quantal* dose-response curves are often

(A) Used for determining the therapeutic index of a drug
(B) Used for determining the maximal efficacy of a drug
(C) Invalid in the presence of inhibitors of the drug being studied
(D) Obtainable from the study of intact subjects but not from isolated tissue preparations
(E) Used to determine the statistical variation (standard deviation) of the maximal response to the drug

3. The results shown in the graph below were obtained in a comparison of positive inotropic agents. Which of the following statements is MOST correct?
- **(A)** Drug A is most effective
- **(B)** Drug B is least potent
- **(C)** Drug C is most potent
- **(D)** Drug B is more potent than drug C and more effective than drug A
- **(E)** Drug A is more potent than drug B and more effective than drug C

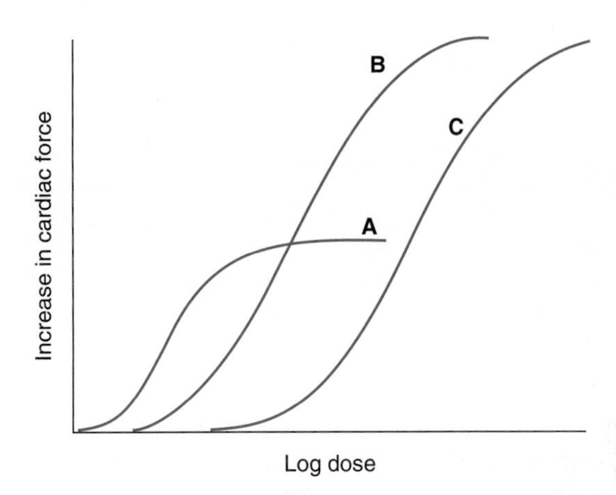

4. In the absence of other drugs, pindolol causes an increase in heart rate by activating beta adrenoceptors. In the presence of highly effective beta stimulants, however, pindolol causes a dose-dependent, reversible decrease in heart rate. Therefore, pindolol is probably
- **(A)** An irreversible antagonist
- **(B)** A physiologic antagonist
- **(C)** A chemical antagonist
- **(D)** A partial agonist
- **(E)** A spare receptor agonist

5. Which of the following statements about spare receptors is MOST correct?
- **(A)** Spare receptors, in the absence of drug, are sequestered in the cytoplasm
- **(B)** Spare receptors will be detected if the intracellular effect of drug-receptor interaction lasts longer than the drug-receptor interaction itself
- **(C)** Spare receptors influence the maximal efficacy of the drug-receptor system
- **(D)** Spare receptors activate the effector machinery of the cell without the need for a drug
- **(E)** Spare receptors may be detected by the finding that the EC_{50} is greater than the K_d for the agonist

6. Two drugs, "A" and "B," were studied in a large group of patients and the percentages of the group showing a specific therapeutic effect were determined. The results are shown in the table:

Drug Dose	Percent Responding to Drug A	Percent Responding to Drug B
0.1 mg	1	10
0.3 mg	5	20
1.0 mg	10	50
3.0 mg	50	70
10.0 mg	70	90
30.0 mg	90	100

Which of the following statements about these results is MOST correct?
(A) Drug A is safer than drug B
(B) Drug B is more effective than drug A
(C) The two drugs act on the same receptors
(D) Drug A is less potent than drug B
(E) The therapeutic index of drug B is 10

7. Which of the following terms best describes the antagonism of leukotriene's bronchoconstrictor effect (mediated at leukotriene receptors) by terbutaline (acting at adrenoceptors) in a patient with asthma?
(A) Pharmacologic antagonist
(B) Partial agonist
(C) Physiologic antagonist
(D) Chemical antagonist
(E) Noncompetitive antagonist

8. Which of the following terms best describes an antagonist that interacts directly with the agonist and not at all, or only incidentally, with the receptor?
(A) Pharmacologic antagonist
(B) Partial agonist
(C) Physiologic antagonist
(D) Chemical antagonist
(E) Noncompetitive antagonist

9. Which of the following terms best describes a drug that blocks the action of epinephrine at its receptors by occupying those receptors without activating them?
(A) Pharmacologic antagonist
(B) Partial agonist
(C) Physiologic antagonist
(D) Chemical antagonist
(E) Noncompetitive antagonist

10. Which of the following provides information about the variation in sensitivity to the drug within the population studied?
(A) Maximal efficacy
(B) Therapeutic index
(C) Drug potency
(D) Graded dose-response curve
(E) Quantal dose-response curve

11. Which of the following most accurately describes the transmembrane signaling process involved in steroid hormone action?
(A) Action on a membrane-spanning tyrosine kinase
(B) Activation of a G protein, which activates or inhibits adenylyl cyclase
(C) Diffusion into the cytoplasm and binding to an intracellular receptor
(D) Diffusion of "STAT" molecules across the membrane
(E) Opening of transmembrane ion channels

12. Which of the following provides information about the largest response a drug can produce, regardless of dose?
(A) Drug potency
(B) Maximal efficacy
(C) Mechanism of receptor action
(D) Therapeutic index
(E) Therapeutic window

DIRECTIONS: (Items 13–15): Each of the curves in the graph below may be considered a concentration-effect curve or a concentration-binding curve. For each numbered item, select the ONE lettered option that is most closely associated with it.
(A) Curve 1
(B) Curve 2
(C) Curve 3
(D) Curve 4
(E) Curve 5

13. Describes the percentage *binding* of a full agonist to its receptors as the concentration of a partial agonist is increased from low to very high levels

14. Describes the percentage *effect* when a full agonist is present throughout the experiment, and the concentration of a partial agonist is increased from low to very high levels

15. Describes the percentage *binding* of the partial agonist whose *effect* is shown by curve 4, if the system has many spare receptors

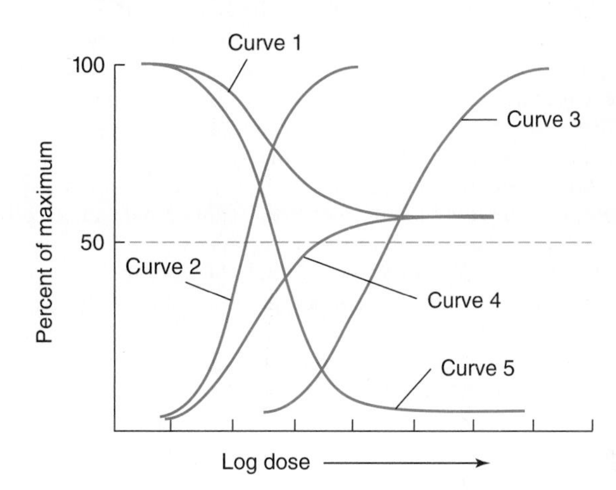

ANSWERS

1. No information is given regarding the magnitude of the maximum diuretic response to either drug. Similarly, no information about toxicity is available. The fact that a given response is achieved with a smaller dose of drug X only indicates that X is more potent than Y in the ratio of 500/5. The answer is **(B).**

2. Graded dose-response curves must be used to determine maximum efficacy (maximal response). Quantal dose-response curves show only the frequency of occurrence of a specified response, which may be therapeutic (ED) or toxic (TD). Dividing the TD_{50} by the ED_{50} gives the therapeutic index. The answer is **(A).**

3. These are straightforward graded dose-response curves. Drug A is the most potent, drug C the least. Drug A is less efficacious than drugs B and C. The answer is **(D).**

4. **(B)** and **(C)** are clearly incorrect, since pindolol is said to act at beta receptors and to block beta stimulants. The drug effect is reversible, so **(A)** is incorrect. "Spare receptor agonist" is a nonsense distracter. The answer is **(D).**

5. While some types of receptors appear to be sequestered in the cytoplasm under certain conditions, there is no difference between "spare" and other receptors. Spare receptors may be defined as those which are not needed for binding drug to achieve the maximal effect. Spare receptors influence the *sensitivity* of the system to an agonist, not the maximal efficacy, since the statistical probability of a drug-receptor interaction increases with the total number of receptors. If they do not bind an agonist molecule, spare receptors do not activate an effector molecule. EC_{50} *less* than K_d is an indication of the presence of spare receptors. The answer is **(B).**

6. No information is presented regarding the safety of these drugs; only the percentage of the population showing the response. Similarly, no information on efficacy is presented and efficacy is not normally obtainable from quantal dose-response data. Although both drugs are said to be producing a "therapeutic effect," no information on their receptor mechanisms is given. Since no data on toxicity are available, the therapeutic index cannot be determined. The answer is **(D),** because the ED_{50} of drug B (1.0 mg) is less than that of drug A (3.0 mg).

7. Because terbutaline interacts with adrenoceptors and leukotriene with leukotriene receptors, terbutaline cannot be a pharmacologic antagonist of leukotriene. Because the results of adrenoceptor activation oppose the effects of leukotriene receptor activation, terbutaline must be a physiologic antagonist. The answer is **(C).**

8. A chemical antagonist interacts directly (chemically) with the agonist drug and not with a receptor. The answer is **(D).**
9. A pharmacologic antagonist occupies the receptors without activating them. The answer is **(A).**
10. Quantal dose-response curves provide information about the statistical distribution of sensitivity to a drug. The answer is **(E).**
11. Steroid hormones (eg, cortisol, sex hormones, and aldosterone) diffuse through the membrane of the cell into the cytoplasm and bind to an intracellular receptor. The hormone-receptor complex then activates gene expression. The answer is **(C).**
12. Maximal efficacy represents the largest response a drug can produce. The answer is **(B).**
13. The binding of a full agonist will *decrease* as the concentration of a partial agonist is increased to very high levels. As the partial agonist displaces more and more of the full agonist, the percentage of receptors that bind the full agonist will drop to zero, ie, curve 5. The answer is **(E).**
14. Curve 1 describes the *response* of the system when combining a large fixed concentration of full agonist and increasing concentrations of partial agonist. This is because the increasing percentage of receptors binding the partial agonist will finally produce the maximum effect typical of the partial agonist. The answer is **(A).**
15. Partial agonists, like full agonists, bind 100% of their receptors when present in high enough concentration. Therefore, the binding curve (but not the effect curve) will go to 100%. If the effect curve is curve 4 and many spare receptors are present, the binding curve must be displaced to the right of curve 4 ($K_d > EC_{50}$). Therefore, curve 3 fits the description better than curve 2. The answer is **(C).**

3 Pharmacokinetics

OBJECTIVES

You should be able to:

- Compute the half-life of a drug based on its clearance and volume of distribution.
- Calculate loading and maintenance dosage regimens for oral or intravenous administration of a drug when given the following information: minimum therapeutic concentration; bioavailability; clearance; and volume of distribution.
- Calculate the dosage adjustment required for a patient with impaired renal function.

Learn the definitions that follow.

Table 3–1. Definitions.

Term	Definition
Volume of distribution (apparent)	The ratio of the amount of a drug in the body to its concentration in the plasma or blood
Clearance	The ratio of the rate of elimination of a drug to its concentration in plasma or blood
Half-life	The time it takes for the amount or concentration of a drug to fall to 50% of an earlier measurement; this number is a constant, regardless of concentration, for drugs eliminated by first-order kinetics (the great majority of drugs). See Chapter 1. Half-life is not a constant and therefore not particularly useful for drugs eliminated by zero-order kinetics (eg, ethanol)
Bioavailability	The fraction (or percentage) of the administered dose of a drug that reaches the systemic circulation
Area under the curve (AUC)	The graphic area under a plot of drug concentration in plasma versus time, after a single dose of a drug or during a single dosing interval; the AUC is important for calculating the bioavailability of a drug given by any route other than intravenous
Peak and trough concentrations	The maximum and minimum drug concentrations—in plasma or blood—measured during cycles of repeated dosing
Minimum effective concentration (MEC)	The plasma concentration below which a patient's response is too small for therapeutic benefit
First-pass effect, presystemic elimination	The elimination of drug that occurs after administration but before it reaches the systemic circulation, eg, during passage through the gut wall, portal blood, and liver for an orally administered drug
Steady state	In pharmacokinetics, the condition in which the total amount of drug in the body does not change over multiple dosing intervals; ie, the rate of drug input equals the rate of elimination
Extraction	The fraction of a drug in the plasma that is removed by an organ as it passes through that organ
Bioequivalence	The equivalence of blood concentrations of two preparations of the same drug measured over time; if the concentration-time plots for the two preparations are nearly superimposable (within certain statistical limits), the preparations are said to be bioequivalent; one preparation may be safely substituted for the other
Biodisposition	Often used as a synonym for pharmacokinetics: the processes of drug absorption, distribution, and elimination

CONCEPTS

A. Effective Drug Concentration: The effective drug concentration is the concentration of a drug at the receptor site (in contrast to drug concentrations that are more readily measured, eg, in blood). Except for topically applied agents, this concentration is often proportionate to the drug's concentration in the plasma. The plasma concentration is a function of the rate of input of the drug (by absorption) into the plasma, the rate of distribution to the peripheral tissues (including the target organ), and the rate of elimination, or loss, from the body. These are all functions of time; but if the rate of input is known, the remaining processes are well-described by two primary parameters: volume of distribution and clearance. These parameters are unique for a particular drug in a particular patient but have average values in large populations that can be used to predict drug concentrations.

B. Volume of Distribution (V_d): The volume of distribution relates the amount of drug in the body to the plasma concentration (Figure 3–1) according to the following equation:

$$V_d = \frac{\text{Amount of drug in the body}}{\text{Plasma drug concentration}} \quad (1)$$

(Units = volume)

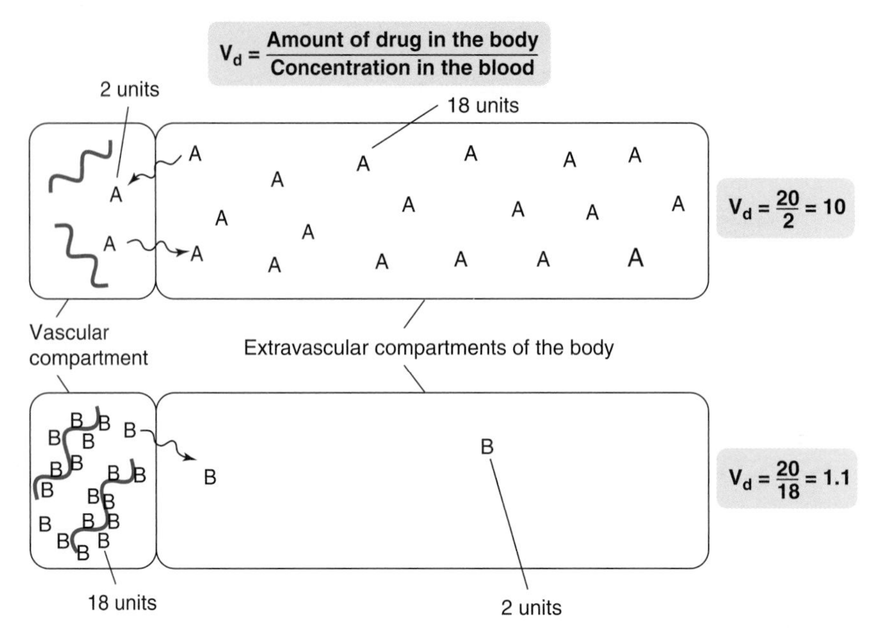

Figure 3–1. Effect of drug binding on volume of distribution. Drug A does not bind to macromolecules (heavy wavy lines) in the vascular or the extravascular compartments of the hypothetical organism in the diagram. Drug A diffuses freely between the two compartments. With 20 units of the drug in the body, the steady-state distribution leaves a blood concentration of 2. Drug B, on the other hand, binds avidly to proteins in the blood. Drug B's diffusion is much more limited. At equilibrium, only 2 units of the total have diffused into the extravascular volume, leaving 18 units still in the blood. In each case the total amount of drug in the body is the same (20 units), but the apparent volumes of distribution are very different.

The calculated parameter for the apparent volume of distribution has no direct physical equivalent. If a drug is avidly bound in peripheral tissues, the drug's concentration in plasma may drop to very low values even though the total amount in the body is large. As a result, the volume of distribution may greatly exceed the total volume of the body. For example, 50 thousand liters is the V_d for the drug quinacrine in a person whose physical body volume is 70 liters. On the other hand, a drug that is completely retained in the plasma compartment will have a volume of distribution equal to the plasma volume (about 4% of body weight). The volume of distribution of drugs that are normally bound to plasma proteins such as albumin can be altered by liver disease (through reduced protein synthesis) and kidney disease (through urinary protein loss).

C. Clearance (CL): Clearance relates the rate of elimination to the plasma concentration:

$$CL = \frac{\textbf{Rate of elimination of drug}}{\textbf{Plasma drug concentration}} \quad \textbf{(2)}$$

(Units = volume per unit time)

For a drug eliminated with first-order kinetics, clearance is a constant, ie, the ratio of rate of elimination to plasma concentration is the same regardless of plasma concentration (Figure 3–2). The magnitudes of clearance for different drugs range from a small fraction of the blood flow to a maximum of the total blood flow to the organ of elimination. Clearance depends upon the drug and the condition of the organs of elimination in the patient. The clearance of a particular drug by an individual organ is equivalent to the extraction capability of that organ for that drug, times the rate of delivery of drug to the organ. Thus the clearance of a drug that is very effectively extracted by an organ is often flow-limited—ie, the blood is completely cleared of the drug as it passes through the organ. For such a drug, the total clearance from the body is a function of blood flow through the eliminating organ, and is limited by the blood flow to the or-

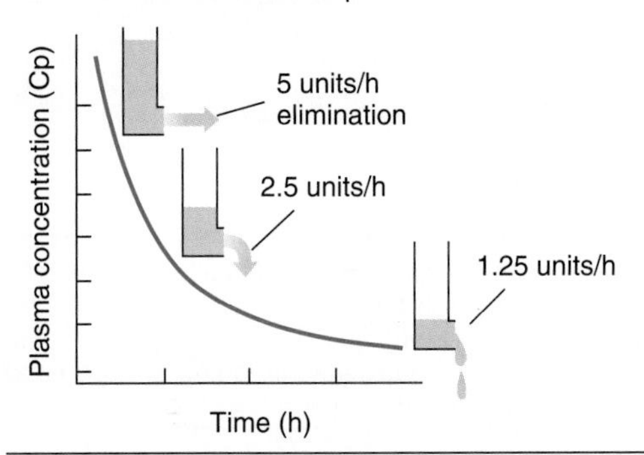

Figure 3–2. The clearance of most drugs is a constant over a broad range of plasma concentrations. Since elimination rate is equal to clearance times plasma concentration, the elimination rate will be rapid at first and slow as the concentration decreases.

gan. In this situation, other conditions—disease or other drugs that change blood flow—may have more dramatic effects on clearance than disease of the organ of elimination.

Skill Keeper: Zero-Order Elimination (see Chapter 1)

The great majority of drugs in clinical use obey the first-order kinetics "rule" described in the text. Can you name three important drugs that do not? *The Skill Keeper Answer appears at the end of the chapter.*

D. Half-life: Half-life ($t_{1/2}$) is a derived parameter, completely determined by volume of distribution and clearance. Half-life can be determined graphically from a plot of the blood level versus time (Figure 1–3), or from the following relationship:

$$t_{1/2} = \frac{0.693 \times V_d}{CL} \tag{3}$$

(Units = time)

One must know both primary variables (V_d and CL) to predict changes in half-life. Disease, age, and other variables usually alter the clearance of a drug much more than its volume of distribution. The half-life of a drug may not change, however, despite a decreased clearance if the volume of distribution decreases at the same time. This occurs, for example, when lidocaine is administered to patients with congestive heart failure. The half-life determines the rate at which blood concentration rises during a constant infusion and falls after administration is stopped (Figure 3–3).

E. Bioavailability: The bioavailability of a drug is the fraction (F) of the administered dose that reaches the systemic circulation. Bioavailability is defined as unity (or 100%) in the case of intravenous administration. After administration by other routes, bioavailability is generally reduced by incomplete absorption (or, in the intestine, expulsion of drug by the intestinal P-glycoprotein transporter), first-pass metabolism, and any distribution into other tissues that occurs before the drug enters the systemic circulation. Even for drugs with equal bioavailabilities, entry into the systemic circulation occurs over varying periods of time, depending on the drug formulation and other factors. To account for such factors, the concentration appearing in the plasma is integrated over time to obtain an integrated total **area under the plasma concentration curve** (**AUC,** Figure 3–4).

F. Extraction: Removal of a drug by an organ can be specified as the extraction ratio, or the fraction of the drug removed from the perfusing blood during its passage through the organ

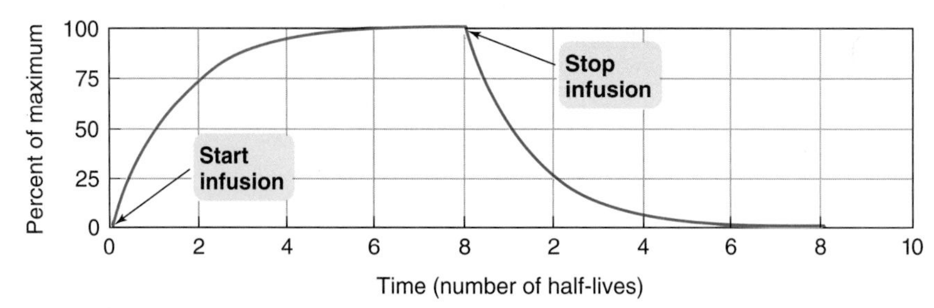

Figure 3–3. Plasma concentration (plotted as percent of maximum) of a drug given by constant IV infusion for eight half-lives and then stopped. The concentration rises smoothly with time, and always reaches 50% of steady state after one half-life, 75% after two half-lives, 87.5% after three half-lives, and so on. The decline in concentration after stopping drug administration follows the same type of curve: 50% is left after one half-life, 25% after two half-lives, etc. The asymptotic approach to steady state on both increasing and decreasing limbs of the curve are characteristic of drugs following first-order kinetics.

(Figure 3–5). After steady-state concentration in plasma has been achieved, the extraction ratio is one measure of the elimination of the drug by that organ. Drugs that have a high hepatic extraction ratio have a large first-pass effect; the bioavailability of these drugs after oral administration will be low.

G. Dosage Regimens: A dosage regimen is a plan for drug administration over a period of time. An appropriate dosage regimen results in the achievement of therapeutic levels of the drug in the blood, without exceeding the minimum toxic concentration. To maintain the plasma concentration within a specified range over long periods of therapy, a schedule of **maintenance doses** is used. If it is necessary to achieve the target plasma level rapidly, a **loading dose** is used to "load" the volume of distribution with the drug. Ideally, the dosing plan is based on knowledge of both the minimum therapeutic and minimum toxic concentrations for the drug, as well as its clearance and volume of distribution.

1. **Maintenance dosage:** Because the maintenance rate of drug administration is equal to the rate of elimination at steady state (this is the definition of steady state), the maintenance dosage is a function of clearance (from equation [2] above).

$$\textbf{Dosing rate} = \frac{\textbf{Clearance} \times \textbf{Desired plasma concentration}}{\textbf{Bioavailability}} \qquad \textbf{(4)}$$

Note that volume of distribution is not directly involved in the above calculation. The dosing rate computed for maintenance dosage is the average dose per unit time. When carrying out

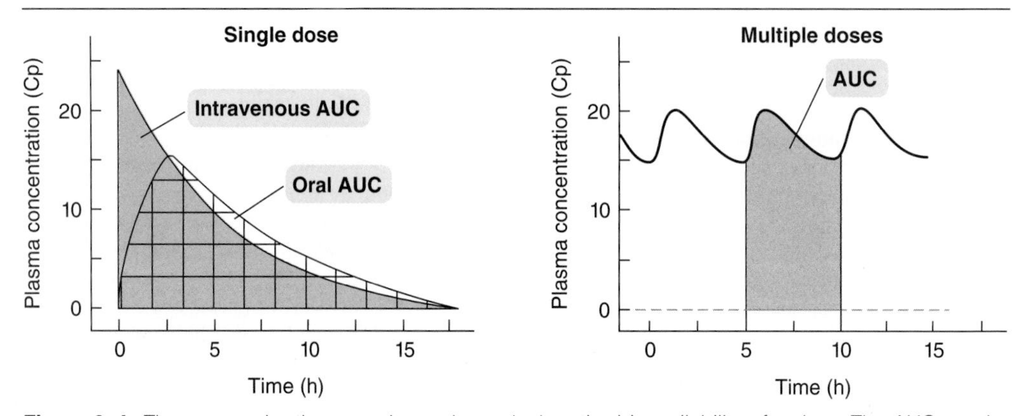

Figure 3–4. The area under the curve is used to calculate the bioavailability of a drug. The AUC can be obtained from either single dose studies (left panel) or multiple dose measurements (right panel). Bioavailability (F) is calculated from $AUC_{(route)}/AUC_{(IV)}$.

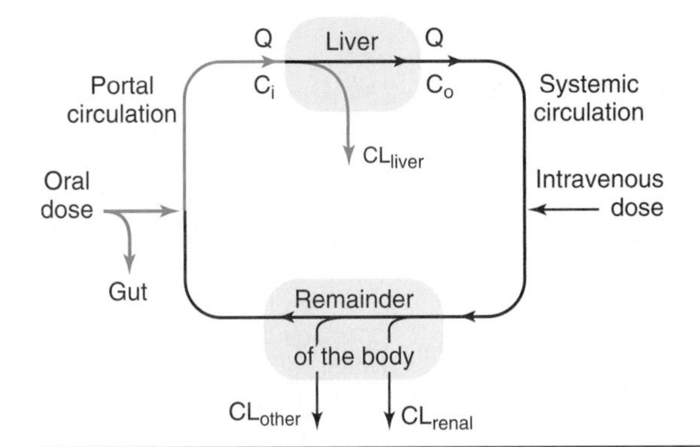

Figure 3–5. The principles of organ extraction and first-pass effect are illustrated. Part of the administered oral dose (color) is lost to metabolism in the gut and the liver before it enters the systemic circulation: this is the first-pass effect. The extraction of drug from the circulation by the liver is equal to blood flow times the difference between entering and leaving drug concentration, ie, $Q \times (C_i - C_o)$. (Reproduced, with permission, from Katzung BG [editor]: *Basic & Clinical Pharmacology,* 8th ed. McGraw-Hill, 2001.)

such calculations, make certain that the units are in agreement throughout. For example, if clearance is given in mL per minute, the resulting dosing rate is a per-minute rate. For chronic therapy, oral administration is desirable; thus doses should be given only once or a few times per day. The size of the daily dose (dose per minute × 60 minutes per hour × 24 hours per day) is a simple extension of the above information. The number of doses to be given per day is usually determined by the half-life of the drug and the difference between the minimum therapeutic and toxic concentrations (see Therapeutic Window, below).

If it is important to maintain a concentration above the minimum therapeutic level at all times, either a larger dose may be given at long intervals or smaller doses at more frequent intervals. If the difference between the toxic and therapeutic concentrations is small, then smaller, more frequent doses must be administered to avoid toxicity.

2. **Loading dosage:** If the therapeutic concentration must be achieved rapidly and the volume of distribution is large, a large loading dose may be needed at the onset of therapy. This is calculated from the following equation:

$$\textbf{Loading dose} = \frac{\textbf{Volume of distribution} \times \textbf{Desired plasma concentration}}{\textbf{Bioavailability}} \quad (5)$$

Note that clearance does not enter into this computation. If the loading dose is very large (V_d much larger than blood volume), the dose should be given slowly to avoid excessively high peak plasma levels during the distribution phase.

H. Therapeutic Window: The therapeutic window is the safe "opening" between the minimum therapeutic concentration and the minimum toxic concentration of a drug. The concept is used to determine the range of plasma levels that is acceptable when designing a dosing regimen. Thus the minimum effective concentration will usually determine the desired **trough** levels of a drug given intermittently, while the minimum toxic concentration determines the permissible **peak** plasma concentration. For example: the drug theophylline has a therapeutic concentration range of 7–10 mg/L, and a toxic concentration range of 15–20 mg/L. The therapeutic window for a given patient might thus be fixed in the range of 8–17 mg/L (Figure 3–6). Unfortunately, for some drugs the therapeutic and toxic concentrations vary so greatly among patients that it is impossible to predict the therapeutic window in a given patient. Such drugs must be titrated individually in each patient.

I. Adjustment of Dosage When Elimination Is Altered by Disease: Renal disease or reduced cardiac output often reduce the clearance of drugs that depend on renal function. Alteration of clearance by liver disease is less common but may occur. The dose in a patient with renal impairment may be corrected by multiplying the average dose for a normal person times the ratio of the patient's altered creatinine clearance to normal creatinine clearance (approximately 100 mL/min or 6 L/h).

$$\textbf{Corrected dose} = \textbf{Average dose} \times \frac{\textbf{Patient's creatinine clearance}}{\textbf{100 mL/min}} \quad (6)$$

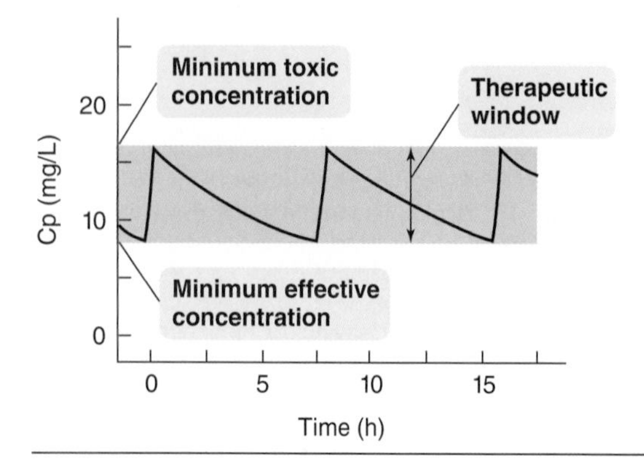

Figure 3–6. The therapeutic window for theophylline in a 13-year-old patient. The minimum effective concentration in this patient was found to be 8 mg/L; the minimum toxic concentration was found to be 16 mg/L. The therapeutic window is indicated by the colored area. In order to maintain the plasma concentration Cp within the window, the drug must be given at least once every half-life (7.5 hours in this patient), since the minimum effective concentration is half the minimum toxic concentration and Cp will decay by 50% in one half-life. (***Note:*** This concept applies to drugs given in the ordinary, prompt-release form. Slow-release formulations can often be given at longer intervals.)

This simplified approach ignores nonrenal routes of clearance that may be significant. If a drug is partly cleared by the kidney and partly by nonrenal clearance, the above equation should be applied to that part of the dose that is eliminated by the kidney. For example, if a drug is 50% cleared by the kidney and 50% by the liver, and the normal dosage is 200 mg/d, the corrected dosage in a patient with a creatinine clearance of 20 mL/min will be:

$$\textbf{Dose} = \textbf{100 mg/d} + \textbf{100 mg/d} \times \frac{\textbf{20 mL/min}}{\textbf{100 mL/min}} \tag{7}$$

$$\textbf{Dose} = \textbf{100 mg/d} + \textbf{20 mg/d} = \textbf{120 mg/d}$$

QUESTIONS

DIRECTIONS: Each of the numbered items or incomplete statements in this section is followed by answers or by completions of the statement. Select the ONE lettered answer or completion that is BEST in each case.

Items 1–2: Mr. Jones is admitted to General Hospital with pneumonia due to gram-negative bacteria. The antibiotic tobramycin is ordered. The CL and V_d of tobramycin in Mr. Jones are 80 mL/min and 40 L, respectively.

1. What maintenance dose should be administered intravenously every 6 hours to eventually obtain average steady-state plasma concentrations of 4 mg/L?
(A) 0.32 mg
(B) 19.2 mg
(C) 115 mg
(D) 160 mg
(E) 230 mg

2. If you wish to give Mr. Jones an IV loading dose to achieve the therapeutic plasma concentration of 4 mg/L rapidly, how much should be given?
(A) 0.1 mg
(B) 10 mg
(C) 115.2 mg
(D) 160 mg
(E) None of the above

3. Despite your careful adherence to basic pharmacokinetic principles, your patient on digoxin therapy has developed digitalis toxicity. The plasma digoxin level is 4 ng/mL. Renal function is normal, and the plasma $t_{1/2}$ for digoxin in this patient is 1.6 days. How long should you withhold digoxin in order to reach a safer yet probably therapeutic level of 1 ng/mL?
(A) 1.6 days
(B) 2.4 days
(C) 3.2 days

(D) 4.8 days
(E) 6.4 days

4. Verapamil and phenytoin are both eliminated from the body by metabolism in the liver. Verapamil has a clearance of 1.5 L/min, approximately equal to liver blood flow, whereas phenytoin has a clearance of 0.1 L/min. When these compounds are administered along with rifampin, a drug that increases hepatic drug-metabolizing enzymes, which of the following is most likely?
(A) The clearance of both verapamil and phenytoin will be increased
(B) The clearance of both verapamil and phenytoin will be decreased
(C) The clearance of verapamil will be unchanged, whereas the clearance of phenytoin will be increased
(D) The clearance of phenytoin will be unchanged, whereas the clearance of verapamil will be increased

5. A 60-year-old man enters the hospital with a myocardial infarction and a severe ventricular arrhythmia. The antiarrhythmic drug chosen has a narrow therapeutic window: the minimum toxic plasma concentration is 1.5 times the minimum therapeutic plasma concentration. The half-life is 6 hours. It is essential to maintain the plasma concentration above the minimum therapeutic level to prevent a possibly lethal arrhythmia. Of the following, the most appropriate dosing regimen would be
(A) Once a day
(B) Twice a day
(C) Three times a day
(D) Four times a day
(E) Constant IV infusion

6. A 50-year-old woman with metastatic breast cancer has elected to participate in the trial of a new chemotherapeutic agent. It is given by constant IV infusion of 8 mg/hour. Plasma concentrations (Cp) are measured with the results shown in the table.

Time After Start of Infusion (hours)	Plasma Concentration (mg/L)	Time After Start of Infusion (hours)	Plasma Concentration (mg/L)
1	0.8	16	3.7
2	1.3	20	3.84
4	2.0	25	3.95
8	3.0	30	4.0
10	3.6	40	4.0

From these data it may be concluded that
(A) Volume of distribution is 30 L
(B) Clearance is 2 L/h
(C) Elimination follows zero-order kinetics
(D) Half-life is 8 hours
(E) Doubling the rate of infusion would result in a plasma concentration of 16 mg/L at 40 hours

7. A city clinic is considering the substitution of generic drugs in order to save money. The clinical pharmacologist is asked to advise on the bioavailability of the generic products. She informs the head of the clinic that the bioavailability of drugs is
(A) Established by FDA regulation at 100% for preparations for intramuscular injection
(B) 100% for oral preparations that are not metabolized in the liver
(C) Calculated from the peak concentration of drug divided by the dose administered
(D) Important because bioavailability determines what fraction of the administered dose reaches the systemic circulation
(E) Equal to 1 (100%) only for drugs administered by any parenteral route

8. A nineteen-year-old woman is brought to the hospital with severe asthmatic wheezing. You decide to use IV theophylline for treatment. The pharmacokinetics of theophylline include the following average parameters: V_d 35 L; CL 48 mL/min; half-life 8 hours. If an IV infusion of

theophylline is started at a rate of 0.48 mg/min, how long will it take to reach 93.75% of the final steady state?
(A) Approximately 48 minutes
(B) Approximately 5.8 hours
(C) Approximately 6 hours
(D) Approximately 8 hours
(E) Approximately 32 hours

Items 9–10: Your 74-year-old patient with a myocardial infarction has a severe cardiac arrhythmia. You have decided to give lidocaine to correct the arrhythmia.

9. A continuous IV infusion of lidocaine, 1.92 mg/min, is started at 8 AM. The average pharmacokinetic parameters of lidocaine are: V_d 77 L; CL 640 mL/min; half-life 1.8 hours. The expected steady-state plasma concentration is approximately
(A) 40 mg/L
(B) 3.0 mg/L
(C) 0.025 mg/L
(D) 7.2 mg/L
(E) 3.46 mg/L

10. Your patient has been receiving lidocaine for 8 hours and you decide to obtain a plasma concentration measurement. When the results come back, the plasma level is exactly half of what you expected. The most probable explanation is
(A) The patient's lidocaine volume of distribution is half the average value
(B) The patient's lidocaine clearance is twice the average value
(C) The patient's lidocaine half-life is four times the average value
(D) The patient's infusion rate was accidentally decreased by half
(E) The laboratory made a mistake in the assay for lidocaine

11. A patient requires an infusion of procainamide. Its half-life is 2 hours. The infusion is begun at 9 AM. At 1 PM the same day a blood sample is taken; the drug concentration is found to be 3 mg/L. What is the probable steady-state drug concentration, eg, after 48 hours of infusion?
(A) 3 mg/L
(B) 4 mg/L
(C) 6 mg/L
(D) 9.9 mg/L
(E) 15 mg/L

12. A narcotics addict is brought to the emergency room in a deep coma. His friends state that he took a large dose of morphine 6 hours earlier. An immediate blood analysis shows a morphine blood level of 0.25 mg/L. Assuming that the pharmacokinetics of morphine in this patient are V_d 200 L and half-life is 3 hours, how much morphine did the patient inject 6 hours earlier?
(A) 25 mg
(B) 50 mg
(C) 100 mg
(D) 200 mg
(E) Too few data to predict

13. A normal volunteer will receive a new drug in a phase I clinical trial. The clearance and volume of distribution of the drug in this subject are 1.386 L/h and 80 L, respectively. The half-life of the drug in this subject will be approximately
(A) 83 hours
(B) 77 hours
(C) 58 hours
(D) 40 hours
(E) 0.02 hours

14. Gentamicin is often given in intermittent IV bolus doses of 100 mg three times a day to achieve target peak plasma concentrations of about 5 mg/L. Gentamicin's clearance (normally 5.4 L/h/70 kg) is almost entirely by glomerular filtration. Your patient, however, is found to have a creatinine clearance one-third of normal. Your initial dosage regimen for this patient would probably be

(A) 20 mg three times a day
(B) 33 mg three times a day
(C) 72 mg three times a day
(D) 100 mg twice a day
(E) 150 mg twice a day

15. Enalapril, an angiotensin converting enzyme inhibitor, has a half-life of 3 hours but is effective and nontoxic in most patients when given once a day. Assuming IV administration, this indicates that the ratio of the minimum toxic concentration to the minimum effective concentration for enalapril is at least
(A) 2 (ie, the toxic concentration is twice the therapeutic concentration)
(B) 8
(C) 21
(D) 256
(E) The data are insufficient to answer

Items 16–18: A new drug was studied in 20 healthy volunteers to determine basic pharmacokinetic parameters. A dose of 100 mg was administered as an intravenous bolus to each volunteer and blood samples were analyzed at intervals as shown in the graph below. The average plasma concentrations at each time are shown by the solid circles at 10 and 30 minutes and at 1, 2, 3, 4, 6, and 8 hours after administration.

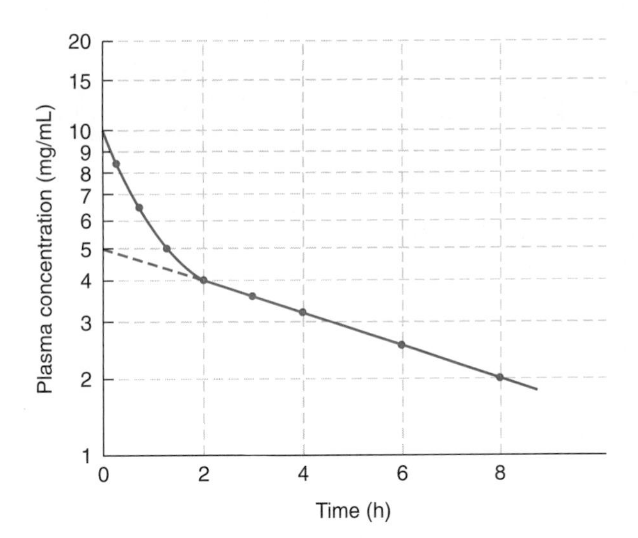

16. The half-life of the new drug is approximately
(A) 1.5 hours
(B) 2 hours
(C) 4 hours
(D) 6 hours
(E) 8 hours

17. The volume of distribution of the new drug is approximately
(A) 0.05 L
(B) 0.1 L
(C) 5 L
(D) 10 L
(E) 20 L

18. The clearance of the new drug is approximately
(A) 0.43 L/h
(B) 0.86 L/h
(C) 1.15 L/h
(D) 2.3 L/h
(E) Too few data to answer

ANSWERS

1. Maintenance dosage is a function of plasma level and clearance only:

$$\text{Rate in} = \text{Rate out at steady state}$$

$$\text{Dosage} = \frac{\text{Plasma level}_{ss} \times \text{Clearance}}{\text{Bioavailability (F)}}$$

$$= \frac{4\ \text{mg/L} \times 0.08\ \text{L/min}}{1.0}$$

$$= 0.32\ \text{mg/min}$$

when given at 6-hour intervals:

$$= 0.32\ \text{mg/min} \times 60\ \text{min/h} \times 6\ \text{hours}$$

$$= 115.2\ \text{mg/dose every 6 hours}$$

The answer is **(B).**

2. Loading dose is a function of volume of distribution and target plasma concentration:

$$\text{Loading dose} = \frac{V_d \times \text{Target concentration}}{\text{Bioavailability}}$$

$$\text{Loading dose} = \frac{40\ \text{L} \times 4\ \text{mg/L}}{1.0} = 160\ \text{mg}$$

The answer is **(D).**

3. Since the blood level for a drug with first-order kinetics drops by 50% during each half-life, the level will be 2 ng/mL after 1.6 days and 1 ng/mL after 3.2 days. The answer is **(C).**
4. Apparently verapamil is metabolized so rapidly that only the rate of delivery to the liver regulates its disappearance, ie, it is blood flow-limited. Further increases in liver enzymes could not increase its elimination. However, the rate of elimination of phenytoin is apparently limited by its rate of metabolism since clearance is much less than hepatic blood flow. Therefore, the clearance of phenytoin can rise if some agent causes an increase in liver enzymes. The answer is **(C).**
5. From the description given, if the minimum therapeutic plasma concentration of the hypothetical drug X is 100 units, the minimum toxic concentration is 150 units. If a dose is given that brings the plasma concentration to 150 units, it will fall to 75 units in one half-life (6 hours). Since 75 units is less than the minimum therapeutic concentration, this dosing interval is too long. Thus none of the intermittent dosing schedules listed would meet the requirement of the question. Thus, a constant IV infusion (which can be visualized as intermittent dosing at infinitely short intervals) would be more appropriate than any of the intermittent schedules. The answer is **(E).**
6. By inspection of the data in the table, it is clear that the steady-state plasma concentration is approximately 4 mg/L. Further inspection shows that 50% of this concentration was reached after 4 hours of infusion. According to the constant infusion principle (Figure 3–3), one half-life is required to reach one half of the final concentration; therefore, the half-life of the drug is 4 hours. Rearranging the equation for maintenance dosing (dosing rate = CL × Cp), it can be determined that the clearance = dosing rate/Cp or 2 L/hour. The volume of distribution can be calculated from the half-life equation ($t_{1/2} = 0.693 \times V_d / CL$) and is equal to 11.5 L. This drug follows first-order kinetics as indicated by the progressive approach to the steady-state plasma concentration. The answer is **(B).**
7. Bioavailability is calculated from the ratio of the area under the curve after oral administration ($AUC_{(PO)}$) to the AUC after intravenous administration of the same dose ($AUC_{(IV)}$, Figure 3–4), not from peak concentration measurements. Many drugs given orally are incompletely absorbed or metabolized in the lumen of the gut; they will have a bioavailability less than 1.0 even if they are not metabolized in the liver. The FDA cannot mandate bioavailability by any particular route, only that the bioavailability by that route be reasonably constant among preparations. Some drugs have a bioavailability of less than 1.0 even when given transdermally or

intramuscularly. This parameter is the ratio of the amount found in the circulating blood to the amount administered. The answer is **(D).**

8. The approach of the drug plasma concentration to steady-state concentration during continuous infusion follows a stereotypical curve (Figure 3–3) that rises rapidly at first and gradually levels off. It reaches 50% of steady state at one half-life, 75% at two half-lives, 87.5% at three, 93.75% at four, and progressively halves the difference between its current level and 100% with each half-life. The answer is **(E),** 32 hours or four half-lives.

9. The drug is being administered continuously; the steady-state concentration for a continuously administered drug is given by the equation in question 1. Thus

$$\textbf{Dosage} = \textbf{Plasma level}_{ss} \times \textbf{Clearance}$$

$$\textbf{1.92 mg/min} = \textbf{Cp}_{ss} \times \textbf{CL}$$

Rearranging:

$$\textbf{Cp}_{ss} = \frac{\textbf{1.92 mg/min}}{\textbf{CL}}$$

$$\textbf{Cp}_{ss} = \frac{\textbf{1.92 mg/min}}{\textbf{640 mL/min}}$$

$$\textbf{Cp}_{ss} = \textbf{0.003 mg/mL or 3 mg/L}$$

The answer is **(B).**

10. If the half-life is 1.8 hours, the plasma concentration should approach steady state after 8 hours (more than four half-lives). As indicated by the equation used in question 9, the steady-state concentration is a function of dosage and clearance, not volume of distribution. If the plasma level is less than predicted, the clearance in this patient must be greater than average. (In questions of this type, do not assume errors of analysis or administration as answers, unless all other possible answers can be positively ruled out.) The answer is **(B).**

11. According to the curve that relates plasma concentration to infusion time (Figure 3–3), a drug will reach 50% of its final steady-state concentration in one half-life, 75% in two half-lives, etc. From 9 AM to 1 PM is 4 hours or two half-lives. Therefore, the measured concentration at 1 PM is 75% of the steady-state value ($0.75 \times Cp_{ss}$). The steady-state concentration will be 3 mg/L divided by 0.75, or 4 mg/L. The answer is **(B).**

12. According to the curve that relates the decline of plasma concentration to time as the drug is eliminated (Figure 3–3), the plasma concentration of morphine was four times higher immediately after administration than at the time of the measurement, which occurred 6 hours or two half-lives later. Therefore the initial plasma concentration was 1 mg/L. Since the amount in the body is equal to $V_d \times Cp$ (text equation [1]), the amount injected was 200 L × 1 mg/L, or 200 mg. The answer is **(D).**

13. Half-life can be estimated from

$$t_{1/2} = \textbf{V}_d \frac{\textbf{0.693}}{\textbf{CL}} \quad \textbf{(text equation [3])}$$

$$= \textbf{80 L} \times \frac{\textbf{0.693}}{\textbf{1.386 L/h}}$$

$$= \textbf{80 L} \times \frac{\textbf{1}}{\textbf{2 L/h}}$$

$$= \textbf{40 hours}$$

The answer is **(D).**

14. If the drug is cleared almost entirely by the kidney and creatinine clearance is reduced to one third of normal, the total daily dose should also be reduced to one-third. The answer is **(B).**

15. If the drug is given only once a day, eight half-lives (24 hours ÷ 3 hours) pass during which it declines in plasma concentration (Figure 3–3). Each half-life results in a decline by half of the preceding level, ie, a power of two (one half-life, to 50%; two half-lives, to 25%; etc). Since the dosing interval is eight times greater than the half-life of the drug, the peak concentration is roughly 2^8 or 256 times higher than the minimum (trough) concentration. If one assumes that the drug is still effective at its trough concentration, the "opening" of the therapeutic window would be at least 256. The answer is **(D).**

16. We are asked to determine the half-life of the drug. Since the *distribution* half-life is not specified, we can assume that the *elimination* half-life is the parameter needed. The elimination phase of the graph of plasma concentration follows a straight line on the semilogarithmic graph, so we can conclude that the new drug follows first-order kinetics, the first requirement for determining the half-life. The straight-line portion of the graph shows a decline of 50% from the 2-hour point (4 mg/L) to the 8-hour sample (2 mg/L). Therefore, the half-life must be 8 minus 2 hours, or 6 hours. The answer is **(D),** 6 hours.

17. By definition, V_d is amount of drug in the body divided by the plasma concentration. To determine the volume of distribution, the drug must have reached equilibrium in its diffusion into the volume of distribution. Equilibrium is not reached until the distribution phase is complete. Therefore, we cannot use any of the data points preceding the start of the elimination phase. On the other hand, the only point at which we know the amount of drug in the body with certainty is immediately after administration, when the amount is equal to the dose administered. We need to determine what the plasma concentration would have been if distribution had been instantaneous. This is the purpose of the extrapolated portion of the straight line that extends to zero time. The dashed line shows the plasma concentration curve that would have been obtained if distribution were instantaneous. From the intercept of the extrapolated line with the plasma concentration axis, we see that the plasma concentration would have been 5 mg/L. Therefore, $V_d = 100$ mg/5 mg/L, or 20 L. The answer is **(E),** 20 L.

18. By definition, CL is equal to the rate of elimination divided by the plasma concentration. However, we are not given direct data for the rate of elimination. On the other hand, we have determined the half-life and the volume of distribution of the drug, so we can calculate the clearance from the relationship $t_{1/2} = 0.693 \times V_d \div CL$. Rearranging this equation, $CL = 0.693 \times V_d \div t_{1/2}$. Using the data from questions 16 and 17, we obtain 0.693×20 L $\div$ 6 h, or 2.3 L/h (approximately). The answer is **(D).**

Skill Keeper Answer: Zero-Order Elimination (see Chapter 1)

The three important drugs that follow zero-order rather than first-order kinetics are ethanol, aspirin, and phenytoin.

4 Drug Metabolism

OBJECTIVES

You should be able to:

- List the major phase I and phase II metabolic reactions.
- Describe the mechanism of hepatic enzyme induction and list three drugs that are known to cause it.
- List three drugs that inhibit the metabolism of other drugs.

- List three drugs for which there are well-defined genetically determined differences in metabolism.
- Discuss the effects of smoking, liver disease, and kidney disease on drug elimination.
- Describe the pathways by which acetaminophen is metabolized (1) to harmless products if normal doses are taken and (2) to hepatotoxic products if an overdose is taken.

Learn the definitions that follow.

Table 4–1. Definitions.

Term	Definition
Phase I reactions	Reactions that convert the parent drug to a more polar (water-soluble) or more reactive product by unmasking or inserting a polar functional group such as –OH, –SH, or $-NH_2$
Phase II reactions	Reactions that increase water solubility by conjugation of the drug molecule with a polar moiety such as glucuronate or sulfate
CYP isozymes	Cytochrome P450 enzyme species, eg, CYP2D6 and CYP3A4, that are responsible for much of drug metabolism. Many species of CYP enzymes have been recognized
Enzyme induction	Stimulation of drug-metabolizing capacity; usually manifested in the liver by increased synthesis of smooth endoplasmic reticulum (which contains a high concentration of phase I enzymes)
P-glycoprotein	An ATP-dependent transport molecule found in many cells, including epithelial cells and cancer cells. The transporter expels drug molecules from the cytoplasm into the extracellular space. Inhibitors of intestinal P-glycoprotein cause increased absorption and decreased fecal excretion of several drugs and mimic drugs that inhibit hepatic drug-metabolizing enzymes

CONCEPTS

A. Need for Drug Metabolism: Many cells that act as portals for entry of external molecules into the body (pulmonary alveoli, intestinal epithelium, etc) contain transporter molecules of the P-glycoprotein family that expel undesired molecules immediately after absorption. However, some foreign molecules manage to evade these gatekeepers and are absorbed. Therefore, all higher organisms require mechanisms for ridding themselves of toxic foreign molecules after they are absorbed as well as for excreting undesirable substances produced within the body. Biotransformation of drugs is one such mechanism. It is an important mechanism by which the body terminates the action of some drugs; in some cases, it serves to activate prodrugs. Most drugs are relatively lipid-soluble, a characteristic favorable to absorption across biomembranes. The same property would result in very slow removal from the body because the molecule would also be readily reabsorbed from the urine in the renal tubule. The body hastens excretion by transforming the drug to a less lipid-soluble, less readily reabsorbed form.

B. Types of Metabolic Reactions:

1. **Phase I reactions:** Phase I reactions include oxidation (especially by the cytochrome P450 group of enzymes, also called mixed-function oxidases), reduction, deamination, and hydrolysis. Examples are listed in Table 4–2.
2. **Phase II reactions:** Phase II reactions are synthetic reactions that involve addition (conjugation) of subgroups to –OH, $-NH_2$, and –SH functions on the drug molecule. The subgroups that are added include glucuronate, acetate, glutathione, glycine, sulfate, and methyl groups. Most of these groups are relatively polar and make the product less lipid-soluble than the original drug molecule. Examples of phase II reactions are listed in Table 4–3.

C. Sites of Drug Metabolism: The most important organ for drug metabolism is the liver. The kidneys play an important role in the metabolism of some drugs. A few drugs (eg, esters) are metabolized in many tissues (liver, blood, intestinal wall, etc) because of the broad distribution of their enzymes.

D. Determinants of Biotransformation Rate: The rate of biotransformation of a drug may vary markedly among different individuals. This variation is most often due to genetic or drug-induced differences. For a few drugs, age or disease-related differences in drug metabolism are

Table 4–2. Examples of phase I drug-metabolizing reactions.

Reaction Type	Typical Drug Substrates
Oxidations, P450-dependent	
Hydroxylation	Barbiturates, amphetamines, phenylbutazone, phenytoin
N-Dealkylation	Morphine, caffeine, theophylline
O-Dealkylation	Codeine
N-Oxidation	Acetaminophen, nicotine, methaqualone
S-Oxidation	Thioridazine, cimetidine, chlorpromazine
Deamination	Amphetamine, diazepam
Oxidations, P450-independent	
Amine oxidation	Epinephrine
Dehydrogenation	Ethanol, chloral hydrate
Reductions	Chloramphenicol, clonazepam, dantrolene, naloxone
Hydrolyses	
Esters	Procaine, succinylcholine, aspirin, clofibrate
Amides	Procainamide, lidocaine, indomethacin

significant. Gender is important for only a few drugs, eg, ethanol. (First-pass metabolism of alcohol is lower in women than in men.) Since the rate of biotransformation is often the primary determinant of clearance, variations in drug metabolism must be considered carefully when designing a dosage regimen. Smoking, a common cause of enzyme induction in the liver and lung, may increase the metabolism of some drugs (eg, theophylline).

1. **Genetic factors:** Several drug-metabolizing systems have been shown to differ among families or populations in genetically determined ways.
   a. **Hydrolysis of esters:** Succinylcholine is an ester that is metabolized by plasma cholinesterase ("pseudocholinesterase" or butyrylcholinesterase). In most individuals, this process occurs very rapidly, and a single dose of the drug has a duration of action of about 5 minutes. Approximately one person in 2500 has an abnormal form of this enzyme that more slowly metabolizes succinylcholine and similar esters. In such individuals, the neuromuscular paralysis produced by a single dose of succinylcholine may last many hours.
   b. **Acetylation of amines:** Isoniazid and some other amines such as procainamide are inactivated by N-acetylation. Individuals deficient in acetylation capacity, termed slow acetylators, may have prolonged or toxic responses to normal doses of these drugs. Slow acetylators constitute about 50% of white and African-American persons in the USA and a much smaller fraction of Asian and Inuit (Eskimo) populations. The slow acetylation trait is inherited as an autosomal recessive gene. There is some evidence linking slow acetylation to increased susceptibility to drug-induced lupus erythematosus.

Table 4–3. Examples of phase II drug-metabolizing reactions.*

Reaction Type	Typical Drug Substrates
Glucuronidation	Acetaminophen, morphine, diazepam, sulfathiazole, digoxin, digitoxin
Acetylation	Sulfonamides, isoniazid, clonazepam, mescaline, dapsone
Glutathione conjugation	Ethacrynic acid, reactive Phase I metabolite of acetaminophen
Glycine conjugation	Salicylic acid, nicotinic acid (niacin), deoxycholic acid
Sulfate conjugation	Acetaminophen, methyldopa, estrone
Methylation	Epinephrine, norepinephrine, dopamine, histamine

*Adapted, with permission, from Katzung BG (editor): *Basic & Clinical Pharmacology,* 8th ed. McGraw-Hill, 2001.

Table 4–4. A partial list of drugs that significantly induce P450-mediated drug metabolism in humans.

CYP Family Induced	Important Inducers	Drugs Whose Metabolism Is Induced
1A2	Benzo[*a*]pyrene (from tobacco smoke), carbamazepine, phenobarbital, rifampin, omeprazole	Acetaminophen, clozapine, haloperidol, theophylline, tricyclic antidepressants, (*R*)-warfarin
2C9	Barbiturates, especially phenobarbital, phenytoin, primidone, rifampin	Barbiturates, chloramphenicol, doxorubicin, ibuprofen, phenytoin, chlorpromazine, steroids, tolbutamide, warfarin
2C19	Carbamazepine, phenobarbital, phenytoin	Tricyclic antidepressants, phenytoin, topiramate, (*R*)-warfarin
2E1	Ethanol, isoniazid	Acetaminophen, ethanol (minor), halothane
3A4	Barbiturates, carbamazepine, corticosteroids, efavirenz, phenytoin, rifampin, troglitazone	Antiarrhythmics, antidepressants, azole antifungals, benzodiazepines, calcium channel blockers, cyclosporine, delavirdine, doxorubicin, efavirenz, erythromycin, estrogens, HIV protease inhibitors, nefazodone, paclitaxel, proton pump inhibitors, HMG-CoA reductase inhibitors, rifabutin, rifampin, sildenafil, SSRIs, tamoxifen, trazodone, vinca anticancer agents

c. **Oxidation:** The rate of oxidation of debrisoquin, sparteine, phenformin, dextromethorphan, metoprolol, and some tricyclic antidepressants by certain P450 isozymes has been shown to be genetically determined.

2. **Other drugs:** Coadministration of certain agents may alter the disposition of many drugs. Mechanisms include the following:

a. **Enzyme induction:** As indicated above, induction usually results from increased synthesis of cytochrome P450-dependent drug-oxidizing enzymes in the liver. Many isozymes of the P450 family exist, and inducers selectively increase subgroups of isozymes. Common inducers of a few of these isozymes and the drugs whose metabolism is increased are listed in Table 4–4. Several days are usually required to reach maximum induction; a similar amount of time is required to regress after withdrawal of the inducer. Some drugs induce their own metabolism.

b. **Metabolism inhibitors:** Common inhibitors and the drugs whose metabolism is diminished are listed in Table 4–5. **Suicide inhibitors** are drugs that are metabolized to products which irreversibly inhibit the metabolizing enzyme. Such agents include

Table 4–5. A partial list of drugs that significantly inhibit P450-mediated drug metabolism in humans.

CYP Family Inhibited	Inhibitor	Drugs Whose Metabolism Is Inhibited
1A2	Cimetidine, fluoroquinolones, grapefruit juice, macrolides, isoniazid, zileuton	Acetaminophen, clozapine, haloperidol, theophylline, tricyclic antidepressants, (*R*)-warfarin
2C9	Amiodarone, chloramphenicol, cimetidine, isoniazid, metronidazole, SSRIs, zafirlukast	Barbiturates, chloramphenicol, doxorubicin, ibuprofen, phenytoin, chlorpromazine, steroids, tolbutamide, (*S*)-warfarin
2C19	Omeprazole, SSRIs	Phenytoin, topiramate, (*R*)-warfarin
2D6	Amiodarone, cimetidine, quinidine, SSRIs	Antidepressants, flecainide, lidocaine, mexiletine, opioids
3A4	Amiodarone, azole antifungals, cimetidine, clarithromycin, cyclosporine, erythromycin, fluoroquinolones, grapefruit juice, HIV protease inhibitors, metronidazole, quinine, SSRIs, tacrolimus	Antiarrhythmics, antidepressants, azole antifungals, benzodiazepines, calcium channel blockers, cyclosporine, delavirdine, doxorubicin, efavirenz, erythromycin, estrogens, HIV protease inhibitors, nefazodone, paclitaxel, proton pump inhibitors, HMG-CoA reductase inhibitors, rifabutin, rifampin, sildenafil, SSRIs, tamoxifen, trazodone, vinca anticancer agents

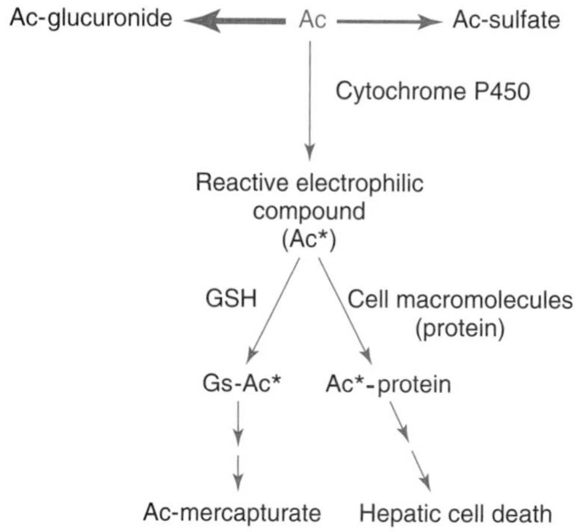

Figure 4–1. Metabolism of acetaminophen to harmless conjugates or to toxic metabolites. Acetaminophen glucuronide, acetaminophen sulfate, and the mercapturate conjugate of acetaminophen are all nontoxic phase II conjugates. Ac* is the toxic, reactive phase I metabolite. Transformation to the reactive metabolite occurs if hepatic stores of sulfate, glucuronide, and glutathione are depleted or overwhelmed or if phase I enzymes have been induced.

Ac-glucuronide ← Ac → Ac-sulfate
Cytochrome P450
Reactive electrophilic compound (Ac*)
GSH
Cell macromolecules (protein)
Gs-Ac*
Ac*-protein
Ac-mercapturate
Hepatic cell death

ethinyl estradiol, norethindrone, spironolactone, secobarbital, allopurinol, fluroxene, and propylthiouracil. Metabolism may also be decreased by pharmacodynamic factors such as a reduction in blood flow to the metabolizing organ (eg, propranolol reduces hepatic blood flow).

c. **Inhibitors of intestinal P-glycoprotein:** P-glycoprotein (P-gp) has been identified as an important modulator of intestinal drug transport and usually functions to expel drugs from the intestinal mucosa into the lumen. (Other members of the P-gp family are found in the blood-brain barrier and in multiply drug-resistant cancer cells.) Drugs that inhibit intestinal P-gp mimic drug metabolism inhibitors by increasing bioavailability and may result in toxic plasma concentrations of drugs given at normally nontoxic dosage. P-gp inhibitors include verapamil, mibefradil (a calcium channel blocker no longer on the market), and certain components of grapefruit juice. Important drugs that are normally expelled by P-gp (and which are therefore potentially more toxic when given with a P-gp inhibitor) include digoxin, cyclosporine, and saquinavir.

E. **Toxic Metabolism:** Drug metabolism is not synonymous with drug inactivation. Some drugs are converted to active products by metabolism. If these products are toxic, severe injury may result under some circumstances. An important example is acetaminophen when taken in large overdoses (Figure 4–1). Acetaminophen is conjugated to harmless glucuronide and sulfate metabolites when it is taken in normal doses. If a large overdose is taken, however, the metabolic pathways are overwhelmed, and a P450-dependent system converts some of the drug to a reactive intermediate (*N*-acetyl-*p*-benzoquinoneimine). This intermediate is conjugated with glutathione to a third harmless product if glutathione stores are adequate. If glutathione stores are exhausted, however, the reactive intermediate combines with essential hepatic cell proteins, resulting in cell death. Prompt administration of other sulfhydryl donors (eg, acetylcysteine) may be life-saving after an overdose. In severe liver disease, stores of glucuronide, sulfate, and glutathione may be depleted, making the patient more susceptible to hepatic toxicity with near-normal doses of acetaminophen. Enzyme inducers (eg, ethanol) may increase acetaminophen toxicity because they increase phase I metabolism more than phase II metabolism, thus resulting in increased production of the reactive metabolite.

QUESTIONS

DIRECTIONS (Items 1–8): Each of the numbered items or incomplete statements in this section is followed by answers or by completions of the statement. Select the ONE lettered answer or completion that is BEST in each case.

1. You have diagnosed asthma in a 19-year-old patient with recurrent, episodic attacks of bronchospasm with wheezing. Avoidance of allergens has been tried unsuccessfully. She is to receive therapy with several drugs. You are concerned about drug interactions caused by changes in drug metabolism in this patient. Drug metabolism usually results in a product that is

(A) More likely to distribute intracellularly
(B) Less lipid-soluble than the original drug
(C) More likely to be reabsorbed by kidney tubules
(D) More lipid-soluble than the original drug
(E) More likely to produce adverse effects

2. If therapy with multiple drugs causes induction of drug metabolism in your asthma patient, it will
(A) Result in increased smooth endoplasmic reticulum
(B) Result in increased rough endoplasmic reticulum
(C) Result in decreased enzymes in the soluble cytoplasmic fraction
(D) Require 3–4 months to reach completion
(E) Be irreversible

3. A factor that is likely to increase the duration of action of a drug that is partially metabolized by CYP3A4 in the liver is
(A) Chronic administration of phenobarbital prior to and during therapy with the drug in question
(B) Chronic therapy with cimetidine prior to and during therapy with the drug in question
(C) Displacement from tissue binding sites by another drug
(D) Increased cardiac output
(E) Chronic administration of rifampin

4. Which of the following is a phase II drug-metabolizing reaction?
(A) Acetylation
(B) Deamination
(C) Hydrolysis
(D) Oxidation
(E) Reduction

5. Reports of cardiac arrhythmias caused by unusually high blood levels of two antihistamines, terfenadine and astemizole, led to their removal from the market. These effects were best explained by
(A) Concomitant treatment with phenobarbital
(B) Use of these drugs by smokers
(C) Use of antihistamines by persons of Asian background
(D) A genetic predisposition to metabolize succinylcholine slowly
(E) Treatment of these patients with ketoconazole, an antifungal agent

6. Which of the following drugs is associated with slower metabolism in Caucasians and African-Americans than in most Asians?
(A) Cimetidine
(B) Procainamide
(C) Quinidine
(D) Rifampin
(E) Succinylcholine

7. Which of the following drugs may inhibit the hepatic microsomal P450 responsible for warfarin metabolism?
(A) Cimetidine
(B) Ethanol
(C) Phenobarbital
(D) Procainamide
(E) Rifampin

8. Which of the following drugs is hydrolyzed by a plazma enzyme that is abnormally low in activity in about one out of every 2500 humans?
(A) Cimetidine
(B) Ethanol
(C) Procainamide
(D) Rifampin
(E) Succinylcholine

DIRECTIONS (Items 9–10): The matching questions in this section consist of a list of seven lettered options followed by several numbered items. For each numbered item, select the ONE lettered option that is most closely associated with it. Each lettered option may be selected once, more than once, or not at all.

(A) Cimetidine
(B) Ethanol
(C) Ketoconazole
(D) Procainamide
(E) Quinidine
(F) Sildenafil
(G) Succinylcholine

9. Pretreatment with this agent for 5–7 days might increase the toxicity of acetaminophen

10. A drug that has higher first-pass metabolism in men than in women

ANSWERS

1. Biotransformation usually results in a product that is less lipid-soluble. The answer is **(B).**
2. The smooth endoplasmic reticulum, which contains the mixed-function oxidase drug-metabolizing enzymes, is selectively increased by "inducers." The answer is **(A).**
3. Phenobarbital can induce drug-metabolizing enzymes and thereby may *reduce* the duration of drug action. Displacement of drug from tissue may transiently increase the intensity of the effect but will decrease the volume of distribution and thereby reduce the half-life. Cimetidine is recognized as an inhibitor of P450 and may also decrease hepatic blood flow under some circumstances. The answer is **(B).**
4. Acetylation is a phase II conjugation reaction. The answer is **(A).**
5. Treatment with phenobarbital and smoking are associated with increased drug metabolism and lower, not higher, blood levels. Persons of Asian origin have a high probability of metabolizing certain amides (isoniazid, procainamide) *more rapidly;* Asians do not appear to metabolize antihistamines differently from other ethnic groups. Ketoconazole, itraconazole, erythromycin, and some substance in grapefruit juice slow the metabolism of certain "nonsedating" antihistamines. The answer is **(E).**
6. Procainamide, like hydralazine and isoniazid, is metabolized by N-acetylation, an enzymatic process that is slower than average in about 20% of Asians and in about 50% of Caucasians and African-Americans. The answer is **(B).**
7. Cimetidine is a very commonly used drug and has well-documented ability to inhibit the hepatic metabolism of many drugs. The answer is **(A).**
8. Succinylcholine is normally hydrolyzed quite rapidly by plasma cholinesterase (pseudocholinesterase). This enzyme is abnormal in about 1/2500 of the human population, resulting in an unusually long duration of action of succinylcholine in these patients. The answer is **(E).**
9. Acetaminophen is normally eliminated by phase II conjugation reactions. The drug's toxicity is dependent on an oxidized reactive metabolite produced by phase I oxidizing P450 enzymes. Drugs that cause induction of P450 enzymes, such as rifampin, may increase the production of this toxic metabolite. Ethanol does this and thus reduces hepatotoxic dose. The answer is **(B).**
10. Ethanol is subject to metabolism in the stomach as well as in the liver. Independently of weight and other factors, men have greater gastric ethanol metabolism than women. The answer is **(B).**

Drug Evaluation & Regulation

5

OBJECTIVES

Learn the definitions that follow.

Table 5–1. Drug evaluation definitions.

Term	Definition
Single-blind study	A clinical trial in which the investigators—but not the subjects—know which subjects are receiving active drug and which are receiving placebos
Double-blind study	A clinical trial in which neither the subjects nor the investigators know which subjects are receiving placebos; the code is held by a third party
IND	Investigational New Drug Exemption; application for FDA approval to carry out new drug trials in humans; requires animal data
NDA	New Drug Application; FDA approval to market a new drug for ordinary medical clinical use
Placebo	An inactive "dummy" medication made up to resemble the active investigational formulation as much as possible
Phases I, II, and III of clinical trials	Three parts of a clinical trial that are usually carried out before submitting an NDA to the FDA
Positive control	A known standard therapy, to be used along with placebo, to fully evaluate the safety and efficacy of a new drug in relation to the others available
Mutagenic	An effect on the inheritable characteristics of a cell or organism—a mutation in the DNA; tested in microorganisms with the Ames test
Teratogenic	An effect on the development of an organism resulting in abnormal structure or function; not generally heritable
Carcinogenic	An effect of inducing malignant characteristics
Orphan drugs	Drugs developed for diseases in which the expected number of patients is small. Some countries bestow certain commercial advantages on companies that develop drugs for uncommon diseases

CONCEPTS

A. Safety and Efficacy: Because society expects prescription drugs to be safe and effective, governments have regulated the development and marketing of new drugs. The **Food & Drug Administration (FDA)** is the regulatory body in the USA that proposes and administers these regulations. The FDA requires evidence of relative safety (derived from acute and subacute toxicity testing in animals) and probable therapeutic action (from the pharmacologic profile in animals) before human testing is permitted. Some information about the pharmacokinetics of a compound is also required before clinical evaluation is begun. Chronic toxicity test results are generally not required before human studies are started. The development of a new drug and its pathway through various levels of testing and regulation are illustrated in Figure 5–1. The cost of development of a new drug, including false starts and discarded molecules, is currently several hundred million dollars.

B. Animal Testing: The amount of animal testing required before human studies begin is a function of the proposed use and the urgency of the application. Thus, a drug proposed for occasional nonsystemic use requires less extensive testing than one destined for chronic systemic

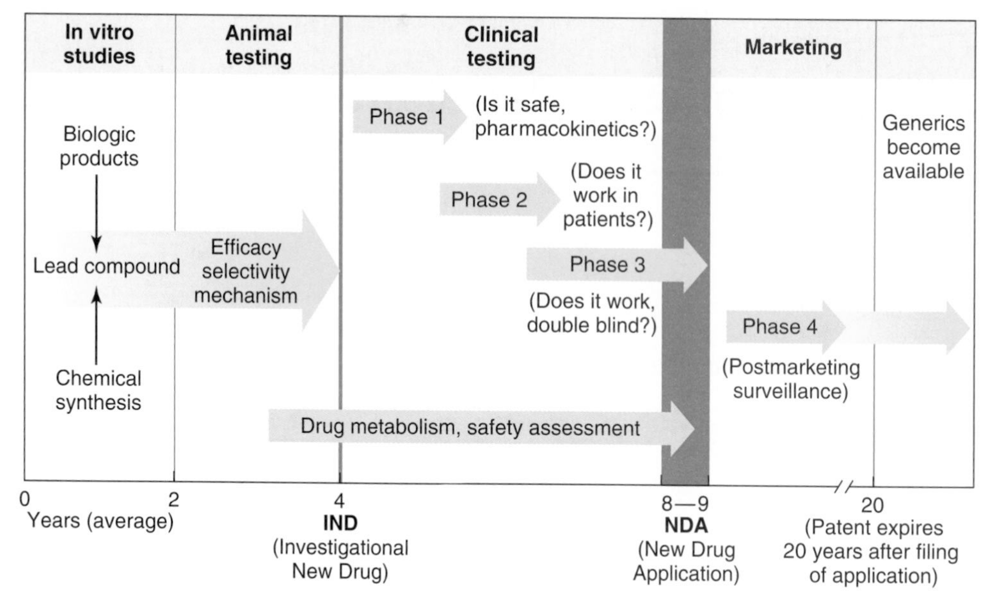

Figure 5–1. The development and testing process required to bring a new drug to market in the USA. Some requirements may be different for drugs used in life-threatening diseases. (Reproduced, with permission, from Katzung BG [editor]: *Basic & Clinical Pharmacology,* 8th ed. McGraw-Hill, 2001.)

administration. Anticancer drugs and drugs proposed for use in AIDS, because of the urgent need for new agents, require less evidence of safety than do drugs used in treatment of less threatening diseases and are often investigated and approved on an accelerated schedule.

1. **Acute toxicity:** Acute toxicity studies are required for all drugs. These studies involve administration of single doses of the agent up to the lethal level in at least two species, eg, one rodent and one nonrodent.
2. **Subacute and chronic toxicity:** Subacute and chronic toxicity testing are required for most agents, especially those intended for chronic use. Tests are usually conducted for at least the amount of time proposed for human application, ie, 2–4 weeks (subacute) or 6–24 months (chronic), in at least two species.

C. Types of Animal Tests: Tests done with animals often include general screening tests for pharmacologic effects, hepatic and renal function monitoring, blood and urine tests, gross and histopathologic examination of tissues, and tests of reproductive effects and carcinogenicity.

1. **Pharmacologic profile:** The pharmacologic profile is a description of all the pharmacologic effects of a drug (eg, effects on blood pressure, gastrointestinal activity, respiration, renal function, endocrine function, the central nervous system).
2. **Reproductive toxicity:** Reproductive toxicity testing involves the study of the fertility effects of the candidate drug and its teratogenic and mutagenic effects. **Teratogenesis** can be defined as the induction of developmental defects in the fetus (by exposure of the fetus to a drug, radiation, etc). Teratogenesis is studied by treating pregnant female animals of at least two species at selected times during early pregnancy when organogenesis is known to take place and later examining the fetuses or neonates for abnormalities. Examples of drugs known to have teratogenic effects include thalidomide, ethanol, glucocorticoids, valproic acid, isotretinoin, warfarin, lithium, and androgens. **Mutagenesis** is induction of changes in the genetic material of animals of any age and therefore induction of heritable abnormalities. The **Ames test,** the standard in vitro test for mutagenicity, uses a special strain of salmonella bacteria that naturally depends on specific nutrients in the culture medium. Loss of this dependence during exposure to the test drug signals a mutation. The **dominant lethal test** is an in vivo mutagenicity test carried out in mice. Male animals are exposed to the test substance before mating. Abnormalities in the results of subsequent mating (loss of embryos, deformed fetuses, etc) signal a mutation in the male's germ cells. Many carcino-

gens (eg, aflatoxin, cancer chemotherapeutic drugs, and other agents that bind to DNA) have mutagenic effects.

3. **Carcinogenesis:** Carcinogenesis is the induction of malignant characteristics in cells. Because carcinogenicity is difficult and expensive to study, the Ames test is often used to screen chemicals, since there is a moderately high degree of correlation between mutagenicity in the Ames test and carcinogenicity in some animal tests. Agents with known carcinogenic effects include coal tar, aflatoxin, dimethylnitrosamine and other nitrosamines, urethane, vinyl chloride, and the polycyclic aromatic hydrocarbons in tobacco smoke, eg, benzo[*a*]pyrene.

D. Clinical Trials: Human testing in the USA requires the prior approval of an **Investigational New Drug Exemption application (IND),** which has been submitted by the manufacturer to the FDA (see Figure 5–1). The major clinical testing process is informally divided into three phases before a **New Drug Application (NDA)** can be submitted. The NDA constitutes the request for approval of general marketing of the new agent for prescription use. A fourth phase of study follows NDA approval.

1. **Phase I:** A phase I trial consists of careful evaluation of the dose-response relationship in a small number of normal human volunteers (eg, 20–30). An exception is in phase I trials of cancer chemotherapeutic agents; these are carried out by administering the agents to patients with cancer. In phase I studies, the acute effects of the agent are studied over a broad range of dosages, starting with one that produces no detectable effect and progressing to one that produces either a significant physiologic response or a very minor toxic effect.
2. **Phase II:** A phase II trial involves evaluation of a drug in a moderate number of patients (eg, 100–300) with the target disease. A placebo or positive control drug is included in a single-blind or double-blind design. The study is carried out under very carefully controlled conditions and patients are very closely monitored, often in a hospital research ward. The goal is to determine whether the agent has the desired therapeutic effects at doses that are tolerated by sick patients.
3. **Phase III:** A phase III trial consists of a large design involving many patients (eg, 1000–5000 or more in many centers) and many clinicians who are using the drug in the manner proposed for its ultimate general use, eg, in outpatients. Such studies usually include placebo and positive controls in a double-blind crossover design. The goal is to explore further the spectrum of beneficial actions of the new drug, to compare it with older therapies, and to discover toxicities, if any, that occur so infrequently as to be undetectable in phase II studies.
4. **Phase IV:** Phase IV represents the postmarketing surveillance phase of evaluation, in which it is hoped that toxicities that occur very infrequently will be detected and reported early enough to prevent major therapeutic disasters. Unlike the first three phases, phase IV is not rigidly regulated by the FDA.

E. Drug Legislation: In the USA, many laws regulating drugs have been passed during this century. Refer to Table 5–2 for a partial list of this legislation.

F. Orphan Drugs: An orphan drug is a drug for a rare disease (one affecting fewer than 200,000 people). The study of such agents has often been neglected because the sales of an effective agent for an uncommon ailment might not pay the costs of development. In the USA, current legislation provides for tax relief and other incentives designed to encourage the development of orphan drugs.

QUESTIONS

DIRECTIONS: Each of the numbered items or incomplete statements in this section is followed by answers or by completions of the statement. Select the ONE lettered answer or completion that is BEST in each case.

1. With regard to clinical trials of new drugs, which of the following is MOST correct?
   (A) Phase I involves the study of a small number of normal volunteers by highly trained clinical pharmacologists
   (B) Phase II involves the use of the new drug in a large number of patients (1000–5000) who have the disease to be treated

Table 5–2. Selected legislation pertaining to drugs in the USA.*

Law	Purpose and Effect
Pure Food & Drug Act of 1906	Prohibited mislabeling and adulteration of drugs
Harrison Narcotics Act of 1914	Established regulations for the use of opium, opioids, and cocaine (marijuana added in 1937)
Food, Drug, & Cosmetic Act of 1938	Required that new drugs be tested for safety as well as purity
Kefauver-Harris Amendment (1962)	Required proof of efficacy as well as safety for new drugs
Comprehensive Drug Abuse Prevention & Control Act (1970)	Outlined strict controls on the manufacture, distribution, and prescribing of habit-forming drugs; established programs for the treatment and prevention of addiction
Drug Price Competition & Patent Restoration Act of 1984	Abbreviated new drug applications for generic drugs; required bioequivalence data; patent life extended by the amount of time drug was delayed by the review process; cannot exceed 5 years or extend to more than 14 years post-NDA

*Modified and reproduced, with permission, from Katzung BG (editor): *Basic & Clinical Pharmacology,* 8th ed, McGraw-Hill, 2001.

(C) Phase III involves the determination of the drug's therapeutic index by the cautious induction of toxicity
(D) Phase IV involves the detailed study of toxic effects that have been discovered in phase III
(E) Phase II requires the use of a positive control (a known effective drug) and a placebo

2. Animal testing of potential new therapeutic agents
(A) Extends over a time period of at least 3 years in order to discover late toxicities
(B) Requires the use of at least two primate species, eg, monkey and baboon
(C) Requires the submission of histopathologic slides and specimens to the FDA for government evaluation
(D) Has good predictability for drug allergy-type reactions
(E) May be abbreviated in the case of some very toxic agents used in cancer

3. The "dominant lethal" test involves the treatment of a male adult animal with a chemical before mating; the pregnant female is later examined for fetal death and abnormalities. The dominant lethal test therefore is a test of
(A) Teratogenicity
(B) Mutagenicity
(C) Carcinogenicity
(D) All of the above
(E) None of the above

4. An optimal phase III clinical trial of a new analgesic drug would not include
(A) A negative control (placebo)
(B) A positive control (current standard therapy)
(C) Double-blind protocol (neither the patient nor immediate observers of the patient know which agent is active)
(D) A group of 2000–3000 subjects with a clinical condition requiring analgesia
(E) Prior submission of an NDA (new drug application) to the FDA

5. In the testing of new compounds (eg, antihypertensive drugs) for potential therapeutic use
(A) Animal tests cannot be used to predict the types of toxicities that may occur because there is no correlation with human toxicity
(B) Human studies in normal individuals will be done before the drug is used in diseased individuals
(C) Degree of risk must be assessed in at least three species of animals, including one primate species
(D) The animal therapeutic index must be known before trial of the agents in humans

6. The Ames test is a method for detecting
(A) Carcinogenesis in rodents
(B) Carcinogenesis in primates

(C) Teratogenesis in any mammalian species
(D) Teratogenesis in primates
(E) Mutagenesis in bacteria

ANSWERS

1. Except for known toxic drugs, eg, cancer chemotherapy drugs, phase I is carried out in 20–30 normal volunteers. Phase II is carried out in several hundred patients with the disease. The therapeutic index is rarely determined in any clinical trial. Phase IV is the general surveillance phase that follows general marketing of the new drug. It is not targeted at specific effects. Positive controls and placebos are not a rigid requirement of any phase of clinical trials, though they are often used in phase II and phase III studies. The answer is **(A).**

2. Drugs proposed for short-term use may not require long-term chronic testing. For some drugs, no primates are used; for other agents, only one species is used. The data from the tests, not the evidence itself, must be submitted to the FDA. Prediction of human drug allergy from animal testing is not very reliable. The answer is **(E).**

3. The description of the test indicates that a chromosomal change (passed from father to fetus) is the toxicity detected. This is a mutation. The answer is **(B).**

4. The first four items **(A–D)** are correct. An NDA cannot be acted upon until the first three phases of clinical trials have been completed. (The IND must be approved before clinical trials can be conducted.) The answer is **(E).**

5. Animal tests in a single species do not always predict human toxicities; but when these tests are carried out in several species, most acute toxicities that occur in humans will also appear in at least one animal species. According to current FDA rules, the "degree of risk" must be determined in at least two species. Use of primates is not always required. The therapeutic index is not required. Except for cancer chemotherapeutic agents, phase I clinical trials are always carried out in normal subjects. The answer is **(B).**

6. The Ames test is carried out in salmonella and detects mutations in the bacterial DNA. Because mutagenic potential is associated with carcinogenic risk for many chemicals, the Ames test is often used to claim that a particular agent may be a carcinogen. However, the test itself only detects mutations. The answer is **(E).**

Part II: Autonomic Drugs

6 Introduction to Autonomic Pharmacology

OBJECTIVES

You should be able to:

- Describe the steps in the synthesis, storage, release, and termination of action of the major autonomic transmitters.
- Name two cotransmitter substances.
- Describe the organ system effects of stimulation of the parasympathetic and sympathetic systems.
- Name examples of inhibitors of acetylcholine and norepinephrine synthesis, storage, and release. Predict the effects of these inhibitors on the function of the major organ systems.
- List the determinants of blood pressure and describe the baroreceptor reflex response for the following perturbations: (1) blood loss, (2) administration of a vasodilator, (3) a vasoconstrictor, (4) a cardiac stimulant, (5) a cardiac depressant.
- Name the major types of receptors found on autonomic effector tissues.
- Describe the differences between the effects of surgical sympathetic ganglionectomy (interruption of ganglionic transmission by surgical removal of the sympathetic ganglia) and the effects of pharmacologic ganglion block.
- Describe the action of several toxins that affect nerve function: tetrodotoxin, saxitoxin, botulinum toxins, and latrotoxin.

Learn the definitions that follow.

Table 6–1. Definitions.

Term	Definition
Adrenergic	A nerve ending that releases norepinephrine as the primary transmitter; also a synapse in which norepinephrine is the primary transmitter
Adrenoceptor	A receptor that binds—and is activated by—one of the catecholamine transmitters (norepinephrine, epinephrine, or dopamine) and related drugs
Autonomic effector cells or tissues	Cells or tissues that have adrenoceptors or cholinoceptors which, when activated, alter the function of those cells or tissues, eg, smooth muscle, heart, glands
Baroreceptor reflex	The neuronal homeostatic mechanism that the body uses to maintain blood pressure constant; the sensory limb originates in the baroreceptors of the carotid sinus
Cholinergic	A nerve ending that releases acetylcholine as the primary transmitter; also a synapse in which acetylcholine is the primary transmitter
Cholinoceptor	A receptor that binds, and is activated by, acetylcholine and related drugs
Dopaminergic	A nerve ending that releases dopamine as the primary transmitter; also a synapse in which dopamine is the primary transmitter
Homeostatic reflex	A neuronal compensatory mechanism for maintaining a body function at a predetermined level, eg, the baroreceptor reflex for blood pressure
Parasympathetic (PANS)	The part of the autonomic nervous system that originates in the cranial nerves and the sacral part of the spinal cord

Table 6–1. Definitions. *(continued)*

Term	Definition
Postsynaptic receptor	Receptor located on the distal side of the synapse, eg, on the effector cell; contrast with presynaptic receptors
Presynaptic receptor	Receptor located on the nerve ending in a synapse; modulates the release of transmitter
Sympathetic (SANS)	The part of the autonomic nervous system that originates in the thoracic and lumbar parts of the spinal cord

CONCEPTS

The autonomic nervous system (ANS) is the major involuntary, unconscious, automatic portion of the nervous system and contrasts in several ways with the somatic (voluntary) nervous system. The anatomy, neurotransmitter chemistry, receptor characteristics, and functional integration of the ANS are discussed below.

A. **Anatomic Aspects of the ANS:** The motor (efferent) portion of the ANS is the major pathway for information transmission from the central nervous system (CNS) to the involuntary effector tissues (smooth muscle, cardiac muscle, and exocrine glands; Figure 6–1). The **enteric nervous system (ENS)** is a semiautonomous part of the ANS, with specific functions for the control of the gastrointestinal tract. The ENS consists of the myenteric plexus (plexus of Auerbach) and the submucous plexus (plexus of Meissner) and includes inputs from the parasympathetic and sympathetic nervous systems.

There are many sensory (afferent) fibers in autonomic nerves. These are of considerable im-

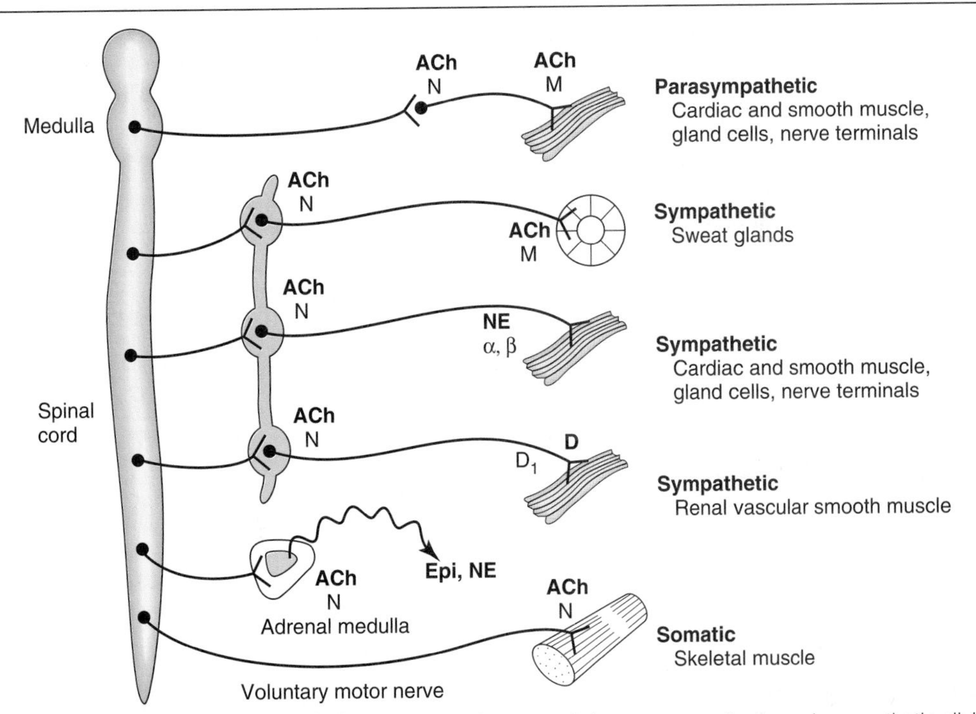

Figure 6–1. Schematic diagram comparing some features of the parasympathetic and sympathetic divisions of the autonomic nervous system with the somatic motor system. Parasympathetic ganglia are not shown as discrete structures because most of them are diffusely distributed in the walls of the organs innervated. ACh, acetylcholine; Epi, epinephrine; NE, norepinephrine; D, dopamine; N, nicotinic; M, muscarinic; α, β, alpha and beta adrenoceptors; D_1, dopamine$_1$ receptors. (Reproduced, with permission, from Katzung BG [editor]: *Basic & Clinical Pharmacology,* 8th ed. McGraw-Hill, 2001.)

portance for the physiologic control of the involuntary organs but are directly influenced by only a few drugs.

1. **Spinal roots of origin:** The parasympathetic preganglionic motor fibers originate in cranial nerve nuclei III, VII, IX, and X and in sacral segments (usually S2–S4) of the spinal cord. The sympathetic preganglionic fibers originate in the thoracic (T1–T12) and lumbar (L1–L5) segments of the cord.
2. **Location of ganglia:** Most of the sympathetic ganglia are located in two paravertebral chains that lie along the spinal column. A few (the prevertebral ganglia) are located on the anterior aspect of the vertebral column. Most of the parasympathetic ganglia are located in the organs innervated, more distant from the spinal cord.
3. **Length of pre- and postganglionic fibers:** Because of the locations of the ganglia noted above, the preganglionic sympathetic fibers are short and the postganglionic fibers are long. The opposite is true for the parasympathetic system: preganglionic fibers are long and postganglionic fibers are short.
4. **Uninnervated receptors:** Some receptors that respond to autonomic transmitters and drugs receive no innervation. These include muscarinic receptors on the endothelium of blood vessels, some presynaptic receptors, and, in some species, the adrenoceptors on apocrine sweat glands and α_2 and β adrenoceptors in some blood vessels.

B. Neurotransmitter Aspects of the ANS: The synthesis, storage, release, and termination of action of the neurotransmitters are very important in the action of autonomic drugs (Figure 6–2).

1. **Cholinergic transmission:** Acetylcholine (ACh) is the primary transmitter in all autonomic ganglia and at the parasympathetic postganglionic neuron-effector cell synapses.

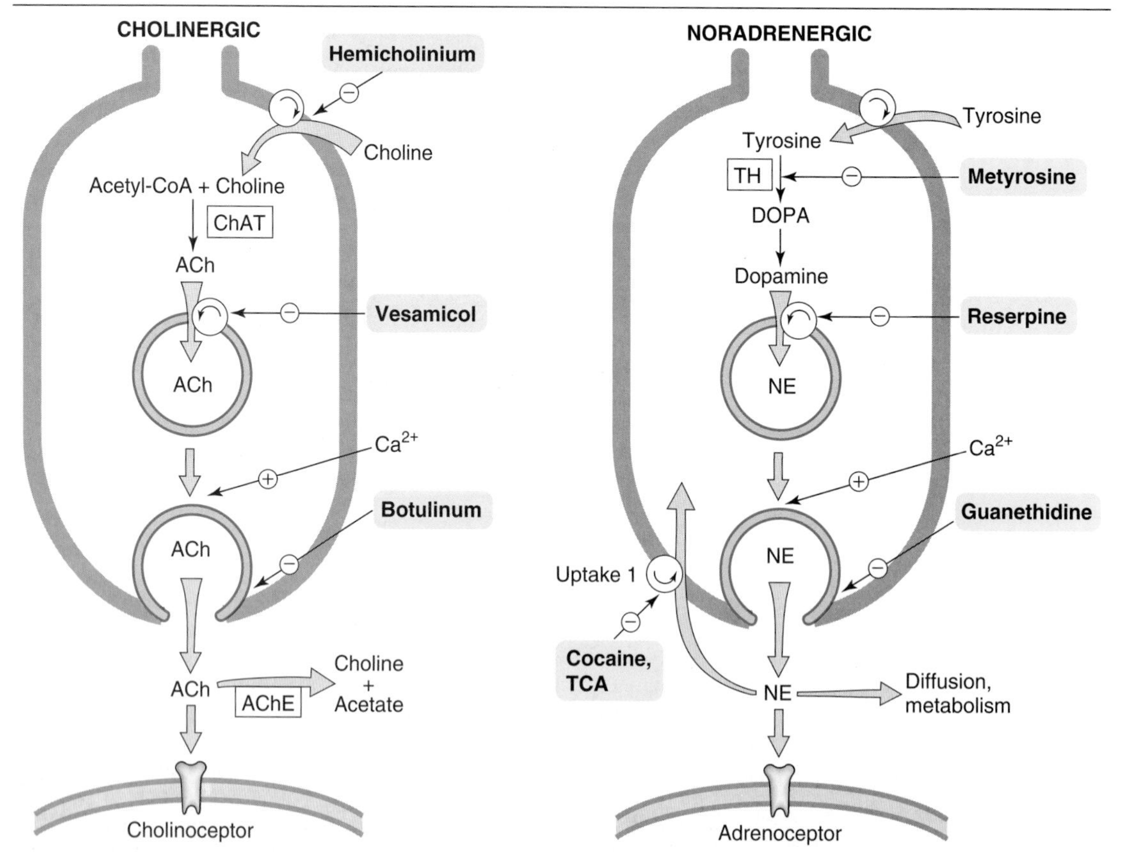

Figure 6–2. Characteristics of transmitter synthesis, storage, release, and termination of action at cholinergic and noradrenergic nerve terminals are shown from the top downward. Circles represent transporters; ACh, acetylcholine; AChE, acetylcholinesterase; ChAT, choline acetate transferase; DOPA, dihydroxyphenylalanine; NE, norepinephrine; TCA, tricyclic antidepressant; TH, tyrosine hydroxylase.

a. **Synthesis and storage:** ACh is synthesized from acetyl-CoA and choline by the enzyme choline acetyltransferase. The rate-limiting step is probably the transport of choline into the nerve terminal. This transport can be inhibited by **hemicholinium.** ACh is actively transported into its vesicles for storage. This process can be inhibited by **vesamicol.**

b. **Release of acetylcholine:** Release of transmitter stores from vesicles in the nerve ending requires the entry of calcium through calcium channels and triggering of an interaction between several proteins associated with the vesicles and the nerve ending membrane (**synaptobrevin, synaptotagmin, synaptosome-associated protein [SNAP],** and others). This interaction results in the fusion of the vesicular and nerve ending membranes, the opening of a pore to the extracellular space, and the release of the stored transmitter. The several types of **botulinum toxins** enzymatically alter synaptobrevin or one of the other docking or fusion proteins to prevent the release process.

Skill Keeper: Drug Permeation (see Chapter 1)

Botulinum toxin is a very large protein molecule and does not diffuse readily when injected into tissue. In spite of this property, it is able to enter cholinergic nerve endings from the extracellular space and block the release of acetylcholine. How might it cross the lipid membrane barrier? *The Skill Keeper Answer appears at the end of the chapter.*

c. **Termination of action of ACh:** The action of acetylcholine in the synapse is normally terminated by metabolism to acetate and choline by the enzyme acetylcholinesterase. The products are not excreted but are recycled in the body. Inhibition of acetylcholinesterase is an important therapeutic (and potentially toxic) effect of several drugs.

d. **Drug effects on synthesis, storage, release, and termination of action of ACh:** Drugs that block the synthesis of ACh (eg, hemicholinium), its storage (eg, vesamicol), or its release (eg, botulinum toxin*) are not very useful in therapy because their effects are not sufficiently selective (ie, PANS and SANS ganglia and somatic neuromuscular junctions may all be blocked).

2. **Adrenergic transmission:** Norepinephrine (NE) is the primary transmitter at the sympathetic postganglionic neuron-effector cell synapses in most tissues. Important exceptions include sympathetic fibers to thermoregulatory (eccrine) sweat glands and probably vasodilator sympathetic fibers in skeletal muscle, which release ACh. Dopamine is an important vasodilator transmitter in renal blood vessels.

   a. **Synthesis and storage:** The synthesis of dopamine and NE is more complex than that of ACh (Figure 6–2). Tyrosine is hydroxylated by **tyrosine hydroxylase** (the rate-limiting step) to DOPA (dihydroxyphenylalanine), decarboxylated to dopamine, and (inside the vesicle) hydroxylated to norepinephrine. Tyrosine hydroxylase can be inhibited by **metyrosine.** NE and dopamine are transported into vesicles and stored there. The vesicular transporter can be inhibited by **reserpine.**

   b. **Release and termination of action:** Dopamine and NE are released from their nerve endings by the same mechanism responsible for ACh release (see above). Termination of action, however, is quite different. Metabolism is not responsible for termination of action of the catecholamine transmitters, norepinephrine and dopamine. Instead, **diffusion** and **reuptake** (especially uptake-1, Figure 6–2) reduce their concentration in the synaptic cleft and stop their action. Outside the cleft, these transmitters can be metabolized—by **monoamine oxidase (MAO)** and **catechol-*O*-methyltransferase (COMT)**—and the products of these enzymatic reactions are excreted. Determination of the 24-hour excretion of **metanephrine, normetanephrine, 3-methoxy-4-hydroxymandelic acid (VMA),** and other metabolites provides a measure of the total body production of

* Botulinum toxin can be used by local injection to achieve a medically useful selective action.

catecholamines, a measure useful in diagnosing conditions such as pheochromocytoma. Inhibition of MAO increases stores of catecholamines and has both therapeutic and toxicologic potential.

c. **Drug effects on adrenergic transmission:** Drugs that block norepinephrine synthesis (eg, metyrosine) or catecholamine storage (eg, reserpine) or release (eg, guanethidine) are useful in several diseases (eg, hypertension) because they block sympathetic but not parasympathetic functions. Other drugs *promote* catecholamine release, eg, the amphetamine-like agents.

3. **Cotransmitters:** Many (perhaps all) autonomic nerves have transmitter vesicles that contain other transmitter molecules in addition to the primary agents (ACh or NE) described above. These cotransmitters may be localized in the same vesicles as the primary transmitter or in a separate population of vesicles. Substances recognized to date as cotransmitters include **ATP, enkephalins, vasoactive intestinal peptide (VIP), neuropeptide Y, substance P, neurotensin, somatostatin,** and others. Their role in autonomic function appears to involve modulation of synaptic transmission. The same substances undoubtedly function as primary transmitters in other synapses.

C. **Receptor Characteristics:** The major receptor systems in the ANS include the following:

1. **Cholinoceptors:** Also referred to as cholinergic receptors, these molecules respond to acetylcholine and its analogs. Cholinoceptors are subdivided as follows (Table 6–2):

a. **Muscarinic receptors:** As their name suggests, these receptors respond to muscarine as well as acetylcholine. The effects of activation of these receptors resemble those of postganglionic parasympathetic nerve stimulation. Muscarinic receptors are located primarily on autonomic effector cells (including heart, vascular endothelium, smooth muscle, presynaptic nerve terminals, and exocrine glands). Evidence has been found for five subtypes, of which three appear to be important in peripheral autonomic transmission.

b. **Nicotinic receptors:** These receptors respond to nicotine, another acetylcholine mimic, but not to muscarine. The two major subtypes are located in ganglia and in skeletal muscle end plates. The nicotinic receptors are the primary receptors for transmission at these sites.

2. **Adrenoceptors:** Also referred to as adrenergic receptors, adrenoceptors are divided into several subtypes (Table 6–3).

a. **Alpha receptors:** Alpha receptors are located on vascular smooth muscle, presynaptic nerve terminals, blood platelets, fat cells (lipocytes), and neurons in the brain. Alpha receptors are further divided into two major types, α_1 and α_2. These two subtypes constitute different families and utilize different G coupling proteins.

b. **Beta receptors:** Beta receptors are located on most types of smooth muscle, cardiac muscle, some presynaptic nerve terminals, and lipocytes as well as in the brain. Beta receptors are divided into three major subtypes, β_1, β_2, and β_3. These subtypes are rather similar and utilize the same G coupling protein.

3. **Dopamine receptors:** Dopamine receptors are a subclass of adrenoceptors but with rather different distribution and function. Dopamine receptors are especially important in the renal and splanchnic vessels and in the brain. Although at least four subtypes exist, the D_1 subtype appears to be the most important peripheral effector-cell dopamine receptor. D_2 receptors are found on presynaptic nerve terminals. D_1, D_2, and other types of dopamine receptors also occur in the CNS.

Table 6–2. Characteristics of the most important cholinoceptors in the peripheral nervous system.

Receptor	Location	Mechanism	Major Functions
M_1	Nerve endings	G_q-coupled	↑ IP_3, DAG cascade
M_2	Heart, some nerve endings	G_i-coupled	↓ cAMP, activates K channels
M_3	Effector cells: smooth muscle, glands, endothelium	G_q-coupled	↑ IP_3, DAG cascade
N_N	ANS ganglia	Ion channel	Depolarizes, evokes action potential
N_M	Neuromuscular end plate	Ion channel	Depolarizes, evokes action potential

Table 6–3. Characteristics of some important adrenoceptors in the ANS.

Receptor	Location	G Protein	Second Messenger	Major Functions
α_1	Effector tissues: smooth muscle, glands	G_q	↑ IP_3, DAG	↑ Ca^{2+}, causes contraction, secretion
α_2	Nerve endings, some smooth muscle	G_i	↓ cAMP	↓ Transmitter release, causes contraction
β_1	Cardiac muscle, juxtaglomerular apparatus	G_s	↑ cAMP	↑ Heart rate, ↑ force; ↑ renin release
β_2	Smooth muscle, cardiac muscle	G_s	↑ cAMP	Relax smooth muscle; ↑ glycogenolysis; ↑ heart rate, force
β_3	Adipose cells	G_s	↑ cAMP	↑ Lipolysis
D_1	Smooth muscle	G_s	↑ cAMP	Relax renal vascular smooth muscle

D. Effects of Activating Autonomic Nerves: Each division of the ANS has specific effects on organ systems. These effects, summarized in Table 6–4, should be memorized.

Dually innervated organs—such as the iris of the eye and the sinoatrial node of the heart—receive both sympathetic and parasympathetic innervation. The pupil has a natural, intrinsic diameter to which it returns if the influence of both divisions of the ANS is removed. Pharmacologic ganglionic blockade will therefore cause it to move to its intrinsic size. Similarly, the cardiac sinus rate has an intrinsic value in the absence of both ANS inputs. How will these variables change (increase or decrease) if the ganglia are blocked? The answer is predictable if one knows which system is dominant. For example, both the pupil and, in young adults, the SA node are dominated by the parasympathetic system. The resting pupil diameter and sinus rate are therefore under considerable PANS influence. Thus, blockade of both systems, with removal of the dominant PANS and nondominant SANS effects, will result in mydriasis and tachycardia.

E. Nonadrenergic, Noncholinergic (NANC) Transmission: Some nerve fibers in autonomic effector tissues do not show the histochemical characteristics of either cholinergic or adrenergic fibers. Some of these are motor fibers that cause the release of ATP and possibly other purines related to it. Purine-evoked responses have been identified in the bronchi, gastrointestinal tract, and urinary tract. Other motor fibers are peptidergic, ie, they release peptides as the primary transmitters (see list above under Cotransmitters).

Other nonadrenergic, noncholinergic fibers have the anatomic characteristics of sensory fibers and contain peptides such as substance P that are stored in and released from the fiber terminals. These fibers have been termed "sensory-efferent" or "sensory-local effector" fibers because when activated by a sensory input they are capable of releasing transmitter peptides from the sensory ending itself, from local axon branches, and from collaterals that terminate in the autonomic ganglia. These peptides are potent agonists in many autonomic effector tissues.

F. Sites of Autonomic Drug Action: Because of the number of steps in the transmission of autonomic commands from the CNS to the effectors, there are many sites at which autonomic drugs may act. These sites include the CNS centers, the ganglia, the postganglionic nerve terminals, the effector cell receptors, and the mechanisms responsible for transmitter synthesis, storage, release, and termination of action. The most selective effect is achieved by drugs acting at receptors that mediate very selective actions (Table 6–5). Many natural and synthetic toxins have significant effects on autonomic and somatic nerve function. Some of these toxins are listed in Table 6–5.

G. Integration of Autonomic Function: Functional integration in the autonomic nervous system is provided mainly through the mechanism of negative feedback. This process utilizes modulatory pre- and postsynaptic receptors at the local level and homeostatic reflexes at the systemic level.

1. Local integration: Local feedback control has been found at the level of the nerve end-

Table 6–4. Direct effects of autonomic nerve activity on some organ systems.*

Organ	Effect of: Sympathetic Action[1]	Sympathetic Receptor[2]	Parasympathetic Action	Parasympathetic Receptor[2]
Eye				
Iris				
Radial muscle	Contracts	α_1	...	...
Circular muscle	...	...	Contracts	M_3
Ciliary muscle	[Relaxes]	β	Contracts	M_3
Heart				
Sinoatrial node	Accelerates	β_1, β_2	Decelerates	M_2
Ectopic pacemakers	Accelerates	β_1, β_2	...	...
Contractility	Increases	β_1, β_2	Decreases (atria)	M_2
Blood vessels				
Skin, splanchnic vessels	Contracts	α	...	...
Skeletal muscle vessels	Relaxes	β_2	...	...
	[Contracts]	α	...	...
	Relaxes	M[3]	...	...
Endothelium			Releases EDRF	M_3[4]
Bronchiolar smooth muscle	Relaxes	β_2	Contracts	M_3
Gastrointestinal tract				
Smooth muscle				
Walls	Relaxes	α_2[5], β_2	Contracts	M_3
Sphincters	Contracts	α_1	Relaxes	M_3
Secretion	...		Increases	M_3
Myenteric plexus			Activates	M_1
Genitourinary smooth muscle				
Bladder wall	Relaxes	β_2	Contracts	M_3
Sphincter	Contracts	α_1	Relaxes	M_3
Uterus, pregnant	Relaxes	β_2	...	...
	Contracts	α	Contracts	M_3
Penis, seminal vesicles	Ejaculation	α	Erection	M
Skin				
Pilomotor smooth muscle	Contracts	α	...	...
Sweat glands			...	...
Thermoregulatory	Increases	M	...	...
Apocrine (stress)	Increases	α	...	...
Metabolic functions				
Liver	Gluconeogenesis	β_2, α	...	...
Liver	Glycogenolysis	β_2, α	...	...
Fat cells	Lipolysis	β_3	...	...
Kidney	Renin release	β_1	...	...
Autonomic nerve endings				
Sympathetic	...	...	Decreases NE release	M[6]
Parasympathetic	Decreases ACh release	α	...	...

*Reproduced, with permission, from Katzung BG (editor): *Basic & Clinical Pharmacology,* 8th ed. McGraw-Hill, 2001.
[1]Less important actions are shown in brackets.
[2]Specific receptor type: α = alpha, β = beta, M = muscarinic.
[3]Vascular smooth muscle in skeletal muscle has sympathetic cholinergic dilator fibers.
[4]The endothelium of most blood vessels releases EDRF (endothelium-derived relaxing factor), which causes marked vasodilation, in response to muscarinic stimuli. However, unlike the receptors innervated by sympathetic cholinergic fibers in skeletal muscle blood vessels, these muscarinic receptors are not innervated and respond only to circulating muscarinic agonists.
[5]Probably through presynaptic inhibition of parasympathetic activity.
[6]Probably M_1, but M_2 may participate in some locations.

ings in all systems investigated. The best-documented of these is the negative feedback of norepinephrine upon its own release from adrenergic nerve terminals. This effect is mediated by α_2 receptors located on the presynaptic nerve membrane (Figure 6–3).

Presynaptic receptors that bind the primary transmitter substance and thereby regulate its release are called autoreceptors. Transmitter release is also modulated by other receptors

Table 6–5. Steps in autonomic transmission: Effects of drugs.*

Process	Drug Example	Site	Action
Action potential propagation	Local anesthetics, tetrodotoxin,[1] saxitoxin[2]	Nerve axons	Block sodium channels; block conduction
Transmitter synthesis	Hemicholinium	Cholinergic nerve terminals: membrane	Blocks uptake of choline and slows synthesis
	α-Methyltyrosine (metyrosine)	Adrenergic nerve terminals and adrenal medulla: cytoplasm	Blocks synthesis
Transmitter storage	Vesamicol	Cholinergic terminals: vesicles	Prevents storage, depletes
	Reserpine	Adrenergic terminals: vesicles	Prevents storage, depletes
Transmitter release	Many[3]	Nerve terminal membrane receptors	Modulate release
	ω-Conotoxin GVIA[4]	Nerve terminal calcium channels	Reduces transmitter release
	Botulinum toxin	Cholinergic vesicles	Prevents release
	Alpha-latrotoxin[5]	Cholinergic and adrenergic vesicles	Causes explosive release
	Tyramine, amphetamine	Adrenergic nerve terminals	Promote transmitter release
Transmitter uptake after release	Cocaine, tricyclic antidepressants	Adrenergic nerve terminals	Inhibit uptake; increase transmitter effect on postsynaptic receptors
	6-Hydroxydopamine	Adrenergic nerve terminals	Destroys the terminals
Receptor activation or blockade	Norepinephrine	Receptors at adrenergic junctions	Binds α receptors; causes contraction
	Phentolamine	Receptors at adrenergic junctions	Binds α receptors; prevents activation
	Isoproterenol	Receptors at adrenergic junctions	Binds β receptors; activates adenylyl cyclase
	Propranolol	Receptors at adrenergic junctions	Binds β receptors; prevents activation
	Nicotine	Receptors at nicotinic cholinergic junctions (autonomic ganglia, neuromuscular end plates)	Binds nicotinic receptors; opens ion channel in postsynaptic membrane
	Tubocurarine	Neuromuscular end plates	Prevents activation
	Bethanechol	Receptors, parasympathetic effector cells (smooth muscle, glands)	Binds and activates muscarinic receptors
	Atropine	Receptors, parasympathetic effector cells	Binds muscarinic receptors; prevents activation
Enzymatic inactivation of transmitter	Neostigmine	Cholinergic synapses (acetylcholinesterase)	Inhibits enzyme; prolongs and intensifies transmitter action
	Tranylcypromine	Adrenergic nerve terminals (monoamine oxidase)	Inhibits enzyme; increases stored transmitter pool

*Reproduced, with permission, from Katzung BG (editor): *Basic & Clinical Pharmacology,* 8th ed. McGraw-Hill, 2001.
[1]Toxin of puffer fish, California newt.
[2]Toxin of *Gonyaulax* (red tide organism).
[3]Norepinephrine, dopamine, acetylcholine, angiotensin II, various prostaglandins, etc.
[4]Toxin of marine snails of the genus *Conus.*
[5]Black widow spider venom.

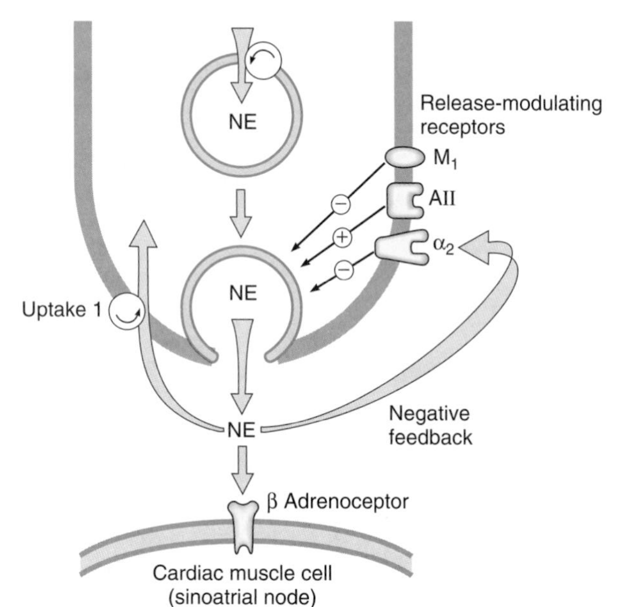

Figure 6–3. Local integration of ANS control via modulation of transmitter release. In the example shown, release of norepinephrine from a sympathetic nerve ending is modulated by norepinephrine itself, acting on presynaptic α_2 autoreceptors, and by acetylcholine and angiotensin II. Many other modulators (see text) influence the release process.

(heteroreceptors); in the case of adrenergic nerve terminals, receptors for acetylcholine (M_1 receptors), histamine, serotonin, prostaglandins, peptides, and other substances have been found. Presynaptic regulation by a variety of endogenous chemicals probably occurs in all nerve fibers.

Postsynaptic receptors, including two types of muscarinic receptors and at least one type of peptidergic receptor, have been found in ganglionic synapses, where nicotinic transmission is primary. These receptors may facilitate or inhibit transmission by evoking slow excitatory or inhibitory postsynaptic potentials (EPSPs or IPSPs).

2. **Systemic reflexes:** Systemic reflexes include mechanisms that regulate blood pressure, gastrointestinal motility, bladder tone, and airway smooth muscle. The control of blood pressure—by the baroreceptor neural reflex and the renin-angiotensin-aldosterone hormonal response—is especially important (Figure 6–4). These homeostatic mechanisms have evolved to maintain mean arterial blood pressure at a level determined by the vasomotor center and renal sensors. Any deviation from this blood pressure "set point" causes a change in ANS activity and renin-angiotensin II-aldosterone levels. These changes are very important in determining the response to conditions or drugs that alter blood pressure. For example, a decrease in blood pressure caused by hemorrhage causes increased SANS discharge and renin release. Peripheral vascular resistance, venous tone, heart rate, and cardiac force are increased by norepinephrine released from sympathetic nerves. Blood volume is replenished by retention of salt and water in the kidney under the influence of increased levels of aldosterone. These compensatory responses may be large enough to overcome some of the actions of drugs. For example, the treatment of hypertension with a vasodilator such as hydralazine will be unsuccessful if the compensatory tachycardia (via the baroreceptor reflex) and the salt and water retention (via the renin system response) are not prevented through the use of additional drugs. It is therefore essential that the student understand this homeostatic system.
3. **Complex organ control—the eye:** The eye contains multiple tissues with various functions, several of them under autonomic control (Figure 6–5). The pupil, discussed above, is under reciprocal control by the SANS (via alpha receptors) and the PANS (via muscarinic receptors) acting on two different muscles in the iris. The ciliary muscle, which controls accommodation, is under primary control of muscarinic receptors innervated by the PANS, with insignificant contributions from the SANS. The ciliary *epithelium,* on the other hand, has important beta receptors that have a permissive effect on aqueous humor secretion.

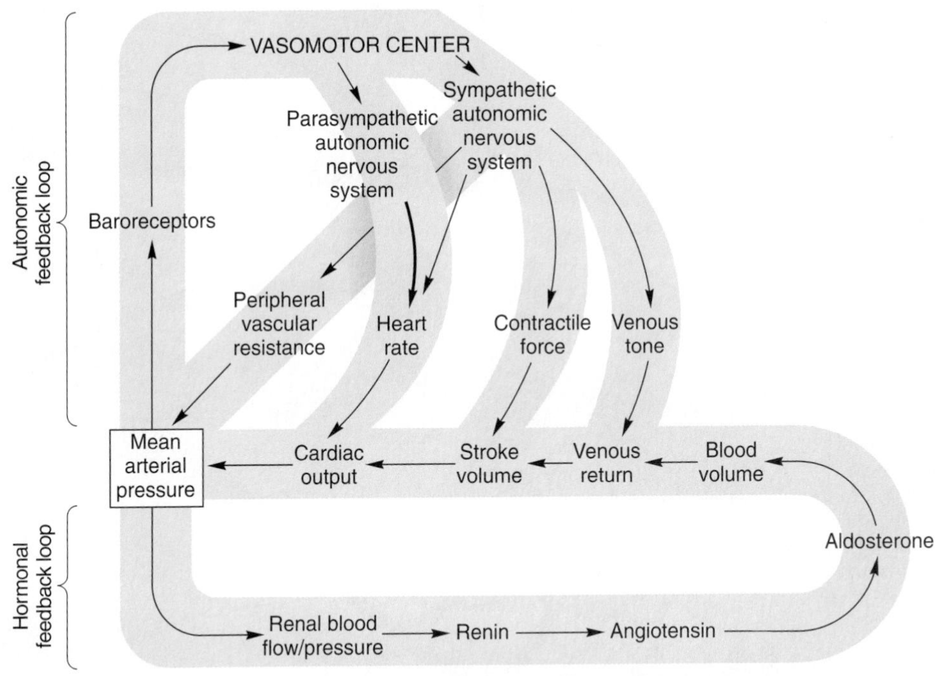

Figure 6–4. Autonomic and hormonal control of cardiovascular function. Note that two feedback loops are present: the autonomic nervous system loop and the hormonal loop. Each major loop has several components. Thus, the sympathetic nervous system directly influences four major variables: peripheral vascular resistance, heart rate, contractile force, and venous tone. The parasympathetic nervous system directly influences heart rate. In addition, angiotensin II directly increases peripheral vascular resistance (not shown), and the sympathetic nervous system directly increases renin secretion (not shown). Because these control mechanisms have evolved to maintain normal blood pressure, the net feedback effect of each loop is negative; feedback tends to compensate for the change in arterial blood pressure that evoked the response. Thus, decreased blood pressure due to blood loss would be compensated by increased sympathetic outflow and renin release. Conversely, elevated pressure due to the administration of a vasoconstricting drug would cause reduced sympathetic outflow and renin release and increased parasympathetic (vagal) outflow.

Each of these receptors is an important target of drugs that are discussed in the following chapters.

DRUG LIST

The following drugs or metabolites mentioned in this chapter are of special significance. It is important to know which ones occur in the normal ANS and what their functions are. For those not normally found in the ANS, it is important to know the effects of their administration.

Acetylcholine	3-Methoxy-4-hydroxymandelic acid (VMA)[1]
Amphetamine	Metyrosine (α-methyltyrosine)
Atropine	Neostigmine
Botulinum toxin[1]	Norepinephrine
Cocaine	Propranolol
DOPA	Reserpine
Dopamine	Saxitoxin[1]
Epinephrine	Tetrodotoxin[1]
Guanethidine	Tyramine
Metanephrine[1]	Vesamicol[1]

[1]Not discussed in succeeding chapters; should be learned with this chapter.

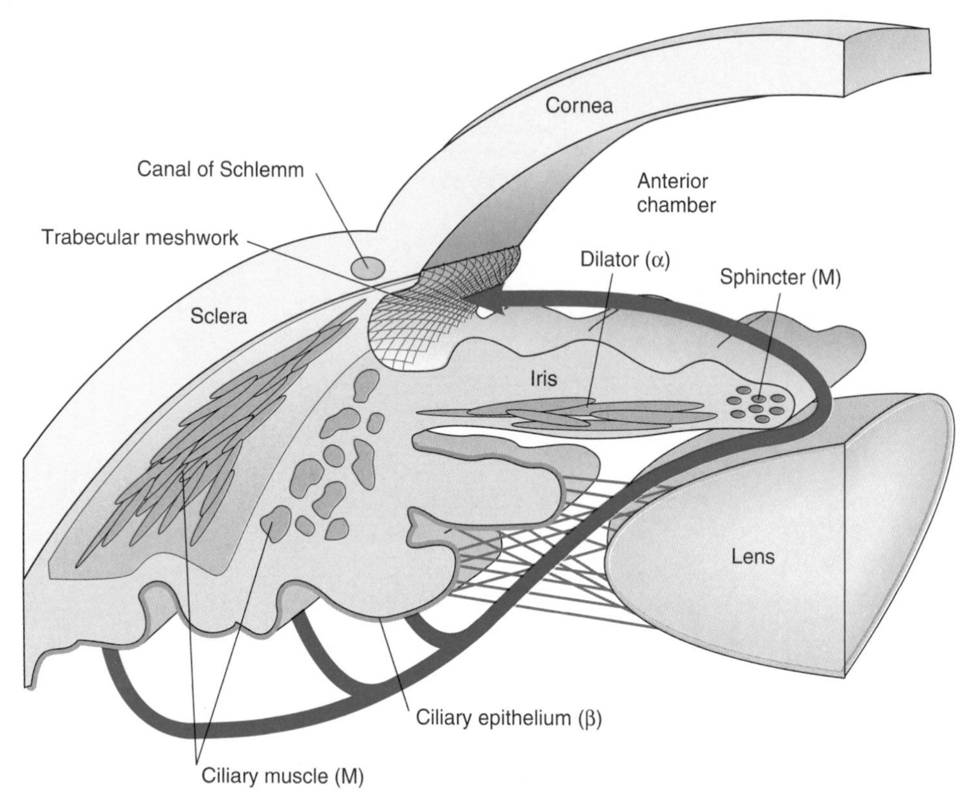

Figure 6–5. Some pharmacologic targets in the eye. The diagram illustrates clinically important structures and their receptors. The heavy arrow (color) illustrates the flow of aqueous humor from its secretion by the ciliary epithelium to its drainage through the canal of Schlemm. (M, muscarinic; α, alpha receptor; β, beta receptor.)

QUESTIONS

DIRECTIONS: Each of the numbered items or incomplete statements in this section is followed by answers or by completions of the statement. Select the ONE lettered answer or completion that is BEST in each case.

1. In the autonomic regulation of blood pressure

(A) Cardiac output is maintained constant at the expense of other hemodynamic variables
(B) Elevation of blood pressure results in elevated aldosterone secretion
(C) Baroreceptor nerve fibers decrease firing rate when arterial pressure increases
(D) Stroke volume and mean arterial blood pressure are the primary direct determinants of cardiac output
(E) A condition that reduces the sensitivity of the sensory baroreceptor nerve endings might cause an increase in sympathetic discharge

2. A child has swallowed the contents of two bottles of a nasal decongestant whose primary ingredient is a potent alpha adrenoceptor agonist drug. The signs of alpha activation that may occur in this patient include

(A) Bronchodilation
(B) Cardioacceleration (tachycardia)
(C) Pupillary dilation (mydriasis)
(D) Vasodepression (vasodilation)
(E) All of the above

3. Ms. Green has severe hypertension and is to receive minoxidil. Minoxidil is a powerful arteriolar vasodilator that does not act on autonomic receptors. When used in severe hypertension, its effects would probably include

(A) Tachycardia and increased cardiac contractility
(B) Tachycardia and decreased cardiac output
(C) Decreased mean arterial pressure and decreased cardiac contractility
(D) No change in mean arterial pressure and decreased cardiac contractility
(E) No change in mean arterial pressure and increased salt and water excretion by the kidney

4. Full activation of the sympathetic nervous system, as in maximal exercise, can produce all of the following responses EXCEPT
(A) Bronchial relaxation
(B) Decreased intestinal motility
(C) Increased renal blood flow
(D) Mydriasis
(E) Increased heart rate (tachycardia)

Items 5–8: For the following questions, use the accompanying diagram. Assume that the diagram can represent either the sympathetic or the parasympathetic system.

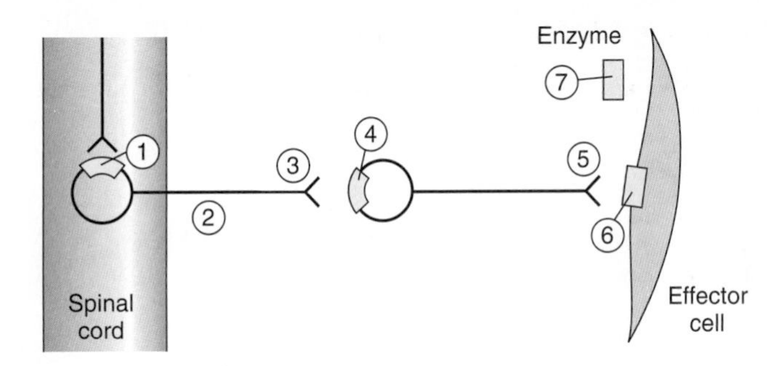

5. Which of the following drugs acts at site 3?
(A) Botulinum toxin
(B) Cocaine
(C) Metyrosine
(D) Reserpine
(E) Tyramine

6. Acetylcholine does not interact at which one of the following sites in the diagram?
(A) Site 2
(B) Site 4
(C) Site 5
(D) Site 6
(E) Site 7

7. Atropine is a useful drug for inducing dilation of the pupil and paralysis of accommodation. These effects of atropine occur at which one of the following sites on the diagram?
(A) Site 3
(B) Site 4
(C) Site 5
(D) Site 6
(E) Site 7

8. If the effector cell in the diagram is a thermoregulatory sweat gland, which of the following compounds is released from structure 5?
(A) Acetylcholine
(B) Dopamine
(C) Hemicholinium
(D) Norepinephrine
(E) Vesamicol

9. "Nicotinic" sites include all of the following EXCEPT
(A) Bronchial smooth muscle
(B) Adrenal medullary cells
(C) Parasympathetic ganglia

(D) Skeletal muscle
(E) Sympathetic ganglia

10. Several children at a summer camp were hospitalized with symptoms thought to be due to ingestion of food containing botulinum toxins. The effects of botulinum toxin are likely to include
(A) Bronchospasm
(B) Cycloplegia
(C) Diarrhea
(D) Skeletal muscle spasms
(E) Hyperventilation

11. The neurotransmitter agent that is normally released in the sinoatrial node of the heart in response to a blood pressure increase is
(A) Acetylcholine
(B) Dopamine
(C) Epinephrine
(D) Glutamate
(E) Norepinephrine

Items 12–14: Assume that the diagram below represents a sympathetic postganglionic nerve ending.

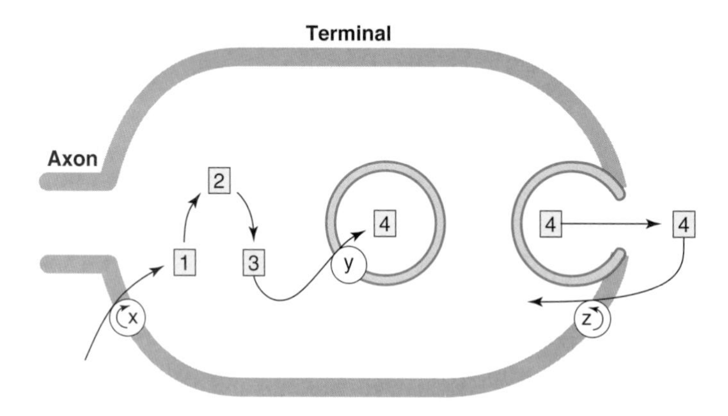

12. The carrier represented by “y” in the diagram can be blocked by
(A) Botulinum toxin
(B) Cocaine
(C) Guanethidine
(D) Hemicholinium
(E) Reserpine

13. The conversion of the intermediate “1” to “2” in the diagram can be inhibited by
(A) Botulinum toxin
(B) Cocaine
(C) Metyrosine
(D) Reserpine
(E) Vesamicol

14. The carrier denoted “z” in the diagram can be inhibited by
(A) Cocaine
(B) Dopamine
(C) Hemicholinium
(D) Metyrosine
(E) Reserpine

DIRECTIONS (Item 15): The matching question in this section consists of a list of lettered options followed by a numbered item. For this numbered item, select the ONE lettered option that is most closely associated with it.

(A) Acetylcholine
(B) Amphetamine
(C) Botulinum toxin
(D) Dopamine
(E) Epinephrine
(F) Metyrosine
(G) Norepinephrine
(H) Reserpine
(I) Tetrodotoxin
(J) Vesamicol

15. Drug that prevents the storage of acetylcholine in synaptic vesicles

ANSWERS

1. Baroreceptors *increase* their firing rate with increased blood pressure. Therefore, a decrease in baroreceptor sensitivity would decrease input to the vasomotor center, which would be interpreted by the vasomotor center as a decrease in blood pressure. This would lead to an increase in sympathetic outflow. The answer is **(E).** (If you chose a different answer, review the components of the autonomic and hormonal feedback loops for the maintenance of blood pressure; Figure 6–4.)

2. Mydriasis can be caused by contraction of the radial fibers of the iris; these smooth muscle cells have alpha receptors. All the other responses are mediated by beta adrenoceptors (Table 6–4). The answer is **(C).**

3. Because of the baroreceptor reflex, a drug that directly decreases peripheral vascular resistance will cause a reflex increase in sympathetic outflow, a decrease in parasympathetic outflow, and an increase in renin release. As a result, heart rate and cardiac force will increase. (In addition, salt and water retention will occur.) The answer is **(A).**

4. Sympathetic discharge causes constriction of the renal resistance vessels and a fall in renal blood flow. This is the typical response in severe exercise or hypotension. The answer is **(C).**

5. Each of these agents has a different mechanism of action, yet all but one act on the sympathetic postganglionic nerve terminal (site 5). Site 3 is a cholinergic nerve ending. The answer is **(A).**

6. Acetylcholine acts at both the nicotinic ganglionic receptor (site 4) and at muscarinic receptors on effector cells (site 6) and presynaptic nerve endings (site 5). ACh also interacts with acetylcholinesterase (site 7) but does not influence electrical transmission in axons (site 2). The answer is **(A).**

7. In the simplified diagram, the muscarinic receptors blocked by atropine are located only at the smooth muscle effector cells and postganglionic nerve terminals. This type of receptor is also found in ganglia, but higher concentrations of atropine are required to block it. Blocking presynaptic muscarinic receptors would not produce mydriasis and cycloplegia. The answer is **(D).**

8. The nerves innervating the thermoregulatory (eccrine) sweat glands are sympathetic *cholinergic* nerves. The answer is **(A).**

9. Both types of ganglia and the neuromuscular junction have nicotinic cholinoceptors, as does the adrenal medulla (a modified form of sympathetic postganglionic neuron tissue). Bronchial smooth muscle contains muscarinic cholinoceptors. The answer is **(A).**

10. Botulinum toxin impairs all types of cholinergic transmission, including preganglionic nerve endings and somatic motor nerve endings. This is particularly important in respiratory muscles because respiratory weakness and paralysis (not hyperventilation) are potentially lethal effects of the toxins. Botulinum toxin prevents discharge of vesicular transmitter content from cholinergic nerve endings. All of the signs listed except cycloplegia indicate increased muscle contraction; cycloplegia (paralysis of accommodation) results in blurred near vision. If not fatal, the effects of this toxin are very long-lasting (signs and symptoms may persist for several months) but are not permanent. The answer is **(B).**

11. Acetylcholine is the transmitter at parasympathetic nerve endings innervating the sinus node (the vagus nerve). When blood pressure increases, the vasomotor center tries to return it to normal by slowing the heart rate. The answer is **(A).**

12. The vesicular carrier in the diagram transports dopamine and norepinephrine into the vesicles for storage. It can be blocked by reserpine. The answer is **(E).**

13. The intermediate "1" in the diagram is tyrosine. It is converted to DOPA ("2"). This rate-limiting step in catecholamine synthesis can be inhibited by the tyrosine analog metyrosine. The answer is **(C).**
14. The reuptake carrier in sympathetic postganglionic nerve endings can be blocked by cocaine or tricyclic antidepressants. The answer is **(A).**
15. Vesamicol prevents the storage of acetylcholine in its vesicles by inhibiting the carrier molecule that normally transports acetylcholine into the vesicle (Figure 6–2). The answer is **(J).**

Skill Keeper Answer: Drug Permeation (see Chapter 1)

Botulinum toxin is too large to cross membranes by means of lipid or aqueous diffusion. It must bind to membrane receptors on susceptible cells and enter by endocytosis. Botulinum-binding receptors are present on cholinergic neurons but not adrenergic ones.

7 Cholinoceptor-Activating & Cholinesterase-Inhibiting Drugs

OBJECTIVES

You should be able to:

- List the locations and types of acetylcholine receptors in the major organ systems (CNS, autonomic ganglia, eye, heart, vessels, bronchi, gut, genitourinary tract, skeletal muscle, exocrine glands).
- Describe the effects of acetylcholine on the major organs.
- Relate the different pharmacokinetic properties of the various choline esters and cholinomimetic alkaloids to their chemical properties.
- List the major clinical uses of cholinomimetic agonists.
- Describe the pharmacodynamic differences between direct-acting and indirect-acting cholinomimetic agents.
- List the major signs and symptoms of (1) organophosphate insecticide poisoning and (2) acute nicotine toxicity.

Learn the definitions that follow.

Table 7–1. Definitions.

Term	Definition
Choline ester	A cholinomimetic drug consisting of choline (an alcohol) esterified with an acidic substance, eg, acetic or carbamic acid
Cholinergic crisis	The clinical condition of excessive activation of cholinoceptors
Cholinomimetic alkaloid	A drug with weakly basic properties (usually of plant origin) whose effects resemble those of acetylcholine
Cyclospasm	Marked contraction of the ciliary muscle; maximum accommodation
Direct-acting cholinomimetic drug	One that binds and activates cholinoceptors; the effects mimic those of acetylcholine
Endothelium-derived relaxing factor (EDRF)	A potent vasodilator substance, largely nitric oxide, that is released from vascular endothelial cells
Indirect-acting cholinomimetic drug	One that amplifies the effects of endogenous acetylcholine by inhibiting acetylcholinesterase
Muscarinic agonist	A cholinomimetic drug with primarily muscarine-like actions
Myasthenic crisis	In patients with myasthenia, an acute condition (especially skeletal muscle weakness) caused by inadequate cholinomimetic treatment
Nicotinic agonist	A cholinomimetic drug with primarily nicotine-like actions
Organophosphate	An ester of phosphoric acid and an organic alcohol that inhibits cholinesterase
Organophosphate aging	A process whereby the organophosphate, after binding to cholinesterase, is chemically modified and becomes more firmly bound to the enzyme
Parasympathomimetic drug	One whose effects resemble those of stimulating the parasympathetic nerves

CONCEPTS

Acetylcholine-like drugs (cholinomimetics) are subdivided in two ways: on the basis of their **mode of action** (ie, whether they act directly at the acetylcholine receptor or indirectly through inhibition of cholinesterase); and for those that act directly, on the basis of their **spectrum of action** (ie, whether they act on muscarinic or nicotinic cholinoceptors; Figure 7–1). Acetylcholine may be considered the prototype that acts directly at both muscarinic and nicotinic receptors. Neostigmine is a prototype for the indirect-acting cholinesterase inhibitors.

DIRECT-ACTING CHOLINOMIMETIC AGONISTS

A group of choline esters (acetylcholine, methacholine, carbachol, and bethanechol) and a second group of naturally occurring alkaloids (muscarine, pilocarpine, nicotine, lobeline) comprise this subclass. Newer drugs are occasionally introduced for special applications. The members differ in their

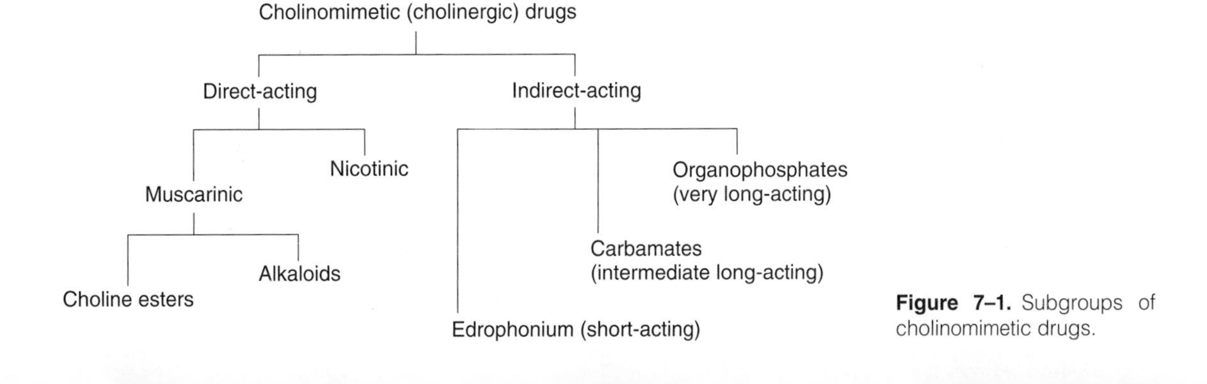

Figure 7–1. Subgroups of cholinomimetic drugs.

spectrum of action (amount of muscarinic versus nicotinic stimulation) and in their pharmacokinetics (Table 7–2). Both factors influence their clinical use.

A. **Classification:** Muscarinic agonists are parasympathomimetic, ie, they mimic the actions of parasympathetic nerve stimulation. Five subgroups of muscarinic receptors have been identified (Table 7–3), but selective agonists for these receptor subtypes are not available for clinical use. Nicotinic agonists are classified on the basis of whether ganglionic or neuromuscular stimulation predominates; however, agonist selectivity is very limited. On the other hand, relatively selective *antagonists* are available for the two nicotinic receptor types (Chapter 8).

Skill Keeper: Drug Metabolism (see Chapter 4)

Acetylcholine and methacholine are metabolized in the body by hydrolysis of the ester bond. Is this a phase I or phase II metabolic reaction? *The Skill Keeper Answer appears at the end of the chapter.*

B. **Molecular Mechanisms of Action:**
   1. **Muscarinic mechanism:** Several molecular mechanisms of muscarinic action have been defined (Table 7–3). One involves G protein coupling of muscarinic receptors (especially M_1 and M_3 receptors) to phospholipase C, a membrane-bound enzyme, leading to the release of the second messengers diacylglycerol (DAG) and inositol-1,4,5-trisphosphate (IP_3). DAG modulates the action of protein kinase C, an enzyme important in secretion, while IP_3 evokes the release of calcium from intracellular storage sites, which results in contraction. A second mechanism couples muscarinic receptors (especially M_2 receptors) to adenylyl

Table 7–2. Cholinomimetics: Spectrum of action and pharmacokinetics.

Drug	Spectrum of Action[1]	Pharmacokinetic Features
Direct-acting		
Acetylcholine	B	Rapidly hydrolyzed by cholinesterase (ChE); duration of action 5–30 seconds
Bethanechol	M	Resistant to ChE, orally active, poor lipid solubility; duration of action 30 minutes to 2 hours
Carbachol	B	Like bethanechol
Pilocarpine	M	Not an ester, good lipid solubility; duration of action 30 minutes to 2 hours
Cevimeline	M	Oral agent, moderate lipid solubility; duration of action 5–8 hours
Nicotine	N	Like pilocarpine; duration of action 1–6 hours
Indirect-acting		
Edrophonium	B	Alcohol, quarternary amine, poor lipid solubility, not orally active; duration of action 5–15 minutes
Neostigmine	B	Carbamate, quarternary amine, poor lipid solubility, orally active, duration of action 30 minutes to 2 hours
Physostigmine	B	Carbamate, tertiary amine, lipid soluble; duration of action 30 minutes to 2 hours
Pyridostigmine, ambenonium	B	Carbamates like neostigmine, but longer duration of action (4–8 hours)
Echothiophate	B	Organophosphate, moderate lipid solubility; duration of action 2–7 days
Parathion	B	Organophosphate, high lipid solubility; duration of action 7–30 days

[1]M, muscarinic; N, nicotinic; B, both

Table 7–3. Identified or cloned cholinoceptors and their mechanisms.

Receptor Type	Other Names	G Protein	Postreceptor Mechanisms
M_1	M_{1a}	G_q	↑ IP_3, DAG cascade
M_2	M_{2a}, cardiac M_2	G_i	↓ cAMP production
M_3	M_{2b}, glandular M_2	G_q	↑ IP_3, DAG cascade
m_4	...	G_i	↓ cAMP production
m_5[1]	...	G_q	↑ IP_3, DAG cascade
N_M	End plate receptor	None	Na^+/K^+ depolarizing current
N_N	Ganglion receptor	None	Na^+/K^+ depolarizing current

[1]Cloned but functional receptors have not been identified conclusively.

cyclase through the inhibitory G_i coupling protein. A third mechanism couples the same receptors directly to potassium channels in the heart and elsewhere; muscarinic agonists facilitate opening of these channels.

2. **Nicotinic mechanism:** The mechanism of nicotinic action has been clearly defined. The ACh receptor is located on a channel protein that is selective for sodium and potassium. When the receptor is activated, the channel opens and depolarization of the cell (an excitatory postsynaptic potential; EPSP) occurs as a direct result of the influx of sodium. These ACh receptors are present on ganglion cells (both sympathetic and parasympathetic) and the neuromuscular end plate. If large enough, the EPSP evokes a propagated action potential in the surrounding membrane.

C. Tissue and Organ Effects: The tissue and organ system effects are summarized in Table 7–4. Note that vasodilation (and decreased blood pressure) is not a parasympathomimetic re-

Table 7–4. Effects of direct-acting cholinoceptor stimulants. Only the direct effects are indicated; homeostatic responses to these direct actions may be important.

Organ	Response
Central nervous system	Complex stimulatory effects; eg, nicotine (elevation of mood), physostigmine (convulsions)
Eye	
Sphincter muscle of iris	Contraction (miosis)
Ciliary muscle	Contraction for near vision (accommodation)
Heart	
Sinoatrial node	Decrease in rate (negative chronotropy), but note important reflex response (see text)
Atria	Decrease in contractile strength (negative inotropy); decrease in refractory period
Atrioventricular node	Decrease in conduction velocity (negative dromotropy); increase in refractory period
Ventricles	Small decrease in contractile strength
Blood vessels	Dilation (via EDRF)
Bronchi	Contraction (bronchoconstriction)
Gastrointestinal tract	
Motility	Increase
Sphincters	Relaxation (via enteric nervous system)
Urinary bladder	
Detrusor	Contraction
Trigone and sphincter	Relaxation
Skeletal muscle	Activation of neuromuscular end plates; contraction of muscle
Glands	Increased secretion: thermoregulatory sweat, lacrimal, salivary, bronchial, gastric, intestinal glands

sponse (ie, it is not evoked by parasympathetic nerve discharge, even though directly acting cholinomimetics cause vasodilation). This action results from the release of endothelium-derived relaxing factor (EDRF; nitric oxide and possibly other substances) in the vessels, mediated by *uninnervated* muscarinic receptors on the endothelial cells. Note also that decreased blood pressure evokes the baroreceptor reflex, resulting in strong compensatory sympathetic discharge to the heart. As a result, injections of small to moderate amounts of direct-acting muscarinic cholinomimetics cause *tachycardia,* not *bradycardia.* Another effect seen with cholinomimetic drugs but not with parasympathetic nerve stimulation is thermoregulatory sweating; this is a *sympathetic cholinergic* effect (see Chapter 6).

The tissue and organ level effects of nicotinic ganglionic stimulation depend on the autonomic innervation of the organ involved. The blood vessels are dominated by sympathetic innervation; therefore, nicotinic receptor activation results in vasoconstriction mediated by sympathetic postganglionic nerve discharge. The gut is dominated by parasympathetic control; nicotinic drugs increase motility and secretion because of increased parasympathetic postganglionic neuron discharge. Nicotinic neuromuscular end plate activation by direct-acting drugs results in fasciculations and spasm of the muscles involved. Prolonged activation results in paralysis (see Chapter 27), which is an important hazard of exposure to nicotine-containing and organophosphate insecticides.

D. Clinical Use: We can predict the major clinical applications of the muscarinic agonists from a consideration of organs and diseases that benefit from an increase in cholinergic activity. They are summarized in Table 7–5. Direct-acting nicotinic agonists have no therapeutic applications except in producing skeletal muscle paralysis (succinylcholine; Chapter 27); indirect-acting agents are used when increased nicotinic activation is needed at the neuromuscular junction (see below).

E. Toxicity: The signs and symptoms of overdosage are readily predicted from the general pharmacology of acetylcholine.

1. **Muscarinic toxicity:** These effects include CNS stimulation (uncommon with direct-acting agonists), miosis, spasm of accommodation, bronchoconstriction, increased gastrointestinal and genitourinary smooth muscle activity, increased secretory activity (sweat glands, airway, gastrointestinal tract), and vasodilation. Transient bradycardia occurs, followed by reflex tachycardia if the drug is administered as an intravenous bolus—reflex tachycardia otherwise.
2. **Nicotinic toxicity:** Nicotine is commonly used in the form of chewing gum and transdermal patches by smokers trying to "kick the habit" and is still used also in some insecticides. Toxic effects include CNS stimulation (including convulsions), ganglionic stimulation, and neuromuscular end plate depolarization leading to fasciculations and paralysis.

Table 7–5. Clinical applications of some cholinomimetics.

Drug	Clinical Applications	Action
Direct-acting agonists		
Bethanechol	Postoperative and neurogenic ileus and urinary retention	Activates bowel and bladder smooth muscle
Carbachol, pilocarpine	Glaucoma	Activates pupillary sphincter and ciliary muscles of eye
Cevimeline	Dry mouth in Sjögren's syndrome	Increases salivation
Indirect-acting agonists		
Neostigmine	Postoperative and neurogenic ileus and urinary retention	Amplifies endogenous acetylcholine
Neostigmine, pyridostigmine, edrophonium	Myasthenia gravis, reversal of neuromuscular blockade	Amplifies endogenous acetylcholine; ↑ skeletal muscle strength
Physostigmine, echothiophate	Glaucoma	Amplifies effects of ACh

INDIRECT-ACTING AGONISTS

A. Classification and Prototypes: The indirect-acting cholinomimetic drugs fall into two major chemical classes: carbamic acid esters (**carbamates;** neostigmine is a prototype) and phosphoric acid esters (**phosphates, organophosphates;** echothiophate is a prototype). A third class has only one member: **edrophonium** is an alcohol (not an ester) with a very short duration of action.

B. Mechanism of Action: Both carbamate and organophosphate inhibitors bind to cholinesterase and undergo prompt hydrolysis. The alcohol portion of the molecule is then released. The acidic portion (carbamate ion or phosphate ion) is released much more slowly, thus preventing the binding and hydrolysis of acetylcholine.

1. **Carbamates:** Carbamates are hydrolyzed and the carbamate residue is released by cholinesterase over a period of 2–8 hours.
2. **Organophosphates:** Organophosphates are long-acting drugs; they form an extremely stable phosphate complex with the enzyme; after initial hydrolysis, the phosphoric acid residue is released over periods of days to weeks.

C. Effects: By inhibiting cholinesterase, the indirect-acting agonists "amplify" the action of endogenous acetylcholine; ie, these agents cause an increase in the concentration and half-life of acetylcholine in synapses where ACh is released physiologically. Therefore, the indirect agents have muscarinic or nicotinic effects depending on which organ system is under consideration. Cholinesterase inhibitors do not have significant actions at uninnervated sites where acetylcholine is not normally released (eg, endothelial cells).

D. Clinical Use: The major clinical applications of the indirect-acting cholinomimetics include both muscarinic and nicotinic effects. These effects are predictable based on a consideration of the organs and the diseases that benefit from an increase in cholinergic activity. The effects are summarized in Table 7–5. Carbamates, which include neostigmine, physostigmine, ambenonium, and pyridostigmine, are used more commonly in therapeutics than are organophosphates. Some carbamates (eg, carbaryl) are used in agriculture as insecticides. Three organophosphates used in medicine are echothiophate (an antiglaucoma drug), malathion (a scabicide), and metrifonate (an anthelmintic agent). A special use of edrophonium is in the diagnosis of myasthenia and in differentiating myasthenic from cholinergic crisis in patients with this disease. Because cholinergic crisis can result in muscle weakness like that of myasthenic crisis, distinguishing the two conditions may be difficult. Administration of a short-acting cholinomimetic such as edrophonium will improve muscle strength in myasthenic crisis but worsen it in cholinergic crisis.

E. Toxicity: In addition to their therapeutic uses, some indirect-acting agents have clinical importance because of accidental exposures to toxic amounts of pesticides. The most toxic of these drugs (eg, parathion) are rapidly fatal if exposure is not immediately recognized and treated. The treatment of first choice is atropine, but this drug has no effect on the nicotinic signs of toxicity. After first binding to cholinesterase, most organophosphate inhibitors can be removed from the enzyme by the use of "regenerator" compounds such as pralidoxime (see Chapter 8), and this may reverse the nicotinic signs. If the enzyme-inhibitor binding is allowed to persist, however, aging (a further chemical change) occurs and regenerator drugs can no longer remove the inhibitor. Treatment is described in more detail in Chapter 8. Because of their toxicity, organophosphates are used extensively in agriculture as insecticides and anthelmintic agents; examples include malathion and parathion. Some of these agents (eg, malathion, dichlorvos) are relatively safe in humans because they are metabolized rapidly to inactive products in mammals (and birds) but not in insects. Some are prodrugs (eg, malathion, parathion) and must be metabolized to the active product (malaoxon from malathion, paraoxon from parathion). The signs and symptoms of poisoning are the same as those described for the direct-acting agents, with the following exceptions: vasodilation is a late and uncommon effect; bradycardia is more common than tachycardia; CNS stimulation is common with organophosphate and physostigmine overdosage and includes convulsions, followed by respiratory and cardiovascular depression. The spectrum of toxicity can be remembered with the aid of the mnemonic "DUMBELS," which stands for diarrhea, urination, miosis, bronchoconstriction, excitation (of skeletal muscle and CNS), lacrimation, and salivation and sweating.

DRUG LIST

The following drugs are important members of the group discussed in this chapter. Prototypes should be learned in detail; the features of major variants should be known well enough to distinguish the variants from prototypes and from each other.

Subclass	Prototypes	Major Variants
Direct-acting drugs		
Muscarinic agonists	Acetylcholine	Muscarine, carbachol, bethanechol, pilocarpine
Nicotinic agonists	Acetylcholine	Nicotine, carbachol, succinylcholine
Indirect-acting drugs		
Alcohol	Edrophonium	
Carbamates	Neostigmine	Pyridostigmine, physostigmine, carbaryl
Organophosphates	Echothiophate	Parathion, DFP, malathion, dichlorvos

QUESTIONS

DIRECTIONS: Each of the numbered items or incomplete statements in this section is followed by answers or by completions of the statement. Select the ONE lettered answer or completion that is BEST in each case.

1. A patient requires mild cholinomimetic stimulation following surgery. Physostigmine and bethanechol in small doses have significantly *different* effects on which one of the following?
(A) Gastric secretion
(B) Neuromuscular junction (skeletal muscle)
(C) Salivary glands
(D) Sweat glands
(E) Ureteral tone

2. Parathion has which one of the following characteristics?
(A) It is inactivated by conversion to paraoxon
(B) It is less toxic to humans than malathion
(C) It is more persistent in the environment than DDT
(D) It is poorly absorbed through skin and lungs
(E) Its toxicity, if treated early, may be partly reversed by pralidoxime

3. Ms. Brown has had myasthenia gravis for several years. She reports to the emergency department complaining of rapid onset of weakness of her hands, diplopia, and difficulty swallowing. She may be suffering from a change in response to her myasthenia therapy, ie, a cholinergic or a myasthenic crisis. The best drug for distinguishing between myasthenic crisis (insufficient therapy) and cholinergic crisis (excessive therapy) is
(A) Atropine
(B) Echothiophate
(C) Edrophonium
(D) Physostigmine
(E) Pralidoxime

4. A crop duster pilot has been accidentally exposed to a high concentration of an agricultural organophosphate insecticide. If untreated, the cause of death from such a poisoning would probably be
(A) Cardiac arrhythmia
(B) Congestive heart failure
(C) Gastrointestinal bleeding
(D) Hypertension
(E) Respiratory failure

5. Mr. Green has just been diagnosed with myasthenia gravis. You are considering different therapies for his disease. Pyridostigmine and neostigmine may cause which one of the following?
(A) Bronchodilation
(B) Cycloplegia
(C) Diarrhea

(D) Irreversible inhibition of acetylcholinesterase
(E) Reduced gastric acid secretion

6. Parasympathetic nerve stimulation and a slow infusion of bethanechol will each increase
(A) Heart rate
(B) Bladder tone
(C) Both (A) and (B) are correct
(D) Neither (A) nor (B) is correct

7. In the human eye, echothiophate causes which one of the following?
(A) Ciliary muscle relaxation
(B) Decrease in the incidence of cataracts
(C) Increase in intraocular pressure
(D) Mydriasis
(E) Reversal of cycloplegia

8. In the comparison of bethanechol and pilocarpine, which one of the following is correct?
(A) Both are hydrolyzed by acetylcholinesterase
(B) Both inhibit nicotinic receptors
(C) Both may decrease sweating
(D) Both may increase gastrointestinal motility
(E) Neither causes tachycardia

9. Actions of cholinoceptor agonists and their clinical uses include which one of the following?
(A) Bronchodilation (asthma)
(B) Cyclospasm, improved aqueous humor drainage (glaucoma)
(C) Decreased gastrointestinal motility with resulting postoperative gastrointestinal relaxation (abdominal surgery)
(D) Decreased neuromuscular transmission and impaired recovery after neuromuscular blockade (surgical anesthesia)
(E) Both (A) and (C) are correct

10. A direct-acting cholinomimetic that is lipid-soluble and often used in the treatment of glaucoma is
(A) Acetylcholine
(B) Bethanechol
(C) Physostigmine
(D) Pilocarpine
(E) Neostigmine

11. Which one of the following is an indirect-acting carbamate cholinomimetic with poor lipid solubility and a duration of action of about 2–4 hours?
(A) Acetylcholine
(B) Bethanechol
(C) Physostigmine
(D) Pilocarpine
(E) Neostigmine

12. Which of the following agents is a prodrug that is much less toxic in mammals than in insects?
(A) Malathion
(B) Nicotine
(C) Parathion
(D) Physostigmine
(E) Pilocarpine

13. Which one of the following is a direct-acting cholinomimetic used for its mood-elevating action and as an insecticide?
(A) Bethanechol
(B) Neostigmine
(C) Nicotine
(D) Physostigmine
(E) Pilocarpine

DIRECTIONS (Item 14): The question in this section consists of a list of lettered options followed by a numbered item. Select the ONE lettered option that is most closely associated with it.

(A) Bethanechol
(B) Malathion

(C) Muscarine
(D) Neostigmine
(E) Nicotine
(F) Parathion
(G) Physostigmine
(H) Pilocarpine

14. A direct-acting cholinomimetic derived from acetylcholine that has a mainly muscarinic spectrum of action

DIRECTIONS (Items 15–17): This case history* is followed by discussion questions. Write out brief answers (two to five sentences) and then compare your answers with those given at the end of the Answers section.

A 55-year-old man was found unconscious by his wife in the greenhouse behind their home. During the past week, he had been complaining of abdominal discomfort and frequent stools. His medical history was restricted to mild hypertension controlled by salt restriction (about 5 years) and type 2 diabetes controlled by diet (about 10 years). He had no history of mental illness or of alcohol or tobacco use, and he was not taking any medication. His last trip outside the country had been to Mexico 5 years earlier. He and his wife operated a small flower shop, and he was an enthusiastic home gardener.

Upon arrival at the emergency room, the patient was unconscious, salivating profusely, and breathing shallowly. His skin was warm and moist. Blood pressure was 140/90 mm Hg, pulse 72/min and regular, respirations 30/min, and temperature normal. There was no evidence of trauma. Both pupils were constricted and did not respond to light. Auscultation of the chest revealed moderate wheezing and numerous rhonchi. The heart was normal. Examination of the abdomen revealed no abnormalities other than hyperactive bowel sounds. The extremities showed subcutaneous muscle fasciculations at the time of admission. These disappeared during the course of the examination, but muscle tone decreased and breathing became shallower during this time. The neurologic examination revealed coma with no response to painful stimuli, no localizing signs, and no abnormal reflexes.

15. What are the possible toxicologic causes of the patient's signs and symptoms?
16. What immediate nonpharmacologic steps must be taken?
17. What drugs may be considered for the treatment of this patient? What are the risks and benefits of their use?

ANSWERS

1. Because physostigmine acts on the enzyme cholinesterase—which is present at all cholinergic synapses—this drug increases acetylcholine effects at the nicotinic junctions as well as muscarinic ones. Bethanechol, on the other hand, is a direct-acting agent that is selective for muscarinic receptors and has no effect on nicotinic junctions such as the skeletal muscle end plate. The answer is **(B).**

2. The "-thion" organophosphates (those containing the P=S bond) are activated, not inactivated, by conversion to "-oxon" (P=O) derivatives. They are less stable than halogenated hydrocarbon insecticides of the DDT type; therefore, they are less persistent in the environment. Parathion is more toxic than malathion. It is very lipid-soluble and rapidly absorbed through the lungs and skin. The answer is **(E).**

3. Since short-acting drugs are usually preferable for diagnostic use, we choose the shortest-acting cholinesterase inhibitor, edrophonium. The answer is **(C).**

4. Respiratory failure, from neuromuscular paralysis or CNS depression, is the most important cause of acute deaths in cholinesterase inhibitor toxicity. The answer is **(E).**

5. Cholinesterase inhibition is typically associated with increased (never decreased) bowel activity. (Fortunately, many patients become tolerant to this effect.) The answer is **(C).**

6. Choice **(A)** is not correct because the vagus slows the heart. The answer is **(B).**

* Modified and reproduced, with permission, from Goldfrank L, Kiersten R: SLUD. Hosp Physician 1976;12:20.

7. The long-acting cholinesterase inhibitors are associated with an *increased* incidence of cataracts in patients who receive them for long periods for glaucoma. The answer is **(E)**.
8. Both bethanechol and pilocarpine may increase gastrointestinal motility. The answer is **(D)**.
9. Cholinomimetics cause cyclospasm, the opposite of paralysis of accommodation (cycloplegia). In open angle glaucoma, this results in increased outflow of aqueous and decreased intraocular pressure. The answer is **(B)**.
10. Pilocarpine is the only direct-acting cholinomimetic on the list that is lipid-soluble and frequently used in the treatment of glaucoma. Physostigmine is also lipid-soluble and used in glaucoma, but it is indirect-acting. The answer is **(D)**.
11. Neostigmine is the prototypical indirect-acting cholinomimetic; it is a quaternary (charged) substance with poor lipid solubility; its duration of action is about 2–4 hours. The answer is **(E)**.
12. Malathion and parathion are prodrug insecticides, but malathion is much less toxic than parathion in mammals. The answer is **(A)**.
13. Nicotine is a direct-acting cholinomimetic alkaloid with the properties noted. The answer is **(C)**.
14. Bethanechol is the carbamic acid ester of β-methylcholine. It has much greater affinity for muscarinic than for nicotinic receptors. The answer is **(A)**.
15. The most probable chemical intoxicants in the case of the 55-year-old gardener are insecticides. The most common constituents of currently available insecticides that produce acute poisoning are the cholinesterase inhibitors and nicotine. This patient's signs of muscarinic excess (abdominal discomfort and diarrhea) developed over a week, suggesting that a long-acting drug was gradually accumulating to a toxic level. Miosis and perspiration are common signs of cholinesterase inhibition. Nicotine toxicity rarely has such a slow onset and usually includes signs of sympathetic as well as parasympathetic discharge. The diagnosis can be confirmed by measuring the patient's blood cholinesterase level and by identifying a carbamate- or organophosphate-containing insecticide among the patient's stock of garden supplies.
16. Immediate measures must be taken to maintain vital signs and to ensure that exposure to the intoxicant has ceased. Because the patient is unconscious, induction of emesis is contraindicated and gastric lavage should not be attempted unless a cuffed endotracheal tube is in place. Since the patient's symptoms developed over a 1-week period, it is unlikely that the present stomach contents are contributing much to his intoxication. Since the organophosphates can be absorbed across the skin, the clothing should be removed and the skin cleansed (with care to avoid contamination of medical personnel). With an endotracheal tube in place, mechanical respiratory assistance can be applied as required to maintain normal blood gases, and gastric lavage may be done if there is any chance that the intoxicant was ingested. An intravenous line should be placed for administration of drugs and fluids for maintenance of good hydration.
17. Drugs to be considered for this patient include atropine for control of muscarinic effects; pralidoxime for regeneration of cholinesterase, especially at the neuromuscular junction; and cardiovascular stimulants, but only if required to maintain normal tissue perfusion. Atropine is the most important agent and should be given as soon as the diagnosis is made. Pralidoxime can be very helpful but is not always effective, and mechanical ventilation may be necessary even if the drug is partially effective. (Cardiovascular stimulants are rarely required.)

Skill Keeper Answer: Drug Metabolism
(see Chapter 4)

The esters acetylcholine and methacholine are hydrolyzed by acetylcholinesterase. Hydrolytic drug metabolism reactions are classified as phase I.

8 Cholinoceptor Blockers & Cholinesterase Regenerators

OBJECTIVES

You should be able to:

- Describe the effects of atropine on the major organ systems (CNS, eye, heart, vessels, bronchi, gut, genitourinary tract, exocrine glands, skeletal muscle).
- List the signs, symptoms, and treatment of atropine poisoning.
- List the major clinical indications and contraindications for the use of muscarinic antagonists.
- Describe the effects of the ganglion-blocking nicotinic antagonists.
- List one antimuscarinic agent promoted for each of the following uses: to produce mydriasis and cycloplegia; to treat parkinsonism, peptic ulcer, and asthma.

Learn the definitions that follow.

Table 8–1. Definitions.

Term	Definition
Anticholinergic	A drug that blocks muscarinic or nicotinic receptors
Atropine fever	Hyperthermia induced by antimuscarinic drugs; caused mainly by inhibition of sweating
Atropine flush	Marked cutaneous vasodilation of the arms and upper torso and head by antimuscarinic drugs; mechanism unknown
Cholinesterase regenerator	A chemical antagonist that binds the phosphorus of organophosphates and displaces acetylcholinesterase
Cycloplegia	Paralysis of accommodation
Depolarizing blockade	Flaccid skeletal muscle paralysis caused by persistent depolarization of the neuromuscular end plate
Miotic	A drug that constricts the pupil
Mydriatic	A drug that dilates the pupil
Nondepolarizing blockade	Flaccid skeletal muscle paralysis caused by blockade of the nicotinic end plate receptor
Organophosphate aging	A chemical change in the organophosphate molecule that occurs 15 minutes to several hours after binding of the organophosphate to cholinesterase; aging renders the enzyme-inhibitor complex less susceptible to regeneration by pralidoxime
Parasympatholytic	A drug that blocks the muscarinic receptors of autonomic effector tissues and reduces the effects of parasympathetic nerve stimulation
Pharmacokinetic selectivity	Selectivity of effect that is achieved by local administration or special distribution of a drug, not by receptor selectivity

pralidoxime is antedote to organophosphate poisons

CONCEPTS

The cholinoceptor antagonists are readily grouped into subclasses on the basis of their spectrum of action (ie, whether they block muscarinic or nicotinic receptors; Figure 8–1). These drugs are pharmacologic antagonists. A special subgroup, the cholinesterase regenerators, are not receptor blockers but rather are chemical antagonists of organophosphate cholinesterase inhibitors.

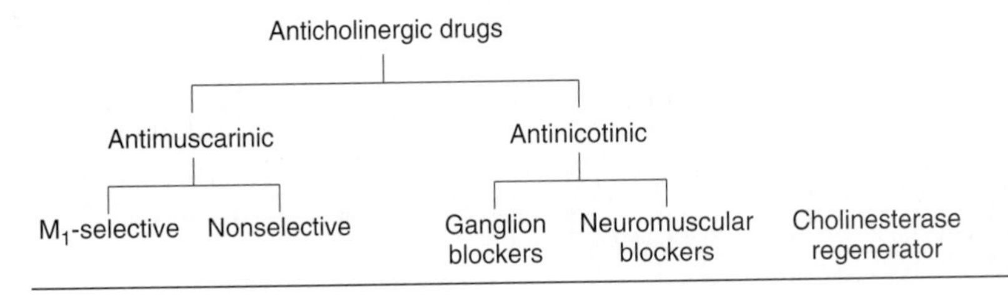

Figure 8–1. Subclasses of anticholinergic drugs and the cholinesterase regenerator discussed in this chapter. (The cholinesterase regenerators are not considered a part of the anticholinergic group.)

MUSCARINIC ANTAGONISTS

A. Classification and Pharmacokinetics:

1. **Classification of the muscarinic antagonists:** Muscarinic antagonists can be subdivided according to their selectivity for M_1 receptors or their lack of such selectivity. Although the division of muscarinic receptors into subgroups is well documented (Chapters 6, 7), only a few receptor-selective antagonists have reached clinical trials in the USA (eg, pirenzepine, telenzepine). All of the drugs in general use in the USA at present are nonselective. These blockers can be further subdivided on the basis of their primary clinical target organs (CNS, eye, bronchi, or gastrointestinal and genitourinary tracts). Drugs used for their effects on the CNS or the eyes must be sufficiently lipid-soluble to cross lipid barriers. A major determinant of this property is the presence or absence of a permanently charged (quaternary) amine group in the drug. This is because charged molecules are more polar and therefore less likely to penetrate a lipid barrier such the blood-brain barrier or the cornea of the eye.
2. **Pharmacokinetics of atropine:** Atropine is the prototypical nonselective muscarinic blocker. This alkaloid is found in *Atropa belladonna* and many other plants. Because it is a tertiary amine, atropine is relatively lipid-soluble and readily crosses membrane barriers. The drug is well distributed into the CNS and other organs and is eliminated partially by metabolism in the liver and partially by renal excretion. The elimination half-life is approximately 2 hours, and the duration of action of normal doses is 4–8 hours except in the eye, where effects last for 72 hours or longer.

> **Skill Keeper: Drug Ionization**
> **(see Chapter 1)**
>
> The pK_a of atropine is 9.7. What fraction of atropine is in the lipid-soluble form in urine of pH 7.7? *The Skill Keeper Answer appears at the end of the chapter.*

3. **Pharmacokinetics of other muscarinic blockers:** In ophthalmology, topical activity (the ability to enter the eye after conjunctival administration) and duration of action are important in determining the usefulness of several antimuscarinic drugs (see Clinical Uses). Similar ability to cross lipid barriers is important for the agents used in parkinsonism. In contrast, the drugs used for their antisecretory or antispastic actions in the gut and the bronchi are often selected for minimum CNS activity; these drugs may incorporate quaternary amine groups to limit penetration through the blood-brain barrier.

B. Mechanism of Action: The muscarinic blocking agents act like competitive (surmountable) pharmacologic antagonists; their blocking effects can be overcome by increased concentrations of muscarinic agonists.

C. Effects: The peripheral actions of muscarinic blockers are mostly predictable effects derived from cholinoceptor blockade (Table 8–2). These include the ocular, gastrointestinal, genitourinary, and secretory effects. The CNS effects are less predictable. Those seen at therapeutic concentrations include sedation, reduction of motion sickness, and, as noted above, reduction of some of the signs of parkinsonism. Cardiovascular effects at therapeutic doses include an initial

Table 8–2. Effects of muscarinic blocking drugs.

Organ	Effect	Mechanism
CNS	Sedation, anti-motion sickness action, antiparkinson action, amnesia, delirium	Block of muscarinic receptors, unknown sub-types
Eye	Cycloplegia, mydriasis	Block of M_3 receptors
Bronchi	Bronchodilation, especially if constricted	Block of M_3 receptors
Gastrointestinal tract	Relaxation, slowed peristalsis	Block of M_1, M_3 receptors
Genitourinary tract	Relaxation of bladder wall, urinary retention	Block of M_3 receptors
Heart	Initial bradycardia, especially at low doses; then tachycardia	Tachycardia from block of M_2 receptors in the heart
Blood vessels	Block of muscarinic vasodilation; not manifest unless a muscarinic agonist is present	Block of M_3 receptors on endothelium of vessels
Glands	Marked reduction of salivation; moderate reduction of lacrimation, sweating; less reduction of gastric secretion	Block of M_1, M_3 receptors
Skeletal muscle	None	

slowing of heart rate caused by central or (more likely) presynaptic vagal effects followed by the tachycardia and decreased atrioventricular conduction time that would be predicted from peripheral vagal blockade.

D. Clinical Uses: The muscarinic blockers have several useful therapeutic applications in the central nervous system, eye, bronchi, gut, and urinary bladder. These uses are summarized in Table 8–3.

1. **CNS:** Scopolamine is standard therapy for motion sickness; this drug is one of the most effective agents available for this condition. A transdermal patch formulation is available. Benztropine, biperiden, and trihexyphenidyl are representative of several antimuscarinic agents used in parkinsonism. Although not as effective as levodopa (see Chapter 28), these agents may be useful as adjuncts or when patients become unresponsive to levodopa. Benztropine is sometimes used parenterally to treat acute dystonias caused by antipsychotic medications.
2. **Eye:** Antimuscarinic drugs are used to dilate the pupil and to paralyze accommodation. They include (in descending order of duration of action) atropine (> 72 hours), homatropine (24 hours), cyclopentolate (2–12 hours), and tropicamide (0.5–4 hours). These agents are all well-absorbed from the conjunctival sac into the eye.

Table 8–3. Some clinical applications of antimuscarinic drugs.

Organ System	Drugs[1]	Application
CNS	Benztropine, trihexyphenidyl, biperiden	To treat the manifestations of Parkinson's disease
	Scopolamine	To prevent or reduce motion sickness
Eye	Atropine, homatropine, cyclopentolate, tropicamide	To produce mydriasis and cycloplegia
Bronchi	Ipratropium	To cause bronchodilation in asthma and COPD[2]
Gastrointestinal tract	Glycopyrrolate, dicyclomine, methscopolamine	To reduce transient hypermotility
Genitourinary tract	Oxybutynin, glycopyrrolate, dicyclomine, tolterodine	To treat transient cystitis, postoperative bladder spasms, or incontinence

[1]Only a few of many drugs are listed.
[2]COPD, chronic obstructive pulmonary disease.

3. **Bronchi:** Parenteral atropine has long been used to reduce airway secretions during surgery. Ipratropium is a quaternary antimuscarinic agent used by inhalation to reduce bronchoconstriction in asthma and chronic obstructive pulmonary disease (COPD). Although not as efficacious as beta agonists, ipratropium is less likely to cause cardiac arrhythmias in sensitive patients. It has very few antimuscarinic effects outside the lungs because it is poorly absorbed and rapidly metabolized.
4. **Gut:** Atropine, methscopolamine, and propantheline were used in acid-peptic disease to reduce acid secretion, but they are not as effective as H_2-blockers such as cimetidine, and they cause far more frequent and severe adverse effects. Pirenzepine is an M_1-selective muscarinic blocker (available in Europe but not the USA) that may be more useful in peptic ulcer. Muscarinic blockers can also be used to reduce cramping and hypermotility in transient diarrheas, but opioids such as diphenoxylate (Chapter 31) are more effective.
5. **Bladder:** Glycopyrrolate, oxybutynin, methscopolamine, tolterodine, or similar agents may be used to reduce urgency in mild cystitis and to reduce bladder spasms following urologic surgery. Tolterodine is promoted for the treatment of stress incontinence. Glycopyrrolate and methscopolamine are quaternary molecules that may have fewer CNS effects.

E. **Toxicity:** A traditional mnemonic for atropine toxicity is "Dry as a bone, red as a beet, mad as a hatter." This description reflects both predictable antimuscarinic effects and some unpredictable actions.
   1. **Predictable toxicities:** Antimuscarinic actions lead to several important and potentially dangerous effects. Blockade of thermoregulatory sweating may result in hyperthermia or "atropine fever." This is the most dangerous effect of the antimuscarinic drugs and is potentially lethal in infants. Atropine toxicity is described as feeling "dry as a bone" because sweating, salivation, and lacrimation are all significantly reduced or stopped. In the elderly, important additional targets of toxicity include the eye (acute angle-closure glaucoma may occur) and the bladder (urinary retention is possible, especially in men with prostatic hyperplasia). Constipation and blurred vision are common adverse effects in all age groups.
   2. **Other toxicities:** Toxicities not predictable from peripheral autonomic actions include the following.
      a. **CNS effects:** CNS toxicity includes sedation, amnesia, and delirium or hallucinations ("mad as a hatter"); convulsions may also occur. Central muscarinic receptors are probably involved.
      b. **Cardiovascular effects:** At toxic doses, intraventricular conduction may be blocked; this action is probably not mediated by muscarinic blockade and is difficult to treat. Dilation of the cutaneous vessels of the arms, head, neck, and trunk also occurs at these doses; the resulting "atropine flush" ("red as a beet") may be diagnostic of overdose with these drugs.

F. **Contraindications:** The antimuscarinic agents should be used cautiously in infants because of the danger of hyperthermia. The drugs are relatively contraindicated in persons with glaucoma, especially the closed-angle form, and in men with prostatic hyperplasia.

NICOTINIC ANTAGONISTS

A. **Classification:** Nicotinic receptor antagonists are divided into ganglion-blocking drugs and neuromuscular-blocking drugs.

B. **Ganglion-Blocking Drugs:** Blockers of ganglionic nicotinic receptors act like competitive pharmacologic antagonists, though there is evidence that they can also block the nicotinic channel pore. These drugs were the first successful agents for the treatment of hypertension. Hexamethonium (C6, a prototype), mecamylamine, and several other ganglion blockers were extensively used for this disease. Unfortunately, the adverse effects of ganglion blockade in hypertension are so severe (both sympathetic and parasympathetic divisions are blocked) that patients were unable to tolerate them for long periods (Table 8–4). Trimethaphan was the ganglion blocker most recently used in clinical practice, but it too has been almost abandoned. It is poorly lipid-soluble, inactive orally, and has a short half-life. It was used intravenously to treat severe accelerated hypertension (malignant hypertension) and to produce controlled hypotension.

Table 8–4. Effects of ganglion-blocking drugs.

Organ	Effects
CNS	Antinicotinic actions may include reduction of nicotine craving and amelioration of Tourette's syndrome (mecamylamine only)
Eye	Moderate mydriasis and cycloplegia
Bronchi	Little effect; asthmatics may note some bronchodilation
Gastrointestinal tract	Markedly reduced motility; constipation may be severe
Genitourinary tract	Reduced contractility of the bladder; impairment of erection and ejaculation
Heart	Slight tachycardia in young adults; reduction in force of contraction and cardiac output
Blood vessels	Reduction in arteriolar tone, marked reduction in venous tone; blood pressure decrease and orthostatic hypotension may be severe
Glands	Reductions in salivation, lacrimation, sweating, and gastric secretion
Skeletal muscle	No significant effect

Recent interest has focussed on nicotinic receptors in the CNS and their relation to nicotine addiction and to Tourette's syndrome. Paradoxically, both nicotine (in the form of nicotine patches) and mecamylamine, a ganglion blocker that enters the CNS, have been shown to have some benefit in these applications.

Because ganglion blockers interrupt sympathetic control of venous tone, they cause marked venous pooling; postural hypotension is a major manifestation of this effect. Other toxicities of ganglion blocking drugs include dry mouth, blurred vision, constipation, and severe sexual dysfunction (see Table 8–4).

C. **Neuromuscular Blocking Drugs:** Neuromuscular blocking drugs are important for producing complete skeletal muscle relaxation in surgery; new ones are frequently introduced. They are discussed in greater detail in Chapter 27.

1. **Nondepolarizing group:** Tubocurarine is the prototype. It produces a competitive block at the end plate nicotinic receptor, causing flaccid paralysis that lasts 30–60 minutes (longer if large doses have been given). Pancuronium, atracurium, vecuronium, and several newer drugs are shorter-acting, nondepolarizing blockers. Gallamine is an older nondepolarizing drug that is no longer used in the USA.
2. **Depolarizing group:** Although these drugs are nicotinic agonists, not antagonists, they cause a flaccid paralysis (see Chapter 27). Succinylcholine, the only member of this group used in the USA, produces fasciculations during induction of paralysis; patients may complain of muscle pain after its use. The drug is hydrolyzed by pseudocholinesterase (plasma cholinesterase) and has a half-life of a few minutes in persons with normal plasma cholinesterase. Approximately one in 2500 individuals produces a genetically determined form of abnormal cholinesterase that does not metabolize succinylcholine effectively. The drug's duration of action is grossly prolonged in such individuals.
3. **Toxicity:** The toxicity of neuromuscular blockers is discussed in Chapter 27.

CHOLINESTERASE REGENERATORS

The cholinesterase regenerators are not receptor antagonists but belong to a class of *chemical* antagonists. These molecules contain an oxime group, which has an extremely high affinity for the phosphorus atom in organophosphate insecticides. Because the affinity of the oxime group for phosphorus exceeds that of the enzyme active site, these agents are able to bind the inhibitor and displace the enzyme (if aging has not occurred). The active enzyme is thus regenerated. **Pralidoxime,** the oxime currently available in the USA, is often used to treat patients exposed to insecticides such as parathion.

DRUG LIST

The following drugs are important members of the group discussed in this chapter. Prototypes should be learned in detail; features of the major variants should be known well enough to distinguish the variants from prototypes and from each other; the other significant agents should be recognized as belonging to a specific subclass.

Subclass	Prototype	Major Variants	Other Significant Agents
Muscarinic blockers Nonselective	Atropine	Scopolamine, glycopyrrolate, ipratropium, cyclopentolate, benztropine	Homatropine, methscopolamine, tropicamide, oxybutynin, tolterodine
M_1-selective	Pirenzepine		Telenzepine
Nicotinic blockers Ganglion blockers	Hexamethonium	Trimethaphan, mecamylamine	
Neuromuscular blockers	Tubocurarine		Pancuronium, atracurium
Cholinesterase regenerator	Pralidoxime		

QUESTIONS

DIRECTIONS: Each of the numbered items or incomplete statements in this section is followed by answers or by completions of the statement. Select the ONE lettered answer or completion that is BEST in each case.

Items 1–2: A 3-year-old child has been admitted to the emergency room. Antimuscarinic drug overdose is suspected.

1. Atropine overdose may cause which one of the following?
(A) Gastrointestinal smooth muscle cramping
(B) Increased cardiac rate
(C) Increased gastric secretion
(D) Pupillary constriction
(E) Urinary frequency

2. In very young children, the most dangerous effect of belladonna alkaloids is
(A) Dehydration
(B) Hallucinations
(C) Hypertension
(D) Hyperthermia
(E) Intraventricular heart block

3. Which of the following pairs of drugs and properties is most correct?
(A) Atropine: Poorly absorbed after oral administration
(B) Benztropine: Quaternary amine, poor CNS penetration
(C) Cyclopentolate: Well-absorbed from conjunctival sac into the eye
(D) Ipratropium: Well-absorbed, long elimination half-life
(E) Scopolamine: Short duration of action when used as anti-motion sickness agent

4. Which one of the following can be blocked by atropine?
(A) Decreased blood pressure caused by hexamethonium
(B) Increased blood pressure caused by nicotine
(C) Increased skeletal muscle strength caused by neostigmine
(D) Tachycardia caused by exercise
(E) Tachycardia caused by infusion of acetylcholine

5. Which of the following best describes the mechanism of action of scopolamine?
(A) Irreversible antagonist at nicotinic receptors
(B) Irreversible antagonist at muscarinic receptors
(C) Physiologic antagonist at muscarinic receptors
(D) Reversible antagonist at muscarinic receptors
(E) Reversible antagonist at nicotinic receptors

Items 6–7: Two new synthetic drugs (X and Y) are to be studied for their cardiovascular effects. The drugs are given to three anesthetized animals while the blood pressure is recorded. The first animal has received no pretreatment (control), the second has received an effective dose of a long-acting ganglion blocker, and the third has received an effective dose of a long-acting muscarinic antagonist.

6. Drug X caused a 50 mm Hg rise in mean blood pressure in the control animal, no blood pressure change in the ganglion-blocked animal, and a 75 mm mean blood pressure rise in the atropine-pretreated animal. Drug X is probably a drug similar to
(A) Acetylcholine
(B) Atropine
(C) Epinephrine
(D) Hexamethonium
(E) Nicotine

7. The net changes induced by drug Y are shown in the graph below. Drug Y is probably a drug similar to
(A) Acetylcholine
(B) Edrophonium
(C) Hexamethonium
(D) Nicotine
(E) Pralidoxime

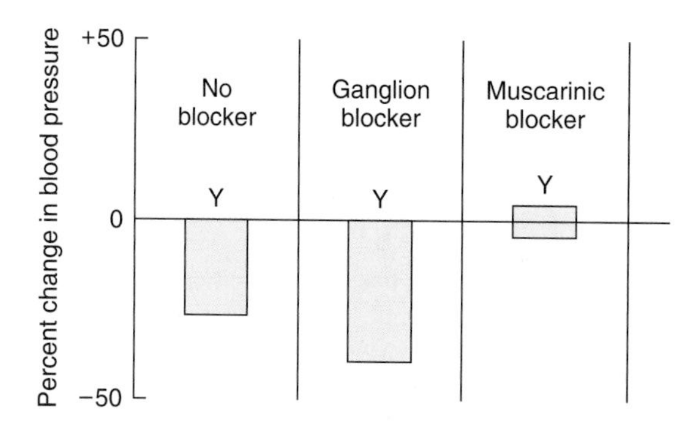

8. A 30-year-old man has been treated with several autonomic drugs for 4 weeks. He is now admitted to the emergency department showing signs of drug toxicity. Which of the following signs would distinguish between an overdose of a ganglion blocker versus a muscarinic blocker?
(A) Mydriasis
(B) Tachycardia
(C) Postural hypotension
(D) Blurred vision
(E) Dry mouth, constipation

9. All of the following may cause cycloplegia (paralysis of accommodation) when used topically in the eye EXCEPT
(A) Atropine
(B) Cyclopentolate
(C) Physostigmine
(D) Scopolamine
(E) Tropicamide

10. You have been asked to consult in the treatment of an 80-year-old patient. An antimuscarinic drug is being considered. Atropine therapy in the elderly may be hazardous because
(A) Atropine can elevate intraocular pressure in patients with glaucoma
(B) Atropine frequently causes ventricular arrhythmias
(C) Urinary retention is often precipitated by atropine in women
(D) The elderly are particularly prone to develop dangerous hyperthermia when given atropine
(E) Atropine often causes excessive vasodilation and hypotension in the elderly

11. When a dose-response study of atropine is carried out in young adults, which of the following effects may be observed?
(A) Bradycardia
(B) Tachycardia

(C) Central nervous system stimulation, eg, hallucinations
(D) Central nervous system depression, eg, sedation
(E) All of the above

12. Accepted therapeutic indications for the use of antimuscarinic drugs include all of the following EXCEPT
(A) Hypertension
(B) Motion sickness
(C) Parkinson's disease
(D) Postoperative bladder spasm
(E) Traveler's diarrhea

13. Which of the following is an expected effect of a therapeutic dose of an antimuscarinic drug?
(A) Decreased cAMP in cardiac muscle
(B) Increased IP_3 in intestinal smooth muscle
(C) Increased sodium influx into skeletal muscle end plate
(D) Decreased DAG in salivary gland tissue
(E) Increased potassium efflux from smooth muscle

DIRECTIONS (Items 14–15): The matching questions in this section consist of lettered options followed by several numbered items. For each numbered item, select the ONE lettered option that is most closely associated with it. Each lettered option may be selected once, more than once, or not at all.

(A) Atropine
(B) Benztropine
(C) Bethanechol
(D) Botulinum
(E) Cyclopentolate
(F) Neostigmine
(G) Pralidoxime
(H) Scopolamine
(I) Trimethaphan
(J) Tubocurarine

14. This drug causes vasodilation that can be blocked by atropine
15. This drug has a very high affinity for the phosphorus atom in parathion and is often used to treat insecticide toxicity

DIRECTIONS (Items 16–18): This case history* is followed by discussion questions. Write out brief answers (two to five sentences) and then compare your answers with those given at the end of the Answers section.

A 15-year-old boy was brought to the emergency room by the police because he "had a flushed face and was acting crazy." He had been found nude, incoherent, and wandering about aimlessly.

Physical examination showed blood pressure 170/100 mm Hg and pulse 144/min. He was comatose. The skin was flushed, dry, and hot to the touch. The pupils were widely dilated and equal, with a minimal response to light. Rectal temperature was 39.8 °C.

At this time, physostigmine salicylate, 2 mg, was given intravenously under electrocardiographic, electroencephalographic, and temperature monitoring. Within 15 minutes, the rectal temperature had fallen to 38.8 °C, while blood pressure and pulse were 160/68 mm Hg and 112/min, respectively. The patient became more alert and responsive to verbal commands but remained agitated. When questioned about ingestion of a toxic agent, the patient said that he had eaten "loco seeds," small black seeds of a weed that grew freely in the area. Remote memory was intact, but recent memory was grossly impaired.

Six hours later, the rectal temperature was 37 °C, and other vital signs were stable. The patient was talking spontaneously in a rapid and garbled manner. Although completely oriented, he continued to speak of imaginary objects and voices.

The patient rapidly improved and was discharged on the eighth hospital day without neurologic deficit.

* Modified and reproduced, with permission, from Mikolich JR, Paulson GW, Cross CJ: Acute anticholinergic syndrome due to Jimson seed ingestion: clinical and laboratory observation in six cases. Ann Intern Med 1975;83:321.

16. Identify the probable drug or drug group contained in "loco seeds"
17. What is the most life-threatening effect of the intoxicant in this case?
18. What are the dangers of physostigmine therapy? What are the risks of other treatments?

ANSWERS

1. Pupillary dilation, not constriction, is a characteristic atropine effect, as indicated by the origin of the name belladonna ("beautiful lady") from the ancient cosmetic use of extracts of the *Atropa belladonna* plant to dilate the pupils. The answer is **(B)**.
2. Choices **(B)**, **(D)**, and **(E)** are possible effects of the atropine group. In small children, however, the most dangerous effect is hyperthermia. Deaths with body temperatures in excess of 42 °C have occurred after the use of atropine-containing eye drops in children. The answer is **(D)**.
3. Atropine is very well absorbed. Scopolamine has a relatively long duration of action, especially when used as an anti-motion sickness transdermal patch. Ipratropium is quaternary and poorly absorbed from the airways. Benztropine is tertiary, lipid-soluble, and penetrates into the CNS well. Only **(C)** is correct.
4. Atropine blocks muscarinic receptors and inhibits parasympathomimetic effects. Nicotine can induce both parasympathomimetic and sympathomimetic effects by virtue of its ganglion-stimulating action. Hypertension and exercise-induced tachycardia reflect sympathetic discharge and therefore would not be blocked by atropine. The answer is **(E)**.
5. All of the muscarinic blockers, including scopolamine, act as reversible, competitive pharmacologic antagonists. The answer is **(D)**.
6. Drug X causes an increase in blood pressure that is blocked by a ganglion blocker but not by a muscarinic blocker. The pressor response is actually increased by pretreatment with a muscarinic blocker, suggesting that compensatory vagal discharge might have blunted the full response. This description fits a ganglion stimulant like nicotine but not epinephrine, since epinephrine's pressor effects are produced at alpha receptors, not in the ganglia. The answer is **(E)**.
7. Drug Y causes a decrease in blood pressure that is blocked by a muscarinic blocker but not by a ganglion blocker. Therefore, the depressor effect must be evoked at a site distal to the ganglia. In fact, the drop in blood pressure is actually greater in the presence of ganglion blockade, suggesting that compensatory sympathetic discharge might have blunted the full depressor action of drug Y in the untreated animal. The description fits a direct-acting muscarinic stimulant such as acetylcholine (given in high dosage). Indirect-acting cholinomimetics (cholinesterase inhibitors) would not produce this pattern because the vascular muscarinic receptors involved in the depressor response are not innervated and are therefore unresponsive to indirectly acting agents. The answer is **(A)**.
8. Ganglion blockers and muscarinic blockers can both cause mydriasis, increase resting heart rate, blur vision, and cause dry mouth and constipation, because these are determined largely by parasympathetic tone. Postural hypotension, on the other hand, is a sign of sympathetic blockade, which would occur with ganglion blockers but not muscarinic blockers (Chapter 6). The answer is **(C)**.
9. All antimuscarinic agents are, in theory, capable of causing cycloplegia. Physostigmine, on the other hand, is an indirect-acting cholinomimetic and has the opposite effect. The answer is **(C)**.
10. The elderly have a much higher incidence of glaucoma than younger people (and may be unaware of the disease until late in its course). Antimuscarinic agents may increase intraocular pressure in individuals with glaucoma. Elderly men (not women) have a much higher probability of developing urinary retention—because they have a high incidence of prostatic hyperplasia. Cardiac and hyperthermic reactions to atropine are not common in the elderly. The answer is **(A)**.
11. All of the effects listed may be observed (see text). The answer is **(E)**.
12. Hypertension is not responsive to antimuscarinic agents. The answer is **(A)**.
13. Muscarinic M_1 and M_3 receptors mediate increases in IP_3 and DAG in target tissues. M_2 receptors mediate a decrease in cAMP and an increase in potassium permeability. Antimuscarinic agents block these effects. The answer is **(D)**.
14. Bethanechol (Chapter 7) causes vasodilation by activating muscarinic receptors on the endothelium of blood vessels. This effect can be blocked by atropine. The answer is **(C)**.

15. Pralidoxime has a very high affinity for the phosphorus atom in organophosphate insecticides. The answer is **(G).**
16. The case description is typical of antimuscarinic drug poisoning. A common source of such agents in nature is Jimson weed *(Datura stramonium).* The patient had ingested several of the 2–3 mm round black seeds from the pods of this plant.
17. The most life-threatening effect of the antimuscarinic agents in many patients, especially small children and infants, is hyperthermia. Unsupervised hallucinating patients may fall or otherwise injure themselves. Convulsions and arrhythmias may occur. In patients with organic heart disease, such arrhythmias may be dangerous. Other effects of these drugs, though uncomfortable, are not life-threatening.
18. The chief danger of physostigmine is its central stimulant effect, which may lead to convulsions. Other anticholinesterase drugs, such as neostigmine, do not enter the CNS as readily as physostigmine; they are less dangerous but also less effective in reversing the central effects of the intoxicant. Symptomatic treatment includes cooling fans or cooling blankets and IV fluids. Cardiac arrhythmias may occasionally require treatment with antiarrhythmic drugs.

Skill Keeper Answer: Drug Ionization
(see Chapter 1)

The pK_a of atropine is 9.7. According to the Henderson-Hasselbalch equation,

$$\text{Log (protonated/unprotonated)} = pK_a - pH$$
$$\text{Log (P/U)} = 9.7 - 7.7$$
$$\text{Log (P/U)} = 2$$
$$\text{P/U} = \text{antilog (2)} = 100/1$$

Therefore, about 99% of the drug is in the protonated form, 1% in the unprotonated form. Since atropine is a weak base, it is the unprotonated form that is lipid-soluble. Therefore, about 1% of the atropine in the urine is lipid-soluble.

9 Sympathomimetics

OBJECTIVES

You should be able to:

- List tissues that contain significant numbers of alpha receptors of the α_1 or α_2 types.
- List tissues that contain significant numbers of β_1 or β_2 receptors.
- Describe the major organ system effects of a pure alpha agonist, a pure beta agonist, and a mixed alpha and beta agonist. Give examples of each type of drug.
- Describe a clinical situation in which the effects of an indirect sympathomimetic would differ from those of a direct agonist.
- List the major clinical applications of the adrenoceptor agonists.

Learn the definitions that follow.

Table 9–1. Definitions.

Term	Definition
Anorexiant	A drug that causes loss of appetite (anorexia)
Catecholamine	A dihydroxyphenylethylamine derivative, eg, norepinephrine, epinephrine
Decongestant	A drug that reduces nasal or oropharyngeal mucosal swelling, usually by constricting blood vessels in the submucosal tissue
Direct agonist, indirect agonist	A direct agonist binds and activates the receptor; an indirect one brings about receptor activation by binding to some other molecule, eg, a reuptake carrier, and causing an increase in the synaptic concentration of the normal transmitter
Mydriatic	A drug that causes dilation of the pupil; opposite of miotic
Phenylisopropylamine	A derivative of phenylisopropylamine, eg, amphetamine, ephedrine. Unlike catecholamines, phenylisopropylamines usually have oral activity, a long half-life, some CNS activity, and an indirect mode of action
Selective alpha agonist, beta agonist	Drugs that have relatively greater effects on alpha or beta adrenoceptors; none are *absolutely* selective
Sympathomimetic	A drug that mimics stimulation of the sympathetic autonomic nervous system
Reuptake inhibitor	An indirectly acting drug that increases the activity of transmitters in the synapse by inhibiting their reuptake into the presynaptic nerve ending. May act selectively on noradrenergic, serotonergic, or both types of nerve endings

CONCEPTS

A. Classification: The sympathomimetics are direct or indirect adrenoceptor agonists and are subdivided in two ways: by mode of action and by spectrum of action (Figure 9–1).

1. Mode of action: Sympathomimetic agonists may directly activate their adrenoceptors, or they may act indirectly to increase the concentration of catecholamine transmitter in the synapse. Amphetamine derivatives and tyramine cause the release of stored catecholamines; these sympathomimetics are therefore mainly indirect in their mode of action. Another form of indirect action is seen with cocaine and the tricyclic antidepressants; these drugs inhibit reuptake of catecholamines by nerve terminals and thus increase the synaptic activity of released transmitter.

Blockade of metabolism (ie, block of catechol-*O*-methyltransferase [COMT] and monoamine oxidase [MAO]) has little direct effect on autonomic activity, but MAO inhibi-

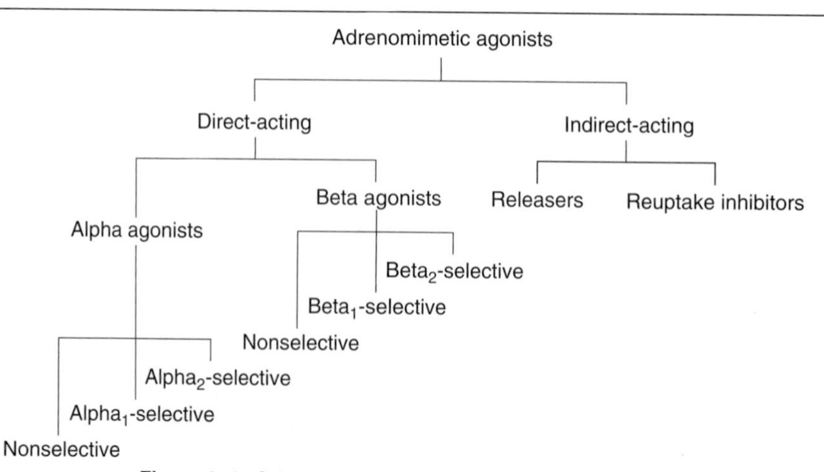

Figure 9–1. Subgroups of drugs discussed in this chapter.

tion increases the stores of catecholamines in adrenergic synaptic vesicles and thus may potentiate the action of indirectly acting sympathomimetics.

2. **Spectrum of action:** Adrenoceptors are classified as alpha or beta receptors; both groups are further subdivided into two (or more) subgroups. The distribution of these receptors is set forth in Table 9–2. Epinephrine may be considered a single prototype with effects at all receptor types (α_1, α_2, β_1, β_2, and β_3). Alternatively, separate prototypes, phenylephrine (alpha) and isoproterenol (beta) may be defined. Dopamine receptors constitute a third class of adrenoceptors. The above-mentioned drugs have relatively little effect on dopamine receptors, but dopamine itself is a potent dopamine receptor agonist and when given as a drug can also activate beta receptors (intermediate doses) and alpha receptors (large doses).

B. Chemistry and Pharmacokinetics: The endogenous adrenoceptor agonists (epinephrine, norepinephrine, and dopamine) are catecholamines and are rapidly metabolized by COMT and MAO. As a result, these adrenoceptor agonists are inactive when given by the oral route. When released from nerve endings, they are subsequently taken up into nerve endings and into perisynaptic cells; this uptake may also occur with norepinephrine, epinephrine, and dopamine given as drugs. These agonists have a short duration of action. When given parenterally, they do not enter the CNS in significant amounts. Isoproterenol, a synthetic catecholamine, is similar to the endogenous transmitters but is not readily taken up into the nerve ending. Phenylisopropylamines, eg, amphetamine, are resistant to MAO; most of them are not catecholamines and are therefore also resistant to COMT. These agents are orally active; they enter the CNS, and their effects last much longer than do those of catecholamines. Tyramine, which is not a phenylisopropylamine, is rapidly metabolized by MAO except in patients who are taking an MAO inhibitor drug. MAO inhibitors are sometimes used in the treatment of depression (Chapter 30).

C. Mechanisms of Action:

1. **Alpha$_1$ receptor effects:** Alpha$_1$ receptor effects are mediated primarily by the coupling protein G_q, which leads to activation of the phosphoinositide cascade and the release of inositol-1,4,5-trisphosphate (IP_3) and diacylglycerol (DAG) from membrane lipids. Calcium is subsequently released from stores in smooth muscle cells, and enzymes are activated. Di-

Table 9–2. Types of adrenoceptors, some of the peripheral tissues in which they are found, and the major effects of their activation. (Adrenoceptor distribution in the CNS is discussed in Chapter 21.)

Type	Tissue	Actions
Alpha$_1$	Most vascular smooth muscle	Contracts (↑ vascular resistance)
	Pupillary dilator muscle	Contracts (mydriasis)
	Pilomotor smooth muscle	Contracts (erects hair)
	Liver (in some species, eg, rat)	Stimulates glycogenolysis
Alpha$_2$	Adrenergic and cholinergic nerve terminals	Inhibits transmitter release
	Platelets	Stimulates aggregation
	Some vascular smooth muscle	Contracts
	Fat cells	Inhibits lipolysis
	Pancreatic B cells	Inhibits insulin release
Beta$_1$	Heart	Stimulates rate and force
	Juxtaglomerular cells	Stimulates renin release
Beta$_2$	Respiratory, uterine, and vascular smooth muscle	Relaxes
	Liver (human)	Stimulates glycogenolysis
	Pancreatic B cells	Stimulates insulin release
	Somatic motor nerve terminals (voluntary muscle)	Causes tremor
Beta$_3$ (β_1, β_2 may also contribute)	Fat cells	Stimulates lipolysis
Dopamine$_1$	Renal and other splanchnic blood vessels	Relaxes (reduces resistance)
Dopamine$_2$	Nerve terminals	Inhibits adenylyl cyclase

rect gating of calcium channels may also play a role in increasing intracellular calcium concentration.

2. **Alpha$_2$ receptor effects:** Alpha$_2$ receptor activation results in inhibition of adenylyl cyclase via the coupling protein G_i.
3. **Beta receptor effects:** Beta receptors (β_1, β_2, and β_3) stimulate adenylyl cyclase via the coupling protein G_s, which leads to an increase in cAMP concentration in the cell.
4. **Dopamine receptor effects:** Dopamine D_1 receptors activate adenylyl cyclase in neurons and vascular smooth muscle. Dopamine D_2 receptors are more important in the brain but probably also play a significant role as presynaptic receptors on peripheral nerves.

D. Organ System Effects:

1. **CNS:** Catecholamines do not enter the CNS effectively. Sympathomimetics that do enter the CNS (eg, amphetamines) have a spectrum of stimulant effects, beginning with mild alerting or reduction of fatigue, and progressing to anorexia, euphoria, and insomnia. These effects probably reflect the release of dopamine in certain dopaminergic tracts. Very high doses lead to marked anxiety or aggressiveness, paranoia, and, rarely, convulsions.
2. **Eye:** The smooth muscle of the pupillary dilator responds to topical phenylephrine and similar alpha agonists with mydriasis. Accommodation is not significantly affected. Outflow of aqueous humor may be facilitated by nonselective alpha agonists, with a subsequent reduction of intraocular pressure. Alpha$_2$-selective agonists also reduce intraocular pressure, apparently by reducing synthesis of aqueous humor.
3. **Bronchi:** The smooth muscle of the bronchi relaxes markedly in response to beta$_2$ agonists. These agents are the most efficacious and reliable drugs available for reversing bronchospasm.
4. **Gastrointestinal tract:** The gastrointestinal tract is well endowed with both alpha and beta receptors, located on both smooth muscle and on neurons of the enteric nervous system. Activation of either alpha or beta receptors leads to relaxation of the smooth muscle. Alpha$_2$ agonists may decrease salt and water secretion into the intestine.
5. **Genitourinary tract:** The genitourinary tract contains alpha receptors in the bladder trigone and sphincter area; the receptors mediate contraction of the sphincter. Sympathomimetics are sometimes used to increase sphincter tone. Beta$_2$ agonists may cause significant uterine relaxation in pregnant women near term, but the doses required also cause significant tachycardia.
6. **Vascular system:**
   a. **Alpha$_1$ agonists:** Alpha$_1$ agonists (eg, phenylephrine) constrict skin and splanchnic blood vessels and increase peripheral vascular resistance and venous pressure. Because these drugs increase blood pressure, they often evoke a compensatory reflex bradycardia.
   b. **Alpha$_2$ agonists:** Alpha$_2$ agonists (eg, clonidine) cause vasoconstriction when administered intravenously or topically (eg, as a nasal spray), but when given orally they accumulate in the CNS and *reduce* sympathetic outflow and blood pressure as described in Chapter 11.
   c. **Beta agonists:** Beta$_2$ agonists (eg, terbutaline) cause significant reduction in arteriolar tone in the skeletal muscle vascular bed and can reduce peripheral vascular resistance and arterial blood pressure. Beta$_1$ agonists have relatively little effect on vessels.
   d. **Dopamine:** Dopamine causes vasodilation in the splanchnic and renal vascular beds by activating D_1 receptors. This effect can be very useful in the treatment of renal failure associated with shock. At higher doses, dopamine activates beta receptors; at still higher doses, alpha receptors are activated.
7. **Heart:** The heart is well supplied with β_1 and β_2 receptors. The β_1 receptors predominate in some parts of the heart; both beta receptors, however, mediate increased rate of cardiac pacemakers (normal and abnormal), increased AV node conduction velocity, and increased cardiac force.
8. **Net cardiovascular actions:** Sympathomimetics with both alpha and beta$_1$ effects (eg, norepinephrine) may cause a reflex increase in vagal outflow because they increase blood pressure and evoke the baroreceptor reflex. This reflex bradycardia often dominates any direct beta effects on the heart rate, so that a slow infusion of norepinephrine typically causes increased blood pressure and bradycardia (Figure 9–2). If the reflex is blocked (eg, by a ganglion blocker), norepinephrine may cause a direct beta$_1$-mediated tachycardia. A pure

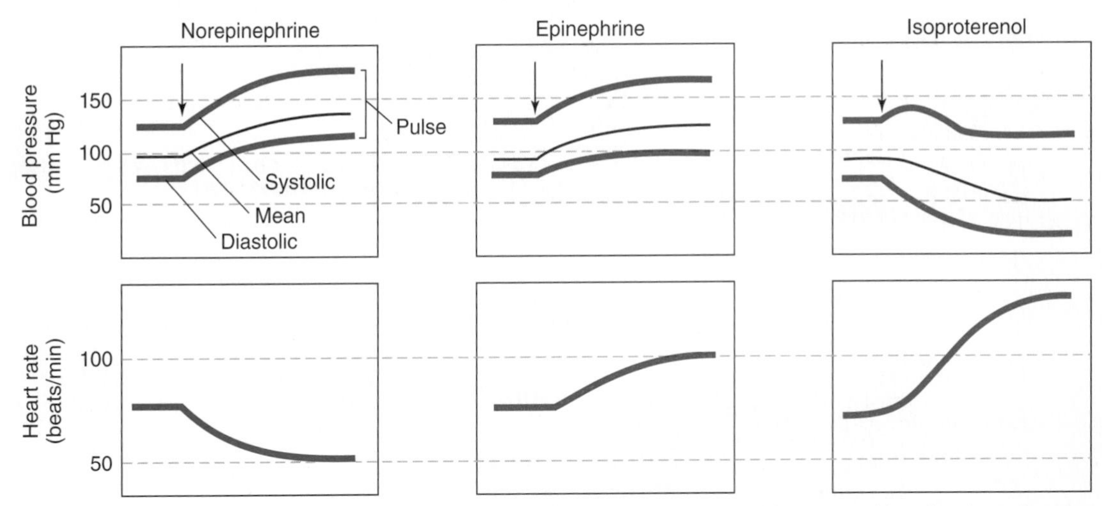

Figure 9–2. Typical effects of the principal catecholamines on blood pressure and heart rate. Note that the pulse pressure ("Pulse") is only slightly increased by norepinephrine but is markedly increased by epinephrine and isoproterenol. The reduction in heart rate caused by norepinephrine is the result of baroreceptor reflex activation of vagal outflow to the heart. The blood pressure effects of epinephrine are typically dose-dependent: small doses exhibit more beta effect (isoproterenol-like); large doses exhibit more alpha effect (norepinephrine-like).

alpha agonist, eg, phenylephrine, will routinely slow heart rate via the baroreceptor reflex, while a pure beta agonist, eg, isoproterenol, almost always increases the heart rate.

The diastolic blood pressure is affected mainly by peripheral vascular resistance and the heart rate. The adrenoceptors with the greatest effects on vascular resistance are alpha and beta$_2$ receptors. The systolic pressure is the sum of the diastolic and the pulse pressures. The pulse pressure is determined mainly by the stroke volume (a function of force of cardiac contraction), which is influenced by beta$_1$ receptors.

9. **Metabolic and hormonal effects:** Beta$_1$ agonists increase renin secretion. Beta$_2$ agonists increase insulin secretion by the pancreas. They also increase glycogenolysis in the liver. The resulting hyperglycemia is countered by the increased insulin levels. Transport of glucose out of the liver is associated initially with hyperkalemia; transport into peripheral organs (especially skeletal muscle) is accompanied by movement of potassium into these cells, resulting in a later hypokalemia. All beta agonists appear to stimulate lipolysis.

Skill Keeper: Blood Pressure Control Mechanisms in Pheochromocytoma (see Chapter 6)

Patients with pheochromocytoma may have this tumor for several months or even years before symptoms or signs lead to a diagnosis. Predict the probable compensatory responses to a chronic increase in blood pressure caused by a tumor releasing large amounts of norepinephrine. *Skill Keeper Answer appears at the end of the chapter.*

E. **Clinical Uses:** Table 9–3.

1. **Anaphylaxis:** Epinephrine is the drug of choice for the immediate treatment of anaphylactic shock. The catecholamine is sometimes supplemented with antihistamines and corticosteroids, but these agents are not as efficacious as epinephrine nor as rapid-acting.
2. **CNS:** The phenylisopropylamines such as amphetamine are widely used and abused for their CNS effects. Legitimate indications include narcolepsy, attention deficit disorder, and, with appropriate controls, weight reduction. The anorexiant effect may be helpful in initiating weight loss but is insufficient to maintain the loss unless patients also receive intensive dietary and psychologic counseling and support. The drugs are abused or misused for the

Table 9–3. Pharmacokinetics and clinical applications of some sympathomimetics.

Drug	Oral Activity	Duration of Action	Clinical Applications
Catecholamines			
Epinephrine	No	Minutes	Anaphylaxis, glaucoma, asthma, and to cause vasoconstriction
Norepinephrine	No	Minutes	To cause vasoconstriction in hypotension
Isoproterenol	Poor	Minutes	Asthma, atrioventricular block (rare)
Dopamine	No	Minutes	Shock, heart failure
Dobutamine	No	Minutes	Shock, heart failure
Other sympathomimetics			
Amphetamine, phenmetrazine, others	Yes	Hours	Narcolepsy, obesity, attention deficit disorder
Ephedrine	Yes	Hours	Asthma (obsolete), urinary incontinence, and to cause vasoconstriction in hypotension
Phenylephrine	Poor	Hours	To cause mydriasis, vasoconstriction, decongestion
Albuterol, metaproterenol, terbutaline	Yes	Hours	Asthma
Oxymetazoline, xylometazoline	Yes	Hours	To cause nasal decongestion (long action)
Cocaine	No	Minutes to hours	To cause vasoconstriction and local anesthesia

purpose of deferring sleep and for their mood-elevating, euphoria-producing action (Chapter 32).

3. **Eye:** The alpha agonists, especially phenylephrine, are often used topically to produce mydriasis and to reduce the conjunctival itching and congestion caused by irritation or allergy. These drugs do not cause cycloplegia. Epinephrine and a prodrug, dipivefrin, are sometimes used topically in the treatment of glaucoma. Phenylephrine has also been used for glaucoma, mainly outside the USA. Newer α_2 agonists introduced for use in glaucoma include apraclonidine and brimonidine. As noted above, the α_2 agonists appear to reduce aqueous synthesis.
4. **Bronchi:** The beta agonists, especially the β_2-selective agonists, are drugs of choice in the treatment of acute asthmatic bronchoconstriction. The short-acting β_2-selective agonists (eg, terbutaline, albuterol, metaproterenol) are not recommended for prophylaxis, but they are safe and effective and may be lifesaving in the treatment of bronchospasm. A much longer-acting β_2-selective agonist, salmeterol, is recommended for prophylaxis (and not for the treatment of acute symptoms).
5. **Cardiovascular applications:**
   a. **Conditions in which an increase in blood flow is desired:** In acute heart failure and some types of shock, an increase in cardiac output and blood flow to the tissues is needed. Beta$_1$ agonists may be useful in this situation because they increase cardiac contractility and reduce afterload (by decreasing the impedance to ventricular ejection through their partial beta$_2$ effect).
   b. **Conditions in which a decrease in blood flow or increase in blood pressure is desired:** Alpha$_1$ agonists are useful in situations in which vasoconstriction is appropriate. These include local hemostatic and decongestant effects as well as spinal shock, in which temporary maintenance of blood pressure may help maintain perfusion of the brain, heart, and kidneys. Shock due to septicemia or myocardial infarction, on the other hand, is usually made worse by vasoconstrictors, since the afterload is increased and tissue perfusion often declines. Alpha agonists are often mixed with local anesthetics to reduce the loss of anesthetic from the area of injection into the circulation. Chronic orthostatic hypotension due to inadequate sympathetic tone can be treated with a newer α_1 agonist, midodrine.

6. **Genitourinary tract:** $Beta_2$ agonists (ritodrine, terbutaline) are used to suppress premature labor, but the cardiac stimulant effect may be hazardous to both mother and fetus. Nonsteroidal anti-inflammatory drugs, calcium channel blockers, and magnesium are also used for this indication.

   Long-acting sympathomimetics such as ephedrine are sometimes used to improve urinary continence in children with enuresis and in the elderly. This action is mediated by alpha receptors in the trigone of the bladder and, in men, the smooth muscle of the prostate.

F. Toxicity:

1. **Catecholamines:** Because of their limited penetration into the brain, these drugs have little CNS toxicity when given systemically. In the periphery, their adverse effects are extensions of their pharmacologic alpha or beta actions: excessive vasoconstriction, cardiac arrhythmias, myocardial infarction, and pulmonary edema or hemorrhage.
2. **Other sympathomimetics:** The phenylisopropylamines may produce mild to severe CNS toxicity, depending on dosage. In small doses, they induce nervousness, anorexia, and insomnia; in higher doses, they may cause anxiety, aggressiveness, or paranoid behavior. Convulsions may occur. Peripherally acting agents have toxicities that are predictable on the basis of the receptors they activate. Thus, α_1 agonists cause hypertension and β_1 agonists cause sinus tachycardia and serious arrhythmias. $Beta_2$ agonists cause skeletal muscle tremor. It is important to note that none of these drugs is perfectly selective; at high doses, β_1-selective agents have β_2 actions and vice versa. Cocaine is of special importance as a drug of abuse: its major toxicities include cardiac arrhythmias or infarction and convulsions. A fatal outcome is far more common with acute cocaine overdose than with any other sympathomimetic.

DRUG LIST

The following drugs are important members of the group discussed in this chapter. Prototypes should be learned in detail; the features of the major variants should be known well enough to distinguish the variants from prototypes and from each other; the other significant agents should be recognized as belonging to a specific subclass.

Subclass	Prototype	Major Variants	Other Significant Agents
General agonists			
Direct (α_1, α_2, β_1, β_2)	Epinephrine		
Indirect, releasers	Amphetamine, tyramine		Ephedrine
Indirect, uptake inhibitors	Cocaine	Tricyclic antidepressants	
Selective agonists			
α_1, α_2, β_1	Norepinephrine		
$\alpha_1 > \alpha_2$	Phenylephrine		Methoxamine, metaraminol, midodrine
$\alpha_2 > \alpha_1$	Clonidine	Methylnorepinephrine[1]	Apraclonidine, brimonidine
$\beta_1 = \beta_2$	Isoproterenol		
$\beta_1 > \beta_2$	Dobutamine		
$\beta_2 > \beta_1$	Terbutaline	Salmeterol	Albuterol, metaproterenol, ritodrine
Dopamine agonist	Dopamine	Bromocriptine[2]	

[1]Active metabolite of methyldopa.
[2]Ergot derivative with CNS dopamine agonist action, discussed in Chapter 28.

QUESTIONS

DIRECTIONS: Each of the numbered items or incomplete statements in this section is followed by answers or by completions of the statement. Select the ONE lettered answer or completion that is BEST in each case.

1. Dilation of vessels in muscle, constriction of cutaneous vessels, and positive inotropic and chronotropic effects on the heart are all actions of
   (A) Acetylcholine
   (B) Epinephrine
   (C) Isoproterenol
   (D) Metaproterenol
   (E) Norepinephrine
2. A 7-year-old boy has a significant bed-wetting problem. A long-acting indirect sympathomimetic agent sometimes used by the oral route for this and other indications is
   (A) Dobutamine
   (B) Ephedrine
   (C) Epinephrine
   (D) Isoproterenol
   (E) Phenylephrine
3. When pupillary dilation—but not cycloplegia—is desired, a good choice is
   (A) Homatropine
   (B) Isoproterenol
   (C) Phenylephrine
   (D) Pilocarpine
   (E) Tropicamide
4. Which of the following act primarily on a receptor located on the membrane of the autonomic effector cell, ie, muscle or glandular tissue?
   (A) Clonidine
   (B) Cocaine
   (C) Norepinephrine
   (D) Tyramine
   (E) All of the above
5. When a moderate pressor dose of norepinephrine is given after pretreatment with a large dose of atropine, which of the following is the most probable response to the norepinephrine?
   (A) A decrease in heart rate caused by direct cardiac effect
   (B) A decrease in heart rate caused by indirect reflex effect
   (C) An increase in heart rate caused by direct cardiac action
   (D) An increase in heart rate caused by indirect reflex action
   (E) No change in heart rate
6. Which of the following may stimulate the central nervous system?
   (A) Antimuscarinic drugs
   (B) Sympathomimetic drugs
   (C) Both **(A)** and **(B)** are correct
   (D) Neither **(A)** nor **(B)** is correct

Items 7–8: Your patient is to receive a selective β_2 stimulant drug.

7. Beta$_2$-selective stimulants are often effective in
   (A) Angina due to coronary insufficiency
   (B) Asthma
   (C) Chronic heart failure
   (D) Delayed or insufficiently strong labor
   (E) Raynaud's syndrome
8. In considering possible drug effects in this patient, you would note that beta$_2$ stimulants frequently cause
   (A) Direct stimulation of renin release
   (B) Increased cGMP in mast cells
   (C) Skeletal muscle tremor
   (D) Vasodilation in the skin
   (E) All of the above
9. Epinephrine increases the concentration of all of the following EXCEPT
   (A) cAMP in heart muscle
   (B) Free fatty acids in blood
   (C) Glucose in blood
   (D) Lactate in blood
   (E) Triglycerides in fat cells

10. Phenylephrine causes
(A) Constriction of vessels in the nasal mucosa
(B) Increased gastric secretion and motility
(C) Increased skin temperature
(D) Miosis
(E) All of the above

Items 11–12: Autonomic drugs X and Y were given in moderate doses as IV boluses to normal volunteers. The systolic and diastolic blood pressure changed as shown in the diagram.

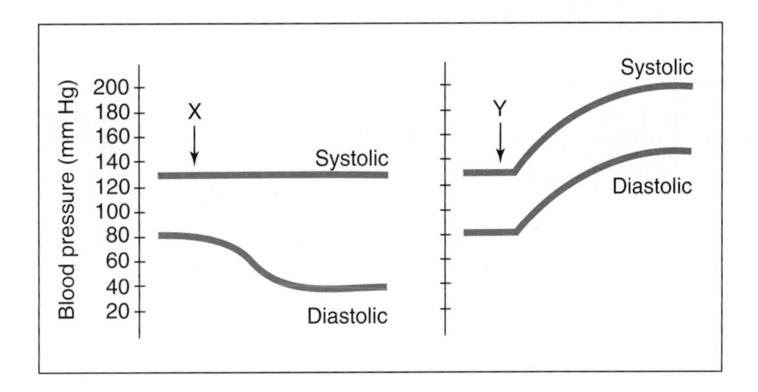

11. Which of the following drugs most resembles drug X?
(A) Acetylcholine
(B) Atropine
(C) Epinephrine
(D) Isoproterenol
(E) Norepinephrine

12. Which of the following most resembles drug Y?
(A) Acetylcholine
(B) Atropine
(C) Epinephrine
(D) Isoproterenol
(E) Norepinephrine

13. A new drug was given by subcutaneous injection to 25 normal subjects in a phase I clinical trial. The cardiovascular effects are summarized in the table below. Which of the following drugs does the new experimental agent most resemble?
(A) Bethanechol
(B) Epinephrine
(C) Isoproterenol
(D) Phenylephrine
(E) Physostigmine

Variable	Control	Peak Drug Effect
Systolic BP (mm Hg)	116	144
Diastolic BP (mm Hg)	76	96
Cardiac output (L/min)	5.4	4.7
Heart rate (beats/min)	71.2	54.3

14. Which of the following drugs will decrease heart rate in a patient with a normal heart but will have little or no effect on heart rate in a cardiac transplant recipient?
(A) Epinephrine
(B) Isoproterenol

(C) Norepinephrine
(D) Phenylephrine
(E) Salmeterol
(F) Terbutaline

15. Which of the following drugs is the drug of choice in anaphylaxis associated with bronchospasm and hypotension?
    (A) Cortisone
    (B) Epinephrine
    (C) Isoproterenol
    (D) Norepinephrine
    (E) Phenylephrine
    (F) Salmeterol
    (G) Terbutaline

ANSWERS

1. The actions describe the effects of activating alpha, β_1, and β_2 receptors. Of the drugs listed, only epinephrine has all of these actions. The answer is **(B)**.
2. Phenylephrine and ephedrine are the only orally effective agents listed. Phenylephrine has a direct and relatively short action. Ephedrine occurs in the herb Ma-huang and in "energy" supplements. The answer is **(B)**.
3. Antimuscarinics (homatropine, tropicamide) are mydriatic and cycloplegic; alpha-sympathomimetic agonists are only mydriatic. Pilocarpine causes *miosis*. The answer is **(C)**.
4. The indirect-acting agents (cocaine and tyramine) act through catecholamines in or released from the nerve terminal; clonidine acts primarily on the α_2 receptor of the presynaptic nerve terminal. The answer is **(C)**.
5. Atropine will prevent the normal reflex bradycardia, since that requires integrity of the vagal pathway. The direct action of norepinephrine on the sinus node will be unmasked. The answer is **(C)**.
6. Phenylisopropylamines such as amphetamine are traditional stimulants with a spectrum of effects from mild alerting to paranoid schizophrenia and convulsions; antimuscarinic agents are capable of inducing hallucinations and convulsions. The answer is **(C)**.
7. Beta agonists increase cardiac rate and force and increase myocardial oxygen demand; they are generally contraindicated in angina. In chronic heart failure, the heart is already subject to excessive sympathetic drive. The absence of β_2 receptors in the cutaneous vascular bed makes beta agonists useless in conditions involving reduced skin blood flow. Uterine and bronchiolar smooth muscle are relaxed by beta$_2$ agonists. The answer is **(B)**.
8. Tremor is a common β_2 effect. Blood vessels in the skin have almost exclusively alpha (vasoconstrictor) receptors. Stimulation of renin release is a β_1 effect. The answer is **(C)**.
9. Epinephrine increases plasma free fatty acids by activating lipolysis of triglycerides in fat cells. The answer is **(E)**.
10. Vasoconstriction in the nasal mucosa is the basis for the widespread use of alpha agonists as topical decongestants. The answer is **(A)**.
11. The drug X infusion caused a decrease in diastolic blood pressure and little change in systolic pressure. Thus, there was a large increase in pulse pressure. The decrease in diastolic pressure suggests that the drug decreased vascular resistance, ie, it must have significant muscarinic or beta agonist effects. The fact that it also markedly increased pulse pressure suggests that it strongly increased stroke volume, also a beta-agonist effect. The drug with these beta effects is isoproterenol (Figure 9–2). The answer is **(D)**.
12. Drug Y caused a marked increase in diastolic pressure, suggesting strong alpha vasoconstrictor effects. It also caused a moderate increase in pulse pressure, suggesting some beta-agonist action. The drug that best matches this description in norepinephrine. The answer is **(E)**.
13. The investigational agent caused a marked increase in diastolic pressure but little increase in pulse pressure (from 40 to 48 mm Hg). These changes suggest a strong alpha effect on vessels but little beta agonist action in the heart. The heart rate decreased markedly, reflecting a baroreceptor reflex compensatory response. Note that the stroke volume increased slightly (cardiac output divided by heart rate; from 75.8 mL to 86.6 mL). This is to be expected even in the absence of beta effects if venoconstriction causes an increase in venous return to the heart. The drug behaves most like a pure alpha agonist. The answer is **(D)**.

14. A pure alpha agonist will cause reflex bradycardia in a subject with intact cardiac innervation, but no change in heart rate if this innervation is severed, eg, in a heart transplant patient. The other drugs listed have direct beta agonist effects and will increase heart rate in the denervated heart. The answer is **(D).**
15. The drug of choice in anaphylaxis is epinephrine. The answer is **(B).**

Skill Keeper Answer: Blood Pressure Control Mechanisms in Pheochromocytoma (see Chapter 6)

Because the control mechanisms that attempt to maintain blood pressure constant are intact in patients with pheochromocytoma (they are reset in patients with ordinary hypertension), a number of compensatory changes are observed in pheochromocytoma patients (see Figure 6–4). These include reduced renin, angiotensin, and aldosterone levels in the blood. With the reduced aldosterone effect on the kidney, more salt and water is excreted, reducing blood volume. Since the red cell mass is not affected, hematocrit is often increased. If the tumor releases only norepinephrine, a compensatory bradycardia may also be present, but most patients release enough epinephrine to maintain heart rate at a normal or even increased level.

10 Adrenoceptor Blockers

OBJECTIVES

You should be able to:

- Describe the effects of an alpha-blocker on the hemodynamic responses to epinephrine.
- Describe the effects of an alpha-blocker on the hemodynamic responses to norepinephrine.
- Compare the effects of propranolol, labetalol, metoprolol, and pindolol.
- Compare the pharmacokinetics of propranolol, atenolol, esmolol, and nadolol.
- Describe the clinical indications and toxicities of typical alpha- and beta-blockers.

Learn the definitions that follow.

Table 10–1. Definitions.

Term	Definition
Competitive blocker	A surmountable antagonist; one that can be overcome by increasing the dose of agonist
Covalently bound inhibitor	An antagonist that binds irreversibly to its receptor or other binding site
Epinephrine reversal	Conversion of the pressor response (typical of large doses of epinephrine) to a blood pressure-lowering effect; caused by alpha blockers
Intrinsic sympathomimetic activity (ISA)	Partial agonist action by adrenoceptor blockers; typical of several beta blockers, eg, pindolol, acebutolol
Irreversible blocker	A nonsurmountable inhibitor, usually because of covalent bond formation; eg, phenoxybenzamine
Membrane stabilizing activity (MSA)	Local anesthetic action; typical of several beta-blockers, eg, propranolol
Orthostatic hypotension	Hypotension that is most marked in the upright position; caused by venous pooling or inadequate blood volume; typical of alpha blockade
Partial agonist	A drug (eg, pindolol) that produces a smaller maximal effect than a full agonist and therefore can inhibit the effect of a full agonist
Pheochromocytoma	A tumor that resembles the adrenal medulla; consisting of cells that release varying amounts of norepinephrine, epinephrine, or both into the circulation
Presynaptic receptor	A receptor located on the presynaptic nerve terminal; the receptor modulates transmitter release from the terminal

CONCEPTS

Alpha- and beta-blocking agents are divided into primary subgroups on the basis of their receptor selectivity (Figure 10–1). All of these agents are pharmacologic antagonists. Because they differ markedly in their effects and clinical applications, these drugs are considered separately in the following discussion.

ALPHA-BLOCKING DRUGS

A. Classification: Subdivisions of the alpha-blockers are based on the presence or absence of selective affinity for α_1 versus α_2 receptors. Other features used to classify the alpha-blocking drugs are their reversibility and duration of action.

1. **Irreversible, long-acting: Phenoxybenzamine** is the prototypical long-acting, irreversible alpha-blocker. It is only slightly α_1-selective.
2. **Reversible, shorter-acting: Phentolamine** (nonselective) and **tolazoline** (slightly α_2-selective) are competitive, reversible blocking agents.
3. **Alpha$_1$-selective: Prazosin** is a selective, reversible pharmacologic α_1-blocker. Doxazosin and terazosin are similar drugs. The advantage of α_1 selectivity is discussed below.

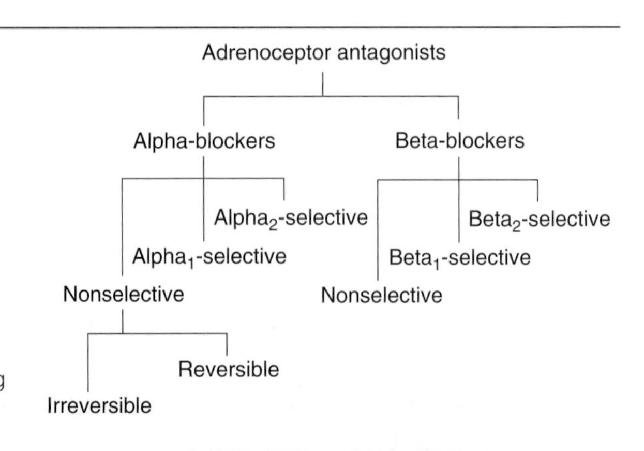

Figure 10–1. Subgroups of adrenoceptor-blocking drugs.

4. **Alpha$_2$-selective:** **Yohimbine** and **rauwolscine** are alpha$_2$-selective competitive pharmacologic antagonists. They are used primarily in research applications.

B. Pharmacokinetics: These drugs are all active by the oral as well as the parenteral route, though phentolamine and tolazoline are rarely given orally. Phenoxybenzamine has a short elimination half-life but a long duration of action—about 48 hours—because it binds covalently to its receptor. Phentolamine and tolazoline have durations of action of 2–4 hours when used orally and 20–40 minutes when given parenterally. Prazosin acts for 8–10 hours.

C. Mechanism of Action: Phenoxybenzamine binds covalently to the alpha receptor, thereby producing an irreversible (insurmountable) blockade. The other agents are competitive pharmacologic antagonists—ie, their effects can be surmounted by increased concentrations of agonist. This difference may be important in the treatment of pheochromocytoma because a massive release of catecholamines from the tumor may overcome a reversible blockade.

D. Effects:

1. **Nonselective blockers:** These agents cause a predictable blockade of alpha-mediated responses to sympathetic nervous system discharge and exogenous sympathomimetics (ie, the alpha responses listed in Table 9–2). The most important effects of nonselective alpha-blockers are those on the cardiovascular system: a reduction in vascular tone with a reduction of both arterial and venous pressures. There are no significant direct cardiac effects. However, the nonselective alpha-blockers do cause baroreceptor reflex-mediated tachycardia as a result of the drop in mean arterial pressure (Figure 6–4). This tachycardia may be exaggerated because the alpha$_2$ receptors on adrenergic nerve terminals in the heart, which normally reduce the net release of norepinephrine, are also blocked (Figure 6–3).

   Epinephrine reversal is a predictable result of the use of this agonist in a patient who has received an alpha-blocker. The term refers to a reversal in the blood pressure effect of moderate to large doses of epinephrine, from a pressor response (mediated by alpha-receptors) to a depressor response (mediated by β_2-receptors) (Figure 10–2). The effect is not observed with phenylephrine or norepinephrine because these drugs lack β_2 effects.

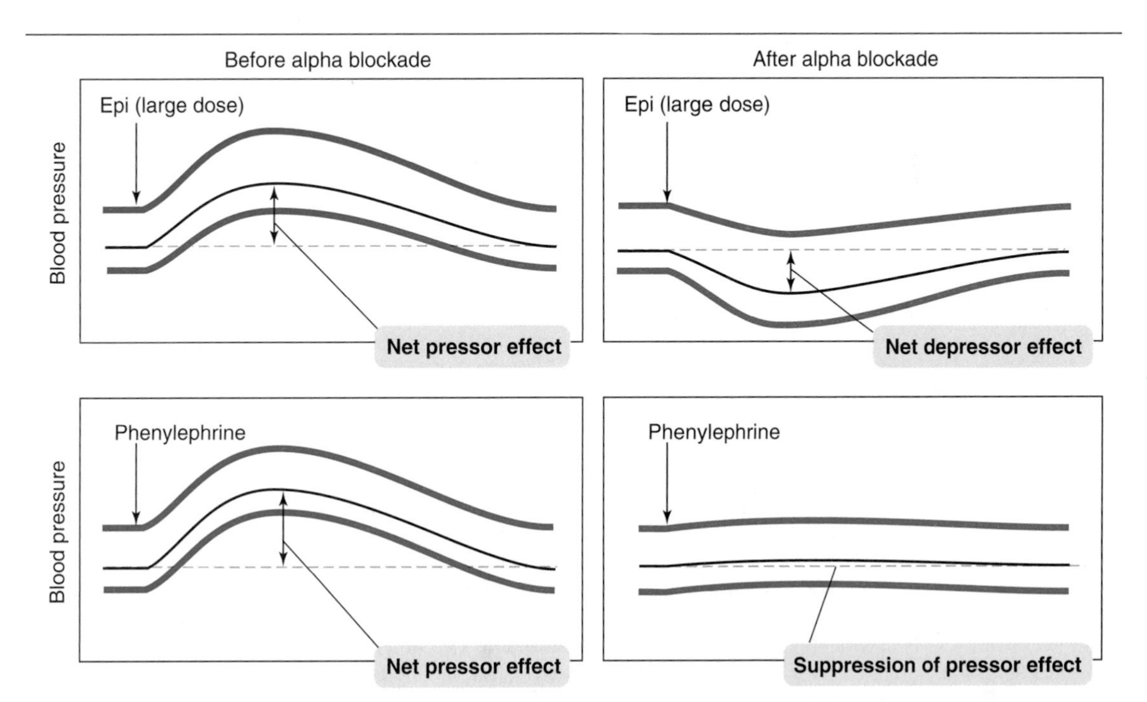

Figure 10–2. The effects of an alpha-blocker, eg, phentolamine, on the blood pressure responses to epinephrine and phenylephrine. The epinephrine response exhibits reversal of the mean blood pressure change from a net increase (the alpha response) to a net decrease (the beta$_2$ response). The response to phenylephrine is suppressed but not reversed, because phenylephrine is a "pure" alpha agonist without beta action.

Epinephrine reversal is occasionally seen as an unexpected (but predictable) effect of drugs for which alpha blockade is an adverse effect (eg, some phenothiazine tranquilizers, antihistamines).

2. **Selective alpha-blockers:** Because prazosin and its analogs block vascular α_1 receptors much more effectively than the α_2-modulatory receptors associated with cardiac sympathetic nerve endings, these drugs cause much less tachycardia than the nonselective alpha-blockers when reducing blood pressure.

E. **Clinical Uses:**

1. **Nonselective alpha-blockers:** Nonselective alpha-blockers have limited clinical applications. The best-documented application is in the presurgical management of pheochromocytoma. Such patients may have severe hypertension and reduced blood volume, which should be corrected before subjecting the patient to the stress of surgery. Phenoxybenzamine is usually used during this preparatory phase; phentolamine is sometimes used during surgery. Phenoxybenzamine also has serotonin receptor-blocking effects, which justify its occasional use in carcinoid tumor; and H_1 antihistamine effects, which lead to its use in mastocytosis.

   Accidental local infiltration of potent alpha agonists such as norepinephrine may lead to tissue ischemia and necrosis if not promptly reversed; infiltration of the ischemic area with phentolamine is sometimes used to prevent tissue damage. Overdose with drugs of abuse such as amphetamine, cocaine, or phenylpropanolamine may lead to severe hypertension because of their indirect sympathomimetic actions. This hypertension will usually respond well to alpha-blockers. Sudden cessation of clonidine therapy leads to rebound hypertension (Chapter 11); this phenomenon is often treated with phentolamine.

   Raynaud's phenomenon sometimes responds to phenoxybenzamine or phentolamine, but their efficacy is not well documented in this condition. Phentolamine or yohimbine is sometimes used by direct injection to cause penile erection in men with impotence.

2. **Selective alpha-blockers:** Prazosin and other α_1 blockers are used in hypertension (see Chapter 11). Selective α_1-blockers have also found increasing use in the management of urinary hesitancy and prevention of urinary retention in men with prostatic hyperplasia.

F. **Toxicity:** The most important toxicities of the alpha-blockers are simple extensions of their alpha-blocking effects. The main manifestations are orthostatic hypotension and, in the case of the nonselective agents, reflex tachycardia. Phentolamine and tolazoline also have some non-alpha-mediated vasodilating effects. In patients with coronary disease, angina may be precipitated by the tachycardia. Oral administration of any of these drugs can cause nausea and vomiting. The α_1-selective agents are associated with an exaggerated orthostatic hypotensive response to the first dose in some patients. Therefore, the first dose is usually small and taken just before going to bed.

BETA-BLOCKING DRUGS

A. **Classification, Subgroups, and Mechanisms:** All of the clinically used beta-blockers are competitive pharmacologic antagonists. Propranolol is the prototype. Drugs in this group are usually classified into subgroups on the basis of β_1 versus β_2 selectivity, partial agonist activity, local anesthetic action, and lipid solubility (Table 10–2).

1. **Receptor selectivity:** Beta$_1$ receptor selectivity (β_1 block > β_2 block), is a property of **acebutolol, atenolol, esmolol, metoprolol,** and several other beta-blockers. This property may be an advantage when treating patients with asthma. **Butoxamine,** a β_2-selective drug, is used only in research. Nadolol, propranolol, and timolol are typical nonselective beta-blockers.

   Labetalol is an unusual agent with combined alpha- and beta-blocking action. This drug has four diastereomers; the alpha-blocking activity resides in the SR enantiomer and the beta-blocking action in the RR enantiomer. The other two enantiomers (RS and SS) are practically inactive. **Carvedilol** has two isomers; one is an alpha blocker while the other is a nonselective beta-blocker.

2. **Partial agonist activity:** Partial agonist activity ("intrinsic sympathomimetic activity") may be an advantage in treating patients with asthma because, even at maximum dosage, these drugs, eg, **pindolol, acebutolol,** will—at least in theory—cause some bronchodila-

Table 10–2. Properties of several beta receptor-blocking drugs.*

Drug	Selectivity	Partial Agonist Activity	Local Anesthetic Action	Lipid Solubility	Elimination Half-Life	Approximate Bioavailability
Acebutolol	β_1	Yes	Yes	Low	3–4 h	50%
Atenolol	β_1	No	No	Low	6–9 h	40%
Esmolol	β_1	No	No	Low	10 min	....
Carvedilol[1]	None	No	No	No data	7–10 h	25–35%
Labetalol[1]	None	Yes[2]	Yes	Moderate	5 h	30%
Metoprolol	β_1	No	Yes	Moderate	3–4 h	50%
Nadolol	None	No	No	Low	14–24 h	33%
Pindolol	None	Yes[2]	Yes	Moderate	3–4 h	90%
Propranolol	None	No	Yes	High	3.5–6 h	30%[3]
Timolol	None	No	No	Moderate	4–5 h	50%

*Modified and reproduced, with permission, from Katzung BG (editor): *Basic & Clinical Pharmacology,* 8th ed. McGraw-Hill, 2001.
[1]Also cause α_1 receptor blockade.
[2]Partial agonist effects at β_2 receptors.
[3]Bioavailability is dose-dependent.

tion. In contrast, the full antagonists such as propranolol may cause severe bronchospasm in patients with airway disease.

Skill Keeper: Partial Agonist Action (see Chapter 2)

Draw a concentration-response graph showing the effect of increasing concentrations of albuterol on airway diameter (as a percentage of maximum) in the presence of a large concentration of pindolol. On the same graph, draw the curves for the percentage of receptors bound to albuterol and to pindolol at each concentration. *The Skill Keeper Answer appears at the end of the chapter.*

3. **Local anesthetic activity:** Local anesthetic activity ("membrane stabilizing activity") is a disadvantage when beta-blockers are used topically in the eye because it decreases protective reflexes and increases the risk of corneal ulceration. Local anesthetic effects are absent from **timolol** and several other beta-blockers.
4. **Pharmacokinetics:** Most of the systemic agents have been developed for chronic oral use, but bioavailability and duration of action vary widely (Table 10–2). Esmolol is a short-acting ester beta-blocker that is only used parenterally. Nadolol is the longest-acting beta-blocker. Acebutolol and atenolol are less lipid-soluble than the older beta-blockers and probably enter the CNS to a lesser extent.

B. **Effects and Clinical Uses:** Most of the organ-level effects of beta-blockers are predictable from blockade of the beta receptor-mediated effects of sympathetic discharge. The clinical applications of beta blockade are remarkably broad (Table 10–3). The treatment of open-angle glaucoma involves the use of several groups of autonomic drugs (Table 10–4). The cardiovascular applications of beta-blockers—especially in hypertension, angina, and arrhythmias—are extremely important and popular. Treatment of chronic (not acute) congestive heart failure is a novel application of beta-blockers, but studies suggest that several, including labetalol and carvedilol, may be beneficial when used in low dosage and titrated very carefully (Chapter 13). It is not certain how much the alpha-blocking action of these two agents contributes to their effect, but other beta-blockers that lack any alpha-blocking action (eg, metoprolol) also appear to be beneficial. Pheochromocytoma is sometimes treated with combined α- and β-blocking

Table 10–3. Clinical applications of beta-blockers.

Application	Drugs	Effect
Hypertension	Propranolol, metoprolol, timolol, others	Reduced cardiac output, reduced renin secretion
Angina pectoris	Propranolol, nadolol, others	Reduced cardiac rate and force
Arrhythmia prophylaxis after myocardial infarction	Propranolol, metoprolol, timolol	Reduced automaticity of all cardiac pacemakers
Supraventricular tachycardias	Propranolol, esmolol, acebutolol	Slowed AV conduction velocity
Hypertrophic cardiomyopathy	Propranolol	Slowed rate of cardiac contraction
Congestive heart failure	Carvedilol, labetalol, others	Mechanism not understood
Migraine	Propranolol	Prophylactic; mechanism uncertain
Familial tremor, other types of tremor, "stage fright"	Propranolol	Reduced β_2 alteration of neuromuscular transmission; possible CNS effects
Thyroid storm, thyrotoxicosis	Propranolol	Reduced cardiac rate and arrhythmogenesis; other mechanisms may be involved
Glaucoma[1]	Timolol, others	Reduced secretion of aqueous humor

[1]See Table 10–4 for additional drugs used in glaucoma.

agents (eg, labetalol), especially if the tumor is producing large amounts of epinephrine as well as norepinephrine.

C. **Toxicity:** Cardiovascular adverse effects, which are extensions of the beta blockade induced by these agents, include bradycardia, atrioventricular blockade, and congestive heart failure. Patients with airway disease may suffer severe asthma attacks. Premonitory symptoms of hypoglycemia from insulin overdosage, eg, tachycardia, tremor, and anxiety, may be masked, and mobilization of glucose from the liver may be impaired. CNS adverse effects include sedation, fatigue, and sleep alterations. Atenolol, nadolol, and several other less lipid-soluble beta-blockers are claimed to have less marked CNS action because they do not enter the CNS as readily as other members of this group.

Table 10–4. Drugs used in glaucoma.*

Group, Drugs	Mechanism	Methods of Administration
Cholinomimetics		
Pilocarpine, carbachol, physostigmine, echothiophate	Ciliary muscle contraction, opening of trabecular meshwork; increased outflow	Topical drops or gel; plastic film slow-release insert
Alpha agonists, nonselective		
Epinephrine, dipivefrin	Increased outflow, probably via the uveoscleral veins	Topical drops
$Alpha_2$-selective		
Apraclonidine, brimonidine	Decreased aqueous secretion	Topical drops
Beta-blockers		
Timolol, betaxolol, carteolol, levobunolol, metipranolol	Decreased aqueous secretion from the ciliary epithelium	Topical drops
Diuretics		
Acetazolamide, dorzolamide	Decreased secretion due to lack of HCO_3^- ion	Oral (acetazolamide) or topical (dorzolamide)
Prostaglandin $PGF_{2\alpha}$		
Latanoprost	Increased outflow	Topical drops

*Modified and reproduced, with permission, from Katzung BG (editor): *Basic & Clinical Pharmacology,* 8th ed. McGraw-Hill, 2001.

DRUG LIST

The following drugs are important members of the group discussed in this chapter. Prototypes should be learned in detail; the features of major variants should be known well enough to distinguish the variants from prototypes and from each other; the other significant agents should be recognized as belonging to a specific subclass.

Subgroup	Prototype	Major Variants	Other Significant Agents
Alpha-blockers Nonselective	Phenoxybenzamine[1]	Phentolamine	
α_1-Selective	Prazosin		Terazosin, doxazosin
α_2-Selective	Yohimbine		Rauwolscine
Beta-blockers Nonselective	Propranolol	Timolol, nadolol	Carvedilol, labetalol
β_1-Selective	Metoprolol	Atenolol, esmolol	
β_2-Selective	Butoxamine		

[1]Compared to prazosin, phenoxybenzamine is only slightly α_1-selective.

QUESTIONS

DIRECTIONS: Each of the numbered items or incomplete statements in this section is followed by answers or by completions of the statement. Select the ONE lettered answer or completion that is BEST in each case.

1. Which of the following effects of epinephrine would be blocked by phentolamine but not by metoprolol?
(A) Cardiac stimulation
(B) Contraction of radial smooth muscle in the iris
(C) Increase of cAMP in fat
(D) Relaxation of bronchial smooth muscle
(E) Relaxation of the uterus

2. Both phentolamine and tolazoline
(A) Are inactive by the oral route
(B) Block both alpha and beta receptors
(C) Cause hypertension
(D) Cause tachycardia
(E) Induce vasospasm in large doses

3. Propranolol is useful in all of the following EXCEPT
(A) Angina
(B) Familial tremor
(C) Hypertension
(D) Idiopathic hypertrophic subaortic cardiomyopathy
(E) Partial atrioventricular heart block

4. Adverse effects that limit the use of adrenoceptor blockers include
(A) Bronchoconstriction from alpha-blocking agents
(B) Congestive heart failure from beta-blockers
(C) Impaired blood sugar response with alpha-blockers
(D) Increased intraocular pressure with beta-blockers
(E) Sleep disturbances from alpha-blocking drugs

Items 5–8: Four new synthetic drugs (designated W, X, Y, and Z) are to be studied for their cardiovascular effects. They are given to four anesthetized rats while the heart rate is recorded. The first animal has received no pretreatment ("control"), the second has received an effective dose of hexamethonium, the third has received an effective dose of atropine, and the fourth has received an effective dose of phenoxybenzamine. The net changes induced by the new drugs (not by the blocking drugs) are described in the following questions.

5. Drug W increased heart rate in the control animal, the atropine-pretreated animal, and the phenoxybenzamine-pretreated animal. However, Drug W had no effect on heart rate in the hexamethonium-pretreated animal. Drug W is probably a drug similar to
   (A) Acetylcholine
   (B) Edrophonium
   (C) Isoproterenol
   (D) Nitric oxide
   (E) Norepinephrine
6. Drug X had the effects shown in the table below.

In the Rat Receiving	Heart Rate Response to Drug X Was
No pretreatment	↓
Hexamethonium	↑
Atropine	↑
Phenoxybenzamine	↑

   Drug X is probably a drug similar to
   (A) Acetylcholine
   (B) Edrophonium
   (C) Isoproterenol
   (D) Nitric oxide
   (E) Norepinephrine
7. Drug Y had the effects shown in the table below.

In the Rat Receiving	Heart Rate Response to Drug Y Was
No pretreatment	↑
Hexamethonium	↑
Atropine	↑
Phenoxybenzamine	↑

   Drug Y is probably a drug similar to
   (A) Acetylcholine
   (B) Edrophonium
   (C) Isoproterenol
   (D) Nitric oxide
   (E) Norepinephrine
8. The results of the test of Drug Z are shown in the graph.

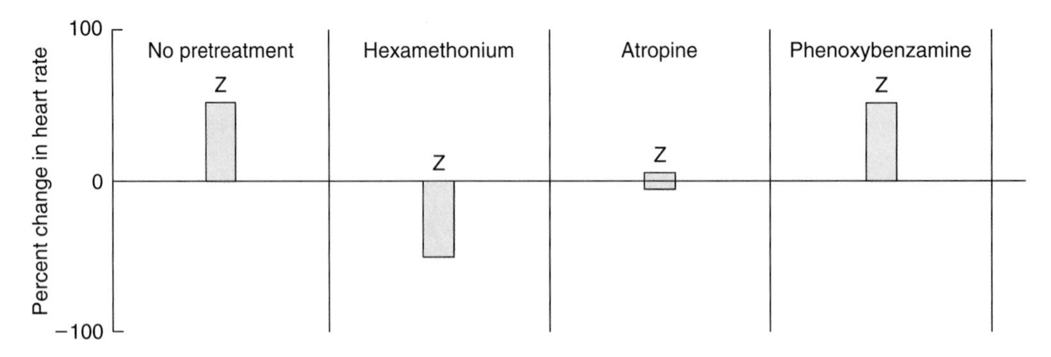

   Drug Z is probably a drug similar to
   (A) Acetylcholine
   (B) Edrophonium

(C) Isoproterenol
(D) Nitric oxide
(E) Norepinephrine

9. A traveler to your city visits you with a request for a renewal of his prescription for phenoxybenzamine. While preparing to telephone his physician, you recall that phenoxybenzamine is used in the treatment of all of the following EXCEPT
(A) Carcinoid
(B) Essential hypertension
(C) Mastocytosis
(D) Pheochromocytoma
(E) Raynaud's phenomenon

10. When given to a patient, phentolamine blocks which one of the following?
(A) Bradycardia induced by phenylephrine
(B) Bronchodilation induced by epinephrine
(C) Increased cardiac contractile force induced by norepinephrine
(D) Miosis induced by acetylcholine
(E) Vasodilation induced by isoproterenol

11. Pretreatment with propranolol will block which one of the following?
(A) Methacholine-induced tachycardia
(B) Nicotine-induced hypertension
(C) Norepinephrine-induced bradycardia
(D) Phenylephrine-induced mydriasis
(E) Pilocarpine-induced miosis

12. Your 55-year-old patient with asthma and glaucoma is to receive a beta-blocking drug. Regarding beta-blocking drugs
(A) Esmolol's pharmacokinetics are compatible with chronic oral use
(B) Metoprolol blocks β_2 receptors selectively
(C) Nadolol lacks β_2-blocking action
(D) Pindolol is a beta antagonist with high membrane-stabilizing (local anesthetic) activity
(E) Timolol lacks the local anesthetic effects of propranolol

13. Which of the following binds covalently to the site specified?
(A) Atenolol—beta receptor
(B) Carvedilol—cardiac beta receptors
(C) Labetalol—alpha and beta receptors
(D) Phenoxybenzamine—alpha receptor
(E) Pindolol—beta receptor

14. A new drug was administered to an anesthetized animal with the results shown. A large dose of epinephrine was administered before and after the new agent for comparison. Which of the following agents does the new drug most closely resemble?

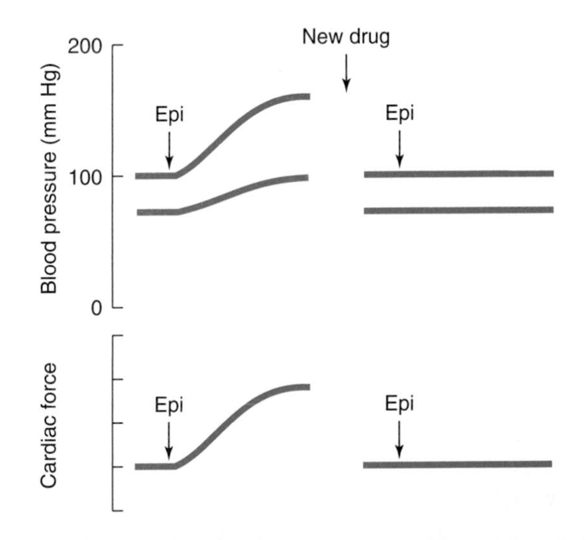

(A) Atenolol
(B) Atropine
(C) Labetalol
(D) Phenoxybenzamine
(E) Propranolol

15. Your 38-year-old patient has symptoms highly suggestive of pheochromocytoma. Her urine VMA and metanephrine levels are markedly elevated, but the normetanephrine level is below normal. She refuses treatment. A month later she enters a local hospital emergency room complaining of severe headache and chest pain. Imaging reveals a small subarachnoid hemorrhage, and electrocardiography indicates a myocardial infarction. Her blood pressure is 230/150 and her heart rate 150. She has been vomiting and is dehydrated. She is immediately given phentolamine intravenously, and an infusion of phenoxybenzamine is prepared. Ten minutes later, her blood pressure is found to be 40/0 and she goes into shock. Vasoconstrictors are ineffective, and she dies after 6 hours. Which of the following statements best explains the exaggerated response to phentolamine in this patient?
(A) The patient had a concurrent familial condition that limited autonomic nervous system control of the blood pressure
(B) The patient had abnormally low secretion of catecholamines from the tumor at the time of admission, so that the recommended dose of phentolamine constituted a major overdose
(C) The patient's tumor secreted almost pure epinephrine with almost no norepinephrine
(D) The tumor had metastasized to the vasomotor center in the medulla

ANSWERS

1. Contraction of the pupillary dilator radial smooth muscle is mediated by alpha receptors. All the other effects are mediated by beta receptors. The answer is **(B).**

2. These alpha-blockers cause hypotension and significant reflex tachycardia. They have no beta-blocking action but do have histaminergic and cholinomimetic properties and never cause vasospasm. The answer is **(D).**

3. Atrioventricular block is an important *contraindication* to the use of beta-blockers. The answer is **(E).**

4. Congestive heart failure can be precipitated by beta blockers. Choices **(A), (C),** and **(E)** reverse the correct pairing of receptor subtype (alpha versus beta) with effect. Choice **(D)** reverses the direction of change of intraocular pressure. The answer is **(B).**

5. In developing a strategy for this type of question, consider first the actions of the known blocking drugs. Hexamethonium blocks reflexes as well as the direct action of nicotine. Atropine would block direct muscarinic effects of an unidentified drug (if it had any) or reflex slowing of the heart mediated by the vagus. Phenoxybenzamine blocks only alpha receptor-mediated processes. If the response produced in the nonpretreated animal is blocked or reversed by hexamethonium, it is probably a reflex response. In that case, consider all the receptors involved in mediating the reflex. Drug W causes tachycardia that is prevented by ganglion blockade and therefore is probably a compensatory reflex tachycardia. We do not have information about beta blockade, but a reflex tachycardia must be mediated by beta receptors in the heart. Two of the choices may cause reflex tachycardia: acetylcholine and nitric oxide. However, the reflex tachycardia evoked by acetylcholine would be blocked by atropine (atropine would prevent the vasodilation that elicited the tachycardia). Thus, drug W must be nitric oxide. The answer is **(D).**

6. Drug X causes slowing of heart rate, but this is converted into tachycardia by hexamethonium and atropine—ie, the bradycardia is caused by reflex vagal discharge. Phenoxybenzamine also reverses the bradycardia to tachycardia, suggesting that alpha receptors are needed to induce the reflex bradycardia and that X has direct beta-agonist actions. The choices that evoke a vagal reflex bradycardia but can also cause direct tachycardia are limited; the answer is **(E).**

7. Drug Y causes tachycardia that is not significantly influenced by any of the blockers; therefore, drug Y must have a direct beta-agonist effect on the heart. The answer is **(C).**

8. Drug Z causes tachycardia that is converted to bradycardia by hexamethonium and blocked completely by atropine. This indicates that the tachycardia is a reflex evoked by vasodilation. Drug Z causes bradycardia when the ganglia are blocked, indicating that it also has a direct muscarinic action on the heart. This is confirmed by the ability of atropine to block both the tachycardia and the bradycardia. The answer is **(A).**

9. Phenoxybenzamine is not useful in essential hypertension because it causes severe tachycardia and marked orthostatic hypotension. The drug is used in Raynaud's phenomenon, but efficacy in this application is controversial. The answer is **(B).**

10. Phenylephrine induces bradycardia through the baroreceptor reflex. Blockade of this drug's alpha-mediated vasoconstrictor effect will prevent the bradycardia. The answer is **(A).**

11. The beta-blocker will not block the vagal slowing induced by norepinephrine hypertension. Nicotine-induced hypertension and phenylephrine-induced mydriasis are mediated by alpha receptors. Pilocarpine is a muscarinic agonist. The answer is **(A).**

12. Esmolol is a short-acting beta-blocker for parenteral use only. Nadolol is a nonselective beta-blocker, and metoprolol is a β_1-selective blocker. Timolol is useful in glaucoma because it does not anesthetize the cornea. The answer is **(E).**

13. Phenoxybenzamine is the only autonomic receptor blocker in clinical use that binds covalently with its receptor. The answer is **(D).**

14. The new drug blocks both the alpha-mediated effects (increased diastolic and mean arterial blood pressure) and beta-mediated action (increased cardiac force). The drug must have *both alpha- and beta-blocking effects.* The answer is **(C).**

15. Note that the original workup of the patient showed highly elevated metanephrine but lower than normal normetanephrine. This suggests that the tumor produces almost pure epinephrine and little or no norepinephrine (recall the metabolites of epinephrine and norepinephrine from Chapter 6). A patient with this type of tumor may have a dramatic *epinephrine reversal* response to any alpha-blocker, plunging the blood pressure to shock levels. This is especially true if the blood volume is low. Although most pheochromocytomas produce a mixture of norepinephrine and epinephrine, cases like the one described have been reported in the literature. The answer is **(C).**

Skill Keeper Answer: Partial Agonist Action (see Chapter 2)

Because pindolol is a partial agonist at beta receptors, the concentration-response curve will show a definite airway-dilating effect at zero albuterol concentration. As albuterol concentration increases, the airway diameter will also increase. The binding curves will show pindolol binding starting at 100% of receptors and going to zero as albuterol concentration increases, with albuterol binding starting at zero and going to 100%.

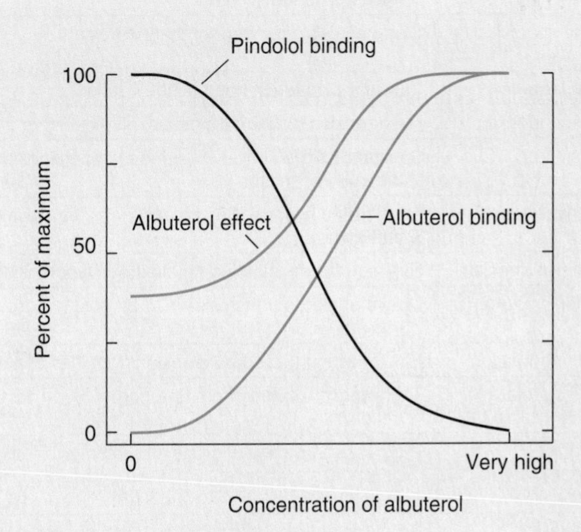

Part III: Cardiovascular Drugs

11 Drugs Used in Hypertension

OBJECTIVES

You should be able to:

- List the four major groups of antihypertensive drugs and give examples of drugs in each group.
- Describe the compensatory responses to each of the four major types of antihypertensive drugs.
- List the major sites of action of sympathoplegic drugs and give examples of drugs that act at each site.
- List the three mechanisms of action of vasodilator drugs.
- List the major antihypertensive vasodilator drugs and describe their effects.
- Describe the differences between the two types of angiotensin antagonists.
- List the major toxicities of the prototype antihypertensive agents.
- Explain why some combinations of antihypertensive drugs are rational and appropriate and others are not.

Learn the definitions that follow.

Table 11–1. Definitions.

Term	Definition
Baroreceptor reflex	Primary autonomic mechanism for blood pressure homeostasis; involves sensory input from carotid sinus to the vasomotor center and output via the parasympathetic and sympathetic motor nerves
Catecholamine reuptake pump	Nerve terminal transporter responsible for recycling catecholamine transmitters after release into the synapse
Catecholamine vesicle pump	Storage vesicle transporter that pumps amine from cytoplasm into vesicle
End organ damage	Vascular damage in heart, kidney, retina, or brain; usually caused by hypertension
Essential hypertension	Hypertension of unknown cause; also called "primary" hypertension
False transmitter	Substance stored in vesicles and released into synaptic cleft but lacking the effect of the true transmitter
Malignant hypertension	Accelerated hypertension causing rapid damage to vessels in end organs; a medical emergency
Orthostatic hypotension	Hypotension on standing up; postural hypotension
Postganglionic neuron blocker	Drug that blocks transmission by an action in the presynaptic postganglionic nerve terminal
Rebound hypertension	Elevated blood pressure resulting from loss of antihypertensive drug effect
Reflex tachycardia	Tachycardia resulting from lowering of blood pressure; mediated by the baroreceptor reflex
Stepped care in hypertension	Progressive addition of drugs to a regimen, starting with one (usually a diuretic) and adding in stepwise fashion a sympatholytic, a vasodilator, and (sometimes) an ACE inhibitor
Sympatholytic, sympathoplegic	Drug that reduces effects of the sympathetic nervous system

CONCEPTS

Antihypertensive drugs are organized around a clinical indication—the need to treat a disease—rather than a receptor type. As a result, the drugs covered in this unit are much more heterogeneous than those in the preceding chapters on autonomic drugs. The antihypertensive drugs include diuretics, sympathoplegics, vasodilators, and angiotensin antagonists (Figure 11–1).

The strategies for treating high blood pressure are based on the determinants of arterial pressure (see Figure 6–4). These strategies include reductions of blood volume, sympathetic tone, vascular smooth muscle tone, and angiotensin concentration. Because of the baroreceptor reflex and the renin response, compensatory homeostatic responses to these drugs may be significant (Table 11–2).

As indicated in Figure 11–2, the compensatory responses can be counteracted with β-blockers or reserpine (for tachycardia) and diuretics or angiotensin antagonists (for salt and water retention).

DIURETICS

Diuretics are covered in greater detail in Chapter 15 but are mentioned in this chapter because of their importance in hypertension. These drugs lower blood pressure by reduction of blood volume and by a direct vascular effect that is not fully understood. The diuretics most important for treating hypertension are the **thiazides** (eg, hydrochlorothiazide) and the **loop diuretics** (eg, furosemide). Thiazides may be adequate in mild hypertension, but the loop agents are used in moderate, severe, and malignant hypertension. Compensatory responses to blood pressure lowering by diuretics are minimal (Table 11–2). When thiazides are given, the maximum antihypertensive effect is often achieved with doses that are below the maximum diuretic doses.

SYMPATHOPLEGICS

Sympathoplegic drugs interfere with sympathetic nerve function in several ways. The result is a reduction of one or more of the following: venous tone, heart rate, contractile force of the heart, cardiac output, and total peripheral resistance. Compensatory responses and adverse effects are marked for some of these agents (Table 11–2). Sympathoplegics are subdivided by anatomic site of action (Figure 11–3).

A. Baroreceptor-Sensitizing Agents: The veratrum alkaloids sensitize the carotid sinus baroreceptors. This leads to a reduction in sympathetic outflow and an increase in parasympathetic outflow. These drugs produce significant adverse effects and are obsolete.

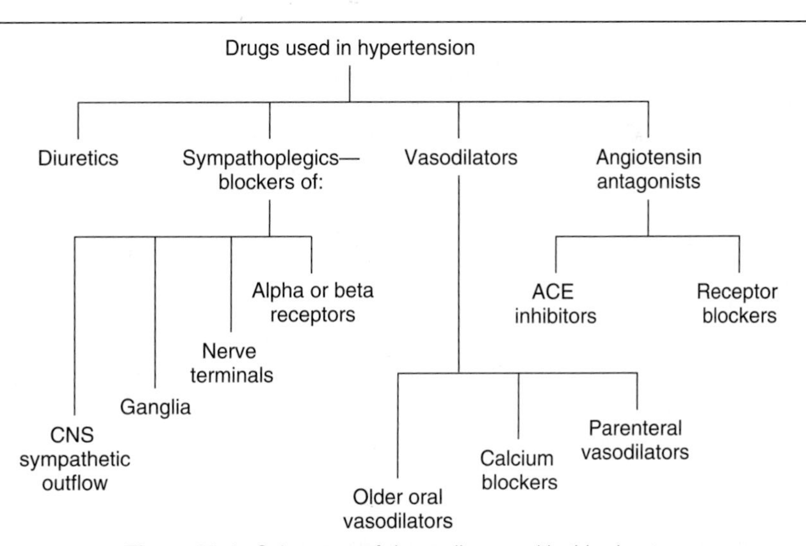

Figure 11–1. Subgroups of drugs discussed in this chapter.

Table 11–2. Compensatory responses to antihypertensive drugs and some of their adverse effects.

Class and Drug	Compensatory Responses	Adverse Effects
Diuretics		
Hydrochlorothiazide	Minimal	Hypokalemia, slight hyperlipidemia, hyperuricemia, hyperglycemia, lassitude, weakness, sexual dysfunction
Sympathoplegics		
Clonidine	Salt and water retention	Dry mouth, severe rebound hypertension if drug is suddenly stopped
Methyldopa	Salt and water retention	Sedation, positive Coombs test, hemolytic anemia
Ganglion blockers	Salt and water retention	Orthostatic hypotension, constipation, blurred vision, sexual dysfunction
Reserpine (low dose)	Minimal	Diarrhea, nasal stuffiness, sedation, depression
Guanethidine	Salt and water retention	Orthostatic hypotension, sexual dysfunction
α_1-Selective blockers	Salt and water retention, slight tachycardia	Orthostatic hypotension (limited to first few doses)
Beta-blockers	Minimal	Sleep disturbances, sedation, sexual dysfunction, cardiac disturbances, asthma
Vasodilators		
Hydralazine	Salt and water retention, marked tachycardia	Lupus-like syndrome (but lacking renal effects)
Minoxidil	Marked salt and water retention, very marked tachycardia	Hirsutism, pericardial effusion
Nifedipine	Minor salt and water retention	Constipation, cardiac disturbances, flushing
Nitroprusside	Salt and water retention	Cyanide toxicity (CN^- released)
Angiotensin antagonists		
ACE inhibitors (eg, captopril)	Minimal	Cough, renal damage in preexisting renal disease and in the fetus
Angiotensin II receptor blockers (eg, losartan)	Minimal	Renal damage in preexisting renal disease and in the fetus

B. CNS-Active Agents: Alpha$_2$-selective agonists (eg, **clonidine, methyldopa**) cause a decrease in sympathetic outflow by a mechanism that involves activation of α_2 receptors in the CNS. These drugs readily enter the CNS when given orally. Methyldopa is a prodrug; it is converted to methylnorepinephrine in the brain. Clonidine and methyldopa both reduce blood pressure by reducing cardiac output, vascular resistance, or both. The major compensatory response is salt retention. Sudden discontinuation of clonidine causes rebound hypertension, which may be quite severe. This rebound increase in blood pressure can be controlled by reinstitution of clonidine therapy or administration of alpha-blockers such as phentolamine. Methyldopa occasionally causes hematologic immunotoxicity, detected initially by test tube agglutination of red blood cells (positive Coombs test) and in some patients progressing to hemolytic anemia. Both drugs may cause sedation—methyldopa more so.

C. Ganglion-Blocking Drugs: Nicotinic blockers that act in the ganglia (eg, trimethaphan) are very efficacious but because of their severe adverse effects (Table 11–2) are now considered obsolete. **Hexamethonium** and **trimethaphan** are extremely powerful blood pressure-lowering drugs. The major compensatory response is salt retention. Toxicities reflect parasympathetic blockade (blurred vision, constipation, urinary hesitancy, sexual dysfunction) and sympathetic blockade (sexual dysfunction, orthostatic hypotension).

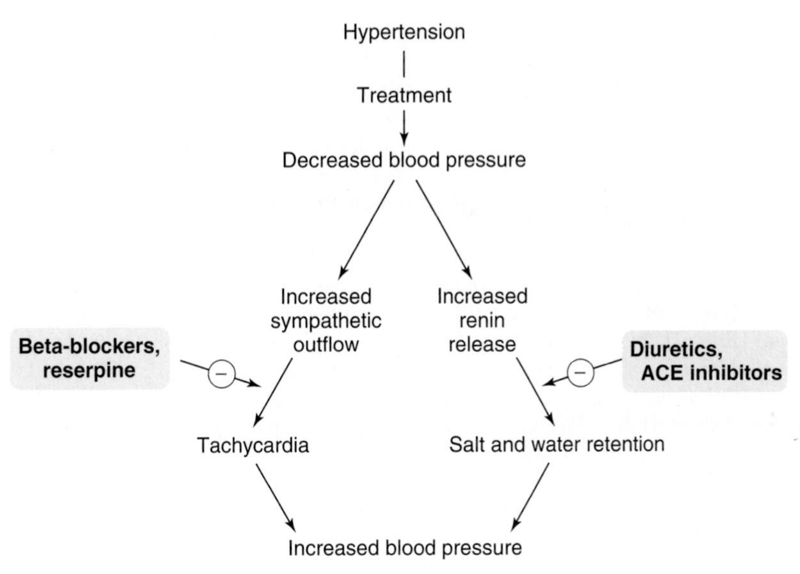

Figure 11–2. Compensatory responses to decreased blood pressure when treating hypertension. Arrows with minus signs indicate drugs used to minimize the compensatory responses.

D. Postganglionic Sympathetic Nerve Terminal Blockers: Drugs that deplete the adrenergic nerve terminal of its norepinephrine stores (eg, **reserpine**) or that deplete and block release of the stores (eg, **guanethidine**) can lower blood pressure. The major compensatory response is salt retention. In high dosages, both reserpine and guanethidine are very efficacious but produce a high incidence of adverse effects. Reserpine is still sometimes used in low doses as an adjunct to other agents. Guanethidine is now rarely used. Reserpine readily enters the CNS; guanethidine does not. Both have long durations of action (days to weeks). The most serious toxicity of reserpine is behavioral depression, which may require discontinuation of the drug. The major

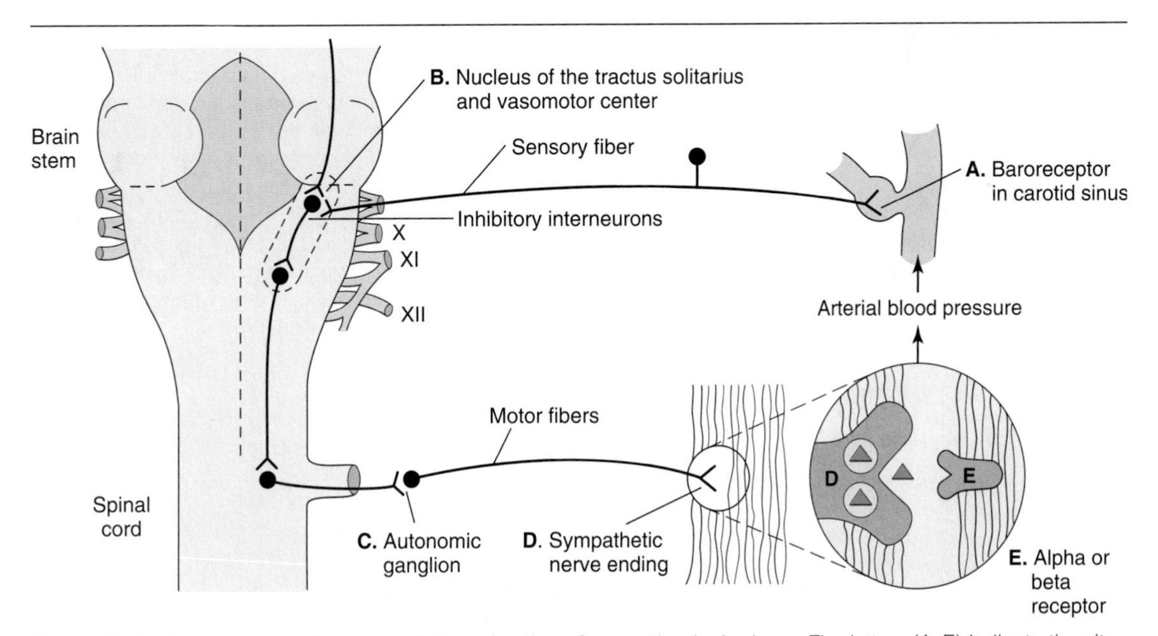

Figure 11–3. Baroreceptor reflex arc and sites of action of sympathoplegic drugs. The letters (A–E) indicate the sites of action of subgroups of sympathoplegics.

toxicities of guanethidine are orthostatic hypotension and sexual dysfunction. Guanethidine requires the catecholamine reuptake pump (uptake 1; see Figure 6–2) to reach its intracellular site of action. Therefore, drugs that inhibit this pump (eg, cocaine, tricyclic antidepressants) will interfere with the action of guanethidine.

MAO inhibitors are of interest in hypertension because they cause the formation of a false transmitter (octopamine) in sympathetic postganglionic neuron terminals and lower blood pressure. Octopamine is stored in the adrenergic vesicles along with reduced amounts (per vesicle) of norepinephrine. Normal nerve action potentials release this weak false transmitter with norepinephrine, resulting in diminished vascular and cardiac responses. However, large doses of indirect-acting sympathomimetics (eg, the tyramine in a meal of fermented foods) may cause release of large amounts of stored norepinephrine and result in a hypertensive crisis. Because of this risk and the availability of better drugs, MAO inhibitors are no longer used in hypertension. However, they are still used for treatment of severe depressive disorder.

E. Adrenoceptor Blockers: Alpha$_1$-selective agents (eg, **prazosin**) and beta-blockers (eg, **propranolol**) are effective antihypertensive drugs. Alpha-blockers reduce vascular resistance and venous return. The nonselective alpha-blockers (phentolamine, phenoxybenzamine) are of no value in chronic hypertension because of excessive compensatory responses, especially tachycardia. Alpha$_1$-selective adrenoceptor blockers are relatively free of the severe adverse effects of the nonselective alpha-blockers and postganglionic nerve terminal sympathoplegic agents.

Beta-blockers initially reduce cardiac output, but after a few days their action may include a decrease in vascular resistance as a contributing effect. The latter effect may result from reduced angiotensin levels (beta-blockers reduce renin release from the kidney). The beta-blockers are among the most heavily used antihypertensive drugs. Beta-blocker therapy is associated with slightly elevated LDL and triglyceride concentrations and diminished HDL levels in the blood; other potential adverse effects are listed in Table 11–2.

VASODILATORS

Drugs that dilate blood vessels by acting directly on smooth muscle cells through nonautonomic mechanisms are useful in treating many hypertensive patients. Three major mechanisms are utilized by vasodilators: release of nitric oxide, opening of potassium channels (which leads to hyperpolarization), and blockade of calcium channels (Table 11–3). Compensatory responses are marked for some vasodilators (especially hydralazine and minoxidil) and include salt retention and tachycardia (Table 11–2).

A. Hydralazine and Minoxidil: These older vasodilators have more effect on arterioles than on veins. They are orally active and suitable for chronic therapy. Hydralazine apparently acts through the release of nitric oxide. However, it is rarely used at high dosage because of its toxicity; therefore, its efficacy is limited. Its toxicities include compensatory responses (tachycardia, salt and water retention; Table 11–2) and drug-induced lupus erythematosus, which is reversible upon stopping the drug. However, this effect is uncommon at dosages below 200 mg/d.

Minoxidil is extremely efficacious and is thus reserved for severe hypertension. Minoxidil is a prodrug; its metabolite, minoxidil sulfate, is a potassium channel opener that hyperpolarizes and relaxes vascular smooth muscle. The toxicity of minoxidil consists of severe compensatory responses (Table 11–2, Figure 11–2), hirsutism, and pericardial abnormalities.

Table 11–3. Mechanisms of action of vasodilators.

Mechanism	Examples
Release of nitric oxide	Nitroprusside, hydralazine
Hyperpolarization of smooth muscle through increased potassium permeability	Minoxidil metabolite (minoxidil sulfate), diazoxide
Reduction of calcium influx	Verapamil, diltiazem, nifedipine

B. Calcium Channel-Blocking Agents: Calcium channel blockers (eg, **nifedipine, verapamil, diltiazem**) are effective vasodilators; because they are orally active, these drugs are suitable for chronic use in hypertension of any severity. Many dihydropyridine analogs of nifedipine are also available. Because they produce fewer compensatory responses, the calcium channel blockers are usually preferred to hydralazine and minoxidil. Their mechanism of action and toxicities are discussed in greater detail in Chapter 12.

C. Nitroprusside and Diazoxide: These parenteral vasodilators are used in hypertensive emergencies. Nitroprusside is a short-acting agent (duration of action is a few minutes) that must be infused continuously. The drug's mechanism of action involves the release of nitric oxide (from the molecule itself, not from the endothelium), which stimulates guanylyl cyclase and increases cGMP concentration in smooth muscle. The toxicity of nitroprusside includes excessive hypotension, tachycardia, and, if infusion is continued over several days, cumulation of cyanide or thiocyanate ions in the blood.

Diazoxide is given as intravenous boluses and has a duration of action of several hours. Diazoxide opens potassium channels, thus hyperpolarizing and relaxing smooth muscle cells. This drug also reduces insulin release and can be used to treat hypoglycemia caused by insulin-producing tumors. The toxicity of diazoxide includes hypotension, hyperglycemia, and salt and water retention.

ANGIOTENSIN ANTAGONISTS

The two primary groups of angiotensin antagonists are the **ACE inhibitors** and the **angiotensin II receptor blockers.** Of these, the more extensively used are the ACE inhibitors (eg, **captopril**), which inhibit the enzyme variously known as angiotensin-converting enzyme, kininase II, and peptidyl dipeptidase. The result is a **reduction** in blood levels of angiotensin II and aldosterone and probably an **increase** in endogenous vasodilators of the kinin family (bradykinin; Figure 11–4). ACE inhibitors have a low incidence of serious adverse effects when given in normal dosage and produce minimal compensatory responses (Table 11–2). The toxicities of ACE inhibitors include cough (up to 30% of patients), renal damage in occasional patients with preexisting renal vascular disease (although they *protect* the diabetic kidney), and renal damage in the fetus. These drugs are absolutely contraindicated in pregnancy.

The second group of angiotensin antagonists, the receptor blockers, are represented by the orally active agents **losartan** and its several analogs plus an older parenteral drug, **saralasin,** which competitively inhibit angiotensin II at its AT_1 receptor site (saralasin is a partial agonist used only in research). Losartan, valsartan, irbesartan, candesartan, and other analogs appear to be as effective in lowering blood pressure as the ACE inhibitors and have the advantage of a much lower incidence of cough. However, they do cause fetal renal toxicity like that of the ACE inhibitors and are thus contraindicated in pregnancy.

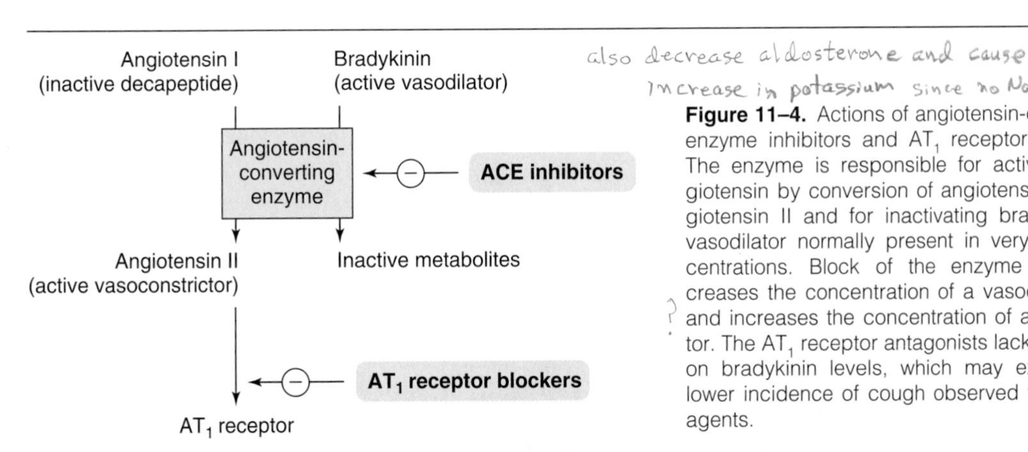

Figure 11–4. Actions of angiotensin-converting enzyme inhibitors and AT_1 receptor blockers. The enzyme is responsible for activating angiotensin by conversion of angiotensin I to angiotensin II and for inactivating bradykinin, a vasodilator normally present in very low concentrations. Block of the enzyme thus decreases the concentration of a vasoconstrictor and increases the concentration of a vasodilator. The AT_1 receptor antagonists lack the effect on bradykinin levels, which may explain the lower incidence of cough observed with these agents.

These drugs reduce aldosterone levels (angiotensin II is a major stimulant of aldosterone release) and cause potassium retention. Potassium accumulation may be marked, especially if the patient has renal impairment, is consuming a high potassium diet, or is taking other drugs that tend to conserve potassium, eg, "potassium sparing" diuretics. Under these circumstances, potassium concentrations may reach toxic levels.

Skill Keeper: Compensatory Responses to Antihypertensive Drugs (see Chapter 6)

If hydralazine in moderate dosage is administered for several weeks, compensatory cardiac and renal responses will be observed. Specify the exact mechanisms and structures involved in these responses. *The Skill Keeper Answer appears at the end of the chapter.*

CLINICAL USES OF ANTIHYPERTENSIVE DRUGS

A. "Stepped Care": Therapy of hypertension is complex because the disease is symptomless until far advanced and because the drugs are expensive and sometimes cause major compensatory responses and significant toxicities. However, overall toxicity can be reduced and compensatory responses minimized by the use of multiple drugs at lower dosages. This approach is usually used in patients with severe hypertension. Typically, drugs are added to a patient's regimen in stepwise fashion; each additional agent is chosen from a different subgroup until adequate blood pressure control has been achieved. The usual steps include (1) lifestyle measures such as salt restriction and weight reduction, (2) diuretics, (3) sympathoplegics, (4) vasodilators, and (5) ACE inhibitors. The ability of drugs in steps 2 and 3 to control the compensatory responses induced by the others should be noted (eg, propranolol reduces the tachycardia induced by hydralazine). Thus, rational polypharmacy minimizes toxicities while producing additive or supra-additive therapeutic effects.

B. Monotherapy: It has been found in large clinical studies that many patients do well on a single drug (eg, an ACE inhibitor, calcium channel blocker, or $alpha_1$-blocker). This approach to the treatment of mild and moderate hypertension has become more popular than stepped care because of its simplicity, better patient compliance, and—with modern drugs—a relatively low incidence of toxicity.

C. Age and Ethnicity: Older patients of most races respond better to diuretics and beta-blockers than to ACE inhibitors. Blacks of all ages respond better to diuretics and calcium channel blockers, less well to ACE inhibitors.

D. Malignant Hypertension: Malignant hypertension is an accelerated phase of severe hypertension associated with rising blood pressure and rapidly progressing damage to vessels and end organs. This condition may be signaled by deterioration of renal function, encephalopathy, and retinal hemorrhages or by angina, stroke, or myocardial infarction. Management of malignant hypertension must be carried out on an emergency basis in the hospital. Powerful vasodilators (nitroprusside or diazoxide) are combined with diuretics (furosemide) and beta-blockers to lower blood pressure to the 140–160/90–110 mm Hg range promptly (within a few hours). Further reduction is then pursued more slowly.

DRUG LIST

The following drugs are important members of the group discussed in this chapter. Prototypes should be learned in detail; features of the major variants should be known well enough to distinguish the variants from prototypes and from each other; the other significant agents should be recognized as belonging to a specific subclass.

Subgroups	Prototypes	Major Variants	Other Significant Agents
Diuretics	Thiazides or loop diuretics, see Chapter 15		
Sympathoplegics Carotid sinus sensitizers	Veratrum alkaloids (obsolete)		
CNS action	Clonidine, methyldopa		
Ganglion blockers	Hexamethonium		Trimethaphan
Postganglionic neuron blockers	Reserpine, guanethidine		
Receptor blockers	Prazosin, propranolol	See Chapter 10	
Vasodilators	Hydralazine, nifedipine, nitroprusside	Minoxidil, verapamil, diazoxide	
Angiotensin antagonists ACE inhibitors	Captopril		Enalapril, others
Angiotensin II receptor blockers	Losartan		Valsartan, saralasin, others

QUESTIONS

DIRECTIONS: Each of the numbered items or incomplete statements in this section is followed by answers or by completions of the statement. Select the ONE lettered answer or completion that is BEST in each case.

1. A friend has very severe hypertension and asks about a drug her doctor wishes to prescribe. Her physician has explained that this drug is associated with tachycardia and fluid retention (which may be marked) and increased hair growth. Which of the following is most likely to produce the effects that your friend has described?
- **(A)** Captopril
- **(B)** Guanethidine
- **(C)** Minoxidil
- **(D)** Prazosin
- **(E)** Propranolol

2. A patient is admitted to the emergency department with severe bradycardia following a drug overdose. His family reports that he has been depressed about his hypertension. Each of the following can slow the heart rate EXCEPT
- **(A)** Clonidine
- **(B)** Guanethidine
- **(C)** Hydralazine
- **(D)** Propranolol
- **(E)** Reserpine

3. In comparing methyldopa and guanethidine, which one of the following is correct?
- **(A)** Guanethidine—but not methyldopa—results in salt and water retention if used alone
- **(B)** Guanethidine causes fewer CNS adverse effects (such as sedation) than methyldopa
- **(C)** Guanethidine causes more immunologic adverse effects (eg, hemolytic anemia) than methyldopa
- **(D)** Guanethidine is less efficacious than methyldopa in severe hypertension
- **(E)** Methyldopa causes more orthostatic hypotension than guanethidine

4. Which one of the following is characteristic of captopril and enalapril?
- **(A)** Competitively blocks angiotensin II at its receptor
- **(B)** Decreases angiotensin II concentration in the blood
- **(C)** Decreases renin concentration in the blood
- **(D)** Increases sodium and decreases potassium in the blood
- **(E)** Decreases sodium and increases potassium in the urine

5. A patient is admitted to the hematology service with moderately severe hemolytic anemia. After a thorough workup, the only positive finding is a history of several months of treatment with an antihypertensive drug. The most likely cause of the patient's blood disorder is

(A) Atenolol
(B) Captopril
(C) Hydralazine
(D) Methyldopa
(E) Minoxidil

6. Postural hypotension is a common adverse effect of which one of the following types of drugs?
(A) ACE inhibitors
(B) Alpha-receptor blockers
(C) Arteriolar dilators
(D) $Beta_1$-selective receptor blockers
(E) Nonselective beta-blockers

7. A visitor from another city comes to your office complaining of incessant cough. He has diabetes and hypertension and has recently started taking a different antihypertensive medication. The most likely cause of his cough is
(A) Enalapril
(B) Losartan
(C) Minoxidil
(D) Propranolol
(E) Verapamil

8. Which one of the following is an important effect of the drug named?
(A) Cyanide toxicity with hydralazine
(B) Hyperglycemia with diazoxide
(C) Lupus erythematosus with nitroprusside
(D) Pericardial abnormalities with verapamil
(E) Reduced cardiac output or atrioventricular block with minoxidil

9. Comparison of prazosin with propranolol shows that
(A) Both decrease cardiac output
(B) Both decrease renin secretion
(C) Both increase heart rate
(D) Both increase sympathetic outflow from the CNS
(E) Both produce orthostatic hypotension

10. Reserpine, an alkaloid derived from the root of *Rauwolfia serpentina,*
(A) Can be used to control hyperglycemia
(B) Can cause severe depression of mood
(C) Can decrease gastrointestinal secretion and motility
(D) Has no cardiac effects
(E) Often causes a reflex increase in heart rate

11. Which of the following is used in severe hypertensive emergencies; is very short acting; and must be given by IV infusion?
(A) Captopril
(B) Cocaine
(C) Diazoxide
(D) Guanethidine
(E) Hydralazine
(F) Minoxidil
(G) Nifedipine
(H) Nitroprusside
(I) Prazosin
(J) Propranolol
(K) Reserpine
(L) Vesamicol

12. Which of the following is not a prodrug and acts by opening potassium channels?
(A) Captopril
(B) Cocaine
(C) Diazoxide
(D) Guanethidine
(E) Hydralazine
(F) Minoxidil

(G) Nifedipine
(H) Nitroprusside
(I) Prazosin
(J) Propranolol
(K) Reserpine
(L) Vesamicol

13. Which of the following is a postganglionic nerve terminal blocker that has insignificant CNS effects?
(A) Captopril
(B) Cocaine
(C) Diazoxide
(D) Guanethidine
(E) Hydralazine
(F) Minoxidil
(G) Nifedipine
(H) Nitroprusside
(I) Prazosin
(J) Propranolol
(K) Reserpine
(L) Vesamicol

DIRECTIONS: The following section consists of a list of lettered options followed by two numbered items. For each numbered item, select the ONE option that is most closely associated with it. Each option may be selected once, more than once, or not at all.

Items 14–15:
(A) Captopril
(B) Cocaine
(C) Diazoxide
(D) Guanethidine
(E) Hydralazine
(F) Minoxidil
(G) Nifedipine
(H) Nitroprusside
(I) Prazosin
(J) Propranolol
(K) Reserpine
(L) Vesamicol

14. A drug that may cause renal damage in the fetus if given during pregnancy
15. A drug that will interfere with the action of guanethidine

ANSWERS

1. Marked tachycardia and fluid retention are compensatory responses usually seen with strong vasodilators. The fact that the unknown drug also increases hair growth points strongly at minoxidil. The answer is **(C).**

2. Except for alpha-blockers, any sympathoplegic can, in sufficient dosage, cause bradycardia. Conversely, any vasodilator may induce tachycardia and, unless it is also sympathoplegic or a calcium channel blocker, will never slow the heart rate. The answer is **(C).**

3. Guanethidine causes many peripheral adverse effects but is poorly distributed into the CNS, so it is relatively free of CNS effects. The answer is **(B).**

4. These converting enzyme inhibitors act on the enzyme, not on the angiotensin receptor. The plasma renin level may increase as a result of the compensatory response to reduced angiotensin II. The answer is **(B).**

5. Methyldopa is the only antihypertensive drug associated with hemolytic anemia (usually preceded by a positive Coombs test). Hydralazine is also associated with autoimmune toxicity, but this takes the form of a lupus-like syndrome with butterfly facial rash, fever, joint and muscle pains, and antinuclear antibodies. The answer is **(D).**

6. Orthostatic hypotension is usually due to venous pooling. Venous pooling is normally prevented by alpha receptor activation. The answer is **(B).**
7. Chronic cough is a common adverse effect of ACE inhibitors. It may be relieved by prior administration of aspirin. These drugs are very commonly used in diabetes. Angiotensin II receptor blockers such as losartan and valsartan have a much lower incidence of cough but do cause renal damage in the fetus. The answer is **(A).**
8. Diazoxide may cause hyperglycemia. It is sometimes used to *treat* hypoglycemia because it can inhibit insulin release. The answer is **(B).**
9. Propranolol—but not prazosin—may decrease cardiac output. Prazosin may increase renin output (a compensatory response), but beta-blockers inhibit its release by the kidney. By reducing blood pressure, both may increase central sympathetic outflow (a compensatory response). Propranolol does not cause orthostatic hypotension. The answer is **(D).**
10. Reserpine is of no value in hyperglycemia. The drug does not induce reflex tachycardia because it reduces sympathetic neurotransmitter release in the heart as well as the vessels. This drug can cause severe depression of mood, including suicidal ideation. The answer is **(B).**
11. Diazoxide, nitroprusside, and (rarely) nifedipine are the drugs in the list that are used in hypertensive emergencies. Diazoxide has a long duration of action and is given by intermittent injection, not by infusion. Nifedipine is almost always given orally. The answer is **(H).**
12. Diazoxide is a potassium channel opener as given. Minoxidil sulfate, a metabolite of minoxidil, also acts by this mechanism. The answer is **(C).**
13. Reserpine and guanethidine are both sympathoplegics that act on the postganglionic sympathetic nerve terminal. Reserpine enters the CNS readily and causes important CNS toxicity. Guanethidine, on the other hand, is too polar to cross the blood-brain barrier easily and is almost devoid of central toxicity. The answer is **(D).**
14. All ACE inhibitors can cause renal damage in patients with preexisting renal vascular disease and in the developing fetus. (The angiotensin II receptor antagonists appear to have similar renal toxicity.) The answer is **(A).**
15. Guanethidine must be transported into the adrenergic nerve ending to exert its effects. Cocaine can block the reuptake carrier. The answer is **(B).**

Skill Keeper Answer: Compensatory Responses to Antihypertensive Drugs (see Chapter 6)

The compensatory responses to hydralazine use are tachycardia and salt and water retention. These responses are generated by the baroreceptor and renin-angiotensin-aldosterone mechanisms summarized in Figure 6–4. The motor limb of the sympathetic response consists of outflow from the vasomotor center to the heart and vessels, as shown in Figure 11–3. You should be able to reproduce these diagrams from memory.

12 Vasodilators & the Treatment of Angina

OBJECTIVES

You should be able to:

- Describe the pathophysiology of effort angina and vasospastic angina.
- List the major determinants of cardiac oxygen consumption.
- List the strategies for relief of anginal pain.
- Contrast the therapeutic and adverse effects of nitrates, beta-blockers, and calcium channel blockers when used for angina.
- Explain why the combination of a nitrate with a beta-blocker or a calcium channel blocker may be more effective than either alone.
- Explain why the combination of a nitrate and sildenafil is potentially dangerous.
- Contrast the effects of medical therapy and surgical therapy of angina.

Learn the definitions that follow.

Table 12–1. Definitions.

Term	Definition
Angina of effort, classic angina, atherosclerotic angina	Angina pectoris (crushing, strangling chest pain) that is precipitated by exertion and caused by increased O_2 demand that cannot be met because of irreversible atherosclerotic obstruction of coronary arteries
Vasospastic angina, variant angina, Prinzmetal's angina	Angina precipitated by reversible spasm of coronary vessels
Coronary vasodilator	Older incorrect name for drugs useful in angina. Drugs that relieve angina of effort do not act primarily through coronary vasodilation; some potent coronary vasodilators are ineffective in angina
Venodilator	Drug that selectively dilates veins, eg, nitroglycerin
"Monday disease"	Industrial disease caused by weekly exposure to vasodilating concentrations of organic nitrates in the workplace; characterized by headache, dizziness, and tachycardia on Mondays, with tolerance developing during the week
Nitrate tolerance, tachyphylaxis	Loss of effect of a nitrate venodilator when exposure is prolonged
Unstable angina	Rapidly progressing increase in frequency and severity of anginal attacks, especially pain at rest; usually heralds imminent myocardial infarction
Preload	Filling pressure of the heart; determines end-diastolic fiber length and tension
Afterload	Resistance to ejection of stroke volume; determined by arterial blood pressure and arterial stiffness
Intramyocardial fiber tension	Force exerted by myocardial fibers, especially ventricular fibers at any given time; a primary determinant of O_2 requirement
Double product	The product of heart rate and systolic blood pressure; an estimate of cardiac work
Myocardial revascularization	Mechanical intervention to improve O_2 delivery to the myocardium by angioplasty or bypass grafting

CONCEPTS

PATHOPHYSIOLOGY OF ANGINA

The name angina pectoris refers to a strangling or pressure-like pain, usually located substernally but sometimes perceived in the neck, shoulder, or epigastrium. The drugs used in angina are diagrammed in Figure 12–1.

A. Types of Angina: There are three major forms of symptomatic angina pectoris.

1. **Atherosclerotic angina:** Atherosclerotic angina is also known as angina of effort or classic angina. It is associated with atheromatous plaques that partially occlude one or more coronaries. When cardiac work increases (eg, in exercise), the obstruction of flow results in the accumulation of acidic metabolites and ischemic changes that stimulate myocardial pain endings. Rest usually leads to prompt relief of the pain within a few minutes. Atherosclerotic angina constitutes about 90% of angina cases and—depending on the rate of progression of the atheromas—may persist for years with little change. However, effort angina may deteriorate into unstable angina.
2. **Vasospastic angina:** Vasospastic angina is also known as rest angina, variant angina, or Prinzmetal's angina. It involves reversible spasm of coronaries, usually at the site of an atherosclerotic plaque. Spasm may occur at any time, even during sleep. Vasospastic angina may deteriorate into unstable angina.
3. **Unstable angina:** The third type of angina, unstable or crescendo angina, also known as acute coronary syndrome, is characterized by increased frequency and severity of attacks caused by repeated episodes of diminished coronary flow that result from a combination of atherosclerotic plaques, platelet aggregation at fractured plaques, and vasospasm. Unstable angina is thought to be the immediate precursor of a myocardial infarction and is treated as a medical emergency.

B. Determinants of Cardiac Oxygen Requirement: The pharmacologic treatment of coronary insufficiency is based on physiologic factors that control the myocardial oxygen requirement. A major determinant is **myocardial fiber tension,** ie, the higher the tension, the greater the oxygen requirement.

Several variables contribute to fiber tension (Figure 12–2):

1. **Preload:** Preload (diastolic filling pressure) is a function of blood volume and venous tone. Because venous tone is mainly controlled by sympathetic outflow, activities that increase sympathetic activity usually increase preload.
2. **Afterload:** Afterload or arterial blood pressure is one of the systolic determinants of oxygen requirement. Arterial blood pressure depends on peripheral vascular resistance, which is determined by sympathetic outflow to the arteriolar vessels.
3. **Heart rate:** Heart rate contributes to time-integrated fiber tension because at fast heart rates, fibers spend more time at systolic tension levels. Furthermore, at faster rates, diastole is abbreviated, and diastole constitutes the time available for coronary flow (coronary blood flow is low or nil during systole). Systolic blood pressure and heart rate may be multiplied to yield the **double product,** a measure of cardiac work and therefore of oxygen requirement. In patients with atherosclerotic angina, effective drugs reduce the double product.

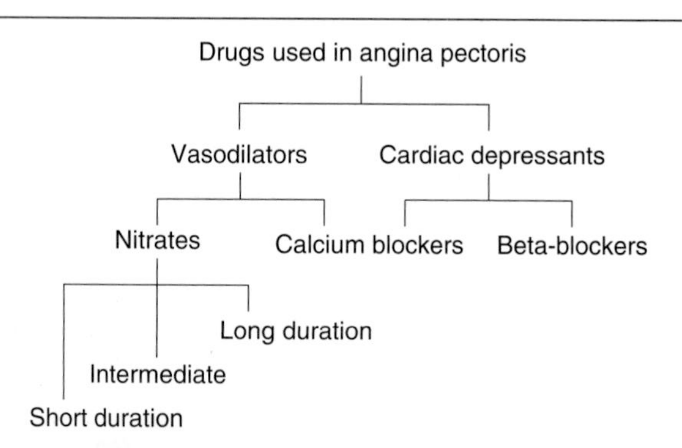

Figure 12–1. Subgroups of drugs discussed in this chapter.

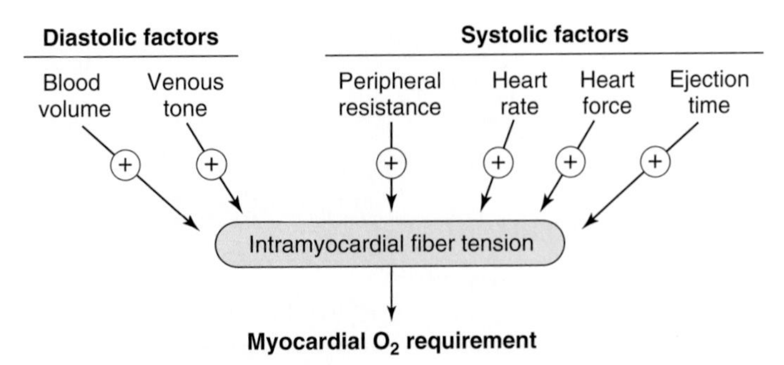

Figure 12–2. Determinants of MVO_2, the minute volume of oxygen required by the heart. Both diastolic and systolic factors contribute to the MVO_2; most of these factors are directly influenced by sympathetic discharge (venous tone, peripheral resistance, heart rate, and heart force).

4. **Cardiac contractility:** Force of cardiac contraction is another systolic factor controlled mainly by sympathetic outflow to the heart. Ejection time for ventricular contraction is inversely related to force of contraction but is also influenced by impedance to outflow. Increased ejection time increases oxygen requirement.

C. **Therapeutic Strategies:** The defect that causes anginal pain is inadequate coronary oxygen delivery relative to the myocardial oxygen requirement. This defect can be corrected in two ways: by **increasing oxygen delivery** or by **reducing oxygen requirement** (Figure 12–3). Pharmacologic therapies include the nitrates, the calcium channel blockers, and the beta-blockers. All three groups reduce the oxygen requirement in atherosclerotic angina; nitrates and calcium channel blockers (but not beta-blockers) can also increase oxygen delivery by reducing vasospasm—but only in vasospastic angina. **Myocardial revascularization** corrects coronary obstruction either by bypass grafting or by angioplasty (enlargement of the lumen by means of a special catheter). Therapy of unstable angina differs from that of stable angina because urgent angioplasty is the treatment of choice in most patients and platelet clotting is the major target of drug therapy. The platelet glycoprotein IIb/IIIa inhibitors—eptifibatide and tirofiban—are used in this condition (see Chapter 34). Intravenous nitroglycerin is sometimes of value.

NITRATES

A. **Classification and Pharmacokinetics:** Nitroglycerin (the active ingredient in dynamite) is the most important of the nitrates and is available in forms that provide a range of durations of action from 10–20 minutes (sublingual) to 8–10 hours (transdermal) (Table 12–2). Because treatment of acute attacks and prevention of attacks are both important aspects of therapy, the pharmacokinetics of these different dosage forms are clinically significant.

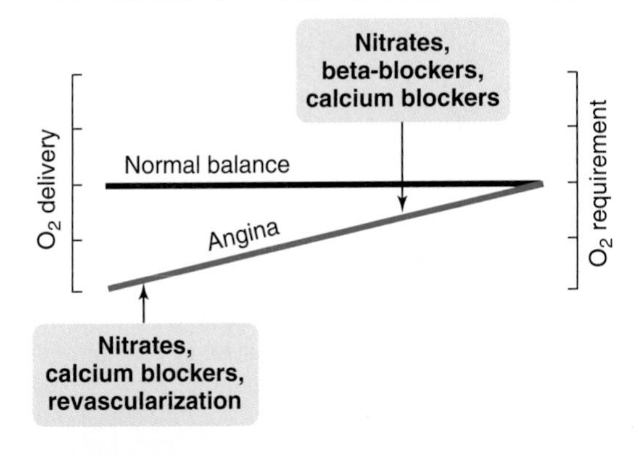

Figure 12–3. Strategies for the treatment of angina pectoris. Angina is characterized by reduced coronary oxygen delivery versus oxygen requirement. In some cases, this can be corrected by increasing oxygen delivery (box on left: revascularization or, in the case of reversible vasospasm, nitrates and calcium channel blockers). More often, drugs are used to reduce oxygen requirement (box on right: nitrates, β-blockers, and calcium channel blockers).

Table 12–2. Pharmacokinetically distinct forms of nitrate and nitrite drugs used in angina.

Category	Example	Duration of Action
Very short	Inhaled amyl nitrite	3–5 minutes
Short	Sublingual nitroglycerin or isosorbide dinitrate	10–30 minutes (isosorbide dinitrate has a somewhat longer half-life than nitroglycerin)
Intermediate	Oral regular or sustained-release nitroglycerin or isosorbide dinitrate	4–8 hours (much of the effect is due to active metabolites)
Long	Transdermal nitroglycerin patch	8–10 hours (blood levels may persist for 24 hours, but tolerance limits the duration of action)

Nitroglycerin (glyceryl trinitrate) is rapidly denitrated in the liver—first to the dinitrate (glyceryl dinitrate), which retains a significant vasodilating effect, and more slowly to the mononitrate, which is much less active. Because of the high enzyme activity in the liver, the first-pass effect for nitroglycerin is large—about 90%. The efficacy of oral (swallowed) nitroglycerin probably results from the high levels of glyceryl dinitrate in the blood. The effects of sublingual nitroglycerin are mainly the result of the unchanged drug.

Other nitrates are similar to nitroglycerin in their pharmacokinetics and pharmacodynamics. Isosorbide dinitrate is another commonly used nitrate; it is available in sublingual and oral forms. Isosorbide dinitrate is rapidly denitrated in the liver to isosorbide mononitrate, which is also active. Isosorbide mononitrate is available as a separate drug for oral use. Several other nitrates are available for oral use and, like the oral nitroglycerin preparation, have an intermediate duration of action (4–6 hours). Amyl nitrite is a volatile and rapidly acting vasodilator that was used for angina by the inhalational route but is now rarely prescribed.

B. **Mechanism of Action:** Denitration of the nitrates within smooth muscle cells releases nitric oxide (NO), which stimulates guanylyl cyclase, causes an increase of the second messenger cGMP, and leads to smooth muscle relaxation, probably by dephosphorylation of myosin light chain phosphate. Note that this mechanism is identical to that of nitroprusside (Chapter 11).

C. **Organ System Effects:**

1. **Cardiovascular:** Smooth muscle relaxation leads to peripheral venodilation, which results in reduced cardiac size and cardiac output through reduced preload. Reduced afterload, from arteriolar dilation, may contribute to an increase in ejection and a further decrease in cardiac size. Some studies suggest that of the vascular beds, the veins are the most sensitive, arteries less so, and arterioles least sensitive. Venodilation leads to decreased diastolic heart size and fiber tension. Arteriolar dilation leads to reduced peripheral resistance and blood pressure. These changes contribute to an overall reduction in myocardial fiber tension, oxygen consumption, and the double product. Thus, the primary mechanism of therapeutic benefit in atherosclerotic angina is reduction of the oxygen requirement. A secondary mechanism—namely, an increase in coronary flow via collateral vessels in ischemic areas—has also been proposed. In vasospastic angina, a reversal of coronary spasm and increased flow can be demonstrated.

   Nitrates have no direct effects on myocardium, but a significant reflex tachycardia and increased force of contraction are predictable when nitroglycerin reduces the blood pressure.
2. **Other organs:** Nitrates relax the smooth muscle of the bronchi, gastrointestinal tract, and genitourinary tract, but these effects are too small to be clinically useful. Intravenous nitroglycerin (sometimes used in unstable angina) reduces platelet aggregation. There are no significant effects on other tissues.

D. **Clinical Uses:** As previously noted, nitroglycerin is available in several formulations (Table 12–2). The standard form for treatment of acute anginal pain is the sublingual tablet, which has a duration of action of 10–20 minutes. Oral (swallowed) normal-release nitroglycerin has a duration of action of 4–6 hours. Sustained-release oral forms have a somewhat longer duration of action (Table 12–2). Transdermal formulations (ointment or patch) can maintain blood levels for up to 24 hours. Tolerance develops after about 8 hours, however, with rapidly diminishing effectiveness thereafter. It is therefore recommended that nitroglycerin patches be removed after 10–12 hours to allow recovery of sensitivity to the drug.

E. Toxicity of Nitrates and Nitrites: The most common toxic effects of nitrates are the responses evoked by vasodilation. These include tachycardia (from the baroreceptor reflex), orthostatic hypotension (a direct extension of the venodilator effect), and throbbing headache from meningeal artery vasodilation.

Nitrates interact with sildenafil, the drug promoted for erectile dysfunction as Viagra. Sildenafil inhibits a phosphodiesterase isoform that metabolizes cGMP in smooth muscle. The increased cGMP in erectile smooth muscle relaxes it, allowing for greater inflow of blood and more effective and prolonged erection. This effect also occurs in vascular smooth muscle. As a result, the combination of nitrates (through increased production of cGMP) and sildenafil (through decreased breakdown of cGMP) causes a synergistic relaxation of vascular smooth muscle with potentially dangerous hypotension and hypoperfusion of critical organs.

Nitrites are of significant toxicologic importance because they cause methemoglobinemia at high blood concentrations. This same effect has a potential antidotal action in cyanide poisoning (see below). The nitrates do not cause methemoglobinemia. In the past, the nitrates were responsible for several occupational diseases in munitions plants in which workplace contamination by these volatile chemicals was severe. The most common of these diseases was "Monday disease," ie, the alternating development of tolerance (during the work week) and loss of tolerance (over the weekend) for the vasodilating action and its associated tachycardia and headache, resulting in headache, tachycardia, and dizziness every Monday.

F. Nitrites in the Treatment of Cyanide Poisoning: Cyanide ion rapidly complexes with the iron in cytochrome oxidase, resulting in a block of oxidative metabolism and cell death. Fortunately, the iron in methemoglobin has a higher affinity for cyanide than does the iron in cytochrome oxidase. Nitrites convert the ferrous iron in hemoglobin to the ferric form, yielding methemoglobin. Therefore, cyanide poisoning can be treated by a three-step procedure: (1) immediate exposure to amyl nitrite, followed by (2) IV administration of sodium nitrite, which rapidly increases the methemoglobin level to the degree necessary to remove a significant amount of cyanide from cytochrome oxidase. This is followed by (3) intravenous sodium thiosulfate, which converts cyanomethemoglobin resulting from step 2 to thiocyanate and methemoglobin. Thiocyanate is much less toxic than cyanide and is excreted by the kidney. (It should be noted that excessive methemoglobinemia is fatal, since methemoglobin is a very poor oxygen carrier.)

CALCIUM CHANNEL-BLOCKING DRUGS

A. Classification and Pharmacokinetics: Several types of calcium channel blockers are approved for use in angina; these drugs are typified by **nifedipine,** a **dihydropyridine,** and several other dihydropyridines; **diltiazem;** and **verapamil.** Although calcium channel blockers differ markedly in structure, all are orally active and most have half-lives of 3–6 hours. Nimodipine is another member of the dihydropyridine family with similar properties, but it is approved only for the management of stroke associated with subarachnoid hemorrhage. Bepridil, a drug that is somewhat similar in structure to verapamil, has a longer duration of action but greater cardiovascular toxicity than the other calcium channel blockers.

B. Mechanism of Action: These drugs block voltage-gated "L-type" calcium channels, the calcium channels most important in cardiac and smooth muscle. By decreasing calcium influx during an action potential in a frequency- and voltage-dependent manner, these agents reduce intracellular calcium concentration and muscle contractility. None of these channel blockers interfere with calcium-dependent neurotransmission or hormone release because these processes do not utilize "L-type" channels.

C. Effects: Calcium blockers relax blood vessels and, to a lesser extent, the uterus, bronchi, and gut. The rate and contractility of the heart are reduced by diltiazem and verapamil. Because

Table 12–3. Predicted effects of nitrates alone and with β-blockers or calcium channel blockers in angina pectoris.[1]

	Nitrates Alone	Beta-Blockers or Calcium Channel Blockers Alone	Combined Nitrate and Beta-Blocker or Calcium Channel Blocker
Heart rate	*Reflex increase*	**Decrease**	**Decrease**
Arterial pressure	Decrease	Decrease	**Decrease**
End-diastolic pressure and fiber tension	**Decrease**	*Increase*	**Decrease**
Contractility	*Reflex increase*	**Decrease**	No effect or **decrease**
Ejection time	Reflex decrease	*Increase*	No effect

[1]Undesirable effects (effects that increase myocardial oxygen requirement) are shown in *italics;* major therapeutic effects are shown in **boldface type.**

they block calcium-dependent conduction in the AV node, verapamil and diltiazem may be used to treat AV nodal arrhythmias (Chapter 14). Nifedipine and other dihydropyridines evoke greater vasodilation, and the resulting sympathetic reflex prevents bradycardia and may actually increase the heart rate. All the calcium channel blockers reduce blood pressure and reduce the double product in patients with angina.

D. Clinical Use: Calcium blockers are effective as prophylactic therapy in both effort and rest angina; nifedipine has also been used to abort acute anginal attacks. In atherosclerotic angina, these drugs are particularly valuable when combined with nitrates (Table 12–3). In addition to well-established uses in angina, hypertension, and supraventricular tachycardia, these agents are used in migraine, preterm labor, stroke, and Raynaud's syndrome. As noted above, nimodipine is approved for use in hemorrhagic stroke.

E. Toxicity: The calcium channel blockers cause constipation, edema, nausea, flushing, and dizziness. More serious adverse effects include congestive heart failure, atrioventricular blockade, and sinus node depression; these are more common with verapamil than with the dihydropyridines. Bepridil may induce **torsade de pointes** and other arrhythmias.

Skill Keeper: Nifedipine Cardiotoxicity (see Chapter 6)

A pair of studies during the 1990s suggested that use of nifedipine was associated with an increased risk of myocardial infarction. What effects of nifedipine might lead to this result? *The Skill Keeper Answer appears at the end of the chapter.*

BETA-BLOCKING DRUGS

A. Classification and Mechanism of Action: These drugs are described in detail in Chapter 10. All beta-blockers are effective in the prophylaxis of atherosclerotic angina attacks.

B. Effects: Actions include both beneficial effects (decreased heart rate, cardiac force, blood pressure) and detrimental effects (increased heart size, longer ejection period; Table 12–3). Like the nitrates and calcium channel blockers, the beta-blockers reduce the double product.

C. Clinical Use: Beta-blockers are used only for prophylactic therapy of angina; they are of no value in an acute attack. They are effective in preventing exercise-induced angina but are ineffective against the vasospastic form. The combination of beta-blockers with nitrates is useful because the adverse undesirable compensatory effects evoked by the nitrates (tachycardia and increased cardiac force) are prevented or reduced by beta blockade. See Table 12–3.

D. Toxicity: See Chapter 10.

NONPHARMACOLOGIC THERAPY

Myocardial revascularization by coronary artery bypass grafting (CABG) and percutaneous transluminal coronary angioplasty (PTCA) have become important in the treatment of severe angina. These are the only methods capable of consistently increasing coronary flow in atherosclerotic angina and increasing the double product.

DRUG LIST

The following drugs are important members of the group discussed in this chapter. Prototypes should be learned in detail; features of the major variants should be known well enough to distinguish the variants from prototypes and from each other; the other significant agents should be recognized as belonging to a specific subclass.

Subclass	Prototype	Major Variants	Other Significant Agents
Nitrates	Nitroglycerin	Different dosage forms (sublingual, oral, transdermal)	Isosorbide dinitrate, isosorbide mononitrate, amyl nitrite
Calcium channel blockers	Nifedipine Verapamil Diltiazem	Nimodipine	Bepridil
Beta-blockers	Propranolol	See Chapter 10	

QUESTIONS

DIRECTIONS: Each of the numbered items or incomplete statements in this section is followed by answers or by completions of the statement. Select the ONE lettered answer or completion that is BEST in each case.

Items 1–3: Mr. Green, 60 years old, has severe chest pain when he attempts to carry parcels upstairs to his apartment. The pain rapidly disappears when he rests. A decision is made to treat him with nitroglycerin.

1. Nitroglycerin, either directly or through reflexes, results in which one of the following effects?
- **(A)** Decreased heart rate
- **(B)** Decreased venous capacitance
- **(C)** Increased afterload
- **(D)** Increased cardiac force
- **(E)** Increased diastolic intramyocardial fiber tension

2. In advising Mr. Green about the adverse effects he may notice, you point out that nitroglycerin in moderate doses often produces certain symptoms. These toxicities result from all of the following EXCEPT
- **(A)** Meningeal vasodilation
- **(B)** Reflex tachycardia
- **(C)** Increased cardiac force
- **(D)** Methemoglobinemia
- **(E)** Sympathetic discharge

3. Two years later, Mr. Green returns complaining that his nitroglycerin works well when he takes it for an acute attack but that he is having frequent attacks now and would like something to *prevent* them. Useful drugs for the prophylaxis of angina of effort include which one of the following?

(A) Amyl nitrite
(B) Diltiazem
(C) Esmolol
(D) Sublingual isosorbide dinitrate
(E) Sublingual nitroglycerin

4. The antianginal effect of propranolol may be attributed to which one of the following?
(A) Block of exercise-induced tachycardia
(B) Decreased end-diastolic ventricular volume
(C) Dilation of constricted coronary vessels
(D) Increased cardiac force
(E) Increased resting heart rate

5. The major common determinant of myocardial oxygen consumption is
(A) Blood volume
(B) Cardiac output
(C) Diastolic blood pressure
(D) Heart rate
(E) Myocardial fiber tension

6. You are considering therapeutic options for a new patient who presents with severe hypertension and angina. In considering adverse effects, you note that an adverse effect which nitroglycerin, guanethidine, and ganglion blockers have in common is
(A) Bradycardia
(B) Impaired sexual function
(C) Lupus erythematosus syndrome
(D) Orthostatic hypotension
(E) Throbbing headache

7. Epidemiologic surveys suggest that, in the past, workers exposed to high levels of organic nitrates in the workplace had
(A) A high incidence of methemoglobinemia on the job
(B) An increased incidence of angina at work as compared with at home
(C) A high incidence of cyanide poisoning in the workplace
(D) An increased incidence of headaches on Mondays as compared with other days
(E) All of the above

8. A patient is admitted to the emergency department following a drug overdose. He is noted to have severe tachycardia. He has been receiving therapy for hypertension and angina. A drug that often causes tachycardia is
(A) Diltiazem
(B) Guanethidine
(C) Isosorbide dinitrate
(D) Propranolol
(E) Verapamil

9. A patient being treated for another condition complains that whenever he takes that medication, his angina becomes worse. Drugs that may precipitate angina when used for other indications include all of the following EXCEPT
(A) Amphetamine
(B) Hydralazine
(C) Isoproterenol
(D) Reserpine
(E) Terbutaline

10. When nitrates are used in combination with other drugs for the treatment of angina, which of the following result in additive effects on the variable specified?
(A) Beta-blockers and nitrates on end-diastolic cardiac size
(B) Beta-blockers and nitrates on heart rate
(C) Calcium channel blockers and beta-blockers on cardiac force
(D) Calcium channel blockers and nitrates on cardiac force
(E) Calcium channel blockers and nitrates on cardiac rate

11. Which of the following is approved for the treatment of hemorrhagic stroke?
(A) Amyl nitrite
(B) Hydralazine
(C) Isosorbide mononitrate

(D) Nifedipine
(E) Nimodipine
(F) Nitroglycerin (sublingual)
(G) Nitroglycerin (transdermal)
(H) Propranolol
(I) Terbutaline
(J) Verapamil

12. Which of the following drugs used for the treatment of angina by inhalation has a very rapid onset and a brief duration of effect (2–5 minutes)?
(A) Amyl nitrite
(B) Hydralazine
(C) Isosorbide mononitrate
(D) Nifedipine
(E) Nimodipine
(F) Nitroglycerin (sublingual)
(G) Nitroglycerin (transdermal)
(H) Propranolol
(I) Terbutaline
(J) Verapamil

13. Which of the following drugs is capable of maintaining blood levels for 24 hours but with useful therapeutic effects lasting only about 10 hours?
(A) Amyl nitrite
(B) Hydralazine
(C) Isosorbide mononitrate
(D) Nifedipine
(E) Nimodipine
(F) Nitroglycerin (sublingual)
(G) Nitroglycerin (transdermal)
(H) Propranolol
(I) Terbutaline
(J) Verapamil

14. Which of the following is a vasodilator drug used for hypertension that lacks a direct effect on autonomic receptors but may provoke anginal attacks?
(A) Amyl nitrite
(B) Hydralazine
(C) Isosorbide mononitrate
(D) Nifedipine
(E) Nimodipine
(F) Nitroglycerin (sublingual)
(G) Nitroglycerin (transdermal)
(H) Propranolol
(I) Terbutaline
(J) Verapamil

DIRECTIONS (Item 15): This matching question consists of a list of ten lettered options followed by item 15. Select the ONE lettered option that is most closely associated with item 15.
(A) Amyl nitrite
(B) Hydralazine
(C) Isosorbide mononitrate
(D) Nifedipine
(E) Nimodipine
(F) Nitroglycerin (sublingual)
(G) Nitroglycerin (transdermal)
(H) Propranolol
(I) Terbutaline
(J) Verapamil

15. An active metabolite of another drug and an active antianginal drug for oral administration in its own right.

ANSWERS

1. Nitroglycerin increases cardiac force because the decrease in blood pressure evokes a compensatory increase in sympathetic discharge. The answer is **(D).**
2. Methemoglobinemia never occurs from the doses of nitroglycerin (or other nitrates) used to treat angina. The *nitrites* (in large doses) cause methemoglobinemia. The answer is **(D).**
3. The calcium channel blockers and the beta-blockers are generally effective in reducing the number of attacks of angina of effort, and most have durations of 4–8 hours. Oral and transdermal nitrates have similar or longer durations. Amyl nitrite, the sublingual nitrates, and esmolol (an IV beta blocker) have short durations of action and are of no value in prophylaxis. The answer is **(B).**
4. Propranolol blocks tachycardia but has none of the other effects listed. The answer is **(A).**
5. The answer is **(E),** fiber tension. The other variables contribute to this determinant.
6. These drugs all reduce venous return sufficiently to cause some degree of postural hypotension (not very prolonged in the case of nitroglycerin). Throbbing headache is a problem only with the nitrates, bradycardia only with guanethidine, sexual problems only with sympathoplegics (ganglion blockers and guanethidine), and lupus with none of them. The answer is **(D).**
7. Nitrites, not nitrates, cause methemoglobinemia in adults. Headache, not angina, increased upon returning to work on Monday. Neither nitrates nor nitrites are related to causation of cyanide poisoning, but nitrites are used as one part of the antidote for cyanide intoxication. The answer is **(D).**
8. Isosorbide dinitrate (like all the nitrates) causes reflex tachycardia, but all the other drugs listed here slow heart rate. The answer is **(C).**
9. In general, drugs that cause hypertension or tachycardia—whether directly or by reflex—tend to precipitate angina in individuals with coronary obstruction unless cardiac work is greatly reduced (as in the case of the nitrates). The answer is **(D).**
10. The effects of beta-blockers (or calcium channel blockers) and nitrates on heart size, force, and rate are opposite. The answer is **(C).**
11. Nimodipine, a dihydropyridine calcium channel blocker, is approved only for the treatment of hemorrhagic stroke. The answer is **(E).**
12. Amyl nitrite, a very volatile liquid, is the only antianginal drug in this list that is usually used by the inhalation route. (Terbutaline is used by aerosol, but it has a longer duration of action and *causes* angina in susceptible patients.) The answer is **(A).**
13. Transdermal formulations of nitroglycerin are capable of maintaining blood concentrations for up to 24 hours. Unfortunately, tolerance develops after about 10 hours of continued exposure, so the beneficial effect is limited to about 8–10 hours. The answer is **(G).**
14. Hydralazine, a direct-acting vasodilator, often precipitates angina in susceptible individuals; the drug should never be used in patients with coronary disease unless heart rate is appropriately controlled. The answer is **(B).**
15. The organic nitrates are denitrated in the liver after oral administration. Glyceryl dinitrate and isosorbide mononitrate are active metabolites. The latter agent is available as a separate drug. The answer is **(C).**

Skill Keeper Answer: Nifedipine Cardiotoxicity (see Chapter 6)

Long-term studies have suggested that patients receiving prompt-release nifedipine may have an increased risk of myocardial infarction. Slow-release formulations do not seem to impose this risk. This surprising result has been explained as follows: Rapidly acting vasodilators—such as nifedipine in its prompt-release formulation—cause significant and sudden reduction in blood pressure. The drop in blood pressure evokes increased sympathetic outflow to the cardiovascular system and increases heart rate and force of contraction as shown in Figure 6–4. These changes can markedly increase cardiac oxygen requirement. If coronary blood flow does not increase sufficiently to match the increased requirement, ischemia and necrosis can result.

Drugs Used in Congestive Heart Failure

13

OBJECTIVES

You should be able to:

- Describe the strategies and list the major drug groups used in the treatment of congestive heart failure.
- Describe the probable mechanism of action of digitalis.
- Describe the nature and mechanism of digitalis's toxic effects on the heart.
- List some positive inotropic drugs that have been investigated as digitalis substitutes.
- Describe the beneficial effects of diuretics, vasodilators, ACE inhibitors, and other drugs that lack positive inotropic effects in congestive heart failure.

Learn the definitions that follow.

Table 13–1. Definitions.

Term	Definition
Bigeminy	An arrhythmia consisting of normal sinus beats coupled with ventricular extrasystoles, ie, "twinned beats"
Cardenolide	The basic chemical structure required for cardiac glycoside action, consisting of a steroid nucleus and a lactone ring at the 17-position
Congestive heart failure	A condition in which cardiac output is insufficient for the needs of the body. Low output failure is the more common form and is more responsive to positive inotropic drugs than high output failure
End diastolic fiber length	The length of the ventricular fibers at the end of diastole; a determinant of the force of the following contraction
PDE inhibitor	Phosphodiesterase inhibitor; a drug that inhibits one or more enzymes that degrade cAMP (and other cyclic nucleotides). Examples: amrinone, high concentrations of theophylline
Premature ventricular beats	An abnormal beat arising from a cell below the AV node; often from a Purkinje fiber, sometimes from a ventricular fiber
Sodium pump (Na^+/K^+ ATPase)	A transport molecule in the membranes of all vertebrate cells; responsible for the maintenance of normal low intracellular sodium and high intracellular potassium concentrations
Sodium-calcium exchanger	A transport molecule in the membrane of many cells (eg, cardiac cells) that pumps one calcium atom against its concentration gradient (outward) in exchange for 3 sodium ions (moving inward, down their concentration gradient)
Ventricular function curve	The graph that relates cardiac output, stroke volume, etc, to filling pressure or end-diastolic fiber length; also known as the Frank-Starling curve
Ventricular tachycardia	An arrhythmia consisting entirely or largely of beats originating below the AV node

CONCEPTS

PATHOPHYSIOLOGY OF CONGESTIVE HEART FAILURE & TREATMENT STRATEGIES

The drugs used in congestive heart failure are shown in Figure 13–1.

A. Pathophysiology: The fundamental physiologic defect in congestive heart failure is a decrease in cardiac contractility. The result of this defect is that cardiac output is inadequate for the needs of the body. This is best shown by the ventricular function curve (Frank-Starling curve; Figure 13–2). The ventricular function curve reflects some compensatory responses of the body and may also be used to demonstrate the response to drugs. As ventricular ejection decreases, the end-diastolic fiber length increases as shown by the shift from point A to point B in Figure 13–2. Operation at point B is intrinsically less efficient than operation at shorter fiber lengths because of the increase in myocardial oxygen requirement associated with increased fiber stretch (see Figure 12–2).

The homeostatic responses of the body to depressed cardiac output are extremely important and are mediated mainly by the sympathetic nervous system and the renin-angiotensin-aldosterone system. They are summarized in Figure 13–3. The major responses include the following: (1) Tachycardia—an early manifestation of increased sympathetic tone. (2) Increased peripheral vascular resistance—another early response, also mediated by increased sympathetic tone. (3) Retention of salt and water by the kidney—an early compensatory response, mediated by the renin-angiotensin-aldosterone system and facilitated by increased sympathetic outflow. Increased blood volume results in edema and pulmonary congestion and contributes to the increased end-diastolic fiber length. (4) Cardiomegaly—enlargement of the heart is a slower compensatory response, mediated at least in part by sympathetic discharge. Angiotensin II also plays an important role. Recent evidence suggests that aldosterone may also play a direct role in cardiac changes. While these compensatory responses may temporarily improve cardiac output (and may be lifesaving), they also increase the load on the heart; the increased load contributes to further long-term decline in cardiac function.

B. Therapeutic Strategies in Congestive Heart Failure: Pharmacologic therapies for congestive heart failure include the removal of retained salt and water with diuretics; direct treatment of the depressed heart with positive inotropic drugs such as digitalis glycosides; reduction of preload or afterload with vasodilators; and reduction of afterload and retained salt and water by angiotensin-converting enzyme inhibitors. In addition, considerable evidence suggests that ACE inhibitors beneficially alter the structural changes that often follow myocardial infarction and lead to congestive failure. Recent clinical results show that beta-adrenoceptor blockers and spironolactone, an aldosterone antagonist, also have long-term beneficial effects. The use of diuretics is discussed in Chapter 15.

Current clinical evidence suggests that acute congestive failure should be treated with a loop diuretic, a prompt-acting positive inotropic agent such as a beta agonist or phosphodiesterase inhibitor, and vasodilators as required to optimize filling pressures and blood pressure. Chronic failure is best treated with diuretics (often a loop agent plus spironolactone) plus an ACE inhibitor and, if tolerated, a beta blocker. Digitalis is used if systolic dysfunction is prominent.

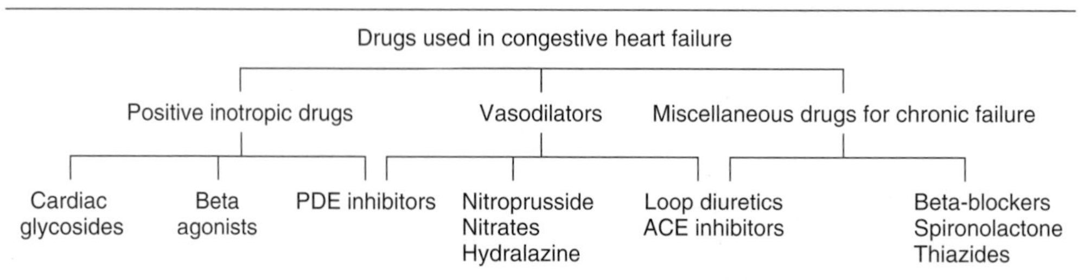

Figure 13–1. Subgroups of drugs discussed in this chapter. PDE, phosphodiesterase.

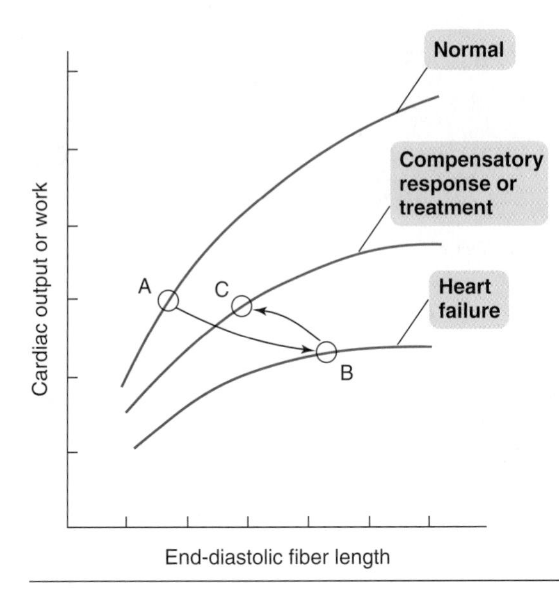

Figure 13–2. Ventricular function (Frank-Starling) curves. The abscissa can be any measure of preload—fiber length, filling pressure, pulmonary capillary wedge pressure, etc. The ordinate is a measure of useful external cardiac work—stroke volume, cardiac output, etc. In congestive heart failure, output is reduced at all fiber lengths and the heart expands because ejection fraction is decreased. As a result, the heart moves from point A to point B. Compensatory sympathetic discharge or effective treatment allows the heart to eject more blood, and the heart moves to point C on the middle curve.

CARDIAC GLYCOSIDES

A. Prototypes and Pharmacokinetics: All cardiac glycosides include a steroid nucleus and a lactone ring; most also have one or more sugar residues. The sugar residues constitute the glycoside portion of the molecule, and the steroid nucleus plus lactone ring comprise the "genin" portion. The cardiac glycosides are often called "digitalis" because several come from the digitalis (foxglove) plant. **Digoxin** is the prototype agent and the one most commonly used in the USA. A very similar molecule, digitoxin, which also comes from the foxglove, is now rarely used. Digitalis-like drugs come from many other plants, and a few come from animals. Ouabain, a shorter-acting glycoside, is derived from a tropical plant, though some evidence suggests that it is synthesized in mammals as well. The pharmacokinetics of digoxin, digitoxin, and ouabain are summarized in Table 13–2.

B. Mechanism of Action: Inhibition of Na^+/K^+ ATPase of the cell membrane by digitalis is well-documented and is considered to be the primary biochemical mechanism of action of digitalis (Figure 13–4). Translation of this effect into an increase in cardiac contractility involves

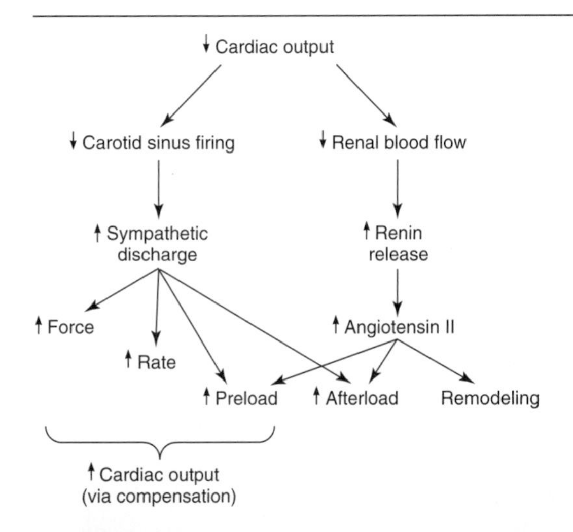

Figure 13–3. Compensatory responses that occur in congestive heart failure. These responses play an important role in the progression of the disease. (Reproduced, with permission, from Katzung BG [editor]: *Basic & Clinical Pharmacology,* 8th ed. McGraw-Hill, 2001.)

Table 13–2. Pharmacokinetic parameters of typical cardiac glycosides in adults. Digoxin is the cardiac glycoside most commonly used in the USA.

	Digitoxin	Digoxin	Ouabain
Oral bioavailability (%)	90–100	60–85	0
Half-life (hours)	168	36–40	20
Primary organ of elimination	Liver	Kidney	Kidney
Volume of distribution (L/kg)	0.6	6–8	18
Protein bound in plasma (%)	> 90	20–40	0

the Na^+/Ca^{2+} exchange mechanism. Inhibition of Na^+/K^+ ATPase results in an increase in intracellular sodium. The increased sodium alters the driving force for sodium-calcium exchange so that less calcium is removed from the cell. The increased intracellular calcium is stored in the sarcoplasmic reticulum and upon release increases contractile force. Other mechanisms of action for digitalis have been proposed, but they are probably not as important as the ATPase effect. The consequences of Na^+/K^+ ATPase inhibition are seen in both the mechanical and the electrical function of the heart. Digitalis also modifies autonomic outflow, and this action has effects on the electrical properties of the heart.

C. Cardiac Effects:

1. **Mechanical effects:** The increase in contractility evoked by digitalis results in increased ventricular ejection, decreased end-systolic and end-diastolic size, increased cardiac output, and increased renal perfusion. These beneficial effects permit a decrease in the compensatory sympathetic and renal responses previously described. The decrease in sympathetic

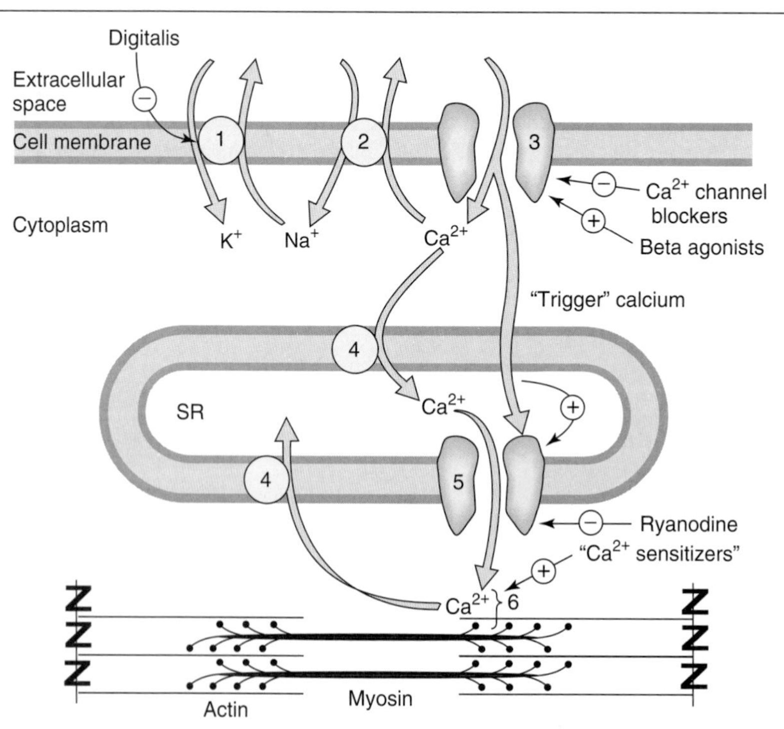

Figure 13–4. Schematic diagram of a cardiac sarcomere with the cellular components involved in excitation-contraction coupling. Factors involved in excitation-contraction coupling are numbered: 1, Na^+/K^+ ATPase; 2, Na^+/Ca^{2+} exchanger; 3, voltage-gated calcium channel; 4, calcium pump in the wall of the sarcoplasmic reticulum (SR); 5, calcium release channel in the SR; 6, site of calcium interaction with the troponin-tropomyosin system. (Reproduced, with permission, from Katzung BG [editor]: *Basic & Clinical Pharmacology,* 8th ed. McGraw-Hill, 2001.)

tone is especially beneficial: reduced heart rate, preload, and afterload permit the heart to function more efficiently (point C in Figure 13–2).

2. **Electrical effects:** Electrical effects include early cardiac parasympathomimetic responses and later arrhythmogenic responses. They are summarized in Table 13–3.
   a. **Early responses:** Increased PR interval, caused by the decrease in atrioventricular conduction velocity, and flattening of the T wave are often seen. The effects on the atria and AV node are largely parasympathetic in origin and can be partially blocked by atropine. The increase in the atrioventricular nodal refractory period is particularly important when atrial flutter or fibrillation is present because the refractoriness of the AV node determines the ventricular rate in these arrhythmias. The effect of digitalis is to slow ventricular rate. Shortened QT, inversion of the T, and ST depression may occur later.
   b. **Toxic responses:** Increased automaticity, caused by intracellular calcium overload, is the most important manifestation of toxicity. It results from delayed afterdepolarizations, which may evoke extrasystoles, tachycardia, or fibrillation in any part of the heart. In the ventricles, the extrasystoles are recognized as premature ventricular beats (PVBs). When PVBs are coupled to normal beats in a 1:1 fashion, the rhythm is called bigeminy (Figure 13–5).

D. Clinical Uses:

1. **Congestive heart failure:** Digitalis is the traditional positive inotropic agent used in the treatment of congestive heart failure. However, careful clinical studies indicate that while digitalis improves functional status (reducing symptoms), it does not prolong life. Other agents (diuretics, ACE inhibitors, vasodilators) may be equally effective and less toxic in some patients, and some of these alternative therapies do prolong life (see below). Because the half-lives of cardiac glycosides are long, the drugs accumulate significantly in the body, and dosing regimens must be carefully designed and monitored.
2. **Atrial fibrillation:** In atrial flutter and fibrillation, it is desirable to reduce the conduction velocity or increase the refractory period of the atrioventricular node so that ventricular rate is decreased. The parasympathomimetic action of digitalis effectively accomplishes this therapeutic objective.

E. Interactions: Quinidine causes a well-documented reduction in digoxin clearance and often increases the serum digoxin level if digoxin dosage is not adjusted. Several other drugs have been shown to have the same effect (amiodarone, verapamil, others), but the interactions with these drugs are not clinically significant. Digitalis effects are inhibited by extracellular potassium and magnesium and facilitated by extracellular calcium. Loop diuretics and thiazides, often used in treating heart failure, may significantly reduce serum potassium and thus precipitate digitalis toxicity. Digitalis-induced vomiting may deplete serum magnesium and similarly facilitate toxicity. These ion interactions are important in treating digitalis toxicity (see below).

F. Digitalis Toxicity: The major signs of digitalis toxicity are arrhythmias, nausea, vomiting, and diarrhea. Rarely, confusion or hallucinations and visual aberrations may occur. The treatment of digitalis arrhythmias is important because this manifestation of digitalis toxicity is

Table 13–3. Major actions of cardiac glycosides on cardiac electrical functions. (PANS, parasympathomimetic actions; direct, direct membrane actions.)

	Tissue		
Variable	**Atrial Muscle**	**AV Node**	**Purkinje System, Ventricles**
Effective refractory period	↓ (PANS)	↑ (PANS)	↓ (Direct)
Conduction velocity	↑ (PANS)	↓ (PANS)	Negligible
Automaticity	↑ (Direct)	↑ (Direct)	↑ (Direct)
Electrocardiogram			
Before arrhythmias	Negligible	↑ PR interval	↓ QT interval; T wave inversion; ST segment depression
Arrhythmias	Atrial tachycardia, fibrillation	AV nodal tachycardia; AV blockade	Premature ventricular contractions, ventricular tachycardia, ventricular fibrillation

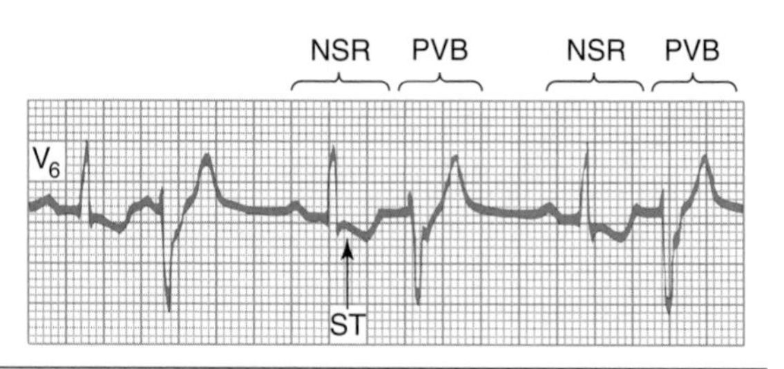

Figure 13–5. Electrocardiographic record showing digitalis-induced bigeminy. The complexes marked NSR are normal sinus rhythm beats; an inverted T wave and depressed ST segment are present. The complexes marked PVB are premature ventricular beats.

common and dangerous. Chronic intoxication is an extension of the therapeutic effect of the drug and is caused by excessive calcium accumulation in cardiac cells (calcium overload). This overload triggers abnormal automaticity and the arrhythmias noted in Table 13–3. Digitalis arrhythmia is more likely if serum potassium or magnesium is lower than normal or if serum calcium is higher than normal.

Severe, acute intoxication is caused by suicidal or accidental extreme overdose and results in cardiac depression leading to cardiac arrest rather than tachycardia or fibrillation.

Treatment of digitalis toxicity includes the following:

1. **Correction of potassium or magnesium deficiency:** Correction of potassium deficiency (caused, for example, by diuretic use) is useful in chronic digitalis intoxication. Mild toxicity may often be managed by omitting one or two doses of digitalis and giving oral or parenteral K^+ supplements. Potassium should not be raised above the normal level of 3.5–5 meq/L. Similarly, if hypomagnesemia is present, it should be treated by normalizing serum magnesium. Severe acute intoxication (as in suicidal overdoses) usually causes marked hyperkalemia and should not be treated with supplemental potassium.
2. **Antiarrhythmic drugs:** Antiarrhythmic drugs may be useful if increased automaticity is prominent and does not respond to normalization of serum potassium. Agents that do not severely impair cardiac contractility (eg, lidocaine or phenytoin) are favored but drugs such as propranolol have also been used successfully. Severe acute digitalis overdose usually causes marked inhibition of all pacemaker cells. Antiarrhythmic drugs are dangerous in such patients.
3. **Digoxin antibodies:** Digoxin antibodies (FAB fragments, Digibind) are extremely effective and should always be used if other therapies appear to be failing. They are effective for poisoning with many cardiac glycosides in addition to digoxin and may save patients who would otherwise die.

Skill Keeper: Maintenance Dose Calculations (see Chapter 3)

Digoxin has a narrow therapeutic window, and its dosing must be carefully managed. The drug's minimum effective concentration is about 1 ng/mL. About 60% is excreted in the urine; the rest is metabolized in the liver. The normal clearance of digoxin is 7 L/h/70 kg; volume of distribution is 500 L/70 kg; and bioavailability is 70%. If your 70-kg patient's renal function is only 30% of normal, what should be the daily oral maintenance dosage in order to achieve a safe plasma concentration of 1 ng/mL? *The Skill Keeper Answer appears at the end of the chapter.*

OTHER DRUGS USED IN CONGESTIVE HEART FAILURE

The other major agents used in heart failure include diuretics, ACE inhibitors, β_1-selective sympathomimetics, β-blockers, phosphodiesterase inhibitors, and vasodilators.

A. **Diuretics:** Diuretics are often used in congestive heart failure before digitalis and other drugs are considered. Furosemide is a very useful agent for immediate reduction of the pulmonary congestion and severe edema associated with acute congestive heart failure or severe chronic failure. Thiazides such as hydrochlorothiazide are often used in the management of mild chronic failure. Recent clinical studies suggest that spironolactone (an aldosterone antagonist diuretic) has particularly significant long-term benefits in chronic failure. The pharmacology of the diuretics is discussed in Chapter 15.

B. Angiotensin-Converting Enzyme Inhibitors: These agents have been shown to reduce morbidity and mortality in chronic heart failure. Although they have no direct positive inotropic action, ACE inhibitors reduce aldosterone secretion, salt and water retention, and vascular resistance. They are now considered among the first line drugs for chronic heart failure, along with diuretics. Angiotensin receptor antagonists (eg, losartan) probably have similar benefits although long-term studies have not been completed with these newer drugs.

C. Beta$_1$-Selective Adrenoceptor Agonists: Dobutamine and dopamine are useful in many cases of *acute* failure, in which systolic function is markedly depressed. However, they are not appropriate for chronic failure because of tolerance, lack of oral efficacy, and significant arrhythmogenic effects.

D. Beta-Adrenoceptor Antagonists: Several beta blockers (carvedilol, labetalol, metoprolol) have been shown in long-term studies to reduce progression of *chronic* heart failure. This benefit of β-blockers had long been recognized in patients with hypertrophic cardiomyopathy but has now been shown to also occur in patients without cardiomyopathy. Beta-blockers are not of value in acute failure and may be detrimental if systolic dysfunction is marked.

E. Phosphodiesterase Inhibitors: Amrinone and milrinone are the major representatives of this infrequently used group, although theophylline (in the form of its salt, aminophylline) was commonly used in the past. These drugs increase cAMP by inhibiting its breakdown by phosphodiesterase and cause an increase in cardiac intracellular calcium similar to that produced by beta adrenoceptor agonists. Phosphodiesterase inhibitors also cause vasodilation, which may be responsible for a major part of their beneficial effect. At sufficiently high concentrations, these agents may increase the sensitivity of the contractile protein system to calcium (site 6 in Figure 13–4). These agents should not be used in chronic failure: they have been shown to increase morbidity and mortality.

F. Vasodilators: Vasodilator therapy with nitroprusside or nitroglycerin is often used for acute severe congestive failure. The use of these vasodilator drugs is based on the reduction in cardiac size and improved efficiency that can be realized with proper adjustment of venous return and reduction of resistance to ventricular ejection. Vasodilator therapy can be dramatically effective, especially in cases in which increased afterload is a major factor in causing the failure (eg, continuing hypertension in an individual who has just had an infarct). Chronic congestive heart failure sometimes responds favorably to oral vasodilators such as hydralazine or isosorbide dinitrate.

DRUG LIST

The following drugs are important members of the group discussed in this chapter. Prototypes should be learned in detail; features of the major variants should be known well enough to distinguish the variants from the prototypes and from each other; the other significant agents should be recognized as belonging to a specific subclass.

Subclass	Prototype	Major Variants	Other Significant Agents
Cardiac glycosides	Digoxin		
Diuretics	Furosemide	Spironolactone	Hydrochlorothiazide
ACE inhibitors	Captopril		Enalapril, lisinopril
Positive inotropic digitalis substitutes	Dobutamine, amrinone		Milrinone, theophylline
Beta-blockers	Carvedilol		Atenolol, labetalol
Vasodilators	Nitroprusside	Nitroglycerin, hydralazine	Isosorbide dinitrate, theophylline

QUESTIONS

DIRECTIONS: Each of the numbered items or incomplete statements in this section is followed by answers or by completions of the statement. Select the ONE lettered answer or completion that is BEST in each case.

1. Drugs that have been found to be useful in one or more types of heart failure include all of the following EXCEPT
(A) Na^+/K^+ ATPase inhibitors
(B) Alpha adrenoceptor agonists
(C) Beta adrenoceptor agonists
(D) Beta adrenoceptor antagonists
(E) ACE inhibitors

2. The biochemical mechanism of action of digitalis is associated with
(A) A decrease in calcium uptake by the sarcoplasmic reticulum
(B) An increase in ATP synthesis
(C) A modification of the actin molecule
(D) An increase in systolic intracellular calcium levels
(E) A block of sodium/calcium exchange

3. A patient who has been taking digoxin for several years for chronic heart failure is about to receive atropine for another condition. A common effect of digoxin (at therapeutic blood levels) that can be almost entirely blocked by atropine is
(A) Decreased appetite
(B) Increased atrial contractility
(C) Increased PR interval on the ECG
(D) Headaches
(E) Tachycardia

4. A 65-year-old woman has been admitted to the coronary care unit with a left ventricular myocardial infarction. If this patient develops acute severe congestive failure with pulmonary edema, which one of the following would be most useful?
(A) Furosemide
(B) Guanethidine
(C) Minoxidil
(D) Propranolol
(E) Spironolactone

5. In a patient given a cardiac glycoside, important effects of the drug on the heart include which of the following?
(A) Decreased atrioventricular conduction velocity
(B) Decreased ejection time
(C) Increased ectopic automaticity
(D) Increased force of contraction
(E) All of the above

6. Which of the following situations constitutes an added risk of digoxin toxicity?
(A) Starting administration of captopril
(B) Starting administration of quinidine
(C) Hyperkalemia
(D) Hypermagnesemia
(E) Hypocalcemia

7. Which row in the following table correctly shows the major effects of full therapeutic doses of digoxin on the AV node and the ECG?

Row	AV Refractory Period	QT Interval	T Wave
(A)	Increased	Increased	Upright
(B)	Increased	Decreased	Inverted
(C)	Decreased	Increased	Upright
(D)	Decreased	Decreased	Upright
(E)	Decreased	Decreased	Inverted

8. Drugs proved to reduce mortality in chronic congestive heart failure include all of the following EXCEPT
- **(A)** Captopril
- **(B)** Carvedilol
- **(C)** Digoxin
- **(D)** Enalapril
- **(E)** Spironolactone

9. Drugs associated with clinically useful or physiologically important positive inotropic effects include all of the following EXCEPT
- **(A)** Amrinone
- **(B)** Captopril
- **(C)** Digoxin
- **(D)** Dobutamine
- **(E)** Norepinephrine

10. Successful therapy of congestive heart failure with digoxin will result in which one of the following?
- **(A)** Decreased heart rate
- **(B)** Increased afterload
- **(C)** Increased aldosterone
- **(D)** Increased renin secretion
- **(E)** Increased sympathetic outflow to the heart

11. Which of the following is a monovalent cation that will decrease or reverse a mild to moderate digitalis-induced arrhythmia?
- **(A)** Digibind antibodies
- **(B)** Digitoxin
- **(C)** Digoxin
- **(D)** Dobutamine
- **(E)** Enalapril
- **(F)** Furosemide
- **(G)** Lidocaine
- **(H)** Magnesium
- **(I)** Potassium
- **(J)** Quinidine

12. Which of the following has been shown to prolong life in patients with chronic congestive failure but has a negative inotropic effect on cardiac contractility?
- **(A)** Carvedilol
- **(B)** Digitoxin
- **(C)** Digoxin
- **(D)** Dobutamine
- **(E)** Enalapril
- **(F)** Furosemide

13. Which of the following is a β_1-selective agonist sometimes used in acute congestive failure?
- **(A)** Atenolol
- **(B)** Digoxin
- **(C)** Dobutamine
- **(D)** Enalapril
- **(E)** Furosemide
- **(F)** Quinidine
- **(G)** Spironolactone

14. Which of the following is the drug of choice in treating suicidal overdose of digitoxin?
- **(A)** Digoxin antibodies
- **(B)** Lidocaine
- **(C)** Magnesium
- **(D)** Potassium
- **(E)** Quinidine

DIRECTIONS (Item 15): The matching question in this section consists of a list of lettered options followed by item 15. Select the ONE lettered option that is most closely associated with item 15.

(A) Digoxin antibodies
(B) Digitoxin
(C) Digoxin
(D) Dobutamine
(E) Enalapril
(F) Furosemide
(G) Lidocaine
(H) Magnesium
(I) Potassium
(J) Quinidine

15. An antiarrhythmic drug that is used to suppress digoxin-induced arrhythmias in some patients

DIRECTIONS (Items 16–18): This case history is followed by questions for discussion. Write out brief answers (two to five sentences) and then compare your answers with those given at the end of the Answers section.

A 39-year-old man with mitral stenosis ingested 90 digoxin tablets (0.25 mg each) in a suicide attempt approximately 2 hours before admission. Upon admission, the blood pressure was 110/70 mm Hg and the pulse was 40–60/min and irregular. The rest of the examination was normal.

Initial laboratory data included a blood ethanol of 190 mg/dL, but electrolytes were normal. An electrocardiogram revealed atrial fibrillation with a high degree of atrioventricular block. The ventricular rate did not exceed 50/min. Atropine had no effect on the ventricular rate and a transvenous pacing catheter was therefore inserted, with ventricular pacing instituted at 60/min.

During the next 8 hours, the spontaneous ventricular rate (determined by briefly halting the transvenous pacemaker) progressively decreased to 33/min and then to 13/min. No atrial activity could be detected on the ECG. The QRS duration reached a maximum of 0.33 s (normal: 0.1 s). Serum potassium increased to 8.7 meq/L (normal: 3.5–5 meq/L). An antidote was administered. Serum potassium rapidly fell to the normal range, and the patient made a complete recovery.

16. What was the cause and the primary source of the elevated serum potassium?
17. Outline the conventional therapy for less severe digitalis intoxication, and explain why it was not used in this case. What antidote was used?
18. This patient ingested digoxin. What treatment is available for severe intoxication with other cardiac glycosides?

ANSWERS

1. All the drug groups listed are commonly used in heart failure except alpha agonists. Alpha-agonist drugs *increase* vascular resistance and would *decrease* the stroke volume of the weakened heart even more. The answer is **(B).**
2. Digitalis does not alter calcium uptake or ATP synthesis; it does not modify actin. Sodium/calcium exchange is not blocked, it is merely altered. The most accurate description of digitalis's mechanism in this list is that it increases intracellular calcium. The answer is **(D).**
3. The parasympathomimetic effects of digitalis can be blocked by muscarinic blockers such as atropine. The only parasympathomimetic effect in the list provided is increased PR interval, representing slowing of AV conduction. The answer is **(C).**
4. Acute severe congestive failure with pulmonary edema often requires a vasodilator that reduces intravascular pressures in the lungs. Furosemide has such vasodilating actions in the context of acute failure. Minoxidil would decrease arterial pressure and increase the heart rate excessively. Spironolactone is useful in chronic failure but not usually in acute pulmonary edema. The answer is **(A).**
5. The effects of digitalis include all of those listed. The answer is **(E).**
6. Digitalis toxicity is facilitated by hypercalcemia, hypokalemia, or hypomagnesemia. It is also more likely if a patient begins taking quinidine after being stabilized on a dose of digitalis, because quinidine reduces the clearance of digoxin. The answer is **(B).**
7. Digitalis increases the AV node refractory period—a parasympathomimetic action. Its effects on the ventricles include shortened action potential and QT interval, and a change in repolarization with inversion of the T wave. The answer is **(B).**

8. All the groups listed *except* digitalis have been shown to reduce mortality. Cardiac glycosides reduce symptoms but not mortality. The answer is **(C).**

9. Although they are extremely useful in congestive heart failure, captopril and the other ACE inhibitors have no positive inotropic effect on the heart. The answer is **(B).**

10. Digoxin reduces sympathetic outflow to the heart and vessels and reduces renin secretion (because the drug replaces the need for compensatory responses). The answer is **(A).**

11. Potassium is the only monovalent cation in the list, and it is used for reversing mild to moderate digitalis toxicity. The answer is **(I).**

12. Several beta-blockers, including carvedilol, have been shown to prolong life in heart failure patients even though these drugs have a negative inotropic action on the heart. Their benefits presumably result from some other effect. The answer is **(A).**

13. Dobutamine is a β_1-selective agonist often used in acute heart failure. The answer is **(C).**

14. The drug of choice in severe, massive overdose with any cardiac glycoside is digoxin antibody, Digibind. These antibodies are sufficiently nonselective to bind a variety of cardiac glycosides. The other drugs are used in moderate overdosage associated with increased automaticity. The answer is **(A).**

15. Although quinidine is an antiarrhythmic drug, it is much more likely than lidocaine to *precipitate* digitalis toxicity. (See Question 14.) The answer is **(G),** lidocaine.

16. The cause of the dramatic rise in serum potassium was the poisoning of membrane Na^+/K^+ ATPase (the sodium pump) in the entire body. The source of the potassium was the intracellular space, particularly that of skeletal muscle (because of the large mass of this organ system).

17. Conventional therapy of mild to moderate cardiac glycoside intoxication consists of the following: (1) Normalization of low serum K^+. In the present case and in most cases of gross overdosage, the serum K^+ is high. However, in many cases of mild to moderate toxicity, the serum K^+ is low (because of concurrent diuretic use) or normal. If it is certain that the overdose is *not* massive and serum K^+ is low, supplemental potassium should be given. However, potassium should *never* be raised above 4–5 meq/L because hyperkalemia is also arrhythmogenic. In some cases (usually involving vomiting, diarrhea, or excessive use of loop diuretics), low serum Mg^{2+} is found, and correction of this deficiency corrects the arrhythmia. (2) Use of antiarrhythmic drugs. Lidocaine is usually tried first. (3) Avoidance of DC cardioversion unless ventricular fibrillation occurs. These approaches were clearly not suitable for this severely intoxicated patient. The antidote used was digoxin antibodies (Digibind).

18. Antidigoxin Fab fragments cross-react sufficiently to be useful in reversing other glycosides' effects, including oleander cardiac glycoside.

Skill Keeper Answer: Maintenance Dose Calculations (see Chapter 3)

Maintenance dosage is equal to CL × Cp ÷ F, so

Maintenance dosage for a patient with normal renal function

$$= 7\ \text{L/h} \times 1\ \text{ng/mL} \div 0.7 = 7\ \text{L/h} \times 1\ \mu\text{g/L} \div 0.7$$
$$= 10\ \mu\text{g/h} = 240\ \mu\text{g/d}$$

But this patient has only 30% of normal renal function, so

$$\text{CL(total)} = 0.3 \times \text{CL (renal [60\% of total])} + \text{CL (liver [40\% of total])}$$
$$\text{CL(total)} = 0.3 \times 0.6 \times 7\ \text{L/h} + 0.4 \times 7\ \text{L/h, and}$$
$$\text{CL(total)} = 1.26\ \text{L/h} + 2.8\ \text{L/h} = 4.06\ \text{L/h, and}$$
$$\text{Maintenance dosage} = 4.06\ \text{L/h} \times 1\ \mu\text{g/L} \div 0.7$$
$$= 5.8\ \mu\text{g/h} = 139\ \mu\text{g/d}$$

14 Antiarrhythmic Drugs

OBJECTIVES

You should be able to:

- Describe the distinguishing features of the four major classes of antiarrhythmic drugs and adenosine.
- List two or three of the most important drugs in each of the four classes.
- List the major toxicities of those drugs.
- Describe the mechanism of selective depression by local anesthetic antiarrhythmic agents.
- Explain how hyperkalemia, hypokalemia, or an antiarrhythmic drug can cause an arrhythmia.

Learn the definitions that follow.

Table 14–1. Definitions.

Term	Definition
Abnormal automaticity	Pacemaker activity that originates anywhere other than in the sinoatrial node
Abnormal conduction	Conduction of an impulse that does not follow the path defined in Figure 14–1 or reenters tissue previously excited
Atrial fibrillation, ventricular fibrillation	Common arrhythmias involving rapid reentry and chaotic movement of impulses through the tissue of the atria or ventricles; ventricular—but not atrial—fibrillation is fatal if not terminated within a few minutes
Effective refractory period	The period that must pass after the upstroke of a conducted impulse in a part of the heart before a new action potential can be propagated in that cell or tissue
Class I, II, III, and IV drugs	A method for classifying antiarrhythmic drugs, sometimes called the Vaughan-Williams classification; based loosely on the channel or receptor affected
Nodal tachycardia	A common reentrant arrhythmia that travels through the AV node; it may also be conducted through atrial and ventricular tissue as part of the reentry circuit
Reentrant arrhythmia	Arrhythmia of abnormal conduction; involves the repetitive passage of an impulse through tissue previously excited by the same impulse
Selective depression	The ability of certain drugs to selectively depress areas of excitable membrane that are most susceptible, leaving other areas relatively unaffected
Ventricular tachycardia	A very common arrhythmia, associated often with myocardial infarction; ventricular tachycardia may involve abnormal automaticity or abnormal conduction, usually impairs cardiac output, and may deteriorate into ventricular fibrillation; for these reasons it requires prompt management

CONCEPTS

Cardiac arrhythmias commonly occur in the presence of preexisting heart disease. They are the most common cause of death in patients who have had a myocardial infarction. They are also the most serious manifestation of digitalis toxicity and are often associated with anesthesia, hyperthyroidism, and electrolyte disorders.

PATHOPHYSIOLOGY

A. **What Is an Arrhythmia?** Normal cardiac function is dependent on generation of an impulse in the normal pacemaker (the sinoatrial [SA] node) and its conduction through the atrial muscle, through the atrioventricular (AV) node, through the Purkinje conduction system, to the ventricular muscle (Figure 14–1). Normal pacemaking and conduction require normal action potentials (dependent on sodium, calcium, and potassium channel activity) under appropriate autonomic control. Arrhythmias are therefore defined by exclusion—ie, any rhythm that is not a normal sinus rhythm (NSR) is an arrhythmia.

B. Arrhythmogenic Mechanisms: Abnormal automaticity and abnormal (reentrant) conduction are the two major mechanisms for arrhythmias. A few of the clinically important arrhythmias are **atrial flutter, atrial fibrillation** (AF), **atrioventricular nodal reentry** (a common type of supraventricular tachycardia [SVT]), **premature ventricular beats** (PVBs), **ventricular tachycardia** (VT), and **ventricular fibrillation** (VF). Examples of electrocardiographic recordings of normal sinus rhythm and some of these common arrhythmias are shown in Figure 14–2. **Torsade de pointes** is a ventricular arrhythmia of great pharmacologic importance because it is often *induced* by antiarrhythmic drugs, especially drugs that prolong the QT interval. It has the electrocardiographic morphology of a polymorphic ventricular tachycardia, often displaying waxing and waning QRS amplitude. Torsade is also associated with **long QT syndrome,** a her-

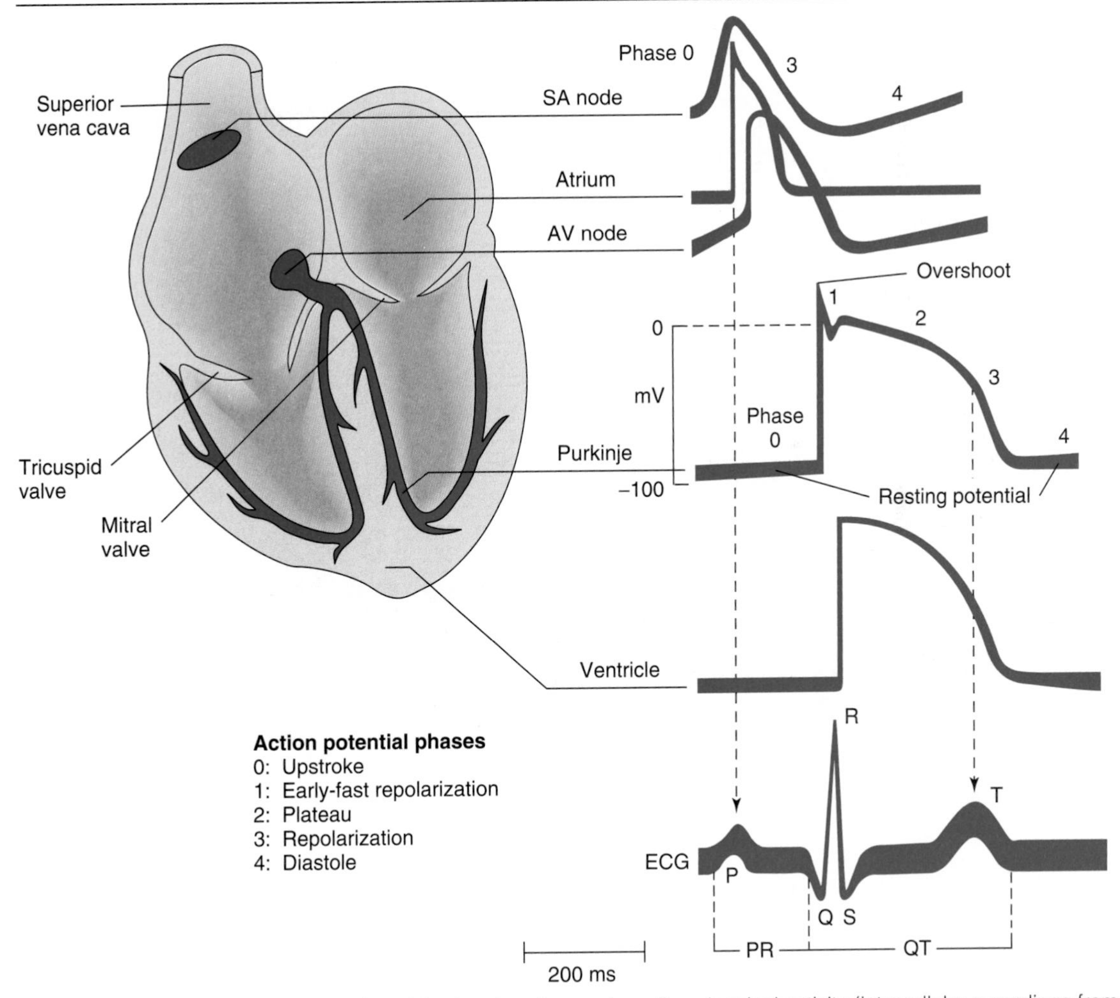

Figure 14–1. Schematic representation of the heart and normal cardiac electrical activity (intracellular recordings from areas indicated and ECG). The ECG is the body surface manifestation of the depolarization and repolarization waves of the heart. The P wave is generated by atrial depolarization, the QRS by ventricular muscle depolarization, and the T wave by ventricular repolarization. The PR interval is a measure of conduction time from atrium to ventricle, and the QRS duration indicates the time required for all of the ventricular cells to be activated (ie, the intraventricular conduction time). The QT interval reflects the duration of the ventricular action potential.

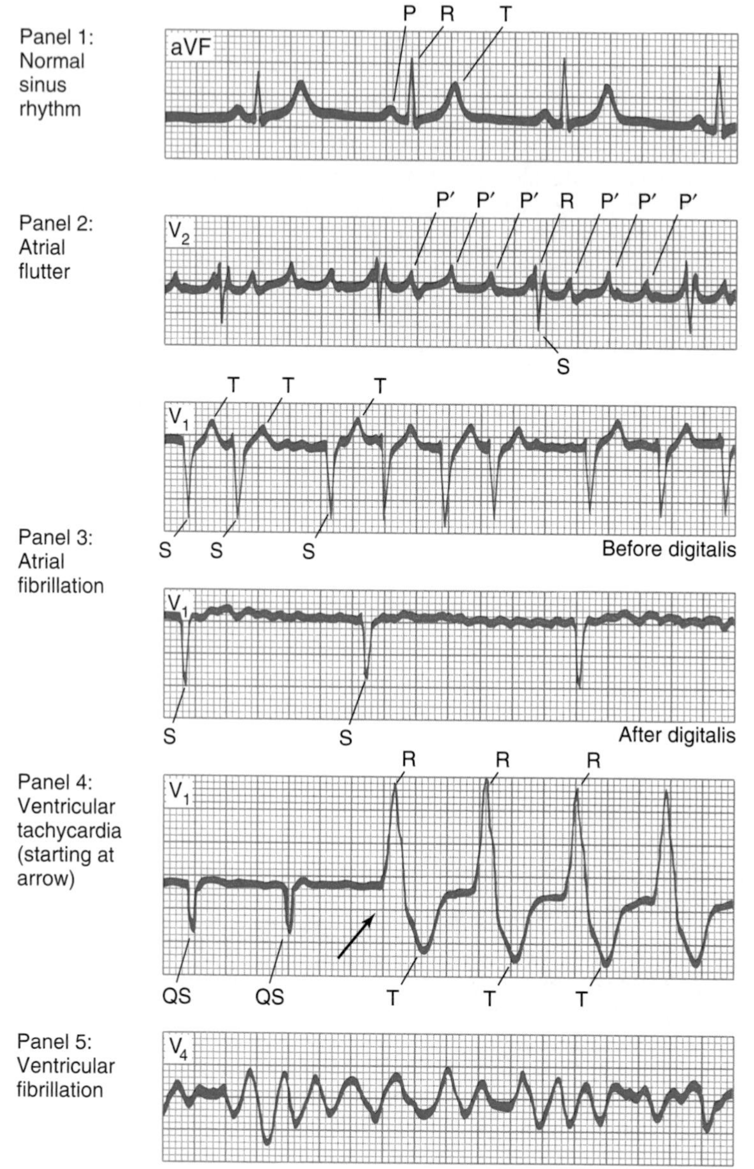

Figure 14–2. Typical ECGs of normal sinus rhythm and some common arrhythmias. Major waves (P, Q, R, S, and T) are labeled in each electrocardiographic record except in panel 5, in which electrical activity is completely disorganized and none of these deflections are recognizable. (Modified and reproduced, with permission, from Goldman MJ: *Principles of Clinical Electrocardiography,* 11th ed. Originally published by Appleton & Lange. Copyright © 1982 by The McGraw-Hill Companies, Inc.)

itable abnormal prolongation of the QT interval caused by mutations in the I_{Kr} or I_{Na} channel molecules.

C. Normal Electrical Activity in the Cardiac Cell: The cellular action potentials shown in Figure 14–1 are the result of ion fluxes through voltage-gated channels and carrier mechanisms. These processes are diagrammed in Figure 14–3. In most parts of the heart, sodium current (I_{Na}) dominates the upstroke of the action potential and is the most important determinant of conduction of that action potential. After a very brief activation, it enters a more prolonged period of inactivation. In the AV node, calcium current (I_{Ca}) dominates the upstroke. The plateau of the action potential is dominated by calcium current (I_{Ca}) and a potassium repolarizing current (I_{Kr}).

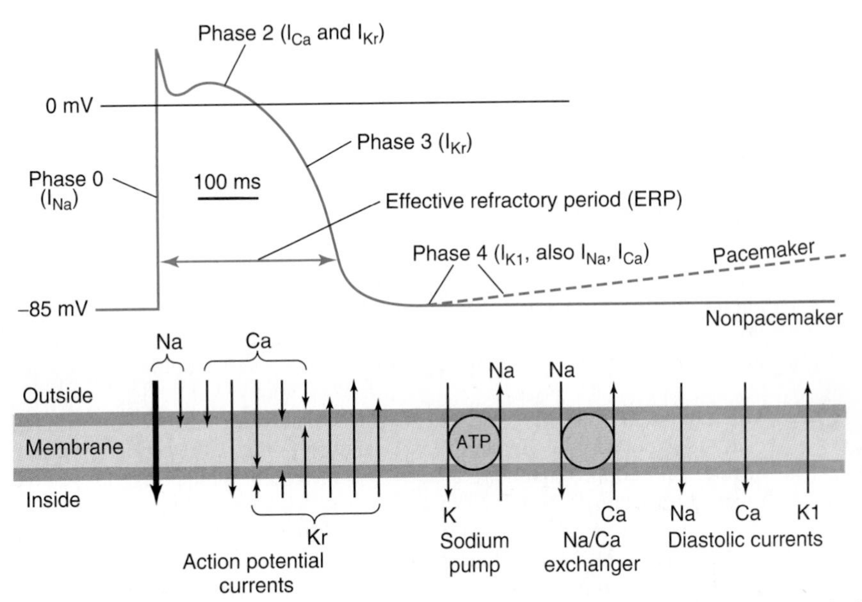

Figure 14–3. Components of the membrane action potential (AP) in a typical Purkinje or ventricular cardiac cell. The deflections of the AP, designated as phases 0–3, are generated by several ionic currents. The actions of the sodium pump and sodium/calcium exchanger are mainly involved in maintaining ionic steady state during repetitive activity. Note that small but significant currents occur during diastole (phase 4) in addition to the pump and exchanger activity. In nonpacemaker cells, the outward potassium current during phase 4 is sufficient to maintain a stable negative resting potential, as shown by the solid line at the right end of the tracing. In pacemaker cells, however, the potassium current is smaller and the depolarizing currents (sodium, calcium, or both) during phase 4 are large enough to gradually depolarize the cell during diastole (shown by the dashed line).

At the end of the plateau, I_{Kr} causes rapid repolarization. The refractory period of the cardiac cell is a function of how rapidly sodium channels recover from inactivation. Recovery from inactivation depends on both the membrane potential (which varies with repolarization time and the extracellular potassium concentration) and the actions of drugs that bind to the sodium channel, ie, sodium channel blockers. The carrier processes (sodium pump and sodium/calcium exchanger) contribute little to the shape of the action potential (but they are critical for the maintenance of the ion gradients on which the sodium, calcium, and potassium currents depend). Antiarrhythmic drugs act on one or more of the three major currents (I_{Na}, I_{Ca}, I_{Kr}) or on the second messenger systems that modulate these currents.

D. Drug Classification: The antiarrhythmic agents are often classified using a system loosely based on the channel or receptor involved (Figure 14–4). This system specifies four classes, usually denoted by roman numerals I–IV:

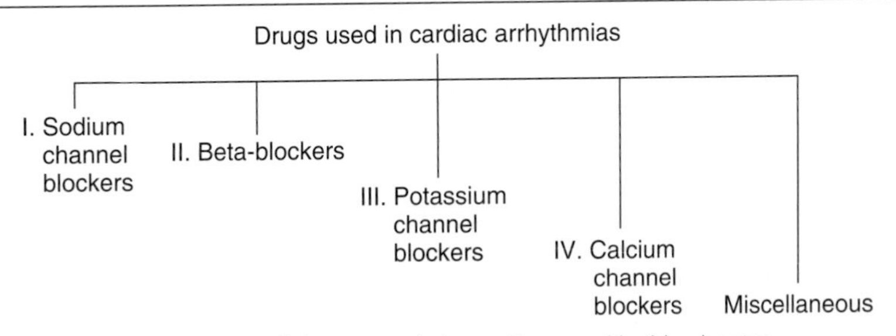

Figure 14–4. Subgroups of drugs discussed in this chapter.

I. Sodium channel blockers
II. Beta adrenoceptor blockers
III. Potassium channel blockers
IV. Calcium channel blockers

A miscellaneous group includes adenosine, digitalis, potassium ion, and magnesium ion.

CLASS I (LOCAL ANESTHETICS)

A. Prototypes: The class I drugs are further subdivided on the basis of their effects on action potential duration. Class IA agents (prototype quinidine) prolong the action potential. Class IB drugs shorten the action potential in some cardiac tissues (prototype lidocaine). Class IC drugs have no effect on action potential duration (prototype flecainide).

B. Mechanism of Action: As local anesthetics, all class I drugs slow or block conduction (especially in depolarized cells) and slow or abolish abnormal pacemakers wherever these processes depend on sodium channels. Useful sodium channel-blocking drugs bind to their receptors much more readily when the channel is open or inactivated than when it is fully repolarized and recovered from its previous activity. Ion channels in arrhythmic tissue spend more time in the open or inactivated states than do channels in normal tissue. Therefore, these antiarrhythmic drugs block channels in abnormal tissue more effectively than channels in normal tissue. As a result, antiarrhythmic sodium channel blockers are **use-dependent** or **state-dependent** in their action—ie, they selectively depress tissue that is frequently depolarizing (eg, during a fast tachycardia) or is relatively depolarized during rest (eg, by hypoxia). The effects of the major class I drugs are summarized in Table 14–2 and in Figure 14–5.

1. **Drugs with class IA action:** Quinidine is the class IA prototype. Other drugs with class IA actions include amiodarone, procainamide, and disopyramide. They affect both atrial and ventricular arrhythmias. These drugs block I_{Na} and therefore slow conduction velocity in the atria, Purkinje fibers, and ventricular cells. The reduction in ventricular conduction results in increased QRS duration in the ECG. In addition, these drugs block I_{Kr}. Therefore, they increase action potential (AP) duration and the effective refractory period (ERP) in ad-

Table 14–2. Properties of the prototype antiarrhythmic drugs.

Drug	Group	Half-Life	Route	PR Interval	QRS Duration	QT Interval
Adenosine	Misc	3 sec	IV	↑	—	—
Amiodarone	IA, III	1–10 weeks	Oral, IV	↑	↑↑	↑↑↑↑
Bretylium	III	4 h	IV	—	—	—[1]
Disopyramide	IA	6–8 h	Oral	↓ or ↑[2]	↑↑	↑↑
Esmolol	II	10 min	IV	↑↑	—	—
Flecainide	IC	20 h	Oral	↑ (slight)	↑↑	—
Ibutilide, dofetilide	III	6–7 h	Oral	—	—	↑↑↑
Lidocaine	IB	1–2 h	IV	—	—[3]	—
Mexiletine, tocainide	IB	12 h	Oral	—	—[3]	—
Procainamide	IA	2–4 h	Oral, IV	↓ or ↑[2]	↑↑	↑↑
Propranolol	II	8 h	Oral, IV	↑↑	—	—
Quinidine	IA	6 h	Oral, IV	↓ or ↑[2]	↑↑	↑↑↑
Sotalol	III	7 h	Oral	↑	—	↑↑↑
Verapamil	IV	7 h	Oral, IV	↑↑	—	—

[1]Bretylium increases action potential duration in ischemic cells.
[2]PR may decrease through antimuscarinic action or increase through channel blocking action.
[3]Lidocaine, mexiletine, and tocainide slow conduction velocity in ischemic, depolarized ventricular cells but not in normal tissue.

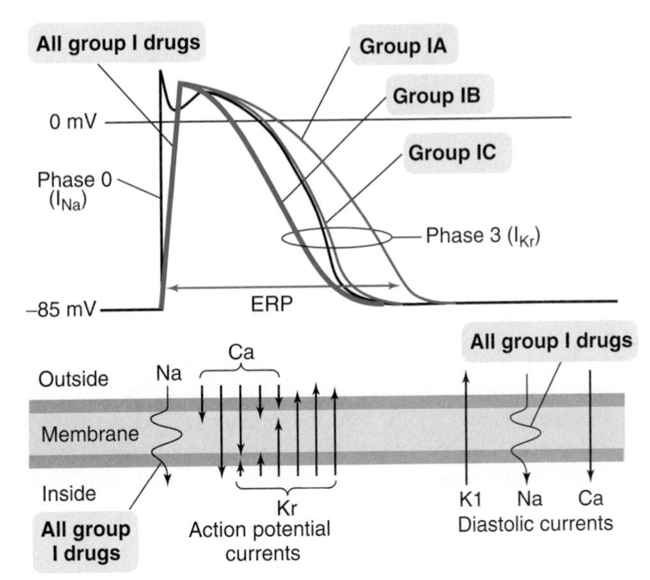

Figure 14–5. Schematic diagram of the effects of class I agents. Note that all class I drugs reduce both phase 0 and phase 4 sodium currents in susceptible cells (shown as wavy lines). Class IA drugs also reduce potassium current (I_{Kr}) and prolong the AP duration. This results in significant prolongation of the effective refractory period. Class IB and class IC drugs have different (or no) effects on potassium current and thus shorten or have no effect on the action potential duration.

dition to slowing conduction velocity and ectopic pacemakers. The increase in action potential duration generates an increase in QT interval (Table 14–2). Amiodarone has similar effects on sodium current and has the greatest AP-prolonging effect. It is often considered a class III drug even though it clearly blocks sodium channels, which is a class I action.

2. **Drugs with class IB actions:** Lidocaine is the prototype IB drug. Mexiletine and tocainide are other IB agents. Lidocaine selectively affects ischemic or depolarized Purkinje and ventricular tissue and has little effect on atrial tissue; the drug reduces action potential duration, but because it slows recovery of sodium channels from inactivation, it does not shorten (and may even prolong) the effective refractory period. Mexiletine and tocainide have similar effects. Because these agents have little effect on normal cardiac cells, they have little effect on the ECG (Table 14–2). Phenytoin, an anticonvulsant and not a true local anesthetic, is sometimes classified with the class IB antiarrhythmic agents because it can be used to reverse digitalis-induced arrhythmias. It resembles lidocaine in lacking significant effect on the normal ECG.
3. **Drugs with class IC action:** Flecainide is the prototype drug with class IC actions. Encainide, moricizine, and propafenone are also members of this class. These drugs have no effect on ventricular action potential duration or the QT interval. They are powerful depressants of sodium current, however, and can markedly slow conduction velocity in atrial and ventricular cells. They increase the QRS duration of the ECG.

C. Pharmacokinetics:

See Table 14–2.

D. Clinical Uses and Toxicities:

1. **Class IA drugs:** Quinidine is used in all types of arrhythmias, especially chronic ones requiring outpatient treatment. Both atrial and ventricular arrhythmias may be responsive. Procainamide and disopyramide have similar uses. Procainamide is also commonly used in arrhythmias during the acute phase of myocardial infarction.

   Quinidine causes cinchonism (headache, vertigo, tinnitus); cardiac depression; gastrointestinal upset; and allergic reactions (eg, thrombocytopenic purpura). As noted in Chapter 13, quinidine reduces the clearance of digoxin and may increase the serum concentration of the glycoside to dangerous levels. Procainamide causes hypotension (especially when used parenterally) and a reversible syndrome similar to lupus erythematosus. Disopyramide has marked antimuscarinic effects and may precipitate congestive heart failure. All class IA drugs may precipitate new arrhythmias. Torsade de pointes is particularly associated with quinidine and other drugs that prolong AP duration (except amiodarone). The toxicities of amiodarone are discussed below.

Hyperkalemia usually exacerbates the cardiac toxicity of class I drugs. Treatment of overdose with these agents is often carried out with sodium lactate (to reverse drug-induced arrhythmias) and pressor sympathomimetics (to reverse drug-induced hypotension) if indicated.

2. **Class IB drugs:** Lidocaine is useful in acute ventricular arrhythmias, especially those involving ischemia, eg, following myocardial infarction. Atrial arrhythmias are not responsive unless caused by digitalis. Mexiletine and tocainide have similar actions and are given orally. Lidocaine is usually given intravenously, but intramuscular administration is also possible. It is never given orally because it has a very high first-pass effect and its metabolites are potentially cardiotoxic.

   Lidocaine, mexiletine, and tocainide rarely cause typical local anesthetic toxicity (ie, CNS stimulation, including convulsions); cardiovascular depression (usually minor); and allergy (usually rashes but may extend to anaphylaxis). Tocainide may cause agranulocytosis. These drugs may also precipitate arrhythmias, but this is less common than with class IA drugs. Hyperkalemia increases cardiac toxicity.

3. **Class IC drugs:** Flecainide is effective in both atrial and ventricular arrhythmias but is approved only for refractory ventricular tachycardias that tend to progress to VF at unpredictable times, resulting in "sudden death," and for certain intractable supraventricular arrhythmias.

   Flecainide and its congeners are more likely than other antiarrhythmic drugs to exacerbate or precipitate arrhythmias (proarrhythmic effect). This toxicity was dramatically demonstrated by the Cardiac Arrhythmia Suppression Trial (CAST), a large clinical trial of class IC drugs in myocardial infarction survivors. The trial results showed that class IC drugs caused greater mortality than placebo. For this reason, the class IC drugs are now restricted to use in arrhythmias that fail to respond to other drugs. These drugs also cause local anesthetic-like CNS toxicity. Hyperkalemia increases the cardiac toxicity of these agents.

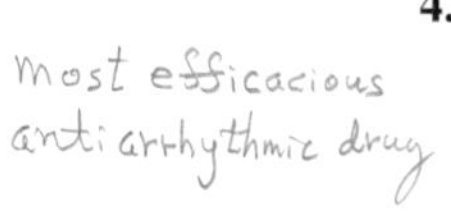

4. **Amiodarone, a special case:** Amiodarone is effective in most types of arrhythmias and is considered the most efficacious of all antiarrhythmic drugs. This may be because it has a broad spectrum: it blocks sodium, calcium, and potassium channels and beta adrenoceptors. Because of its toxicities, however, amiodarone is usually reserved for use in arrhythmias that are resistant to other drugs.

   Amiodarone causes microcrystalline deposits in the cornea and skin, thyroid dysfunction (hyper- or hypothyroidism), paresthesias, tremor, and pulmonary fibrosis. Amiodarone rarely causes new arrhythmias, perhaps because it blocks calcium channels and beta receptors as well as sodium and potassium channels.

CLASS II (BETA-BLOCKERS)

A. **Prototypes, Mechanisms, and Effects:** Beta-blockers are discussed in more detail in Chapter 10. Propranolol and esmolol are the prototype antiarrhythmic beta-blockers. Their mechanism in arrhythmias is primarily cardiac beta blockade and reduction in cAMP, which results in the reduction of both sodium and calcium currents and the suppression of abnormal pacemakers. The AV node is particularly sensitive to beta-blockers; the PR interval is usually prolonged by class II drugs (Table 14–2). Under some conditions, these drugs may have some direct local anesthetic (sodium channel-blocking) effect in the heart, but this is probably rare at the concentrations achieved clinically.

B. **Clinical Uses and Toxicities:** Esmolol, a very short-acting beta-blocker for intravenous administration, is used exclusively in acute arrhythmias. Propranolol, metoprolol, and timolol are commonly used as prophylactic drugs in patients who have had a myocardial infarction. These drugs provide a protective effect for 2 years or longer after the infarct.

   The toxicities of beta-blockers are the same in patients with arrhythmias as in patients with other conditions. While patients with arrhythmias are often more prone to β-blocker-induced depression of cardiac output than are patients with normal hearts, it must be noted that judicious use of these drugs reduces progression of chronic congestive heart failure (Chapter 13) and reduces the incidence of potentially fatal arrhythmias in this condition.

Skill Keeper: Characteristics of Beta-Blockers (see Chapter 10)

Describe the important subgroups of beta-blockers and their major pharmacokinetic and pharmacodynamic features. *The Skill Keeper Answer appears at the end of the chapter.*

CLASS III (POTASSIUM CHANNEL BLOCKERS)

A. Prototypes: Sotalol and ibutilide are the prototypical class III drugs. Sotalol is a chiral compound—ie, it has two optical isomers. One isomer is an effective beta-blocker, and both isomers contribute to the antiarrhythmic action. The clinical preparation contains both isomers. Dofetilide is a newer potassium channel-blocking drug. Amiodarone is often classified as a class III drug because it markedly prolongs AP duration as well as blocking sodium channels. Bretylium is an older drug that combines general sympathoplegic actions and a potassium channel-blocking effect in ischemic tissue.

B. Mechanism and Effects: The hallmark of class III drugs is prolongation of the action potential duration. This AP prolongation is caused by blockade of I_{Kr} potassium channels that are responsible for the repolarization of the action potential (Figure 14–6). AP prolongation results in an increase in effective refractory period and reduces the ability of the heart to respond to rapid tachycardias. Sotalol, ibutilide, dofetilide, and amiodarone (and quinidine; see above) produce this effect on most cardiac cells; the action of these drugs is therefore apparent in the ECG as an increase in QT interval. *N*-acetylprocainamide (NAPA), a metabolite of procainamide, also significantly prolongs the action potential and the QT interval. Bretylium, on the other hand, produces AP prolongation mainly in ischemic cells and causes little change in the ECG.

C. Clinical Uses and Toxicities: Bretylium is used only in the treatment of refractory post-myocardial infarction arrhythmias, eg, recurrent ventricular fibrillation. This rarely used drug may

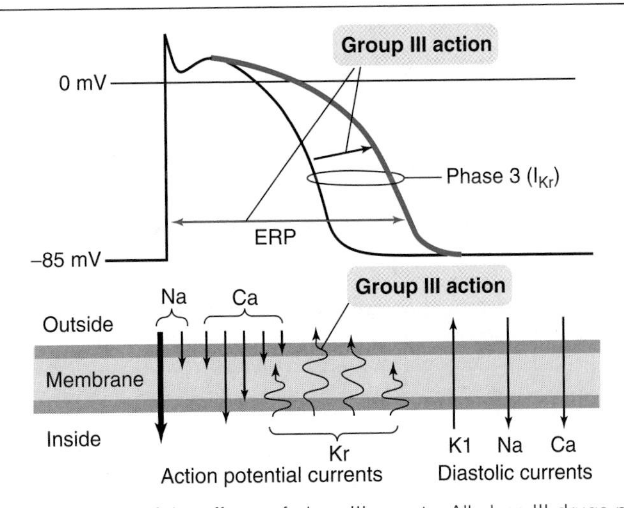

Figure 14–6. Schematic diagram of the effects of class III agents. All class III drugs prolong the AP duration in susceptible cardiac cells by reducing the outward phase 3 potassium current (I_{Kr}, wavy lines). The main effect is to prolong the effective refractory period. Note that the phase 4 diastolic potassium current (I_{K1}) is not affected by these drugs.

precipitate new arrhythmias or marked hypotension. Sotalol is more commonly used and is available by the oral route (Table 14–2). Sotalol may precipitate torsade de pointes arrhythmia as well as signs of excessive beta blockade such as sinus bradycardia or asthma. Ibutilide and dofetilide are recommended for atrial flutter and fibrillation. Their most important toxicity is induction of torsade de pointes. The toxicities of amiodarone and other class IA drugs (which share the I_{Kr} potassium channel-blocking action of class III agents) are discussed with the class IA drugs.

CLASS IV (CALCIUM CHANNEL BLOCKERS)

A. Prototype: Verapamil is the prototype. Diltiazem is also an effective antiarrhythmic drug though it is not approved for this purpose. Nifedipine and the other dihydropyridines are not useful as antiarrhythmics, probably because they decrease arterial pressure sufficiently to evoke a compensatory sympathetic discharge to the heart. The latter effect facilitates rather than suppresses arrhythmias.

B. Mechanism and Effects: Verapamil and diltiazem are effective in arrhythmias that must traverse calcium-dependent cardiac tissue (eg, the atrioventricular node). These agents cause a state- and use-dependent selective depression of calcium current in tissues that require the participation of L-type calcium channels (Figure 14–7). Conduction velocity is decreased and effective refractory period is increased by these drugs. PR interval is consistently increased (Table 14–2).

C. Clinical Use and Toxicities: Calcium channel blockers are effective for converting atrioventricular nodal reentry (also known as nodal tachycardia) to normal sinus rhythm. Their major use is in the prevention of these nodal arrhythmias in patients prone to recurrence. These drugs are orally active; verapamil is also available for parenteral use (Table 14–2). The most important toxicity of verapamil is excessive pharmacologic effect, since cardiac contractility, AV conduction, and blood pressure can be significantly depressed. See Chapter 12 for additional discussion of toxicity. Amiodarone has moderate calcium channel-blocking activity.

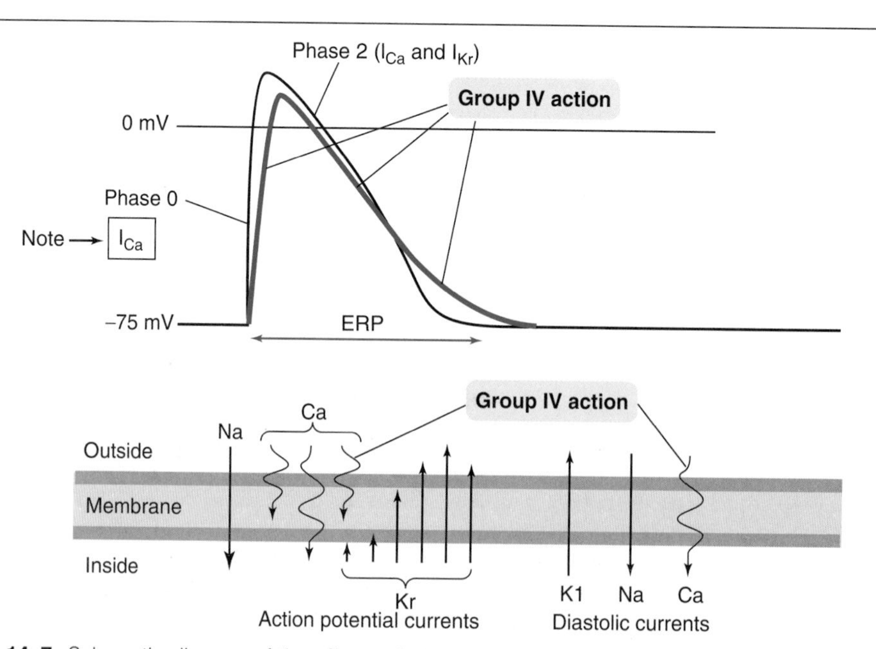

Figure 14–7. Schematic diagram of the effects of class IV drugs in a calcium-dependent cardiac cell in the AV node (note that the AP upstroke is due mainly to calcium current). Class IV drugs reduce inward calcium current during the action potential and during phase 4 (wavy lines). As a result, conduction velocity is slowed in the AV node and refractoriness is prolonged. Pacemaker depolarization during phase 4 is slowed as well if caused by excessive calcium current.

MISCELLANEOUS ANTIARRHYTHMIC DRUGS

A. Adenosine: Adenosine is a normal component of the body, but when it is given in high doses (6–12 mg) as an intravenous bolus the drug markedly slows conduction in the atrioventricular node (Table 14–2), probably by hyperpolarizing this tissue (through increased I_{K1}) and by reducing calcium current. Adenosine is extremely effective in abolishing AV nodal arrhythmias and because of its very low toxicity has become the drug of choice for this arrhythmia. Adenosine has an extremely short duration of action (about 15 seconds). Toxicity includes flushing and hypotension, but because of their short duration these effects do not limit the use of the drug. Chest pain and dyspnea may also occur.

B. Digitalis: The actions of digitalis were discussed in Chapter 13. The cardiac parasympathomimetic action of digoxin is sometimes exploited in the treatment of rapid atrial or AV nodal arrhythmias. In atrial flutter or fibrillation, digitalis slows AV conduction sufficiently to protect the ventricles from excessively high rates. In AV nodal reentrant arrhythmias, digitalis may exert enough depressant effect to abolish the arrhythmia. The latter use of digitalis has become less common since the introduction of calcium channel blockers and adenosine as antiarrhythmic drugs.

C. Potassium Ion: Potassium depresses ectopic pacemakers, including those caused by digitalis toxicity. Hypokalemia is associated with an increased incidence of arrhythmias, especially in patients receiving digitalis. Conversely, excessive potassium levels depress conduction and can cause reentry arrhythmias. Therefore, when treating arrhythmias, serum potassium should be measured and, if abnormal, normalized.

D. Magnesium Ion: Magnesium has not been as well studied as potassium but appears to have similar depressant effects on digitalis-induced arrhythmias. Magnesium also appears to be effective in some cases of torsade de pointes arrhythmia.

DRUG LIST: See Table 14–2.

QUESTIONS

DIRECTIONS: Each of the numbered items or incomplete statements in this section is followed by answers or by completions of the statement. Select the ONE lettered answer or completion that is BEST in each case.

Items 1–3: An elderly patient with rheumatoid arthritis and chronic heart disease is being considered for treatment with procainamide. She is already receiving digoxin, hydrochlorothiazide, and potassium supplements for her cardiac condition.

1. In making your decision to treat with procainamide, which of the following statements would be relevant?
- **(A)** Procainamide may worsen or precipitate hyperthyroidism
- **(B)** Procainamide is not effective for atrial arrhythmias
- **(C)** Procainamide prolongs the effective refractory period in atrial and ventricular cells
- **(D)** Procainamide commonly induces thrombocytopenia
- **(E)** Procainamide commonly induces nausea, headache, and tinnitus

2. In deciding on a treatment regimen with procainamide for this patient, which of the following statements is MOST correct?
- **(A)** A possible drug interaction with digoxin suggests that digoxin blood levels should be obtained before and after starting procainamide
- **(B)** Hyperkalemia should be avoided to reduce the likelihood of procainamide toxicity
- **(C)** Procainamide cannot be used if the patient has asthma because it has a beta-blocking effect
- **(D)** Procainamide has a duration of action of 20–30 hours
- **(E)** Procainamide is not active by the oral route

3. If this patient should manifest severe procainamide toxicity from an overdose, rational therapy would entail the immediate administration of

(A) A calcium chelator such as EDTA
(B) Digitalis
(C) KCl
(D) Nitroprusside
(E) Sodium lactate

4. When used as an antiarrhythmic drug, lidocaine typically
(A) Increases action potential duration
(B) Increases contractility
(C) Increases PR interval
(D) Reduces abnormal automaticity
(E) Reduces resting potential

5. All of the following can be used for chronic oral therapy of arrhythmias EXCEPT
(A) Amiodarone
(B) Disopyramide
(C) Esmolol
(D) Quinidine
(E) Verapamil

6. A 16-year-old girl is found to have paroxysmal attacks of rapid heart rate. The antiarrhythmic of choice in most cases of *acute* AV nodal tachycardia is
(A) Adenosine
(B) Amiodarone
(C) Flecainide
(D) Propranolol
(E) Quinidine

7. A patient is admitted to the emergency department for evaluation of an abnormal ECG. Overdose of an antiarrhythmic drug is considered. Which of the following drugs is correctly paired with its ECG effects?
(A) Quinidine: Increased PR and decreased QT intervals
(B) Flecainide: Increased PR, QRS, and QT intervals
(C) Verapamil: Increased PR interval
(D) Lidocaine: Decreased QRS and PR interval
(E) Metoprolol: Increased QRS duration

8. Drugs that consistently reduce potassium (I_{Kr}) current and thereby prolong the action potential duration include all of the following EXCEPT
(A) Amiodarone
(B) Ibutilide
(C) Lidocaine
(D) Quinidine
(E) Sotalol

9. Recognized adverse effects of quinidine include which one of the following?
(A) Cinchonism
(B) Constipation
(C) Lupus erythematosus
(D) Increase in digoxin clearance
(E) Precipitation of hyperthyroidism

10. A drug that hyperpolarizes and prevents conduction of impulses in the AV node is
(A) Adenosine
(B) Digoxin
(C) Lidocaine
(D) Quinidine
(E) Verapamil

11. Which of the following is an orally active drug that blocks sodium channels and decreases action potential duration?
(A) Adenosine
(B) Amiodarone
(C) Disopyramide
(D) Esmolol
(E) Flecainide
(F) Lidocaine

(G) Mexiletine
(H) Procainamide
(I) Quinidine
(J) Verapamil

12. Which of the following slows conduction through the atrioventricular node and has its primary action directly on L-type calcium channels?
(A) Adenosine
(B) Amiodarone
(C) Disopyramide
(D) Esmolol
(E) Flecainide
(F) Lidocaine
(G) Mexiletine
(H) Procainamide
(I) Quinidine
(J) Verapamil

13. Which of the following has the longest half-life of all antiarrhythmic drugs?
(A) Adenosine
(B) Amiodarone
(C) Disopyramide
(D) Esmolol
(E) Flecainide
(F) Lidocaine
(G) Mexiletine
(H) Procainamide
(I) Quinidine
(J) Verapamil

14. A drug was tested in the electrophysiology laboratory to determine its effects on the cardiac action potential in ventricular cells. The results are shown in the diagram. Which of the following drugs does this agent most resemble?

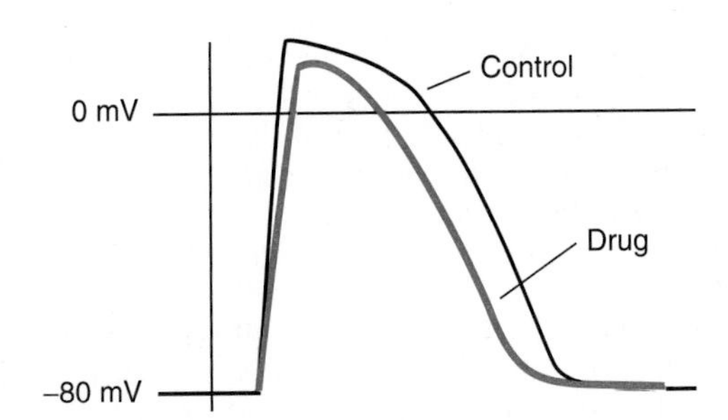

(A) Adenosine
(B) Disopyramide
(C) Flecainide
(D) Lidocaine
(E) Verapamil

DIRECTIONS (Items 15–20): The matching questions in this section consist of a list of lettered options followed by numbered items. For each numbered item, select the ONE lettered option that is most closely associated with it. Each lettered option may be selected once, more than once, or not at all.

(A) Adenosine
(B) Amiodarone
(C) Disopyramide
(D) Esmolol
(E) Flecainide
(F) Lidocaine

(G) Mexiletine
(H) Procainamide
(I) Quinidine
(J) Verapamil

15. Very useful in supraventricular tachycardia; duration of action is 10–15 seconds
16. Beta blocker, used only by the IV route
17. Orally active drug that may cause purpuric rash
18. Derived from the bark of the cinchona tree; may cause tinnitus and diarrhea
19. Causes reversible lupus erythematosus
20. Sodium channel blocker with little effect on AP duration; high incidence of arrhythmia induction

ANSWERS

1. Procainamide prolongs refractory period by blocking sodium channels and by prolonging the action potential. All of the other statements are false. The answer is **(C).**
2. Hyperkalemia facilitates procainamide toxicity. Procainamide is active by the oral route and has a duration of action of 2–4 hours (in the prompt-release form). Procainamide has no documented interaction with digoxin and little or no beta-blocking action. The answer is **(B).**
3. The most effective therapy for procainamide toxicity appears to be concentrated sodium lactate. This drug may (1) increase sodium current by increasing the ionic gradient and (2) reduce drug-receptor binding by alkalinizing the tissue. The answer is **(E).**
4. Lidocaine reduces automaticity in the ventricles; the drug does not alter resting potential or AP duration and does not increase contractility. The answer is **(D).**
5. Esmolol is an ester that is rapidly metabolized even when given intravenously; it is inactive by the oral route. Therefore, esmolol would not be suitable for chronic therapy. The answer is **(C).**
6. Calcium channel blockers are effective in supraventricular tachycardias. However, adenosine is just as effective in most acute nodal tachycardias and is less toxic because of its extremely short duration of action. The answer is **(A).**
7. All the associations listed are incorrect except verapamil. This class IV drug increases PR interval. The answer is **(C).**
8. All of the IA drugs and class III agents reduce potassium current during phase 3 and prolong the action potential. Lidocaine, the prototype IB drug, actually shortens the duration under some circumstances. The answer is **(C).**
9. Quinidine has a wide spectrum of adverse effects but causes increased—not decreased—gastrointestinal motility and often results in diarrhea. Procainamide causes lupus; quinidine causes thrombocytopenia; amiodarone causes thyroid dysfunction. The answer is **(A).**
10. The only antiarrhythmic agent that consistently alters the resting potential of the AV node is adenosine. It apparently activates I_{K1} potassium channels in the AV node, thus forcing the membrane potential closer to the Nernst potassium potential; thus, adenosine significantly hyperpolarizes this tissue, preventing the conduction of action potentials. The answer is **(A).**
11. Class IB drugs such as lidocaine and mexiletine typically block sodium channels and decrease the action potential duration. Mexiletine, but not lidocaine, is orally active. The answer is **(G).**
12. Verapamil is the calcium channel blocker in this list. (Adenosine and beta-blockers also slow AV conduction but do not act primarily on calcium channels.) The answer is **(J).**
13. Amiodarone has the longest half-life of all the antiarrhythmics (Table 14–2). The answer is **(B).**
14. The drug effect shown in the diagram includes slowing of the upstroke of the action potential and shortening of the repolarization phase. This is typical of class IB drugs. The answer is **(D),** lidocaine.
15. The only drug in the list with a half-life of seconds is adenosine. The answer is **(A).**
16. Esmolol is the only beta-blocker in the list. The answer is **(D).**
17. Quinidine may cause thrombocytopenia; this can lead to punctate hemorrhages under the skin (purpura). The answer is **(I).**
18. Quinidine is derived, along with quinine, from cinchona bark. The answer is **(I).**
19. Procainamide frequently results in a positive antinuclear antibody (ANA) test after prolonged

therapy; this may progress to typical signs of drug-induced lupus (joint, skin, and systemic but not renal changes). The answer is **(H).**

20. The IC antiarrhythmic drugs have little effect on AP duration; they have been associated with a high incidence of drug-induced arrhythmias. The answer is **(E).**

Skill Keeper Answer: Characteristics of Beta-Blockers (see Chapter 10)

The major subgroups of beta-blockers and their pharmacologic features are conveniently listed in a table:

Beta-Blocker Subgroup	Features
Nonselective	Propranolol and timolol are typical
β_1-Selective	Atenolol, acebutolol, and metoprolol are typical; possibly less hazardous in asthmatic patients
Partial agonist	Acebutolol and pindolol are typical; possibly less hazardous in asthmatic patients
Lacking local anesthetic effect	Timolol is the prototype; important for use in glaucoma
Low lipid solubility	Atenolol is the prototype; may reduce CNS toxicity
Very short- and long-acting	Esmolol (an ester) is the shortest-acting and used only IV; nadolol is the longest-acting
Combined β and α blockade	Carvedilol, labetalol

15 Diuretic Agents

OBJECTIVES

You should be able to:

- List five major types of diuretics and relate them to their sites of action.
- Describe two drugs that reduce potassium loss during sodium diuresis.
- Describe a therapy that will reduce calcium excretion in patients who have recurrent urinary stones.
- Describe a treatment for severe hypercalcemia in a patient with advanced carcinoma.
- Describe a method for reducing urine volume in nephrogenic diabetes insipidus.
- List the major applications and the toxicities of thiazides, loop diuretics, and potassium-sparing diuretics.

Learn the definitions that follow.

Table 15–1. Definitions.

Term	Definition
Bicarbonate diuretic	A diuretic that selectively increases sodium bicarbonate excretion. Example: a carbonic anhydrase inhibitor
Diluting segment	A segment of the nephron that removes solute without water; the thick ascending limb and the distal convoluted tubule are active salt-absorbing segments that are not permeable by water
Hyperchloremic metabolic acidosis	A shift in body electrolyte and pH balance involving elevated chloride, diminished bicarbonate concentration, and a decrease in pH in the blood. Typical result of bicarbonate diuresis
Hypokalemic metabolic alkalosis	A shift in body electrolyte balance and pH involving a decrease in serum potassium and an increase in blood pH. Typical result of loop and thiazide diuretics
Nephrogenic diabetes insipidus	Loss of urine-concentrating ability in the kidney caused by lack of responsiveness to antidiuretic hormone (ADH is present)
Pituitary diabetes insipidus	Loss of urine-concentrating ability in the kidney caused by lack of antidiuretic hormone (ADH is absent)
Potassium-sparing diuretic	A diuretic that reduces the exchange of potassium for sodium in the collecting tubule; a drug that increases sodium and reduces potassium excretion. Example: aldosterone antagonist
Uricosuric diuretic	A diuretic that increases uric acid excretion, usually by inhibiting uric acid reabsorption in the proximal tubule. Example: ethacrynic acid

CONCEPTS

RENAL TRANSPORT MECHANISMS & DIURETIC DRUG GROUPS

A. **Renal Transport Mechanisms:** Each segment of the nephron—proximal convoluted tubule (PCT), thick ascending limb of the loop of Henle (TAL), distal convoluted tubule (DCT), and cortical collecting tubule (CCT)—has a different mechanism for reabsorbing sodium and other ions. The subgroups of the diuretics are based upon these sites and processes in the nephron (Figure 15–1). The effects of the diuretic agents are predictable from a knowledge of the function of the segment of the nephron in which they act (Figure 15–2).

1. **Proximal convoluted tubule (PCT):** This segment carries out isosmotic reabsorption of amino acids, glucose, and numerous cations. This is also the major site for sodium chloride and sodium bicarbonate reabsorption. The mechanism for bicarbonate reabsorption is shown in Figure 15–3. Bicarbonate itself is poorly reabsorbed through the luminal mem-

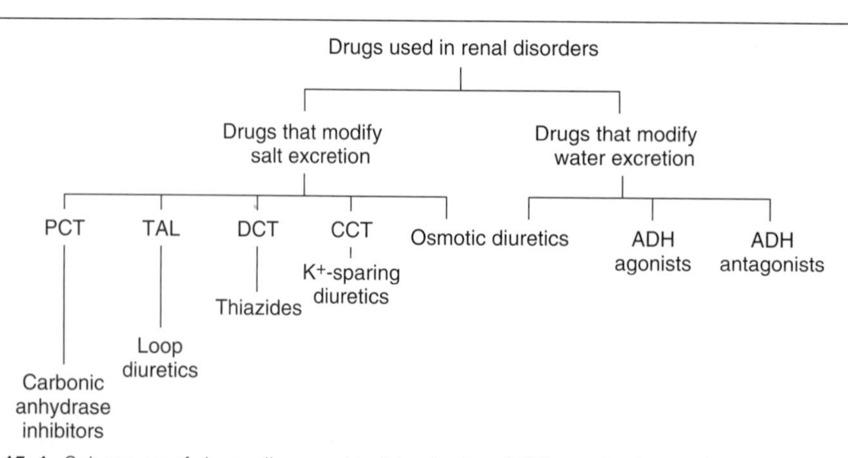

Figure 15–1. Subgroups of drugs discussed in this chapter. (PCT, proximal convoluted tubule; TAL, thick ascending limb of the loop of Henle; DCT, distal convoluted tubule; CCT, cortical collecting tubule.)

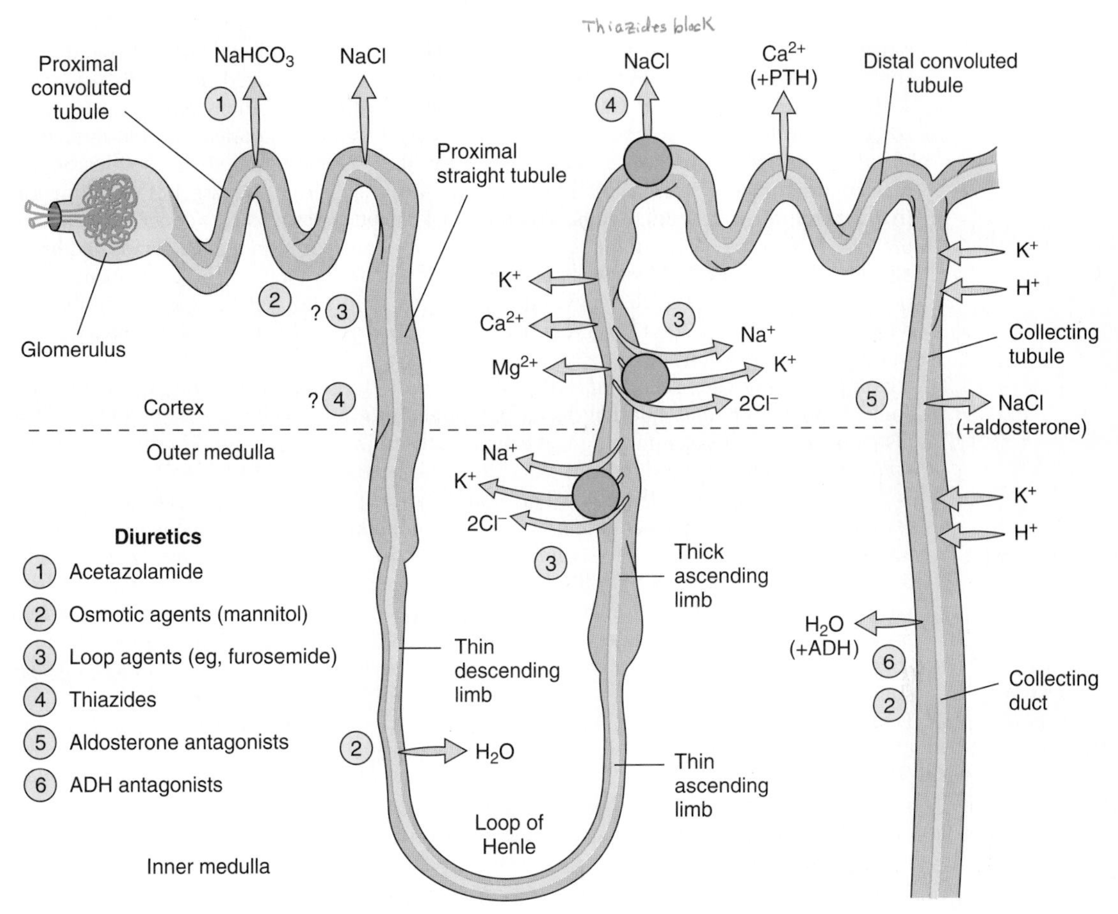

Figure 15–2. Tubule transport systems and sites of action of diuretics. Circles with arrows denote known ion cotransporters that are targets of the diuretics indicated by the numerals. Question marks denote preliminary or incompletely documented suggestions for the location of certain drug effects. (Reproduced, with permission, from Katzung BG [editor]: *Basic & Clinical Pharmacology,* 8th ed. McGraw-Hill, 2001.)

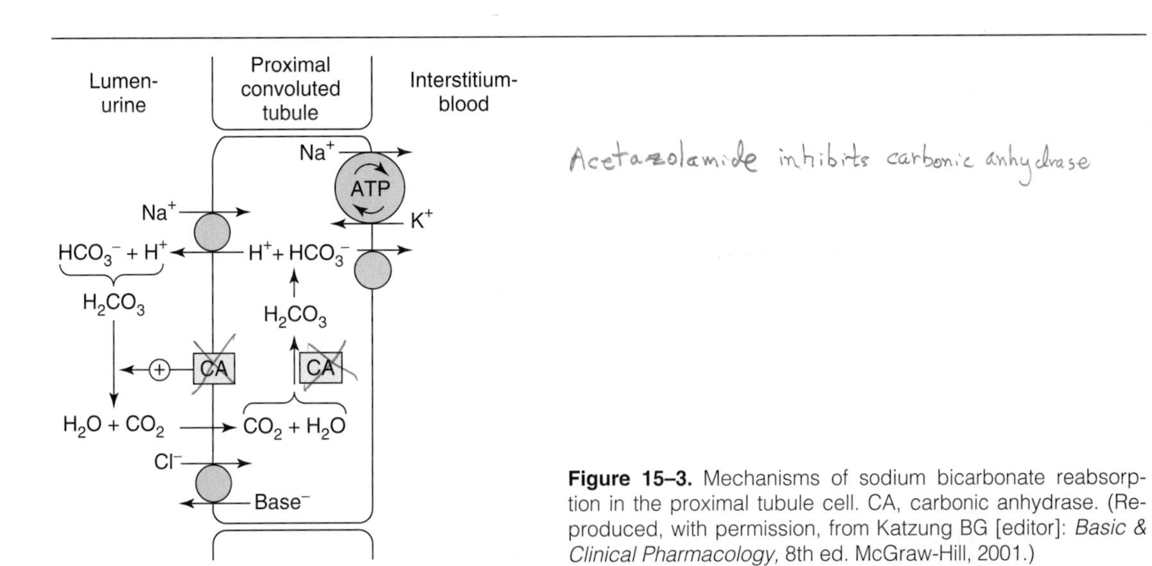

Figure 15–3. Mechanisms of sodium bicarbonate reabsorption in the proximal tubule cell. CA, carbonic anhydrase. (Reproduced, with permission, from Katzung BG [editor]: *Basic & Clinical Pharmacology,* 8th ed. McGraw-Hill, 2001.)

brane, but conversion of bicarbonate to carbon dioxide via carbonic acid permits rapid reabsorption of the carbon dioxide. Bicarbonate can then be regenerated from carbon dioxide within the tubular cell and transported into the interstitium. Sodium is separately reabsorbed from the lumen in exchange for hydrogen ions and transported into the interstitial space by the sodium pump. Carbonic anhydrase, the enzyme required for the bicarbonate reabsorption process on the brush border and in the cytoplasm, is the target of **carbonic anhydrase inhibitor diuretic drugs.** The proximal tubule is responsible for 50% or more of the total reabsorption of sodium. Active secretion and reabsorption of weak acids and bases also occurs in the PCT. Most weak acid transport occurs in the straight S_2 segment of the proximal tubule, distal to the convoluted part. Uric acid transport is especially important and is targeted by some of the drugs used in treating gout (Chapter 35). Weak bases are transported in the S_1 and S_2 segments.

2. **Thick portion of the ascending limb of the loop of Henle (TAL):** This segment pumps sodium, potassium, and chloride out of the lumen into the interstitium of the kidney. It is also a major site of calcium and magnesium reabsorption, as shown in Figure 15–4. Reabsorption of sodium, potassium, and chloride are all accomplished by a single carrier, which is the target of the **loop diuretics.** This cotransporter provides the concentration gradient for the countercurrent-concentrating mechanism in the kidney and is responsible for the reabsorption of 30–40% of the sodium filtered at the glomerulus. Because potassium is pumped into the cell from both the luminal and basal sides, an escape route must be provided; this occurs into the lumen via a potassium-selective channel. Since the potassium diffusing through these channels is not accompanied by an anion, a net positive charge is set up in the lumen. This positive potential drives the reabsorption of calcium and magnesium.
3. **Distal convoluted tubule (DCT):** This segment actively pumps sodium and chloride out of the lumen of the nephron via the carrier shown in Figure 15–5. This cotransporter is the target of the **thiazide diuretics.** The distal convoluted tubule is responsible for approximately 10% of sodium reabsorption. Calcium is also reabsorbed in this segment under the control of parathyroid hormone (PTH). Removal of the reabsorbed calcium back into the blood requires the sodium-calcium exchange process discussed in Chapter 13.
4. **Cortical collecting tubule (CCT):** The final segment of the nephron is the last tubular site of sodium reabsorption and is controlled by aldosterone (Figure 15–6). This segment is responsible for reabsorbing 2–8% of the total filtered sodium. The reabsorption of sodium occurs via channels (not a transporter) and is accompanied by an equivalent loss of potassium or hydrogen ions. The collecting tubule is thus the primary site of acidification of the urine and of potassium excretion. The aldosterone receptor and the sodium channels are sites of action of the **potassium-sparing diuretics.** Reabsorption of water occurs in the medullary collecting tubule under the control of antidiuretic hormone (ADH).

B. Diuretic Drug Groups: Because the mechanisms for reabsorption of salt and water differ in each of the four segments discussed above, the diuretics acting in these segments each have differing mechanisms of action. Most diuretics act from the luminal side of the membrane and

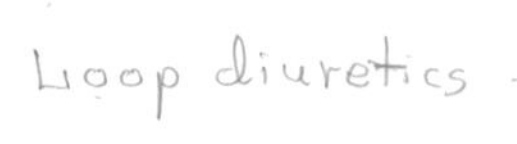

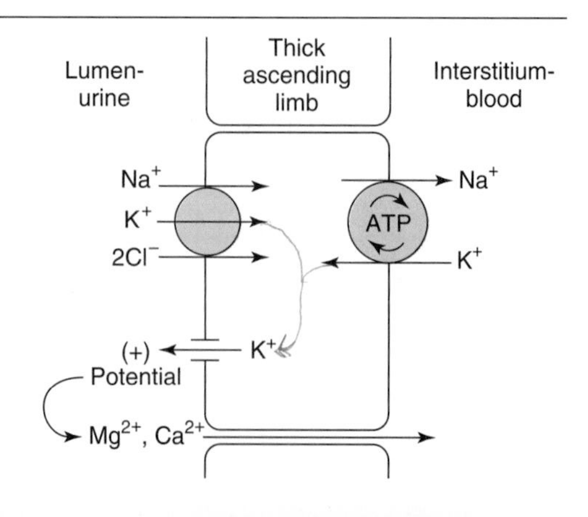

Figure 15–4. Mechanisms of sodium, potassium, and chloride reabsorption in the thick ascending limb of the loop of Henle. Note that pumping of potassium into the cell from both the lumen and the interstitium would result in unphysiologically high intracellular K^+ concentration. This is avoided by movement of K^+ down its concentration gradient back into the lumen, carrying with it excess positive charge. This positive charge drives the reabsorption of calcium and magnesium. (Reproduced, with permission, from Katzung BG [editor]: *Basic & Clinical Pharmacology,* 8th ed. McGraw-Hill, 2001.)

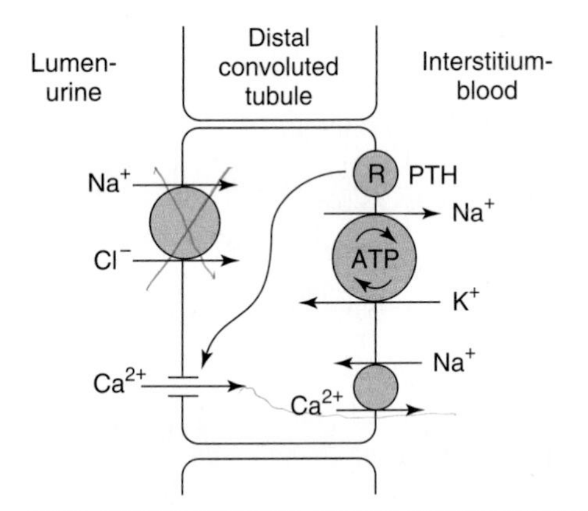

Figure 15–5. Mechanism of sodium and chloride reabsorption in the distal convoluted tubule. A separate reabsorptive mechanism, modulated by parathyroid hormone, is present for movement of calcium into the cell from the urine. This calcium must be transported via the sodium-calcium exchanger back into the blood. (Reproduced, with permission, from Katzung BG [editor]: *Basic & Clinical Pharmacology,* 8th ed. McGraw-Hill, 2001.)

must be present in the urine. They are filtered at the glomerulus and some are also secreted by the weak acid-secretory carrier in the proximal tubule. An exception is the aldosterone receptor antagonist spironolactone, which enters the collecting tubule cell from the basolateral side and binds to the cytoplasmic aldosterone receptor.

CARBONIC ANHYDRASE INHIBITORS

A. Prototypes and Mechanism of Action: **Acetazolamide** is the prototypical agent. These diuretics are sulfonamide derivatives. The mechanism of action is inhibition of carbonic anhydrase in the brush border and intracellular carbonic anhydrase in the PCT cells (Figure 15–3). Inhibition of carbonic anhydrase by acetazolamide occurs in other tissues of the body as well as in the kidney.

B. Effects: The major renal effect is bicarbonate diuresis (ie, sodium bicarbonate is excreted); body bicarbonate is depleted, and metabolic acidosis results. As increased sodium is presented to the cortical collecting tubule, some of the excess sodium is reabsorbed and potassium is se-

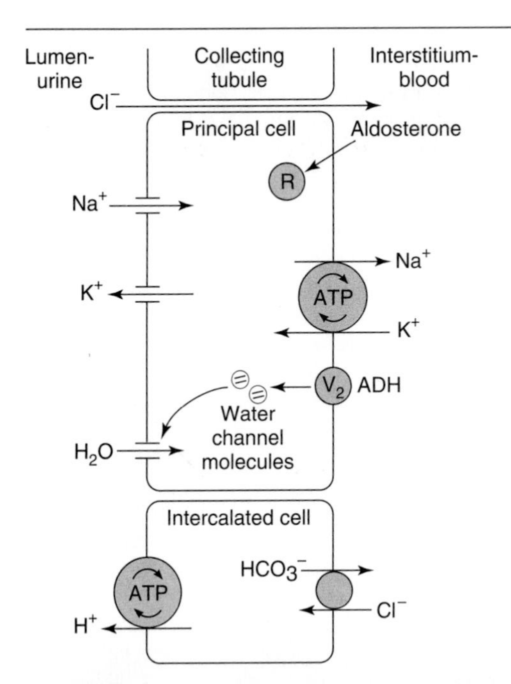

Figure 15–6. Mechanisms of sodium, potassium, and hydrogen ion movement and water reabsorption in the collecting tubule cells. Synthesis of Na^+/K^+ ATPase and sodium and potassium channels is under the control of aldosterone, which combines with an intracellular receptor, *R,* before entering the nucleus. ADH acts on its receptor, V_2, to facilitate the insertion of water channels from storage vesicles into the luminal membrane. (Reproduced, with permission, from Katzung BG [editor]: *Basic & Clinical Pharmacology,* 8th ed. McGraw-Hill, 2001.)

Table 15–2. Electrolyte changes produced by diuretic drugs.

Drug Group	Urine NaCl	Urine $NaHCO_3$	Urine K^+	Body pH
Carbonic anhydrase inhibitors	↑	↑↑↑	↑	Acidosis
Loop diuretics	↑↑↑↑	—	↑	Alkalosis
Thiazides	↑↑	—	↑	Alkalosis
Potassium-sparing diuretics	↑	—	↓	Acidosis

creted, resulting in significant potassium "wasting" (Table 15–2). As a result of bicarbonate depletion, sodium bicarbonate excretion slows—even with continued diuretic administration—and the diuresis is self-limiting within 2–3 days. The inhibitory effect of acetazolamide occurs throughout the body; secretion of bicarbonate into aqueous humor by the ciliary epithelium in the eye and into the cerebrospinal fluid by the choroid plexus is reduced. In the eye, a useful reduction in intraocular pressure can be achieved. This effect is not self-limiting. In the CNS, acidosis of the cerebrospinal fluid results in hyperventilation, which can protect against high-altitude sickness.

C. **Clinical Uses:** The major application of carbonic anhydrase inhibitors is in the treatment of glaucoma. Acetazolamide must be administered orally, but topical analogs are now available (dorzolamide, brinzolamide) for use in the eye. Carbonic anhydrase inhibitors are also used to prevent acute mountain (high-altitude) sickness. These agents are used for their diuretic effect only if edema is accompanied by significant metabolic alkalosis.

D. **Toxicity:** Drowsiness and paresthesias are commonly reported after oral therapy. Cross allergenicity between these and all other sulfonamide derivatives (other sulfonamide diuretics, hypoglycemic agents, antibacterial sulfonamides) is uncommon but does occur. Alkalinization of the urine by these drugs may cause precipitation of calcium salts and formation of renal stones. Renal potassium wasting may be marked. Patients with hepatic impairment may develop hepatic encephalopathy because of increased ammonia reabsorption.

LOOP DIURETICS

block Ca^{2+} reabsorption

A. **Prototypes and Mechanism of Action: Furosemide** is the prototypic loop agent. Furosemide, bumetanide, and torsemide are sulfonamide derivatives. Ethacrynic acid is a phenoxyacetic acid derivative; it is not a sulfonamide but acts by the same mechanism. Loop diuretics inhibit the cotransport of sodium, potassium, and chloride (Figure 15–4). The loop diuretics are relatively short-acting (diuresis usually occurs over a 4-hour period following a dose).

B. **Effects:** The loop of Henle is responsible for a significant fraction of total renal sodium chloride reabsorption; therefore, a full dose of a loop diuretic produces a massive sodium chloride diuresis. If tissue perfusion is adequate, edema fluid is rapidly excreted and blood volume may be significantly reduced. The diluting ability of the nephron is reduced because the loop of Henle is the site of significant dilution of urine. Inhibition of the $Na^+/K^+/2Cl^-$ transporter also results in loss of the lumen-positive potential, which reduces reabsorption of divalent cations as well. As a result, calcium excretion is significantly increased. Ethacrynic acid is a moderately effective uricosuric drug if blood volume is maintained. The presentation of large amounts of sodium to the collecting tubule may result in significant potassium wasting and excretion of protons; hypokalemic alkalosis may result (Table 15–2). The loop diuretics also have potent pulmonary vasodilating effects; the mechanism is not known.

Prostaglandins are important in maintaining glomerular filtration and substrate for diuretic action. When synthesis of prostaglandins is inhibited, as with nonsteroidal anti-inflammatory drugs (Chapter 36), the efficacy of diuretics—especially loop diuretics—decreases.

C. **Clinical Use:** The major application of loop diuretics is in the treatment of edematous states (eg, congestive heart failure and ascites). They are particularly valuable in acute pulmonary edema, in which the pulmonary vasodilating action plays a useful role. They are sometimes used in hypertension if response to thiazides is inadequate, but the short duration of action of loop diuretics is a disadvantage in this condition. A less common but important application is in the treatment of severe hypercalcemia (eg, that induced by malignancy). This life-threatening condition can often be managed with large doses of furosemide coupled with parenteral volume and electrolyte (sodium and potassium chloride) supplementation. It should be noted that diuresis *without* volume replacement will result in hemoconcentration; serum calcium concentration then will not diminish and may even increase further.

D. Toxicity: Loop diuretics usually induce hypokalemic metabolic alkalosis. Because large amounts of sodium are presented to the collecting tubules, wasting of potassium (which is excreted by the kidney in an effort to conserve sodium) may be severe. Because they are so efficacious, the loop diuretics can cause hypovolemia and cardiovascular complications. Ototoxicity is an important toxic effect of the loop agents. The sulfonamides in this group may cause typical sulfonamide allergy.

THIAZIDE DIURETICS

A. Prototypes and Mechanism of Action: Hydrochlorothiazide, the prototypical agent, and all the other members of this group are sulfonamide derivatives. A few derivatives that lack the typical thiazide ring in their structure nevertheless have effects identical to those of thiazides and are therefore considered thiazide-like. Indapamide is one of these thiazide-like agents and has a significant vasodilating effect in addition to its diuretic effect. Thiazides are active by the oral route and have a duration of action of 6–12 hours, considerably longer than the loop diuretics. The major action of thiazides is to inhibit sodium chloride transport in the early segment of the distal convoluted tubule (Figure 15–5).

B. Effects: In full doses, thiazides produce moderate but sustained sodium and chloride diuresis. Hypokalemic metabolic alkalosis may occur (Table 15–2). Reduction in the transport of sodium into the tubular cell reduces intracellular sodium and promotes sodium-calcium exchange. As a result, reabsorption of calcium from the urine is increased and urine calcium content is decreased—the *opposite* of the effect of loop diuretics. Because they act in a diluting segment of the nephron, thiazides may interfere with excretion of water and cause dilutional hyponatremia.

Thiazides reduce the blood pressure (Chapter 11). Initially, the reduction reflects the reduction of blood volume, but with continued use these agents appear to reduce vascular resistance as well. The antihypertensive effect is modest but significant and is maximal at doses lower than the maximal diuretic dosage. Compared with older thiazides and thiazide-like agents, indapamide may have a greater ratio of vasodilating effect relative to its sodium diuretic effect.

When a thiazide is used with a loop diuretic, a synergistic effect occurs with marked diuresis.

C. Clinical Use: The major application of thiazides is in hypertension, for which their long duration and moderate intensity of action are particularly useful. Chronic therapy of edematous conditions such as congestive heart failure is another common application. Chronic renal calcium stone formation can sometimes be controlled with thiazides because of their ability to reduce urine calcium concentration.

D. Toxicity: Massive sodium diuresis with hyponatremia is an uncommon but dangerous early effect of thiazides. Chronic therapy is often associated with potassium wasting, since an increased sodium load is presented to the collecting tubules. Diabetic patients may have significant hyperglycemia. Serum uric acid and lipid levels are also increased in some individuals. Thiazides are sulfonamides and share potential sulfonamide allergenicity.

POTASSIUM-SPARING DIURETICS

A. Prototypes and Mechanism of Action: Spironolactone, a steroid derivative, is a pharmacologic antagonist of aldosterone in the collecting tubules. By combining with and blocking the intracellular aldosterone receptor, spironolactone reduces the expression of genes controlling synthesis of sodium ion channels and Na^+/K^+ ATPase. **Amiloride** and **triamterene** act by blocking the sodium channels in the same portion of the nephron (Figure 15–6). Spironolactone has a slow onset and offset of action (24–72 hours). Amiloride and triamterene have durations of action of 12–24 hours.

B. Effects: All three drugs in this class cause an increase in sodium clearance and a decrease in potassium and hydrogen ion excretion and therefore qualify as "potassium-sparing" diuretics. They may cause hyperkalemic metabolic acidosis (Table 15–2).

C. Clinical Use: Potassium wasting caused by chronic therapy with loop or thiazide diuretics, if not controlled by dietary potassium supplements, will usually respond to these drugs. The most common use is in the form of products that combine a thiazide with a potassium-sparing agent in a single pill.

Aldosteronism (eg, the elevated serum aldosterone levels that occur in cirrhosis) is an important indication for spironolactone. Aldosteronism is also a feature of heart failure, and spironolactone has been shown to have significant long-term benefits in this condition (Chapter 13). Some of this effect may occur in the heart, an action that is not yet understood.

D. Toxicity: The most important toxic effect is hyperkalemia. These drugs should never be given with potassium supplements. Other aldosterone antagonists (such as ACE inhibitors and angiotensin receptor inhibitors), if used at all, should be used with great caution. Spironolactone may cause endocrine abnormalities, including gynecomastia and anti-androgenic effects.

Skill Keeper: Diuretic Combinations & Electrolytes (see Chapter 11)

Describe the possible interactions of ACE inhibitors with diuretics of the thiazide and the potassium-sparing groups. Are such interactions likely to be beneficial or toxic? *The Skill Keeper Answer appears at the end of the chapter.*

OSMOTIC DIURETICS

A. Prototypes and Mechanism of Action: Mannitol, the prototypical osmotic diuretic, is given intravenously. Other drugs often classified with mannitol (but rarely used) include glycerin, isosorbide, and urea. Because it is freely filtered at the glomerulus but poorly reabsorbed from the tubule, mannitol remains in the lumen and "holds" water by virtue of its osmotic effect. The major location for this action is the proximal convoluted tubule, where the bulk of isosmotic reabsorption normally takes place. Reabsorption of water is also reduced in the descending limb of the loop of Henle and the collecting tubule.

B. Effects: The volume of urine is increased. Most filtered solutes will be excreted in larger amounts unless they are actively reabsorbed. Sodium excretion is usually increased because the rate of urine flow through the tubule is greatly accelerated and sodium transporters cannot handle the volume rapidly enough. Mannitol can also reduce brain volume and intracranial pressure by osmotically extracting water from the tissue into the blood. A similar effect occurs in the eye.

C. Clinical Use: These drugs are used to maintain high urine flow (eg, when renal blood flow is reduced and in conditions of solute overload from severe hemolysis or rhabdomyolysis). Mannitol and several other osmotic agents are useful in reducing intraocular pressure in acute glaucoma and intracranial pressure in neurologic conditions.

D. Toxicity: Removal of water from the intracellular compartment may cause hyponatremia and pulmonary edema. As the water is excreted, hypernatremia may follow. Headache, nausea, and vomiting are common.

ANTIDIURETIC HORMONE AGONISTS & ANTAGONISTS

A. Prototypes and Mechanism of Action: Antidiuretic hormone (ADH) and **desmopressin** are prototypical antidiuretic hormone agonists. They are peptides and must be given parenterally. **Demeclocycline** and **lithium** ion are ADH *antagonists* that are administered orally.

ADH facilitates water reabsorption from the collecting tubule by activation of adenylyl cyclase. The increased cAMP causes the insertion of additional water channels into the luminal membrane in this part of the tubule (Figure 15–6). Demeclocycline and lithium inhibit the action of ADH at some point distal to the generation of cAMP and presumably interfere with the insertion of water channels into the membrane.

B. Effects and Clinical Uses: ADH and desmopressin reduce urine volume and increase its concentration. ADH and desmopressin are useful in pituitary diabetes insipidus. They are of no value in the nephrogenic form of the disease, but salt restriction, thiazides, and loop diuretics may be used. These therapies reduce blood volume, a very strong stimulus to proximal tubular reabsorption. The proximal tubule thus substitutes—in part—for the deficient concentrating function of the collecting tubule.

ADH antagonists oppose the actions of ADH and other naturally occurring peptides that act on the same V_2 receptor. Such peptides are produced by certain tumors (eg, small cell carcinoma of the lung) and can cause significant water retention and dangerous hyponatremia. This **syndrome of inappropriate ADH secretion (SIADH)** can be treated with demeclocycline. Lithium also works but has greater toxicity.

C. Toxicity: In the presence of ADH or desmopressin, a large water load may cause dangerous hyponatremia. Large doses of either peptide may cause hypertension in some individuals.

In children under 8 years of age, demeclocycline (like other tetracyclines) causes bone and teeth abnormalities. Lithium causes nephrogenic diabetes insipidus as a toxic effect; the drug is never used to treat SIADH because of its other toxicities.

DRUG LIST

The following drugs are important members of the group discussed in this chapter. Prototypes should be learned in detail; the features of major variants should be known well enough to distinguish the variants from prototypes and from each other; the other significant agents should be recognized as belonging to a specific subclass.

Subclass	Prototype	Major Variants	Other Significant Drugs
Carbonic anhydrase inhibitors	Acetazolamide		Dorzolamide
Loop diuretics	Furosemide	Ethacrynic acid	Bumetanide, torsemide
Thiazides and thiazide-like drugs	Hydrochlorothiazide	Indapamide	Metolazone
Potassium-sparing diuretics	Spironolactone, amiloride		Triamterene
Osmotic diuretics	Mannitol		
ADH agonists	Vasopressin (ADH)	Desmopressin	
ADH antagonists	Demeclocycline	Lithium	

QUESTIONS

DIRECTIONS: Each of the numbered items or incomplete statements in this section is followed by answers or by completions of the statement. Select the ONE lettered answer or completion that is BEST in each case.

1. A 70-year-old man is admitted with a history of heart failure and an acute left ventricular myocardial infarction. He has severe pulmonary edema. Which of the following drugs is LEAST likely to prove useful in the treatment of acute pulmonary edema?
(A) Bumetanide
(B) Ethacrynic acid
(C) Furosemide
(D) Hydrochlorothiazide
(E) Torsemide

2. A 50-year-old man has a history of frequent episodes of renal colic with high-calcium renal stones. The most useful agent in the treatment of recurrent calcium stones is
(A) Mannitol
(B) Furosemide
(C) Spironolactone
(D) Hydrochlorothiazide
(E) Acetazolamide

3. When used chronically to treat hypertension, thiazide diuretics have all of the following properties or effects EXCEPT
(A) Reduce blood volume or vascular resistance, or both
(B) Have maximal effects on blood pressure at doses below the maximal diuretic dose
(C) May cause an elevation of plasma uric acid and triglyceride levels
(D) Decrease the urinary excretion of calcium
(E) Cause ototoxicity

4. Which of the following drugs is correctly associated with its site of action and maximal diuretic efficacy?
(A) Thiazides—distal convoluted tubule—10% of filtered Na^+
(B) Spironolactone—proximal convoluted tubule—40%
(C) Bumetanide—thick ascending limb—15%
(D) Metolazone—collecting tubule—2%
(E) All of the above

5. A patient with long-standing diabetic renal disease and hyperkalemia and recent-onset congestive heart failure requires a diuretic. Which of the following agents would be LEAST harmful in a patient with severe hyperkalemia?
(A) Amiloride
(B) Hydrochlorothiazide
(C) Losartan
(D) Spironolactone
(E) Triamterene

6. Which of the following diuretics would be most useful in a patient with cerebral edema?
(A) Acetazolamide
(B) Amiloride
(C) Ethacrynic acid
(D) Furosemide
(E) Mannitol

7. Which of the following is not a complication of therapy with thiazide diuretics?
(A) Hypercalciuria
(B) Hyponatremia
(C) Hypokalemia
(D) Hyperuricemia
(E) Metabolic alkalosis

8. Which of the following therapies would be most useful in the management of severe hypercalcemia?
(A) Amiloride plus saline infusion
(B) Furosemide plus saline infusion
(C) Hydrochlorothiazide plus saline infusion
(D) Mannitol plus saline infusion
(E) Spironolactone plus saline infusion

9. A 60-year-old patient complains of paresthesias and occasional nausea associated with one of her drugs. She is found to have hyperchloremic metabolic acidosis. She is probably taking

(A) Acetazolamide for glaucoma
(B) Amiloride for edema associated with aldosteronism
(C) Furosemide for severe hypertension and congestive failure
(D) Hydrochlorothiazide for hypertension
(E) Mannitol for cerebral edema

10. A 70-year-old woman is admitted to the emergency room because of a "fainting spell" at home. She appears to have suffered no trauma from her fall, but her blood pressure is 110/60 when lying down and 60/40 when she sits up. Neurologic examination and an ECG are within normal limits when she is lying down. Questioning reveals that she has recently started taking "water pills" (diuretics) for a heart condition. Which of the following drugs is the most likely cause of her fainting spell?
(A) Acetazolamide
(B) Amiloride
(C) Furosemide
(D) Hydrochlorothiazide
(E) Spironolactone

11. A 55-year-old patient with severe post-hepatitis cirrhosis is started on a diuretic for another condition. Two days later he is found in a coma. The drug most likely to cause coma in a patient with cirrhosis is
(A) Acetazolamide
(B) Amiloride
(C) Furosemide
(D) Hydrochlorothiazide
(E) Spironolactone

12. A drug that has its major effect in the distal convoluted tubule is
(A) Acetazolamide
(B) Amiloride
(C) Demeclocycline
(D) Desmopressin
(E) Ethacrynic acid
(F) Furosemide
(G) Metolazone
(H) Mannitol
(I) Spironolactone
(J) Triamterene

13. A drug that increases the formation of dilute urine in water-loaded subjects and is used to treat SIADH is
(A) Acetazolamide
(B) Amiloride
(C) Demeclocycline
(D) Desmopressin
(E) Ethacrynic acid
(F) Furosemide
(G) Metolazone
(H) Mannitol
(I) Spironolactone
(J) Triamterene

14. A drug that is useful in glaucoma and high-altitude sickness is
(A) Acetazolamide
(B) Amiloride
(C) Demeclocycline
(D) Desmopressin
(E) Ethacrynic acid
(F) Furosemide
(G) Metolazone
(H) Mannitol
(I) Spironolactone
(J) Triamterene

DIRECTIONS (Items 15–16): Different diuretic drugs act at different sites in the nephron. The diagram below denotes such potential sites of action with the letters A–E. For questions 15 and 16, select the lettered site of action that applies to the description given.

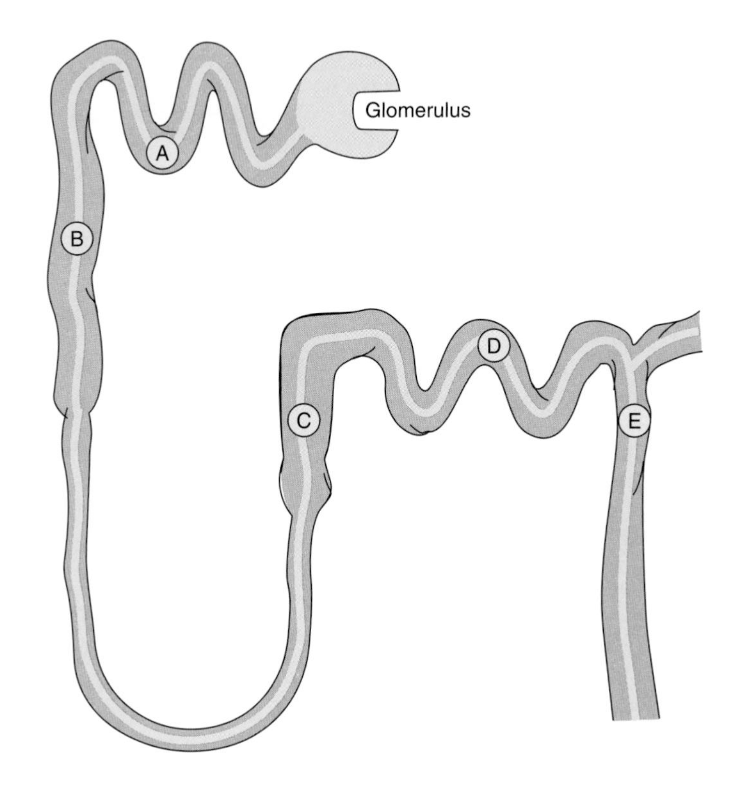

15. Site of action of a drug that blocks a steroid receptor and causes potassium retention.

16. Site of action of a drug that blocks a sodium, potassium, and chloride cotransporter and increases calcium excretion.

DIRECTIONS (Items 17–20): The diagram below shows some of the steps involved in the reabsorption of bicarbonate. For each of the numbered items in the diagram, identify the substance denoted.

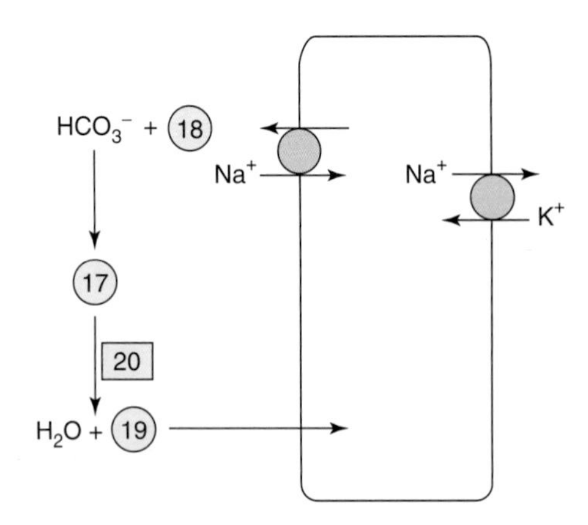

17. Identify the substance denoted 17.

(A) Bicarbonate

(B) Carbon dioxide

(C) Carbonic acid
(D) Carbonic anhydrase
(E) Hydrogen ion

18. Identify the substance denoted 18.
(A) Bicarbonate
(B) Carbon dioxide
(C) Carbonic acid
(D) Carbonic anhydrase
(E) Hydrogen ion

19. Identify the substance denoted 19.
(A) Bicarbonate
(B) Carbon dioxide
(C) Carbonic acid
(D) Carbonic anhydrase
(E) Hydrogen ion

20. Identify the substance denoted 20.
(A) Bicarbonate
(B) Carbon dioxide
(C) Carbonic acid
(D) Carbonic anhydrase
(E) Hydrogen ion

ANSWERS

1. Loop diuretics have a rapid onset of action, are very efficacious, and appear to have significant direct smooth muscle-relaxing effects in the pulmonary vessels. They are therefore drugs of choice in acute pulmonary edema. The only drug in the list that is *not* a loop agent is hydrochlorothiazide. The answer is **(D).**

2. The thiazides are useful in the prevention of calcium stones because these drugs inhibit the renal excretion of calcium. In contrast, the loop agents facilitate calcium excretion. The answer is **(D).**

3. Thiazides do not cause ototoxicity; loop diuretics do. The answer is **(E).**

4. Spironolactone acts in the collecting tubule, not the proximal convoluted tubule. This drug is not usually capable of causing a 40% sodium diuresis. Bumetanide, a loop diuretic, can produce a 30–40% increase in sodium excretion. Metolazone, a thiazide-like drug, acts in the distal convoluted tubule, not in the collecting tubule. The answer is **(A).**

5. Hyperkalemia should not be treated with drugs that interfere with aldosterone production (eg, losartan, an angiotensin II receptor blocker) or collecting tubule potassium excretion (eg, amiloride, spironolactone, triamterene). These agents are all capable of increasing serum potassium. Hydrochlorothiazide would not reduce serum potassium rapidly, but it would not increase it. The answer is **(B).**

6. An osmotic agent is needed to remove water from the cells of the edematous brain and reduce intracranial pressure. The answer is **(E).**

7. Thiazides produce all of the effects listed except hypercalciuria. They *reduce* urine calcium and for this reason are useful in chronic stone-formers. The answer is **(A).**

8. Diuretic therapy of hypercalcemia requires a reduction in calcium reabsorption in the thick ascending limb. However, a loop diuretic alone would reduce blood volume around the remaining calcium so that serum calcium would not decrease appropriately. Therefore, saline infusion should accompany the loop diuretic. The answer is **(B).**

9. Paresthesias and gastrointestinal distress are common adverse effects of acetazolamide, especially when it is taken chronically, as in glaucoma. The observation that the patient has metabolic acidosis also suggests the use of acetazolamide. The answer is **(A).**

10. The case history suggests that the syncope (fainting) is associated with diuretic use. Complications of diuretics that can result in syncope include both postural hypotension (which this patient exhibits) due to excessive reduction of blood volume and arrhythmias due to excessive potassium loss. Potassium wasting is more common with thiazides (because of their long duration of action), but these drugs rarely cause reduction of blood volume sufficient to result in orthostatic hypotension. The answer is **(C).**

11. The carbonic anhydrase inhibitors cause metabolic acidosis and urinary alkalosis. Patients with severe impairment of liver function are unable to synthesize urea efficiently and become dependent on renal excretion of ammonium ion to rid the body of nitrogenous wastes. However, in alkaline urine the ammonium ion is rapidly converted to ammonia gas, which is very rapidly reabsorbed. Hyperammonemia results, with severe neurologic consequences. The answer is **(A).**
12. Metolazone, though not a thiazide, is a sulfonamide that is often used as a thiazide substitute. Metolazone's site of action, effects, and toxicities (including sulfonamide allergy) are indistinguishable from the true thiazides. The answer is **(G).**
13. Inability to form dilute urine in the fully hydrated condition is characteristic of SIADH. Antagonists of ADH are needed to treat this condition. The answer is **(C).**
14. Carbonic anhydrase inhibitors are useful in glaucoma and altitude sickness. The answer is **(A).**
15. Spironolactone is an aldosterone receptor antagonist, acts intracellularly in the cortical collecting tubule, and causes potassium retention. The answer is **(E).**
16. Loop diuretics block the $Na^+/K^+/2Cl^-$ cotransporter. The answer is **(C).**
17. The substance denoted 17 results from the combination of bicarbonate ion with a proton; this is carbonic acid. The answer is **(C).**
18. The substance denoted 18 is countertransported against sodium in the PCT cell and combines with bicarbonate ion to yield carbonic acid; it is a proton. The answer is **(E).**
19. Substance 19 and water are the products of the dissociation of carbonic acid; this is carbon dioxide. The answer is **(B).**
20. The substance denoted 20 is the enzyme that catalyzes the dissociation of carbonic acid into water and carbon dioxide. The answer is **(D).**

Skill Keeper Answer: Diuretic Combinations & Electrolytes (see Chapter 11)

ACE inhibitors reduce angiotensin II production, so aldosterone secretion will be reduced. Sodium excretion may increase, and potassium retention is facilitated. These actions will interact beneficially with thiazides because the latter drugs are used when sodium excretion is desired and cause potassium wasting as an undesirable effect.

When used with potassium-sparing diuretics, the potassium-retaining action of ACE inhibitors (and angiotensin receptor blockers) may result in dangerous hyperkalemia. In general, ACE inhibitors should not be used with any drug that increases serum potassium, including potassium-sparing diuretics and oral potassium chloride supplements. (See Chapter 11 for angiotensin antagonists.)

Part IV. Drugs with Important Actions on Smooth Muscle

Histamine, Serotonin, & the Ergot Alkaloids

16

OBJECTIVES

You should be able to:

- List the major organ system effects of histamine and serotonin.
- Describe the pharmacology of the two generations and three subgroups of H_1 antihistamines; list prototypical agents for each subgroup.
- Describe the pharmacology of the H_2 antihistamines; identify the four members of this group.
- Describe the action, indication, and toxicity of sumatriptan.
- Describe one 5-HT_2 and one 5-HT_3 antagonist and their major applications.
- List the major organ system effects of the ergot alkaloids.
- Describe the major clinical applications and toxicities of the ergot drugs.

Learn the definitions that follow.

Table 16–1. Definitions.

Term	Definition
Acid-peptic disease	Disease of the upper digestive tract caused by acid and pepsin; includes erosions and ulcers
Autacoids	Endogenous substances with complex physiologic and pathophysiologic functions; commonly interpreted to include histamine, serotonin, prostaglandins, and vasoactive peptides
Carcinoid	A neoplasm of the bronchi or gastrointestinal tract that may secrete serotonin and a variety of peptides
Ergotism ("St. Anthony's Fire")	Disease caused by excess ergot alkaloids; classically caused by consumption of grain (in bread, etc) that is contaminated by the ergot fungus
Gastrinoma	A tumor that produces large amounts of gastrin; associated with hypersecretion of gastric acid and pepsin leading to ulceration
IgE-mediated immediate reaction	An allergic response caused by interaction of an antigen with IgE antibodies on mast cells; results in the release of histamine and other mediators of allergy
Oxytocic	A drug that causes contraction of the uterus
Prolactinoma	A tumor of the anterior pituitary that produces large amounts of prolactin and leads to the amenorrhea-galactorrhea syndrome
Zollinger-Ellison syndrome	Syndrome of hypersecretion of gastric acid and pepsin, often caused by gastrinoma; it is associated with severe acid-peptic ulceration and diarrhea

CONCEPTS

Autacoids are endogenous molecules with powerful pharmacologic effects but poorly defined physiologic roles. Histamine and serotonin (5-hydroxytryptamine; 5-HT) are two of the most important autacoids. Both are synthesized in the body from amino acid precursors and then eliminated by amine oxidation; the pathways of synthesis and metabolism are very similar to those used for catecholamine synthesis and metabolism. The ergot alkaloids are a heterogeneous group of drugs that interact with serotonin receptors, dopamine receptors, and alpha receptors. They are included in this chapter because of their effects on serotonin receptors and on smooth muscle.

HISTAMINE

Histamine is formed from the amino acid histidine and is stored in high concentrations in vesicles in mast cells. Histamine is metabolized by the enzymes monoamine oxidase and diamine oxidase. Excess production of histamine in the body (by, for example, systemic mastocytosis) can be detected by measurement of imidazoleacetic acid (its major metabolite) in the urine. Because it is released from mast cells in response to IgE-mediated (immediate) allergic reactions, this autacoid plays an important pathophysiologic role in seasonal rhinitis (hay fever), urticaria, and angioneurotic edema. Histamine also plays an important physiologic role in the control of acid secretion in the stomach and as a neurotransmitter.

A. Receptors and Effects: Two receptors for histamine, H_1 and H_2, mediate most of the well-defined peripheral actions; a third (H_3) has also been identified (Table 16–2).

1. **H_1 receptor:** This G_q-coupled receptor is important in smooth muscle effects, especially those caused by IgE-mediated responses. IP_3 and DAG are the second messengers. Typical responses include bronchoconstriction and vasodilation, the latter by release of nitric oxide, the major component of endothelium-derived relaxing factor (EDRF). Capillary endothelium, in addition to releasing EDRF, also contracts, opening gaps in the permeability barrier and leading to the formation of local edema. These effects are manifest in allergic reactions and in mastocytosis.
2. **H_2 receptor:** This G_s-coupled receptor mediates gastric acid secretion by parietal cells in the stomach. It also has a cardiac stimulant effect. A third action is to reduce histamine release from mast cells—a negative feedback effect. These actions are mediated by activation of adenylyl cyclase, which increases intracellular cAMP.
3. **H_3 receptor:** This receptor appears to be involved mainly in presynaptic modulation of histaminergic neurotransmission in the central nervous system. In the periphery, it appears to be a presynaptic heteroreceptor with modulatory effects on the release of other transmitters (see Chapter 6).

B. Clinical Use: Histamine has no therapeutic applications, but drugs that block histamine's effects are very important in clinical medicine.

Table 16–2. Histamine and some serotonin receptor subtypes.[1]

Receptor Subtype	Distribution	Postreceptor Mechanisms	Prototype Antagonist
H_1	Smooth muscle	G_q; ↑ IP_3, DAG	Diphenhydramine
H_2	Stomach, heart, mast cells	G_s; ↑ cAMP	Cimetidine
H_3	Nerve endings, CNS	G protein-coupled	Impromidine[2]
$5\text{-}HT_{1D}$	Brain	G_i; ↓ cAMP	—
$5\text{-}HT_2$	Smooth muscle, platelets	G_q; ↑ IP_3, DAG	Ketanserin
$5\text{-}HT_3$	Area postrema (CNS), sensory and enteric nerves	Gated cation channel	Ondansetron

[1]Many other serotonin receptors are recognized in the CNS. They are discussed in Chapter 21.
[2]Research use only.

HISTAMINE H_1 ANTAGONISTS

A. Classification and Prototypes: A wide variety of antihistaminic H_1 blockers are available from several different chemical families. Two major subgroups or "generations" have been developed (Figure 16–1). The older members of the first-generation, typified by **diphenhydramine** and **doxylamine,** are highly sedating agents with significant autonomic receptor-blocking effects. A newer subgroup of first-generation agents are less sedating and have much less autonomic effect. **Chlorpheniramine** and **cyclizine** may be considered prototypes. The second-generation H_1 blockers, typified by **fexofenadine, loratadine,** and **cetirizine,** are far less lipid-soluble than the first-generation agents and are mostly free of sedating and autonomic effects. Because they have been developed for use in chronic conditions, all H_1 blockers are active by the oral route. Most are metabolized extensively in the liver. Half-lives of the older H_1 blockers vary from 4 hours to 12 hours. Most newer agents (eg, fexofenadine, cetirizine, loratadine) have half-lives of 12–24 hours.

B. Mechanism and Effects: H_1 blockers are competitive pharmacologic antagonists at the H_1 receptor; these drugs have no effect on histamine release from storage sites. They are more effective if given before histamine release occurs.

Because their structure closely resembles that of muscarinic blockers and α-adrenoceptor blockers, many of the first-generation agents are potent pharmacologic antagonists at these autonomic receptors. A few also block serotonin receptors. As noted above, most older first-generation agents are sedating, and some—not all—first generation agents have anti-motion sickness effects. Many H_1 blockers are potent local anesthetics.

H_1-blocking drugs have negligible effects at H_2 receptors.

C. Clinical Use: H_1 blockers have major applications in allergies of the immediate type (ie, those caused by antigens acting on IgE antibody-sensitized mast cells). These conditions include hay fever and urticaria.

Diphenhydramine, dimenhydrinate, cyclizine, meclizine, and promethazine are used as anti-motion sickness drugs. Diphenhydramine is also used for management of chemotherapy-induced vomiting.

The drugs' adverse effects are sometimes exploited therapeutically, as in their use as hypnotics in institutions and in over-the-counter sleep aids.

D. Toxicity and Interactions: Sedation is common, especially with diphenhydramine, doxylamine, and promethazine. It is much less common with second-generation agents, which do not enter the CNS readily. Antimuscarinic effects such as dry mouth and blurred vision occur with some first-generation drugs in some patients. Alpha-blocking actions may cause orthostatic hypotension.

Interactions occur between older antihistamines and other drugs with sedative effects, eg, benzodiazepines and alcohol. Drugs that inhibit hepatic metabolism may result in dangerously high levels of certain antihistaminic drugs that are taken concurrently. For example, azole antifungal drugs and certain other CYP3A4 inhibitors interfere with the metabolism of astemizole and terfenadine, two second-generation agents that have been withdrawn from the United States market. Excessively high plasma concentrations of either antihistamine can precipitate lethal arrhythmias.

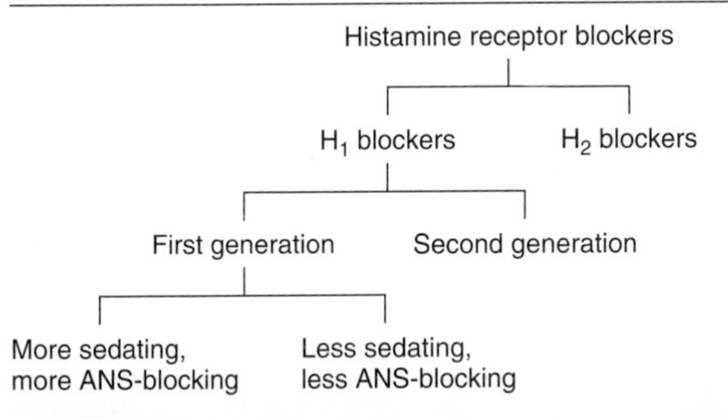

Figure 16–1. Subgroups of histamine receptor blockers.

HISTAMINE H_2 ANTAGONISTS

A. Classification and Prototypes: Four H_2 blockers are available; **cimetidine** is the prototype. **Ranitidine, famotidine,** and **nizatidine** differ only in being slightly less toxic than cimetidine. These drugs do not resemble H_1 blockers structurally. They are orally active, with half-lives of 1–3 hours. Because they are relatively nontoxic, they can be given in large doses, so that the duration of action of a single dose may be 12–24 hours.

B. Mechanism and Effects: These drugs produce a surmountable pharmacologic blockade of histamine H_2 receptors. They are relatively selective and have no significant blocking actions at H_1 or autonomic receptors.

The only therapeutic effect of clinical importance is the reduction of gastric acid secretion, but this is a *very* useful action. Blockade of cardiovascular and mast cell H_2 receptor-mediated effects can be demonstrated but has no clinical significance.

C. Clinical Use: In acid-peptic disease, especially duodenal ulcer, these drugs reduce symptoms, accelerate healing, and prevent recurrences. Acute ulcer is usually treated with two or more doses per day, while recurrence of the ulcer can often be prevented with a single bedtime dose. H_2 blockers are also effective in accelerating healing and preventing recurrences of gastric peptic ulcers. In Zollinger-Ellison syndrome, which is characterized by acid hypersecretion, severe recurrent peptic ulceration, gastrointestinal bleeding, and diarrhea, these drugs are very helpful (though large doses are required, and they are not as effective as proton pump inhibitors). Similarly, the H_2 blockers have been used in gastroesophageal reflux disease (GERD), but they are not as effective as proton pump inhibitors (see Chapter 60).

D. Toxicity: Cimetidine is a potent inhibitor of hepatic drug-metabolizing enzymes and may also reduce hepatic blood flow. Cimetidine also has significant antiandrogen effects in patients receiving high doses. Ranitidine has a weaker inhibitory effect on hepatic drug metabolism; neither it nor the other H_2 blockers appear to have endocrine effects.

Skill Keeper: Antihistamine Adverse Effects (see Chapters 8 and 10)

A young dental patient was given promethazine intravenously to reduce anxiety before undergoing an extraction in the dental office. Promethazine is an older first-generation antihistamine. Predict the CNS and autonomic effects of this drug when given intravenously. *The Skill Keeper Answer appears at the end of the chapter.*

SEROTONIN (5-HYDROXYTRYPTAMINE; 5-HT) & RELATED AGONISTS

Serotonin is produced from tryptophan and stored in vesicles in the enterochromaffin cells of the gut and neurons of the CNS. After release, it is metabolized by monoamine oxidase. Excess production in the body can be detected by measuring its major metabolite, 5-hydroxyindoleacetic acid (5-HIAA), in the urine. Serotonin plays a physiologic role as a neurotransmitter in both the central nervous system and the enteric nervous system and perhaps has a role as a local hormone that modulates gastrointestinal activity. Serotonin is also stored (but synthesized to only a minimal extent) in platelets. In spite of the very large number of serotonin receptors (14 identified to date), the only serotonin *agonists* in clinical use act at 5-HT_{1D} receptors. Serotonin *antagonists* in use or under investigation act at 5-HT_2 and 5-HT_3 receptors (Figure 16–2).

A. Receptors and Effects:

1. **5-HT_1 receptors:** 5-HT_1 receptors are most important in the brain and mediate synaptic inhibition via increased potassium conductance (Table 16–2). Peripheral 5-HT_1 receptors mediate both excitatory and inhibitory effects in various smooth muscle tissues. 5-HT_1 receptors are G_i protein-coupled receptors.

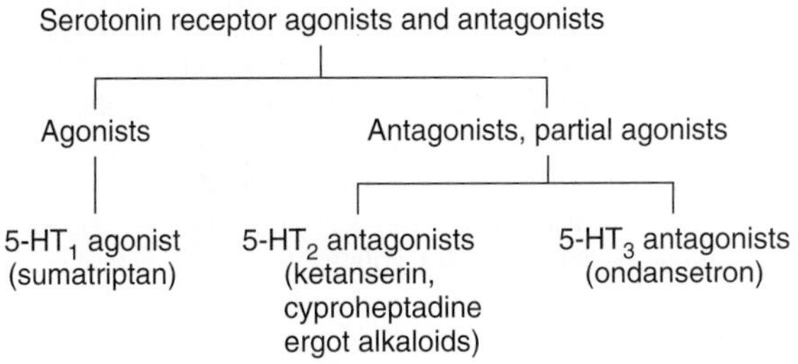

Serotonin receptor agonists and antagonists

- Agonists
  - 5-HT_1 agonist (sumatriptan)
- Antagonists, partial agonists
  - 5-HT_2 antagonists (ketanserin, cyproheptadine ergot alkaloids)
  - 5-HT_3 antagonists (ondansetron)

Figure 16–2. Subgroups of drugs acting at serotonin receptors and nerve endings.

2. **5-HT_2 receptors:** 5-HT_2 receptors are important in both brain and peripheral tissues. These receptors mediate synaptic excitation in the CNS and smooth muscle contraction (gut, bronchi, uterus, vessels) or dilation (vessels). The mechanism involves (in different tissues) increased IP_3, decreased potassium conductance, and decreased cAMP. This receptor probably mediates some of the vasodilation, diarrhea, and bronchoconstriction that occur as symptoms of carcinoid tumor, a neoplasm that releases serotonin and other substances.
3. **5-HT_3 receptors:** 5-HT_3 receptors are found in the CNS, especially in the chemoreceptive area and vomiting center, and in peripheral sensory and enteric nerves. These receptors mediate excitation via a 5-HT-gated cation channel. Antagonists acting at this receptor have proved to be extremely useful antiemetic drugs.

B. Clinical Use: Serotonin has no clinical applications.

C. Other Serotonin Agonists:

1. **5-HT_{1D} agonists:** **Sumatriptan,** a substituted indole compound, is the prototype. **Naratriptan** and **rizatriptan** are similar. They are effective in the treatment of acute migraine and cluster headache attacks, an observation that strengthens the association of serotonin abnormalities with these headache syndromes. These drugs are active orally; sumatriptan is also available for parenteral administration.

   Ergot alkaloids, discussed below, are partial agonists at 5-HT receptors.
2. **Serotonin reuptake inhibitors:** A number of important antidepressant drugs act to increase activity at serotonergic synapses by inhibiting the reuptake carrier for 5-HT. These drugs are discussed in Chapter 29. **Dexfenfluramine** (now withdrawn) was a reuptake inhibitor used exclusively for its appetite-reducing effect. Dexfenfluramine was combined with phentermine, an amphetamine-like anorexiant, in a weight-loss product known as "fen-phen." While effective as an anorexiant, dexfenfluramine caused important cardiac toxicity in the form of subendocardial fibroplasia and valve dysfunction in patients. Neurologic damage was also reported.

SEROTONIN ANTAGONISTS

A. Classification and Prototypes: **Ketanserin** is a 5-HT_2 and alpha-adrenoceptor blocker. **Phenoxybenzamine** (an alpha-adrenoceptor blocker) and **cyproheptadine** (an H_1 blocker) are also good 5-HT_2 blockers. **Ondansetron, granisetron, dolasetron,** and **alosetron** are 5-HT_3 blockers. The **ergot alkaloids** are partial agonists at 5-HT and other receptors (see below).

B. Mechanisms and Effects: Ketanserin and cyproheptadine are competitive pharmacologic antagonists. Phenoxybenzamine is an irreversible blocker.

Ketanserin, cyproheptadine, and phenoxybenzamine are weakly selective agents. In addition to inhibition of serotonin effects, they also have alpha-blocking effects (ketanserin, phenoxybenzamine) or H_1 blocking effects (cyproheptadine).

Ondansetron, granisetron, and dolasetron are selective 5-HT_3 receptor blockers and have a central antiemetic action in the area postrema of the medulla and also on peripheral sensory and enteric nerves.

C. Clinical Uses: Ketanserin has been studied as an antihypertensive drug. Ketanserin, cyproheptadine, and phenoxybenzamine may be of value (separately or in combination) in the treatment of carcinoid tumor, a neoplasm that secretes large amounts of serotonin (and peptides) and causes diarrhea, bronchoconstriction, and flushing.

Ondansetron and its congeners are extremely useful in the control of vomiting associated with cancer chemotherapy and postoperative vomiting. **Alosetron,** another 5-HT_3 antagonist, was used in irritable bowel syndrome in women but has been withdrawn.

D. Toxicity: Adverse effects of ketanserin are those of alpha blockade and H_1 blockade. The toxicities of ondansetron, granisetron, and dolasetron include diarrhea and headache. Dolasetron has been associated with QRS and QT_c prolongation in the ECG and should not be used in patients with heart disease. Alosetron caused significant constipation in some patients.

ERGOT ALKALOIDS

These complex molecules are produced by a fungus found in wet or spoiled grain. They are responsible for the epidemics of "St. Anthony's fire" (ergotism) described during the Middle Ages. There are at least 20 naturally occurring members of the family, but only a few of these and a handful of semisynthetic derivatives are used as therapeutic agents. The ergot alkaloids are partial agonists at α adrenoceptors and 5-HT receptors. The balance of α adrenoceptor versus 5-HT affinity and agonist versus antagonist effect varies from compound to compound and even differs among tissues. Some ergot alkaloids are also agonists at the dopamine receptor.

A. Classification and Prototypes: The ergot alkaloids may be divided into three major subgroups on the basis of the organ or tissue in which they have their primary effects (Figure 16–3). This division is not absolute, since most of the alkaloids have some effects on several tissues.

The brain is a target organ for several natural ergot alkaloids that cause the hallucinations and chemical psychoses associated with epidemics of ergotism. The most important derivatives acting in the CNS, however, are the semisynthetic drugs **LSD** and **bromocriptine.** The uterus is very sensitive to ergot alkaloids as term pregnancy nears but less so at other times. **Ergonovine** is a prototypical oxytocic ergot alkaloid. Blood vessels are sensitive to another subgroup of ergot drugs of which **ergotamine** is the prototype.

B. Effects: The receptor effects of the ergot alkaloids are summarized in Table 16–3 and include the following:

1. **Vessels:** Ergot alkaloids can produce marked and prolonged α receptor-mediated vasoconstriction. An overdose can cause ischemia and gangrene of the limbs.
2. **Uterus:** A powerful contraction occurs in this tissue near term. This is sufficient to cause abortion or miscarriage. Earlier in pregnancy (and in the nonpregnant uterus) much higher doses of ergot alkaloids are needed to produce this effect. After delivery of the placenta, ergonovine or ergotamine can produce a useful contraction of the uterus that reduces blood loss.
3. **Brain:** Hallucinations may be prominent with the naturally occurring ergots and with LSD but are uncommon with the therapeutic ergot derivatives. Although LSD is a potent 5-HT_2 blocker in peripheral tissues, its actions in the CNS are believed to be due to agonist actions at dopamine receptors. In the pituitary, some ergot alkaloids are potent dopamine-like agonists and inhibit prolactin secretion. Bromocriptine and pergolide are among the

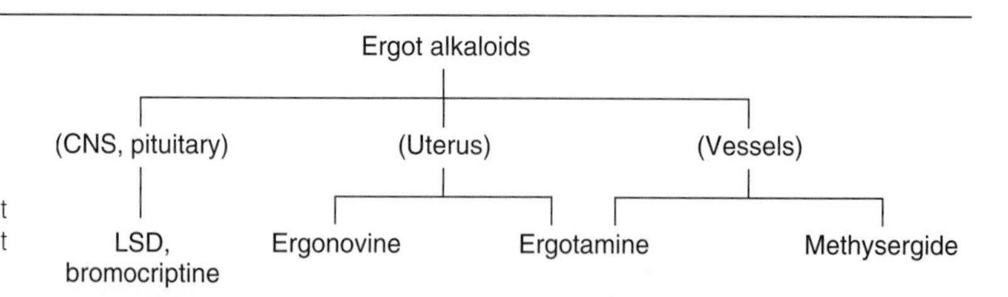

Figure 16–3. Subgroups of ergot alkaloids based on primary target organs.

Table 16–3. Effects of ergot alkaloids at several receptors.*[1]

Ergot Alkaloid	Alpha Adrenoceptor	Dopamine Receptor (D_2)	Serotonin Receptor (5-HT_2)	Uterine Smooth Muscle Stimulation
Bromocriptine	–	+++	–	0
Ergonovine	+	+	– (PA)	+++
Ergotamine	– – (PA)	0	+ (PA)	+++
Lysergic acid diethylamide (LSD)	0	+++	– – (++ in CNS)	+
Methysergide	+/0	+/0	– – – (PA)	+/0

*Reproduced, with permission, from Katzung BG (editor): *Basic & Clinical Pharmacology,* 8th ed. McGraw-Hill, 2001.
[1]Agonist effects are indicated by +, antagonist by –, no effect by 0. Relative affinity for the receptor is indicated by the number of + or – signs. PA means partial agonist.

most potent of the semisynthetic ergot derivatives at these dopamine D_2 receptors in the pituitary. Bromocriptine has similar effects on the dopamine receptors in the basal ganglia.

C. Clinical Uses:

1. **Migraine:** Ergotamine is a mainstay of treatment of acute attacks. Methysergide and ergonovine are used for prophylaxis.
2. **Obstetric bleeding:** Ergonovine and ergotamine are effective agents for the reduction of postpartum bleeding.
3. **Hyperprolactinemia and parkinsonism:** Bromocriptine and pergolide are used to reduce prolactin secretion (dopamine is the physiologic prolactin release inhibitor). Bromocriptine also appears to reduce the size of pituitary tumors of the prolactin-secreting cells. This drug is also useful in the treatment of Parkinson's disease (Chapter 27).

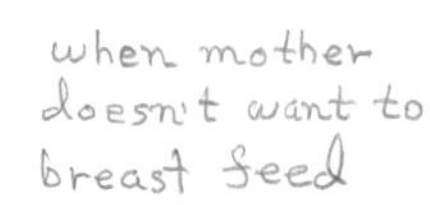

4. **Other uses:** Methysergide has been used in carcinoid tumor.

D. Toxicity: The toxic effects of ergot alkaloids are quite important, both from a public health standpoint (epidemics of ergotism from spoiled grain) and from the toxicity resulting from overdose or abuse by individuals.

1. **Vascular effects:** Severe prolonged vasoconstriction can result in ischemia and gangrene. The only consistently effective antagonist is nitroprusside. When used for long periods, methysergide produces an unusual hyperplasia of connective tissue. This fibroplasia may be retroperitoneal, retropleural, or subendocardial and can cause hydronephrosis or cardiac valvular and conduction system malfunction. Similar lesions are found in some patients with carcinoid, suggesting that this action is probably mediated by agonist effects at serotonin receptors.
2. **Gastrointestinal effects:** Most ergot alkaloids cause gastrointestinal upset (nausea, vomiting, diarrhea) in many individuals.
3. **Uterine effects:** Marked uterine contractions may be produced. The uterus becomes progressively more sensitive to ergot alkaloids during pregnancy. Although abortion due to use of ergot for migraine is rare, most obstetricians recommend avoidance or very conservative use of these drugs as pregnancy progresses.
4. **CNS effects:** Hallucinations resembling psychosis are common with LSD but less so with the other ergot alkaloids. Methysergide has occasionally been used as an LSD substitute by users of "recreational drugs."

DRUG LIST

The following drugs are important members of the group discussed in this chapter. Prototypes should be learned in detail; features of the major variants should be known well enough to distinguish them from the prototypes and from each other; the other significant agents should be recognized as belonging to a specific subclass.

Subclass	Prototype	Major Variants	Other Significant Agents
Histamine agonists	Histamine		
H_1 blockers	Diphenhydramine Chlorpheniramine Fexofenadine		Doxylamine, cyproheptadine, promethazine, cyclizine, loratadine, cetirizine
H_2 blockers	Cimetidine		Ranitidine, famotidine, nizatidine
5-HT agonists	Serotonin, sumatriptan		Naratriptan, rizatriptan
5-HT antagonists	Ketanserin		Cyproheptadine, ergot alkaloids
	Ondansetron		Granisetron, dolasetron
Ergot alkaloids	Bromocriptine	LSD, methysergide	Pergolide
	Ergonovine		
	Ergotamine		

QUESTIONS

DIRECTIONS: Each of the numbered items or incomplete statements in this section is followed by answers or by completions of the sentence. Select the ONE lettered answer or completion that is BEST in each case.

Items 1–2: Your patient has been diagnosed with a rare metastatic carcinoid tumor. This neoplasm is releasing serotonin, bradykinin, and several unknown peptides.

1. The effects of serotonin in this patient are MOST likely to include which one of the following?
(A) Constipation
(B) Episodes of bronchospasm
(C) Hypersecretion of gastric acid
(D) Hypotension
(E) Urinary retention

2. In recommending treatment for your carcinoid patient, you will consider all of the following EXCEPT
(A) Cyproheptadine
(B) Ketanserin
(C) Methysergide
(D) Phenoxybenzamine
(E) Sumatriptan

3. Which of the following drugs can reverse one or more smooth muscle effects of circulating histamine in humans?
(A) Dolasetron
(B) Epinephrine
(C) Granisetron
(D) Ranitidine
(E) Sumatriptan

4. Many antihistamines (H_1 blockers) have additional nonhistamine-related effects; these are likely to include all of the following EXCEPT
(A) Antimuscarinic reduction in bladder tone
(B) Local anesthetic effects if the drug is injected
(C) Anti-motion sickness effect
(D) Increase in total peripheral resistance
(E) Sedation

5. Which of the following will result from blockade of H_2 receptors?
(A) Decreased cAMP in cardiac muscle
(B) Increased cAMP in cardiac muscle
(C) Decreased IP_3 in gastric mucosa
(D) Increased IP_3 in gastric mucosa
(E) Increased IP_3 in smooth muscle

6. Toxicities of H_2 antihistamines include which one of the following?
- **(A)** Blurred vision
- **(B)** Diarrhea
- **(C)** Orthostatic hypotension
- **(D)** P450 inhibition
- **(E)** Sleepiness

7. All of the following statements about possible pharmacologic causes of 16th and 17th century accounts of witchcraft are reasonable EXCEPT
- **(A)** Ingestion of bread made with flour from spoiled grain could cause painful burning sensations in the limbs, leading naive individuals to suspect supernatural evil forces
- **(B)** Similar ingestion could cause "epidemics" of abortions, with similar interpretations
- **(C)** Similar ingestion by elderly women might cause them to have hallucinations and exhibit behaviors interpretable by others as "casting spells"
- **(D)** The major substance now known to occur in spoiled grain is methysergide, a substance similar to PCP

8. A patient undergoing cancer chemotherapy is vomiting frequently. A drug that might help in this situation is
- **(A)** Bromocriptine
- **(B)** Cimetidine
- **(C)** Ketanserin
- **(D)** Loratadine
- **(E)** Ondansetron

9. Which of the following descriptions of H_2 histamine blockers is MOST correct?
- **(A)** All have long half-lives of 12–24 hours
- **(B)** All available H_2 blockers have approximately equal efficacy
- **(C)** Famotidine is associated with more drug interactions than other H_2 blockers as a result of inhibition of hepatic P450 systems
- **(D)** Ranitidine is associated with antiandrogenic effects in some patients
- **(E)** H_2 blockers must be given four or five times a day for therapeutic effect

10. Which of the following is a correct application of the drug mentioned?
- **(A)** Cetirizine: for hay fever
- **(B)** Ergonovine: for Alzheimer's disease
- **(C)** Methysergide: for acute migraine headache
- **(D)** Ondansetron: for acute migraine headache
- **(E)** Ranitidine: for Parkinson's disease

11. Which of the following is most useful in the treatment of hyperprolactinemia?
- **(A)** Bromocriptine
- **(B)** Cimetidine
- **(C)** Ergotamine
- **(D)** Ketanserin
- **(E)** LSD
- **(F)** Methysergide
- **(G)** Nitroprusside
- **(H)** Ondansetron
- **(I)** Phenoxybenzamine
- **(J)** Sumatriptan

12. Which of the following is most effective in the treatment of peptic ulcer disease?
- **(A)** Bromocriptine
- **(B)** Cimetidine
- **(C)** Ergotamine
- **(D)** Ketanserin
- **(E)** LSD
- **(F)** Methysergide
- **(G)** Nitroprusside
- **(H)** Ondansetron
- **(I)** Phenoxybenzamine
- **(J)** Sumatriptan

13. Which of the following is a serotonin agonist useful for aborting an acute migraine headache and is not derived from a fungus?

(A) Bromocriptine
(B) Cimetidine
(C) Ergotamine
(D) Ketanserin
(E) LSD
(F) Methysergide
(G) Nitroprusside
(H) Ondansetron
(I) Phenoxybenzamine
(J) Sumatriptan

14. Which of the following is the most useful for reversing severe ergot-induced vasospasm?
(A) Bromocriptine
(B) Cimetidine
(C) Ergotamine
(D) Ketanserin
(E) LSD
(F) Methysergide
(G) Nitroprusside
(H) Ondansetron
(I) Phenoxybenzamine
(J) Sumatriptan

DIRECTIONS (Items 15 and 16): The matching questions in this section consist of a list of options followed by two numbered items. For each numbered item, select the ONE lettered option that is most closely associated with it.
(A) Bromocriptine
(B) Cimetidine
(C) Ergotamine
(D) Ketanserin
(E) LSD
(F) Methysergide
(G) Nitroprusside
(H) Ondansetron
(I) Phenoxybenzamine
(J) Sumatriptan

15. Causes inhibition of hepatic metabolism of many drugs; some antiandrogenic effects
16. Useful irreversible antagonist for treatment of some carcinoid tumors

ANSWERS

1. Serotonin causes bronchospasm, but the other effects listed are not observed. The answer is **(B).**
2. All of the drugs listed have significant blocking effects on 5-HT receptors except sumatriptan, which is an *agonist* at 5-HT_{1D} receptors. The answer is **(E).**
3. Dolasetron and granisetron are 5-HT_3 antagonists. Sumatriptan is a 5-HT_{1D} agonist. Ranitidine is a histamine antagonist but blocks the H_2 receptor in the stomach and the heart, not H_1 receptors in smooth muscle. Epinephrine has a *physiologic* antagonist action that reverses histamine's effects on smooth muscle. The answer is **(B).**
4. H_1 blockers do not activate receptors that mediate vasoconstriction; some of these drugs actually block α adrenoceptors, causing significant vasodilation. The answer is **(D).**
5. H_2 receptors are G_s protein-coupled receptors, like β adrenoceptors. Blockade of this system will cause a *decrease* in cAMP. The answer is **(A).**
6. The H_1 blockers, not H_2 blockers, cause blurred vision, orthostatic hypotension, and sleepiness. Neither group typically causes diarrhea. Cimetidine is a potent CYP3A4 inhibitor. The answer is **(D).**
7. Historians have noted that many of the behaviors described for accused "witches" and their purported victims during the Salem witch trials period of American history resemble signs of ergotism. Ergotism is caused by a mixture of naturally occurring ergot alkaloids, not methy-

sergide, a semisynthetic ergot derivative. Methysergide is not similar to PCP (phencyclidine). The answer is **(D).**

8. Ondansetron has significant antiemetic effects. The answer is **(E).**
9. H_2 blockers have equal efficacies, though their potencies vary. Cimetidine has significant antiandrogenic and CYP3A4-inhibiting effects. The answer is **(B).**
10. Methysergide is useful in the prophylaxis of migraine headache but is of no value for acute attacks. Cetirizine is useful for the treatment of hay fever. The answer is **(A).**
11. Bromocriptine is an effective dopamine agonist in the CNS with the advantage of oral activity. The drug inhibits prolactin secretion by activating pituitary dopamine receptors. The answer is **(A).**
12. An H_2 blocker is appropriate treatment for peptic ulcer; cimetidine is such a drug. The answer is **(B).**
13. Sumatriptan, an agonist at 5-HT_{1D} receptors, is indicated for parenteral treatment of migraine. Ergotamine is also effective for acute migraine but is produced by the fungus *Claviceps purpurea.* The answer is **(J).**
14. A very powerful vasodilator is necessary to reverse ergot-induced vasospasm; nitroprusside is such a drug. The answer is **(G).**
15. Cimetidine is well known for causing drug interactions because of its ability to inhibit hepatic P450 isozymes. The drug also has weak antiandrogenic effects. The answer is **(B).**
16. Phenoxybenzamine is the only irreversible blocker in this list. The drug has significant affinity for histamine and 5-HT_2 receptors as well as for alpha receptors and has been found useful in some patients with carcinoid, presumably because of this agent's ability to block 5-HT_2 receptors. The answer is **(I).**

Skill Keeper Answer: Antihistamine Adverse Effects (see Chapters 8 and 10)

Promethazine very effectively alleviated the anxiety of this young man. However, when he attempted to get out of the dental chair following the procedure, he experienced severe orthostatic hypotension and fainted. In the horizontal position on the floor and later on a couch, he rapidly regained consciousness. Supine blood pressure was low normal, and heart rate was elevated. When he sat up, blood pressure dropped and heart rate increased. Promethazine and several other first-generation agents are effective α (and M_3) blockers (Chapters 8 and 10). After 30 minutes supine, he was able to stand without fainting and experienced only a slight tachycardia. Older antihistaminic agents readily enter the CNS, causing sedation. This young man felt somewhat sleepy for 2 hours but had no further signs or symptoms.

17 Vasoactive Peptides

OBJECTIVES

You should be able to:

- Name an antagonist of angiotensin at its receptor and at least two drugs that reduce the formation of angiotensin II.
- Outline the major effects of bradykinin and atrial natriuretic peptide.
- Describe the functions of converting enzyme (peptidyl dipeptidase, kininase II).
- List two potent vasoconstrictor peptides.
- Describe the effects of vasoactive intestinal peptide, substance P, and calcitonin gene-related peptide.

CONCEPTS

A. Classification and Prototypes: Vasoactive peptides comprise a large class of endogenous substances that function as neurotransmitters as well as local and systemic hormones. The better-known peptides include angiotensin, bradykinin, atrial natriuretic peptide, endothelin, vasoactive intestinal peptide, substance P, calcitonin gene-related peptide, vasopressin, glucagon, and several opioid peptides. Vasopressin is discussed in Chapters 15 and 37, the opioid peptides in Chapter 31, and glucagon in Chapter 41. The peptides discussed in this chapter and their effects are summarized in Table 17–1.

B. Mechanisms: These agents probably all act on cell surface receptors. As indicated in Table 17–1, most act via G protein-coupled receptors and cause the production of second messengers; a few may open ion channels.

ANGIOTENSIN & ITS ANTAGONISTS

A. Source and Disposition: **Angiotensin I** is produced from angiotensinogen by **renin,** an enzyme released from the juxtaglomerular apparatus of the kidney. An inactive decapeptide, angiotensin I is converted into **angiotensin II (AII),** an octapeptide, by **angiotensin-converting**

Table 17–1. Some vasoactive peptides and their properties.

Peptide	Properties
Angiotensin II (AII)	↑ IP_3, DAG. Constricts arterioles, increases aldosterone secretion
Atrial natriuretic peptide (ANP)	↑ cGMP. Dilates vessels, inhibits aldosterone secretion and effects, increases glomerular filtration
Bradykinin	↑ IP_3, DAG; ↑ cAMP, ↑ NO. Dilates arterioles, increases capillary permeability, stimulates sensory pain endings
Calcitonin gene-related peptide (CGRP)	Causes hypotension and tachycardia by unknown mechanisms
Endothelins	↑ IP_3, DAG. Synthesized in vascular endothelium. Constrict most vessels and contract other smooth muscle
Neuropeptide Y (NPY)	Causes vasoconstriction and stimulates the heart. Effects mediated in part by IP_3
Substance P	Dilates arterioles, contracts veins, intestinal, and bronchial smooth muscle, causes diuresis; and is a transmitter in sensory pain neurons
Vasoactive intestinal peptide (VIP)	Dilates vessels, relaxes bronchi and intestinal smooth muscle

enzyme (ACE), also known as peptidyl dipeptidase or kininase II (Figure 11–4). Angiotensin II, the active form of the peptide, is rapidly degraded by peptidases (angiotensinases).

B. Effects: Angiotensin II is a potent arteriolar vasoconstrictor and stimulant of aldosterone release. AII directly increases peripheral vascular resistance and, through aldosterone, causes renal sodium retention. AII also facilitates the release of norepinephrine from adrenergic nerve endings via presynaptic heteroreceptor action. All of these effects are mediated by the angiotensin AT_1 receptor, a G_q-coupled receptor.

C. Clinical Role: Angiotensin II was used in the past by intra-arterial infusion to control bleeding in difficult-to-access sites. The peptide is no longer used for this indication. Its major clinical significance is as a pathophysiologic mediator in some cases of hypertension (high-renin hypertension) and in congestive heart failure. Therefore, AII antagonists are of considerable clinical importance.

D. Antagonists: As noted in Chapter 11, two types of antagonists are available. **Angiotensin-converting enzyme (ACE) inhibitors** (eg, **captopril, enalapril,** others) are important agents for the treatment of hypertension and heart failure. Angiotensin II receptor-blockers (eg, **losartan, valsartan,** others) are orally active nonpeptide inhibitors at the angiotensin II AT_1 receptor. **Saralasin,** a peptide partial agonist at this receptor, is not used clinically. Block of angiotensin's effects by either of these drug types is often accompanied by a compensatory increase in renin and angiotensin I.

BRADYKININ

A. Source and Disposition: Bradykinin is one of several vasodilator **kinins** produced from kininogen by a family of enzymes, the kallikreins. Bradykinin is rapidly degraded by various peptidases, including angiotensin-converting enzyme.

B. Effects: Bradykinin acts through at least two receptors (B_1 and B_2) and causes the production of IP_3, DAG, cAMP, nitric oxide, and prostaglandins in tissues (Table 17–1). It is one of the most potent vasodilators known. The peptide is involved in inflammation and causes edema and pain when released or injected into tissue. Bradykinin can be found in saliva and may play a role in stimulating its secretion.

C. Clinical Role: Although it has no therapeutic application, bradykinin may play a role in the antihypertensive action of angiotensin-converting enzyme inhibitors, as previously noted (Chapter 11; Figure 11–4). At present there are no clinically important bradykinin antagonists.

ATRIAL NATRIURETIC PEPTIDE

A. Source and Disposition: Atrial natriuretic peptide (ANP; also known as atrial natriuretic factor [ANF]) is synthesized and stored in the cardiac atria of mammals. Atrial natriuretic peptide is released from the atria in response to distension of the chambers. Two similar peptides, brain natriuretic peptide (BNP) and C-type natriuretic peptide (CNP), have been isolated from brain, heart, and other tissues.

B. Effects: Atrial natriuretic peptide activates guanylyl cyclase in many tissues (Table 17–1). ANP is a vasodilator as well as a natriuretic (sodium excretion-enhancing) agent. Its renal action includes increased glomerular filtration, decreased proximal tubular sodium reabsorption, and inhibitory effects on renin secretion. The peptide also inhibits the actions of angiotensin II and aldosterone. Although it lacks positive inotropic action, endogenous atrial natriuretic peptide may play an important compensatory role in congestive heart failure by limiting sodium retention.

C. Clinical Role: ANP has been studied for possible use in the treatment of congestive heart failure, but results have been mixed. BNP has showed some benefit in small studies in patients with heart failure. At present there are no clinically important products that act as agonists or antagonists at atrial natriuretic peptide receptors.

ENDOTHELINS

Endothelins are peptide vasoconstrictors formed in and released by endothelial cells in blood vessels. Endothelins are believed to function as autocrine and paracrine hormones in the vasculature. Three different endothelin peptides (ET-1, ET-2, and ET-3) with minor variations in amino acid sequence have been identified in humans. Two receptors have been identified, both of which are G protein-coupled.

Endothelins are much more potent than norepinephrine as vasoconstrictors and have a relatively long-lasting effect. The peptides also stimulate the heart, increase atrial natriuretic peptide release, and activate smooth muscle proliferation. The peptides may be involved in some forms of hypertension and other cardiovascular disorders. Antagonists have recently become available for research use.

VASOACTIVE INTESTINAL PEPTIDE, SUBSTANCE P, CALCITONIN GENE-RELATED PEPTIDE, & NEUROPEPTIDE Y

Vasoactive intestinal peptide (VIP) is an extremely potent vasodilator but is probably more important as a neurotransmitter. It is found in the central and peripheral nervous systems and in the gastrointestinal tract. No clinical application has been found for this peptide.

Substance P is another neurotransmitter peptide with potent vasodilator action on arterioles. However, substance P is a potent *stimulant* of veins and of intestinal and airway smooth muscle. The peptide may also function as a local hormone in the gastrointestinal tract. Highest concentrations of substance P are found in those parts of the nervous system that contain neurons subserving pain. At the present time, there are no clinical applications for substance P or its antagonists. However, **capsaicin,** the "hot" component of chili peppers, releases substance P from its stores in nerve endings and depletes the peptide. Capsaicin has been approved for topical use on arthritic joints and for postherpetic neuralgia.

Calcitonin gene-related peptide (CGRP) is found (along with calcitonin) in high concentrations in the thyroid but is also present in most smooth muscle tissues. The presence of CGRP in smooth muscle suggests a function as a cotransmitter in autonomic nerve endings. CGRP is the most potent hypotensive agent discovered to date and causes reflex tachycardia. There is no clinical application for this peptide at present.

Unlike the three preceding peptides in this section, neuropeptide Y (NPY) is a potent *vasoconstrictor* that also stimulates the heart. NPY is found in both the CNS and the peripheral nerves. In the periphery, NPY is most commonly localized as a cotransmitter in adrenergic nerve endings. Several receptor subtypes have been identified.

Skill Keeper: Angiotensin Antagonists
(see Chapter 11)

Discuss the differences between ACE inhibitors and AT_1-receptor blockers in the context of the peptides described in this chapter. *The Skill Keeper Answer appears at the end of the chapter.*

DRUG LIST: See Table 17–1.

QUESTIONS

DIRECTIONS: Each of the numbered items or incomplete statements in this section is followed by answers or by completions of the statement. Select the ONE lettered answer or completion that is BEST in each case.

1. Regarding peptides,

(A) Angiotensin I is the most potent of the series that includes angiotensinogen and angiotensin II

(B) Bradykinin is a potent vasodilator with pain- and edema-inducing effects

(C) Atrial natriuretic peptide increases cardiac contractility in congestive heart failure
(D) Because they cannot cross the blood-brain barrier, peptides are not found in the brain
(E) Bradykinin is inactivated by the enzyme kallikrein

2. Which of the following—if given intravenously—will cause increased gastrointestinal motility and diarrhea?
(A) Angiotensin II
(B) Bethanechol
(C) Bradykinin
(D) Renin
(E) All of the above

3. A peptide that causes increased capillary permeability and edema is
(A) Angiotensin II
(B) Bradykinin
(C) Captopril
(D) Histamine
(E) Losartan

4. Agents that produce arteriolar vasoconstriction include all of the following EXCEPT
(A) Angiotensin II
(B) Endothelin-1
(C) Epinephrine
(D) Serotonin
(E) Substance P

5. A vasodilator that can be inactivated by proteolytic enzymes is
(A) Angiotensin I
(B) Isoproterenol
(C) Histamine
(D) Neuropeptide Y
(E) Vasoactive intestinal peptide

6. Which of the following is released in traumatized tissue; causes pain and edema; and is inactivated by angiotensin converting enzyme?
(A) Angiotensin I
(B) Angiotensin II
(C) Atrial natriuretic peptide
(D) Bradykinin
(E) Calcitonin gene-related peptide
(F) Endothelin
(G) Neuropeptide Y
(H) Renin
(I) Substance P
(J) Vasoactive intestinal peptide

7. Which of the following is a decapeptide precursor of a vasoconstrictor substance?
(A) Angiotensin I
(B) Angiotensin II
(C) Atrial natriuretic peptide
(D) Bradykinin
(E) Calcitonin gene-related peptide
(F) Endothelin
(G) Neuropeptide Y
(H) Renin
(I) Substance P
(J) Vasoactive intestinal peptide

8. Which of the following is an arterial vasodilator found in peripheral and CNS nerves; causes contraction of veins and airway smooth muscle; and is found in afferent pain fibers?
(A) Angiotensin I
(B) Angiotensin II
(C) Atrial natriuretic peptide
(D) Bradykinin
(E) Calcitonin gene-related peptide
(F) Endothelin

(G) Neuropeptide Y
(H) Renin
(I) Substance P
(J) Vasoactive intestinal peptide

9. Which of the following is an octapeptide vasoconstrictor that increases in the blood of hypertensive patients treated with large doses of diuretics?
(A) Angiotensin I
(B) Angiotensin II
(C) Atrial natriuretic peptide
(D) Bradykinin
(E) Calcitonin gene-related peptide
(F) Endothelin
(G) Neuropeptide Y
(H) Renin
(I) Substance P
(J) Vasoactive intestinal peptide

10. Which of the following is a vasodilator that increases in the blood or tissues of patients treated with captopril?
(A) Angiotensin I
(B) Angiotensin II
(C) Atrial natriuretic peptide
(D) Bradykinin
(E) Calcitonin gene-related peptide
(F) Endothelin
(G) Neuropeptide Y
(H) Renin
(I) Substance P
(J) Vasoactive intestinal peptide

11. Which of the following is the most potent vasodilator discovered to date and is found in high concentration in the thyroid?
(A) Angiotensin I
(B) Angiotensin II
(C) Atrial natriuretic peptide
(D) Bradykinin
(E) Calcitonin gene-related peptide
(F) Endothelin
(G) Neuropeptide Y
(H) Renin
(I) Substance P
(J) Vasoactive intestinal peptide

12. Which of the following is a peptide cotransmitter in many autonomic nerve endings and directly relaxes vascular, airway, and gastrointestinal smooth muscle?
(A) Angiotensin I
(B) Angiotensin II
(C) Atrial natriuretic peptide
(D) Bradykinin
(E) Calcitonin gene-related peptide
(F) Endothelin
(G) Neuropeptide Y
(H) Renin
(I) Substance P
(J) Vasoactive intestinal peptide

DIRECTIONS (Items 13–14): These matching questions consist of a list of lettered options followed by the numbered items. For each numbered item, select the ONE lettered option that is most closely associated with it.

(A) Angiotensin I
(B) Angiotensin II
(C) Atrial natriuretic peptide

(D) Bradykinin
(E) Calcitonin gene-related peptide
(F) Endothelin
(G) Neuropeptide Y
(H) Renin
(I) Substance P
(J) Vasoactive intestinal peptide

13. Peptide cotransmitter found in autonomic nerve endings; a vasoconstrictor
14. A potent vasoconstrictor peptide synthesized in the endothelium of blood vessels

ANSWERS

1. Angiotensin I is an inactive precursor. Atrial natriuretic peptide has no effect on cardiac contractility. Peptides are found in high concentrations in parts of the brain because they are synthesized there. The answer is **(B).**
2. The peptides listed here are not associated with marked increases in gastrointestinal motility. Bethanechol, a muscarinic cholinoceptor agonist, is an effective stimulant of the gut. The answer is **(B).**
3. Histamine and bradykinin both cause a marked increase in capillary permeability that is often associated with edema, but histamine is not a peptide. The answer is **(B).**
4. Substance P is a potent arterial *vasodilator.* The answer is **(E).**
5. A peptide, but not an amine, would be altered by proteolytic enzymes. Vasoactive intestinal peptide is the only peptide in the list that is a vasodilator. The answer is **(E).**
6. Bradykinin is a mediator of tissue damage, pain, and edema. The answer is **(D).**
7. Angiotensin I is a decapeptide. The answer is **(A).**
8. Substance P is an arteriolar vasodilator that is also a pain-mediating neurotransmitter. The answer is **(I).**
9. Angiotensin II, an octapeptide, increases when blood volume decreases because the compensatory response causes an increase in renin secretion. The answer is **(B).**
10. Bradykinin increases because the enzyme inhibited by captopril, converting enzyme, normally degrades kinins in addition to synthesizing angiotensin II (see Figure 11–4). The answer is **(D).**
11. The most potent vasodilator discovered to date is calcitonin gene-related peptide. The answer is **(E).**
12. Vasoactive intestinal peptide is a general smooth muscle relaxant that is also an important cotransmitter in ANS nerves. The answer is **(J).**
13. Neuropeptide Y is found in many sympathetic postganglionic nerve endings as a cotransmitter. Unlike vasoactive intestinal peptide (another autonomic cotransmitter), neuropeptide Y is a vasoconstrictor. The answer is **(G).**
14. Endothelins are synthesized in vascular endothelium and are powerful vasoconstrictors. The answer is **(F).**

Skill Keeper Answer: Angiotensin Antagonists (see Chapter 11)

Both ACE inhibitors (captopril, etc) and AT_1-receptor blockers (losartan, etc) reduce the effects of the renin-angiotensin-aldosterone system and thereby reduce blood pressure. Both result in a compensatory increase in the release of renin and angiotensin I. The major difference between the two types of drugs results from the fact that ACE inhibitors increase the circulating levels of bradykinin because bradykinin is normally eliminated by angiotensin-converting enzyme. The increase in bradykinin contributes to the hypotensive action of ACE inhibitors but is probably also responsible for the high incidence of cough associated with ACE inhibitor use. The cough is believed to result from prostaglandins synthesized as a result of the increased bradykinin. AT_1-receptor blockers lack this effect.

18 Prostaglandins & Other Eicosanoids

OBJECTIVES

You should be able to:

- List the major effects of PGE_2, $PGF_{2\alpha}$, LTB_4, LTC_4, and LTD_4.
- List important sites of synthesis and the effects of thromboxane and prostacyclin in the vascular system.
- List the currently available therapeutic antagonists of leukotrienes and prostaglandins and their targets (receptors or enzymes).
- Explain the different effects of aspirin on prostaglandin synthesis and on leukotriene synthesis.

Learn the definitions that follow.

Table 18–1. Definitions.

Term	Definition
Abortifacient	A drug used to cause an abortion. *Example:* Prostaglandin $F_{2\alpha}$
Cyclooxygenase	Enzyme that converts arachidonic acid to PGG and PGH, the precursors of the prostaglandins
Dysmenorrhea	Painful uterine cramping activated by prostaglandins released during menstruation
Endoperoxide	General term for prostaglandin precursors, eg, PGG, PGH
Great vessel transposition	Congenital anomaly in which the pulmonary artery exits from the left ventricle and the aorta from the right ventricle. Incompatible with life unless a large patent ductus or ventricular septal defect is present
Lipoxygenase	Enzyme that converts arachidonic acid to leukotriene precursors (HPETEs)
NSAID	Nonsteroidal anti-inflammatory drug, eg, aspirin, ibuprofen, celecoxib. Inhibitor of cyclooxygenase
Patent ductus arteriosus	Persistence after birth of the fetal connection between the pulmonary artery and the aorta
Phospholipase A_2	Enzyme in the cell membrane that generates arachidonic acid from membrane lipid constituents
Slow-reacting substance of anaphylaxis (SRS-A)	Material originally identified by bioassay from tissues of animals undergoing anaphylactic shock; now recognized as a mixture of leukotrienes, especially LTB_4, LTC_4, and LTD_4

CONCEPTS

The eicosanoids are an important group of endogenous fatty acid derivatives that are produced from arachidonic acid. Arachidonic acid is derived from cell membrane lipids.

EICOSANOID AGONISTS

A. Classification: The principal eicosanoid subgroups are the prostaglandins, prostacyclin, thromboxanes, and leukotrienes. Prostacyclin and thromboxane are often considered members of the prostaglandin group since they are also cyclized derivatives. The leukotrienes retain the straight chain configuration of arachidonic acid. There are several series for most of the principal subgroups, based on different substituents (indicated by A, B, C, etc) and different numbers of double bonds (indicated by a subscript 2, 3, 4, etc) in the molecule.

B. **Synthesis:** (Figure 18–1) Active eicosanoids are synthesized in response to various stimuli, eg, physical injury, immune reactions. These stimuli activate phospholipases in the cell membrane or cytoplasm, and arachidonic acid is released from membrane phospholipids. Arachidonate is then metabolized by one of several possible mechanisms. The two most important mechanisms are as follows: First, metabolism to straight-chain products is carried out by **lipoxygenase,** finally producing leukotrienes. Second, cyclization by the enzyme **cyclooxygenase** may occur, resulting in the production of prostacyclin, prostaglandins, or thromboxane. Cyclooxygenase (COX) exists in at least two forms. **COX-1** is found in many tissues; the prostaglandins produced in these tissues by COX-1 appear to be important for a variety of normal physiologic processes (see below). In contrast, **COX-2** is found primarily in inflammatory cells; the products of its actions play a major role in tissue injury, eg, inflammation. Thromboxane is preferentially synthesized in platelets, whereas prostacyclin is synthesized in the endothelial cells of vessels. Naturally occurring eicosanoids have very short half-lives (seconds to minutes) and are inactive when given by the oral route.

C. **Mechanism of Action:** Most eicosanoid effects appear to be brought about by activation of cell surface receptors that are coupled by G proteins to adenylyl cyclase (producing cAMP) or the phosphatidylinositol cascade (producing IP_3 and DAG second messengers).

D. **Effects:** A vast array of effects are produced in smooth muscle, platelets, the CNS, and other tissues. Some of the most important effects are summarized in Table 18–2. Eicosanoids most directly involved in pathologic processes include $PGF_{2\alpha}$, thromboxane A_2 (TXA_2), and the leukotrienes LTC_4 and LTD_4. LTC_4 and LTD_4 comprise the important mediator of bronchoconstriction, **slow-reacting substance of anaphylaxis (SRS-A).** Leukotriene LTB_4 is a chemotactic factor important in inflammation. PGE_2 and prostacyclin may play important roles as endogenous vasodilators. PGE_1 and its derivatives have significant protective effects on the gastric mucosa. The mechanism may involve increased secretion of bicarbonate and mucus, decreased acid secretion, or both. PGE_1 and PGE_2 relax vascular and other smooth muscle. PGE_2 is believed to be the natural vasodilator that maintains patency of the ductus arteriosus during fetal development. PGE_2 and $PGF_{2\alpha}$ are released in large amounts from the endometrium during menstruation and may play a physiologic role in labor. PGE_2 appears to be involved in the physiologic ripen-

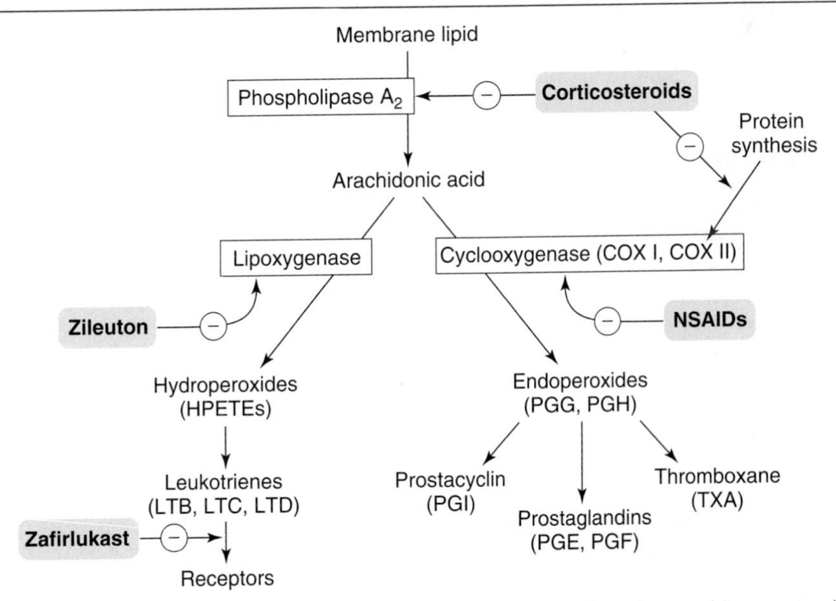

Figure 18–1. Synthesis of eicosanoids and sites of inhibitory effects of corticosteroids, nonsteroidal anti-inflammatory drugs (NSAIDs), and leukotriene antagonist drugs.

Table 18–2. Effects of some important eicosanoids.

Effect	PGE_2	PGF_{2a}	PGI_2	TXA_2	LTB_4	LTC_4	LTD_4
Vascular tone	↓	↑↑	↓↓	↑↑↑	?	↑ or ↓	↑ or ↓
Bronchial tone	↓↓	↑	↓	↑↑↑	?	↑↑↑↑	↑↑↑↑
Uterine tone	↑↑	↑↑↑	↓		?	?	?
Platelet aggregation	↑ or ↓	?	↓↓↓	↑↑↑	?	?	?
Leukocyte chemotaxis	?	?	?	?	↑↑↑↑	?	?

? = unknown effect.

ing of the cervix at term. Dysmenorrhea is associated with uterine contractions induced by prostaglandins, especially $PGF_{2\alpha}$. Platelet clotting is strongly activated by thromboxane. $PGF_{2\alpha}$ reduces intraocular pressure (see below), but it is not known whether this is a physiologic effect of endogenous $PGF_{2\alpha}$. Therapeutic effects of prostaglandins are described below.

E. Clinical Uses:

1. **Obstetrics:** PGE_2 and $PGF_{2\alpha}$ are involved in contraction of the uterus. PGE_2 (as **dinoprostone**) is approved for use to ripen the cervix at term before induction of labor with oxytocin. Both PGE_2 and $PGF_{2\alpha}$ have been used as abortifacients in the second trimester of pregnancy. Although effective in inducing labor at term, they produce more adverse effects (nausea, vomiting, diarrhea) than do other oxytocics used for this application. In Europe, the PGE_1 analog **misoprostol** has been used with the progesterone antagonist mifepristone (RU 486) as an extremely effective and safe abortifacient combination. Misoprostol has been used for this purpose in combination with methotrexate in the USA. In 2000, the FDA approved mifepristone for the same application.
2. **Pediatrics:** PGE_1 is given as an infusion to maintain patency of the ductus arteriosus in infants with transposition of the great vessels until surgical correction can be undertaken.
3. **Dialysis:** Prostacyclin (PGI_2) is approved for use (as **epoprostenol**) in severe pulmonary hypertension. It has occasionally been used to prevent platelet aggregation in dialysis machines.
4. **Peptic ulcer associated with NSAID use:** Misoprostol is approved in the USA for the prevention of peptic ulcers in patients who must take high doses of nonsteroidal anti-inflammatory drugs for arthritis and have a history of ulcer associated with this use.
5. **Urology:** PGE_1 (as **alprostadil**) is used in the treatment of impotence. Preparations are available for injection as well as for insertion into the urethra.
6. **Ophthalmology:** **Latanoprost**, a $PGF_{2\alpha}$ derivative, is used for the treatment of glaucoma. **Unoprostone** is a newer related drug. These agents apparently increase the outflow of aqueous humor, thus reducing intraocular pressure.

EICOSANOID ANTAGONISTS

Phospholipase A_2 and cyclooxygenase can be inhibited by drugs; these inhibitors are mainstays in the treatment of inflammation (Figure 18–1; Chapter 36). **Zileuton** is a selective inhibitor of lipoxygenase; some cyclooxygenase inhibitors exert a mild inhibitory effect on leukotriene synthesis. Inhibitors of the receptors for the prostaglandins and the leukotrienes are being actively sought. **Zafirlukast** and **montelukast,** inhibitors at the LTD_4 receptor, are currently available for the treatment of asthma (Chapter 20).

A. Corticosteroids: As indicated in Figure 18–1, corticosteroids inhibit the production of arachidonic acid by phospholipases in the membrane. This effect is mediated by intracellular steroid receptors that, when activated by an appropriate steroid, increase expression of specific proteins capable of inhibiting phospholipase. Steroids also inhibit the synthesis of COX-2. These actions are thought to be the major mechanisms of the important anti-inflammatory action of corticosteroids.

B. NSAIDs: Aspirin and other nonsteroidal (ie, noncorticosteroid) anti-inflammatory drugs inhibit cyclooxygenase and the production of the thromboxane, prostaglandin, and prostacyclin branch of the synthetic path (Figure 18–1). Most of the currently available NSAIDs nonselectively inhibit both COX-1 and COX-2. In fact, most inhibit COX-1 somewhat more effectively than COX-2, the isoform thought to be responsible for synthesis of inflammatory eicosanoids. Selective COX-2 inhibitors include **celecoxib** and **rofecoxib** (see Chapter 36).

Inhibition of cyclooxygenase by aspirin, unlike that of other NSAIDs, is irreversible. It is thought that some cases of aspirin allergy result from diversion of arachidonic acid to the leukotriene pathway when the cyclooxygenase-catalyzed prostaglandin pathway is blocked. The resulting increase in leukotriene synthesis causes the bronchoconstriction that is typical of aspirin allergy. For unknown reasons, this form of aspirin allergy is more common in individuals with nasal polyps.

The antiplatelet action of aspirin results from the fact that inhibition of thromboxane synthesis is essentially permanent in platelets; they lack the machinery for new protein synthesis. In contrast, inhibition of prostacyclin synthesis in the vascular endothelium is temporary because these cells can synthesize new enzyme. Inhibition of prostaglandin synthesis also results in important anti-inflammatory effects. Inhibition of synthesis of fever-inducing prostaglandins in the brain produces the antipyretic action of NSAIDs. Closure of a patent ductus arteriosus in an otherwise normal infant can be accelerated with a potent NSAID such as indomethacin.

C. Leukotriene Antagonists: As noted above, an inhibitor of lipoxygenase (zileuton) and LTD_4 (and LTE_4) receptor antagonists (zafirlukast, montelukast) have become available for clinical use. At present, these agents are approved only for use in asthma.

DRUG LIST

The following drugs are important members of the group discussed in this chapter. Prototypes should be learned in detail; features of the major variants should be known well enough to distinguish the variants from prototypes and from each other; the other significant agents should be recognized as belonging to a specific subclass.

Subclass	Prototype	Major Variants	Other Significant Agents
Prostaglandins	PGE_2 (dinoprostone), $PGF_{2\alpha}$	PGE_1 (misoprostol)	Latanoprost
Prostacyclin	PGI_2 (epoprostenol)		
Thromboxane	TXA_2		
Leukotrienes	LTC_4	LTB_4	LTD_4
Leukotriene inhibitors	Zafirlukast, zileuton		Montelukast
Phospholipase inhibitors	Prednisone, hydrocortisone	(See Chapter 39)	
Cyclooxygenase inhibitors	Aspirin	Ibuprofen, celecoxib, etc (see Chapter 36)	

QUESTIONS

DIRECTIONS: Each of the numbered items or incomplete statements in this section is followed by answers or by completions of the statement. Select the ONE lettered answer or completion that is BEST in each case.

1. Your patient calls the office complaining that your last prescription has caused severe diarrhea. Which of the following is frequently associated with increased gastrointestinal motility and diarrhea?

(A) Corticosteroids
(B) Leukotriene LTB_4
(C) Misoprostol
(D) Timolol
(E) Zileuton

2. Which of the following drugs inhibits cyclooxygenase irreversibly?
   - (A) Aspirin
   - (B) Hydrocortisone
   - (C) Ibuprofen
   - (D) Indomethacin
   - (E) Zileuton
3. Agents that often cause vasoconstriction include all of the following EXCEPT
   - (A) Angiotensin II
   - (B) Methysergide
   - (C) $PGF_{2\alpha}$
   - (D) Prostacyclin
   - (E) Thromboxane
4. A patient complains of severe dysmenorrhea. A uterine stimulant derived from membrane lipid in the endometrium is
   - (A) Angiotensin II
   - (B) Histamine
   - (C) Prostacyclin (PGI_2)
   - (D) Prostaglandin E_2
   - (E) Serotonin
5. Inflammation is a complex tissue reaction that includes the release of cytokines, leukotrienes, prostaglandins, and peptides. Prostaglandins involved in inflammatory processes are produced from arachidonic acid by
   - (A) Cyclooxygenase 1
   - (B) Cyclooxygenase 2
   - (C) Glutathione-*S*-transferase
   - (D) Lipoxygenase
   - (E) Phospholipase A_2
6. Recognized clinical indications for eicosanoids or their inhibitors include all of the following EXCEPT
   - (A) Abortion
   - (B) Hypertension
   - (C) Patent ductus arteriosus
   - (D) Primary dysmenorrhea
   - (E) Transposition of the great arteries
7. A 60-year-old woman has glaucoma following cataract surgery. Which of the following can be used to reduce intraocular pressure?
   - (A) Leukotriene LTD_4 or its analogs
   - (B) Prostaglandin E_2 or its analogs
   - (C) Prostaglandin $F_{2\alpha}$ or its analogs
   - (D) Slow-reacting substance of anaphylaxis (SRS-A)
   - (E) Thromboxane A_2 or its analogs
8. Which of the following is a reversible inhibitor of platelet cyclooxygenase?
   - (A) Alprostadil
   - (B) Aspirin
   - (C) Ibuprofen
   - (D) LTC_4
   - (E) Misoprostol
   - (F) Prednisone
   - (G) Prostacyclin
   - (H) Zafirlukast
   - (I) Zileuton
9. Which of the following is a component of SRS-A (slow-reacting substance of anaphylaxis)?
   - (A) Alprostadil
   - (B) Aspirin
   - (C) Ibuprofen
   - (D) LTC_4
   - (E) Misoprostol
   - (F) Prednisone
   - (G) Prostacyclin

(H) Zafirlukast
(I) Zileuton

10. Which of the following reduces the activity of phospholipase A_2?
(A) Alprostadil
(B) Aspirin
(C) Ibuprofen
(D) LTC_4
(E) Misoprostol
(F) Prednisone
(G) Prostacyclin
(H) Zafirlukast
(I) Zileuton

11. A 17-year-old patient complains that he gets severe shortness of breath whenever he takes aspirin for headache. Increased levels of which of the following may be responsible, in part, for some cases of aspirin hypersensitivity?
(A) Alprostadil
(B) Aspirin
(C) Ibuprofen
(D) LTC_4
(E) Misoprostol
(F) Prednisone
(G) Prostacyclin
(H) Zafirlukast
(I) Zileuton

12. Which of the following is used to accelerate closure of patent ductus arteriosus in a newborn?
(A) Alprostadil
(B) Aspirin
(C) Ibuprofen
(D) LTC_4
(E) Misoprostol
(F) Prednisone
(G) Prostacyclin
(H) Zafirlukast
(I) Zileuton

13. Which of the following is a leukotriene receptor blocker?
(A) Alprostadil
(B) Aspirin
(C) Ibuprofen
(D) LTC_4
(E) Misoprostol
(F) Prednisone
(G) Prostacyclin
(H) Zafirlukast
(I) Zileuton

DIRECTIONS (Items 14–15): The two matching questions in this section follow a list of lettered options. For each numbered item, select the ONE lettered option that is most closely associated with it. Each lettered option may be selected once, more than once, or not at all.

(A) Alprostadil
(B) Aspirin
(C) Ibuprofen
(D) LTC_4
(E) Misoprostol
(F) Prednisone
(G) Prostacyclin
(H) Zafirlukast
(I) Zileuton

14. Used in the treatment of impotence
15. Lipoxygenase inhibitor

ANSWERS

1. Beta-blockers (eg, timolol), corticosteroids, and zileuton do not cause diarrhea. LTB_4 is a chemotactic factor. The answer is **(C).**
2. Hydrocortisone and other corticosteroids inhibit phospholipase. Ibuprofen and indomethacin inhibit cyclooxygenase reversibly, while zileuton inhibits lipoxygenase. The answer is **(A),** aspirin.
3. Prostacyclin PGI_2 is a very potent vasodilator. The answer is **(D).**
4. While serotonin and, in some species, histamine may cause uterine stimulation, these substances are not derived from membrane lipid. Prostacyclin relaxes the uterus (Table 18–2). The answer is **(D).**
5. Phospholipase A_2 converts membrane phospholipid to arachidonic acid. Cyclooxygenases convert arachidonic acid to prostaglandins. COX-2 is the enzyme believed to be responsible for this reaction in inflammatory cells. The answer is **(B).**
6. None of the vasodilator eicosanoids have a long enough duration of action or sufficient bioavailability to be useful in hypertension. The answer is **(B).**
7. $PGF_{2\alpha}$ and its analogs reduce intraocular pressure. The answer is **(C).**
8. NSAIDs other than aspirin are reversible inhibitors of cyclooxygenase. The answer is **(C).**
9. The leukotriene C and D series are major components of SRS-A. The answer is **(D).**
10. Corticosteroids cause inhibition of phospholipase A_2, the enzyme that releases arachidonic acid from membrane lipids. The answer is **(F).**
11. It is thought that the leukotrienes may be produced in increased amounts when cyclooxygenase is blocked; in patients with aspirin hypersensitivity, this might precipitate the bronchoconstriction often observed in this condition. The answer is **(D).**
12. Ibuprofen has been shown to be effective in accelerating closure of the ductus arteriosus. The answer is **(C).**
13. Zafirlukast is a blocker of LTD_4 receptors. The answer is **(H).**
14. Alprostadil is used by injection into the corpus cavernosa or by absorption from the urethra in impotence. The answer is **(A).**
15. Zileuton is an inhibitor of lipoxygenase. The answer is **(I).**

19 Nitric Oxide, Donors, & Inhibitors

Objectives

You should be able to:

- Name the enzyme responsible for the synthesis of nitric oxide in tissues.
- List the major beneficial and toxic effects of endogenous nitric oxide.
- List two drugs that cause release of endogenous nitric oxide.
- List two drugs that spontaneously or enzymatically break down in the body to release nitric oxide.

Learn the definitions that follow.

Table 19–1. Definitions.

Term	Definition
Endothelium-derived relaxing factor, EDRF	A mixture of nitric oxide and other vasodilator substances synthesized in vascular endothelium
Nitric oxide donor	A molecule from which nitric oxide can be released, eg, arginine, nitroprusside, nitroglycerin
cNOS, iNOS, eNOS	Naturally occurring isoforms of nitric oxide synthase: respectively, constitutive, inducible, and endothelial isoforms

CONCEPTS

Nitric oxide (NO) is a common product of the metabolism of arginine in many tissues. It is thought to be an important paracrine vasodilator, and it may also play a role in cell death and in neurotransmission. Nitric oxide is also released from several important vasodilator drug molecules (see below).

A. Endogenous Nitric Oxide: Endogenous nitric oxide is synthesized by a family of enzymes collectively called **nitric oxide synthase (NOS).** These intracellular enzymes are activated by calcium influx or by cytokines. Arginine, the primary substrate, is converted by NOS to citrulline and nitric oxide. Three forms of nitric oxide synthase are known: isoform I (bNOS, cNOS, or nNOS, a constitutive form found in epithelial and neuronal cells); isoform II (iNOS or mNOS, an inducible form found in macrophages and smooth muscle cells); and isoform III (eNOS, a constitutive form found in endothelial cells). Nitric oxide synthase can be inhibited by arginine analogs such as N^{G}-monomethyl-L-arginine (L-NMMA). Under some circumstances (eg, ischemia), nitric oxide may be formed from endogenous nitrate ion. Nitric oxide is not stored in cells. Because it is a gas at body temperature, nitric oxide *very* rapidly diffuses from its site of synthesis to surrounding tissues. Drugs that cause endogenous nitric oxide release do so by stimulating its synthesis by nitric oxide synthase. Such drugs include acetylcholine, other muscarinic agonists, and histamine.

B. Exogenous Nitric Oxide Donors: Nitric oxide is released from several important drugs, including **nitroprusside** (Chapter 11), **nitrates,** (Chapter 12), and **nitrites.** Release from nitroprusside occurs spontaneously in the blood in the presence of oxygen, while release from nitrates and nitrites is enzymatic, intracellular, and requires the presence of thiol compounds such as cysteine. Tolerance may develop to nitrates and nitrites if endogenous thiol compounds are depleted.

Skill Keeper: Noninnervated Receptors (see Chapter 6)

List the noninnervated receptors found in blood vessels and describe their second-messenger mechanisms of action. *The Skill Keeper Answer appears at the end of the chapter.*

C. Effects of Nitric Oxide:

1. **Smooth muscle:** Nitric oxide is a powerful vasodilator in all vascular beds and a potent relaxant in most other smooth muscle tissues. The mechanism of this effect involves activation of guanylyl cyclase and the synthesis of cGMP. cGMP in turn facilitates the dephosphorylation and inactivation of myosin light chains, which results in relaxation of the muscle cells. Nitric oxide plays a physiologic role in erectile tissue function, in which smooth muscle relaxation is required to bring about the influx of blood that causes erection.

2. **Cell adhesion:** Nitric oxide has effects on cell adhesion that result in reduced platelet aggregation and reduced neutrophil adhesion to vascular endothelium. The latter effect is probably due to reduced expression of adhesion molecules by endothelial cells.
3. **Inflammation:** Nitric oxide appears to *facilitate* inflammation, both directly and through the stimulation of prostaglandin synthesis by cyclooxygenase II.

D. Clinical Applications of Nitric Oxide Inhibitors and Donors: While *inhibitors* of nitric oxide synthesis are of great research interest, none are currently in clinical use. Nitric oxide can be *inactivated* by heme, but application of this approach is in preclinical research.

In contrast, drugs that *release* endogenous nitric oxide and *donors* of the molecule were in use long before nitric oxide was discovered and continue to be very important in clinical medicine. The cardiovascular applications of nitroprusside (Chapter 11) and the nitrates and nitrites (Chapter 12) have been discussed. The treatments of preeclampsia and of pulmonary hypertension and acute respiratory distress syndrome are currently under clinical investigation. Early results from the pulmonary disease studies appear promising, and one preparation of nitric oxide gas (INOmax) has been approved for use in neonates with hypoxic respiratory failure.

Preclinical studies suggest that nitric oxide donor drugs or dietary supplementation with arginine may assist in slowing atherosclerosis, especially in grafted organs. In contrast, *acute rejection* of grafts may involve up-regulation of nitric oxide synthase enzymes, and inhibition of these enzymes may prolong graft survival.

QUESTIONS

DIRECTIONS: Each of the numbered items or incomplete statements in this section is followed by answers or by completions of the statement. Select the ONE lettered answer or completion that is BEST in each case.

1. Molecules from which nitric oxide can be released in vivo include all of the following EXCEPT
   (A) Amyl nitrite
   (B) Arginine
   (C) Histamine
   (D) Isosorbide dinitrate
   (E) Nitroprusside
2. A molecule that stimulates nitric oxide synthase, especially the eNOS isoform, is
   (A) Acetylcholine
   (B) Citrulline
   (C) Isoproterenol
   (D) Nitroglycerin
   (E) Nitroprusside
3. The inducible isoform of nitric oxide synthase (iNOS, isoform II) is found primarily in
   (A) Cartilage
   (B) Eosinophils
   (C) Macrophages
   (D) Platelets
   (E) Vascular endothelial cells
4. The primary endogenous substrate for nitric oxide synthase is
   (A) Acetylcholine
   (B) Angiotensinogen
   (C) Arginine
   (D) Citrulline
   (E) Heme
5. Which of the following is a recognized effect of nitric oxide?
   (A) Arrhythmia
   (B) Bronchoconstriction
   (C) Constipation
   (D) Inhibition of acute graft rejection
   (E) Pulmonary vasodilation

6. Which of the following is an approved application for nitric oxide administered as a gas?
(A) Asthma
(B) Dysmenorrhea
(C) Neonatal hypoxic respiratory failure
(D) Patent ductus arteriosus
(E) Rejection following renal transplant

ANSWERS

1. Nitroprusside and organic nitrites (eg, amyl nitrite) and nitrates (eg, isosorbide dinitrate) contain NO groups that can be released as nitric oxide. Arginine is the normal source of endogenous nitric oxide. Histamine stimulates the production of nitric oxide from arginine. The answer is **(C)**.
2. Acetylcholine is the only molecule in this list that stimulates the endogenous production of nitric oxide by nitric oxide synthase. The answer is **(A)**.
3. The inducible form of nitric oxide synthase is associated with inflammation and the enzyme is found in macrophages. The answer is **(C)**.
4. Arginine is the substrate and citrulline (along with nitric oxide) is the product of nitric oxide synthase. The answer is **(C)**.
5. Nitric oxide does not cause arrhythmias or constipation. It causes bronchodilation and may hasten graft rejection. Nitric oxide does cause pulmonary vasodilation. The answer is **(E)**.
6. Thus far, nitric oxide gas has been approved for use by inhalation only in neonatal hypoxic respiratory failure. The answer is **(C)**.

Skill Keeper Answer: Noninnervated Receptors (see Chapter 6)

Endothelial cells lining blood vessels have noninnervated muscarinic receptors. These M_3 receptors utilize the G_q-coupling protein to activate phospholipase C, which releases IP_3 and DAG from membrane lipids. Other noninnervated (or poorly innervated) receptors found in blood vessels include α_2 and β_2 receptors. Alpha$_2$ receptors utilize G_i to inhibit adenylyl cyclase, reducing cAMP and causing contraction in the vessel. (Recall that the blood pressure-lowering action of α_2 agonists is mediated by actions in the CNS, not in the vessels.) Conversely, β_2 receptors activate adenylyl cyclase via G_s and increase cAMP, resulting in relaxation.

20 Bronchodilators & Other Drugs Used in Asthma

OBJECTIVES

You should be able to:

- Describe the strategies of drug treatment of asthma.
- List the major classes of drugs used in asthma.
- Describe the mechanisms of action of these drug groups.
- List the major adverse effects of the prototype asthma drugs.

Learn the definitions that follow.

Table 20–1. Definitions.

Term	Definition
Bronchial hyperreactivity	Pathologic increase in the bronchoconstrictor response to antigens and irritants; caused by bronchial inflammation
IgE-mediated disease	Disease caused by excessive or misdirected immune response mediated by IgE antibodies. *Example:* asthma
Mast cell degranulation	Exocytosis of granules from mast cells with release of mediators of inflammation and bronchoconstriction
Phosphodiesterase (PDE)	Enzyme that degrades cAMP (active) to AMP (inactive)
Tachyphylaxis	Rapid loss of responsiveness to a stimulus, eg, a drug

CONCEPTS

A. Pathophysiology of Asthma: Asthma is a disease characterized by airway inflammation and episodic, reversible bronchospasm. The immediate cause of the bronchial smooth muscle contraction is the release of several mediators from sensitized mast cells and other cells involved in immunologic responses (Figure 20–1). These mediators include the leukotrienes LTC_4 and LTD_4. In addition, chemoattractant mediators such as LTB_4 attract inflammatory cells to the airways. Finally, several cytokines and some enzymes are released, leading to chronic inflammation. Chronic inflammation leads to marked bronchial hyperreactivity to various inhaled substances, including antigens, histamine, muscarinic agonists, and irritants such as SO_2 and cold air. This reactivity is partially mediated by vagal reflexes.

B. Subgroups of Antiasthmatic Drugs: Drugs useful in asthma include bronchodilators (smooth muscle relaxants) and anti-inflammatory drugs (Figure 20–2). Leukotriene antagonists may have both bronchodilator and anti-inflammatory properties.

Bronchodilators include sympathomimetics, especially β_2-selective agonists, muscarinic antagonists, methylxanthines, and leukotriene receptor blockers.

The most important anti-inflammatory drugs in the treatment of asthma are the corticosteroids and drugs such as cromolyn and nedocromil that inhibit release of mediators from mast cells and other inflammatory cells. The lipoxygenase inhibitor zileuton probably also exerts an anti-inflammatory effect in asthma.

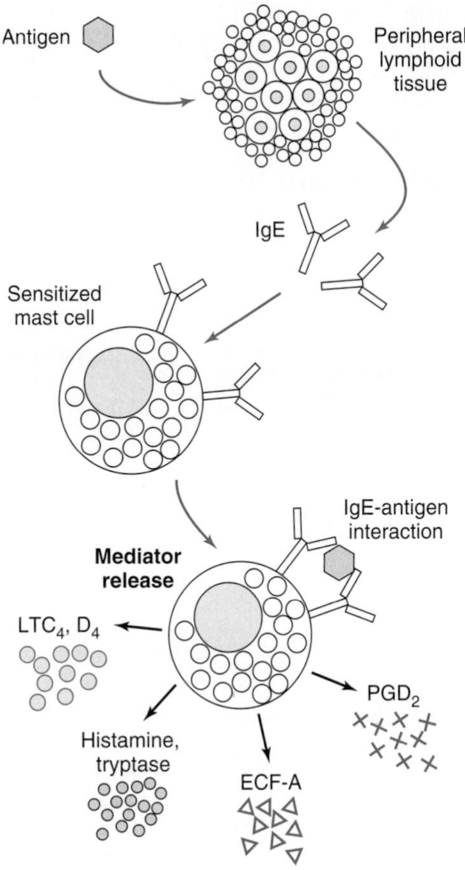

Figure 20–1. Immunologic model for the pathogenesis of asthma. Exposure to antigen causes synthesis of IgE, which binds to and sensitizes mast cells and other inflammatory cells. When such sensitized cells are challenged with antigen, a variety of mediators are released that can account for most of the signs of the early bronchoconstrictor response in asthma. (Modified and reproduced, with permission, from Gold WW: Cholinergic pharmacology in asthma. In: *Asthma Physiology, Immunopharmacology, and Treatment.* Austen KF, Lichtenstein LM [editors]. Academic Press, 1974.)

BETA-ADRENOCEPTOR AGONISTS

A. Prototypes and Pharmacokinetics: The most important sympathomimetics used to reverse asthmatic bronchoconstriction are the β_2-selective agonists, though epinephrine and isoproterenol are still used occasionally (see Chapter 9). Of the selective agents, **terbutaline, albuterol,** and **metaproterenol** are the most important in the USA. **Salmeterol** is a long-acting β_2-selective agonist that is available in the USA. Formoterol is a similar long-acting drug avail-

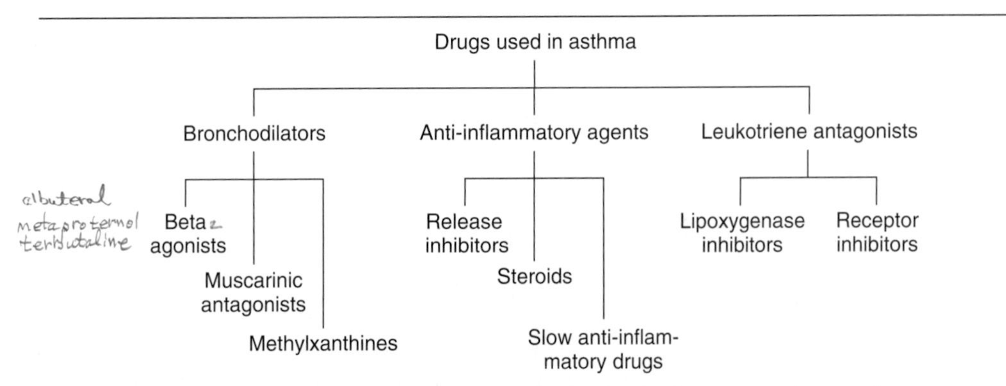

Figure 20–2. Subgroups of drugs discussed in this chapter. Leukotriene antagonists are shown as a separate category because it is not yet clear whether their benefits are primarily as bronchodilators or as anti-inflammatory agents.

able outside the USA. Beta agonists are given almost exclusively by inhalation, usually from pressurized aerosol canisters but occasionally by nebulizer. The inhalational route decreases the systemic dose (and adverse effects) while delivering an effective dose locally to the airway smooth muscle. The older drugs have durations of action of 6 hours or less; salmeterol acts for 12 hours or more.

B. Mechanism and Effects: These agents act by stimulating adenylyl cyclase and increasing cAMP in smooth muscle cells (Figure 20–3). The increase in cAMP results in a powerful bronchodilator response.

C. Clinical Use: Sympathomimetics are used very extensively in asthma. Shorter-acting sympathomimetics (albuterol, metaproterenol, terbutaline) should be used only for acute episodes of bronchospasm (not for prophylaxis), whereas the long-acting agents (salmeterol, formoterol) should be used for prophylaxis, not for acute episodes. In almost all patients, the shorter-acting beta agonists are the most effective bronchodilators available for acute asthma and therefore the drugs of choice.

D. Toxicity: Skeletal muscle tremor is a common adverse β_2 effect. Beta$_2$-selectivity is relative. At high clinical dosage, these agents have significant β_1 effects. Even when they are given by inhalation, some cardiac effect (tachycardia) is common. Other adverse effects are rare. When the agents are used excessively, arrhythmias may occur. Loss of responsiveness (tolerance, tachyphylaxis) is an unwanted effect of excessive use of the short-acting sympathomimetics.

Skill Keeper: Sympathomimetics in Asthma (see Chapter 9)

The sympathomimetic bronchodilators are drugs of choice in acute asthma. Compare the properties of direct- and indirect-acting sympathomimetics relative to the therapeutic goals in asthma. Which type is superior and why? *The Skill Keeper Answer appears at the end of the chapter.*

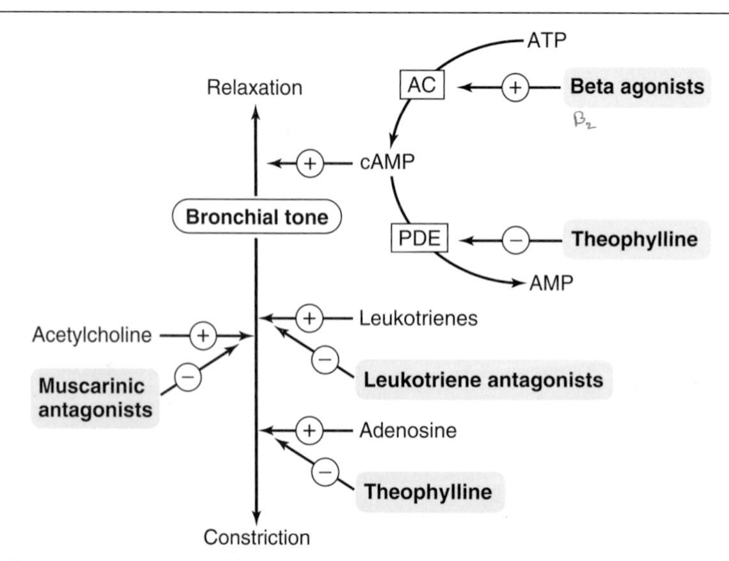

Figure 20–3. Possible mechanisms of beta agonists, muscarinic antagonists, theophylline, and leukotriene antagonists in altering bronchial tone in asthma. AC, adenylyl cyclase; PDE, phosphodiesterase.

METHYLXANTHINES

A. Prototypes and Pharmacokinetics: The methylxanthines are purine derivatives. Three major methylxanthines are found in plants and provide the stimulant effects of three common beverages: **caffeine** (in coffee), **theophylline** (tea), and **theobromine** (cocoa). Theophylline is the only member of this group important in the treatment of asthma. The drug and several analogs are orally active and available as various salts and as the base. Theophylline is provided in both rapid-release and slow-release forms. Theophylline is eliminated by P450 drug-metabolizing enzymes in the liver. Clearance varies with age (highest in young adolescents), smoking status (higher in smokers), and concurrent use of other drugs that inhibit or induce hepatic enzymes.

B. Mechanism of Action: The methylxanthines inhibit phosphodiesterase (PDE), the enzyme that degrades cAMP to AMP (Figure 20–3), and thus increase cAMP. This anti-PDE effect, however, requires high concentrations of the drug. Methylxanthines also block adenosine receptors in the CNS and elsewhere, but a relationship between this action and the bronchodilating effect has not been clearly established. It is possible that bronchodilation is caused by a third as yet unrecognized action.

C. Effects: In asthma, bronchodilation is the most important therapeutic action. Increased strength of contraction of the diaphragm has been demonstrated in some patients. Other effects of therapeutic doses include CNS stimulation, cardiac stimulation, vasodilation, a slight increase in blood pressure (probably caused by the release of norepinephrine from adrenergic nerves), and increased gastrointestinal motility.

D. Clinical Use: The major clinical indication for the use of methylxanthines is asthma; theophylline is the most important methylxanthine in clinical use. Another methylxanthine derivative, **pentoxifylline,** is promoted as a remedy for intermittent claudication; this effect is said to result from decreased viscosity of the blood. Of course, the nonmedical use of the methylxanthines in coffee, tea, and cocoa is far greater, in total quantities consumed, than the medical uses of the drugs.

E. Toxicity: The common adverse effects include gastrointestinal distress, tremor, and insomnia. Severe nausea and vomiting, hypotension, cardiac arrhythmias, and convulsions may result from overdosage. Very large overdoses (eg, in suicide attempts) are potentially lethal because of the arrhythmias and convulsions. Beta-blockers are useful antidotes for severe cardiovascular toxicity from theophylline.

MUSCARINIC ANTAGONISTS

A. Prototypes and Pharmacokinetics: Atropine and other naturally occurring belladonna alkaloids were used for many years in the treatment of asthma with only modest benefits. A quaternary antimuscarinic agent designed for aerosol use, **ipratropium,** has achieved much greater success. This drug is delivered to the airways by pressurized aerosol. When absorbed, ipratropium is rapidly metabolized and has little systemic action.

B. Mechanism of Action: When given as an aerosol, ipratropium competitively blocks muscarinic receptors in the airways and effectively prevents bronchoconstriction mediated by vagal discharge. If given systemically (not an approved use), the drug is indistinguishable from other short-acting muscarinic blockers.

C. Effects: Ipratropium reverses bronchoconstriction in some asthma patients (especially children) and in many patients with chronic obstructive pulmonary disease (COPD). It has no effect on the inflammatory aspects of asthma.

D. Clinical Use: Asthma. Muscarinic blockers are useful in one-third to two-thirds of asthmatic patients; β_2 agonists are effective in almost all. For acute bronchospasm, therefore, the beta agonists are usually preferred. However, in chronic obstructive pulmonary disease (which is often associated with acute episodes of bronchospasm), the antimuscarinic agents may be more effective and less toxic than beta agonists.

E. Toxicity: Because ipratropium is delivered directly to the airway and is minimally absorbed, systemic effects are small. When given in excessive dosage, minor atropine-like toxic effects may occur (Chapter 8). In contrast to the β_2 agonists, ipratropium does not cause tremor or arrhythmias.

CROMOLYN & NEDOCROMIL

A. Prototypes and Pharmacokinetics: Cromolyn (disodium cromoglycate) and nedocromil are unusual chemicals: they are extremely insoluble, so that even massive doses given orally or by aerosol result in minimal systemic blood levels. They are given by aerosol for asthma. Cromolyn is the older compound and is the prototype of this group.

B. Mechanism of Action: The mechanism of action of these drugs is poorly understood but appears to involve a decrease in the release of mediators (such as the leukotrienes and histamine) from mast cells. The drugs have no bronchodilator action but can prevent bronchoconstriction caused by a challenge with antigen to which the patient is allergic. Cromolyn and nedocromil are capable of preventing both early and late responses to challenge (Figure 20–4).

C. Effects: Because they are not absorbed from the airway, cromolyn and nedocromil have only local effects. When administered orally, cromolyn has some efficacy in preventing food allergy. Similar actions have been demonstrated after local application in the conjunctiva and the nasopharyngeal tract.

D. Clinical Uses: Asthma (especially in children) is by far the most important use for cromolyn and nedocromil. Nasal and eyedrop formulations of cromolyn are available for hay fever, and an oral formulation is used for food allergy.

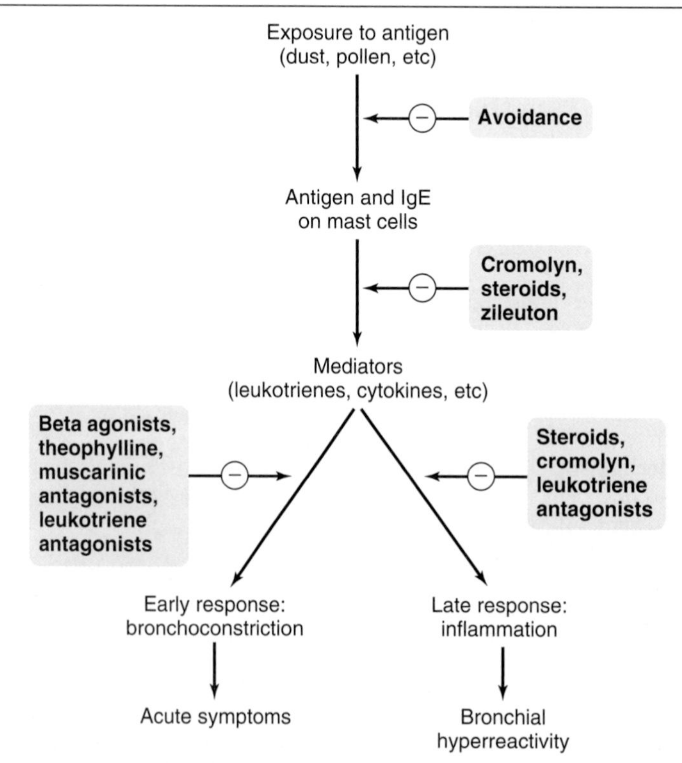

Figure 20–4. Summary of treatment strategies in asthma. (Modified and redrawn from Cockcroft DW: The bronchial late response in the pathogenesis of asthma and its modulation by therapy. Ann Allergy 1985;55:857.)

E. Toxicity: These drugs may cause cough and irritation of the airway when given by aerosol. Rare instances of drug allergy have been reported.

CORTICOSTEROIDS

A. Prototypes and Pharmacokinetics: All of the corticosteroids are potentially beneficial in severe asthma (see Chapter 39). However, because of their toxicity, systemic (oral or intravenous) corticosteroids are used only if other therapies are unsuccessful. In contrast, local aerosol administration of surface-active corticosteroids (eg, **beclomethasone, budesonide, dexamethasone, flunisolide, fluticasone, mometasone**) is relatively safe; inhaled corticosteroids have become common first-line therapy for individuals with moderate to severe asthma.

B. Mechanism of Action: Corticosteroids reduce the synthesis of arachidonic acid by phospholipase A_2 and inhibit the expression of COX-2, the inducible form of cyclooxygenase (see Chapter 18 and Figure 18–1). It has also been suggested that corticosteroids increase the responsiveness of beta adrenoceptors in the airway.

C. Effects: See Chapter 39 for details. Glucocorticoids bind to intracellular receptors and activate glucocorticoid response elements (GREs) in the nucleus, resulting in synthesis of substances that prevent the full expression of inflammation and allergy. Reduced activity of phospholipase A_2 is thought to be particularly important in asthma because the leukotrienes that result from eicosanoid synthesis are extremely potent bronchoconstrictors and may also participate in the late inflammatory response (Figure 20–4).

D. Clinical Use: Inhaled glucocorticoids are now considered appropriate (even for children) in most cases of moderate asthma that are not fully responsive to aerosol beta agonists. It is believed that such early use may prevent the severe, progressive inflammatory changes characteristic of long-standing asthma. This is a shift from earlier beliefs that steroids should be used only in severe refractory asthma. In such cases of severe asthma, patients are usually hospitalized and stabilized on daily systemic prednisone and then switched to inhaled or alternate-day oral therapy before discharge. (See Chapter 39 for other uses.) In status asthmaticus, parenteral steroids are lifesaving and apparently act more promptly than in ordinary asthma. Their mechanism of action in this condition is not fully understood.

E. Toxicity: Local aerosol administration can occasionally result in a very small degree of adrenal suppression, but this is rarely significant. More commonly, changes in oropharyngeal flora result in candidiasis. If oral therapy is required, adrenal suppression can be reduced by using alternate-day therapy—ie, by giving the drug in slightly higher dosage every other day rather than smaller doses every day. The major systemic toxicities of the glucocorticoids described in Chapter 39 are much more likely to occur if systemic treatment is required for more than 2 weeks, as in severe refractory asthma. Regular use of inhaled steroids *does* cause mild growth retardation in children, but these children eventually reach full predicted adult stature.

LEUKOTRIENE ANTAGONISTS

Recognition of the importance of leukotrienes in the pathophysiology of asthma has led to the introduction of drugs that interfere with the synthesis or the action of these arachidonic acid derivatives (see also Chapter 18). Although their value has been documented, these agents are not as effective as corticosteroids in severe asthma.

A. Zileuton: Zileuton is an orally active drug that selectively inhibits 5-lipoxygenase, a key enzyme in the conversion of arachidonic acid to leukotrienes. The drug is effective in preventing both exercise- and antigen-induced bronchospasm. It is also effective against "aspirin allergy," the bronchospasm that results from ingestion of aspirin by individuals who apparently divert all eicosanoid production to leukotrienes when the cyclooxygenase pathway is blocked (Chapter 18). The toxicity of zileuton includes occasional elevation of liver enzymes.

B. Leukotriene Receptor Blockers: Zafirlukast and **montelukast** are antagonists at the LTD_4 leukotriene receptor. The LTE_4 receptor is also blocked. Like zileuton, these drugs are orally active and have been shown to be effective in preventing exercise-, antigen-, and aspirin-induced bronchospastic attacks. They are not recommended for acute episodes of asthma. Toxicity is generally low, but rare reports of Churg-Strauss syndrome, allergic granulomatous angiitis, have appeared.

DRUG LIST

The following drugs are important members of the group discussed in this chapter. Prototypes should be learned in detail; features of the major variants should be known well enough to distinguish the variants from prototypes and from each other; the other significant agents should be recognized as belonging to a specific subclass.

Subclass	Prototype	Major Variants	Other Significant Agents
Beta agonists	Terbutaline	Salmeterol	Metaproterenol, albuterol, formoterol
Methylxanthines	Theophylline	Aminophylline (a theophylline salt)	Caffeine, theobromine
Muscarinic antagonist	Ipratropium		
Release inhibitors	Cromolyn		Nedocromil
Glucocorticoids	Beclomethasone	Prednisone	Prednisolone
Leukotriene antagonists	Zileuton, zafirlukast		Montelukast

QUESTIONS

DIRECTIONS: Each of the numbered items or incomplete statements in this section is followed by answers or by completions of the statement. Select the ONE lettered answer or completion that is BEST in each case.

1. One effect that theophylline, nitroglycerin, isoproterenol, and histamine have in common is
(A) Direct stimulation of cardiac contractile force
(B) Tachycardia
(C) Increased gastric acid secretion
(D) Postural hypotension
(E) Throbbing headache

2. A 23-year-old woman is using a terbutaline inhaler for frequent acute episodes of asthma and describes symptoms that she ascribes to the terbutaline. Which of the following is not a recognized action of terbutaline?
(A) Diuretic effect
(B) Positive inotropic effect
(C) Skeletal muscle tremor
(D) Smooth muscle relaxation
(E) Tachycardia

3. A 10-year-old child has severe asthma and was hospitalized five times between the ages of 7 and 9. He is now receiving outpatient medications that have greatly reduced the frequency of severe attacks. Which of the following is most likely to have adverse effects when used daily over long periods for severe asthma?
(A) Albuterol by aerosol
(B) Beclomethasone by aerosol
(C) Cromolyn by inhaler
(D) Prednisone by mouth
(E) Theophylline in long-acting oral form

4. Cromolyn has as its major action
(A) Block of calcium channels in lymphocytes
(B) Block of mediator release from mast cells
(C) Block of phosphodiesterase in mast cells and basophils
(D) Smooth muscle relaxation in the bronchi
(E) Stimulation of cortisol release by the adrenals

Items 5–6: A 16-year-old patient is in the emergency room receiving nasal oxygen. She has a heart rate of 135/min, a respiratory rate of 40/min, and a peak expiratory flow (PEF) less than 50% of the predicted value. Wheezing and rales are audible without a stethoscope.

5. Drugs that can dilate bronchi during an acute asthmatic attack include all of the following EXCEPT
(A) Epinephrine
(B) Terbutaline
(C) Nedocromil
(D) Theophylline
(E) Ipratropium

6. After successful treatment of the acute attack, the patient was referred to the outpatient clinic for follow-up treatment of her asthma. Successful strategies currently in use for asthma include all of the following EXCEPT
(A) Avoidance of antigen exposure
(B) Blockade of histamine receptors
(C) Blockade of leukotriene receptors
(D) Inhibition of phospholipase A_2
(E) Inhibition of release of mediators from mast cells and leukocytes

7. Mr. Green is a 60-year-old former smoker with severe chronic obstructive pulmonary (COPD) and cardiac disease associated with frequent episodes of bronchospasm. Which of the following is a bronchodilator useful in COPD and least likely to cause cardiac arrhythmia?
(A) Aminophylline
(B) Cromolyn
(C) Epinephrine
(D) Ipratropium
(E) Metaproterenol
(F) Metoprolol
(G) Prednisone/prednisolone
(H) Salmeterol
(I) Zafirlukast
(J) Zileuton

8. Which of the following is a nonselective but very potent and efficacious bronchodilator that is not active by the oral route?
(A) Aminophylline
(B) Cromolyn
(C) Epinephrine
(D) Ipratropium
(E) Metaproterenol
(F) Metoprolol
(G) Prednisone/prednisolone
(H) Salmeterol
(I) Zafirlukast
(J) Zileuton

9. Which of the following is a prophylactic agent that appears to stabilize mast cells?
(A) Aminophylline
(B) Cromolyn
(C) Epinephrine
(D) Ipratropium
(E) Metaproterenol
(F) Metoprolol
(G) Prednisone/prednisolone
(H) Salmeterol

(I) Zafirlukast
(J) Zileuton

10. Which of the following is a direct bronchodilator that is most often used in asthma by the oral route?
(A) Aminophylline
(B) Cromolyn
(C) Epinephrine
(D) Ipratropium
(E) Metaproterenol
(F) Metoprolol
(G) Prednisone/prednisolone
(H) Salmeterol
(I) Zafirlukast
(J) Zileuton

11. Which of the following in its parenteral form is lifesaving in severe status asthmaticus and acts, at least in part, by inhibiting phospholipase A_2?
(A) Aminophylline
(B) Cromolyn
(C) Epinephrine
(D) Ipratropium
(E) Metaproterenol
(F) Metoprolol
(G) Prednisone/prednisolone
(H) Salmeterol
(I) Zafirlukast
(J) Zileuton

12. Which of the following has overdose toxicity that includes insomnia, arrhythmias, and convulsions?
(A) Aminophylline
(B) Cromolyn
(C) Epinephrine
(D) Ipratropium
(E) Metaproterenol
(F) Metoprolol
(G) Prednisone/prednisolone
(H) Salmeterol
(I) Zafirlukast
(J) Zileuton

13. Which of the following is a very long-acting β_2-selective agonist that is used for asthma prophylaxis?
(A) Aminophylline
(B) Cromolyn
(C) Epinephrine
(D) Ipratropium
(E) Metaproterenol
(F) Metoprolol
(G) Prednisone/prednisolone
(H) Salmeterol
(I) Zafirlukast
(J) Zileuton

DIRECTIONS (Items 14–15): The two matching questions in this section consist of a list of lettered options followed by two numbered items. For each numbered item, select the ONE lettered option that is most closely associated with it. Each lettered option may be selected once, more than once, or not at all.
(A) Aminophylline
(B) Cromolyn
(C) Epinephrine
(D) Ipratropium

(E) Metaproterenol
(F) Metoprolol
(G) Prednisone/prednisolone
(H) Salmeterol
(I) Zafirlukast
(J) Zileuton

14. A drug that directly inhibits 5-lipoxygenase and reduces leukotriene synthesis
15. Inhibitor of LTD_4 receptors

DIRECTIONS (Items 16–18): This case history* is followed by discussion questions. Write out brief answers (two to five sentences) and then compare your answers with those given at the end of the Answers section.

A businesswoman with a history of mild asthma attacks had onset of symptoms of bronchoconstriction in a restaurant. Repeated self-medication with an inhaler did not provide relief, and symptoms progressed until she became cyanotic. Paramedics administered a subcutaneous drug upon arrival and nasal oxygen during transport. She was admitted to the hospital emergency room in severe respiratory distress. Her pulse was 100/min, respiratory rate 32/min, and blood pressure 140/90 mm Hg on nasal oxygen. Severe wheezing was present.

After this evaluation, she was given another dose of the subcutaneous medication that had been previously administered by the paramedics. Fifteen minutes later, her symptoms had decreased markedly, but she still had some respiratory wheezing. Use of a bronchodilator administered by handheld nebulizer abolished the wheezing, and oxygen could be discontinued. She was discharged 3 hours later.

16. What are the probable mediators of the bronchoconstriction noted in this woman's asthma attack?
17. What medications are commonly used for the outpatient treatment of mild and moderate asthma? What are their mechanisms of action?
18. What drug was administered subcutaneously by the paramedics and later in the emergency room? Which agents are suitable for nebulizer use?

ANSWERS

1. Theophylline does not cause headache. Nitroglycerin does not increase gastric acid secretion. Isoproterenol does not cause either. Histamine may cause all of the effects listed. The answer is **(B)**.
2. Terbutaline is a "selective" β_2-receptor agonist, but in moderate to high doses it induces β_1 cardiac effects as well as β_2-mediated smooth and skeletal muscle effects. The answer is **(A)**.
3. If oral corticosteroids must be used, alternate-day therapy is preferred because it interferes less with normal growth in children. The answer is **(D)**.
4. The answer is **(B)**, inhibition of mediator release from mast cells. The mechanism for this effect is not known.
5. Neither nedocromil nor cromolyn is capable of reversing bronchospasm; their action is prophylactic. The answer is **(C)**.
6. Histamine does not appear to play a significant role in asthma, and antihistaminic drugs, even in high doses, are of little or no value. The answer is **(B)**.
7. Ipratropium is the bronchodilator that is most likely to be useful in COPD without causing arrhythmias. The answer is **(D)**.
8. Epinephrine is still one of the most potent and efficacious agents available for asthma. However, because it is nonselective, β_2-selective agents are preferred. The answer is **(C)**.
9. Cromolyn is useful only for prophylaxis. The drug stabilizes mast cells, ie, prevents mediator release. The answer is **(B)**.
10. Aminophylline, a salt of theophylline, is a bronchodilator that is active by the oral route. The answer is **(A)**.

* Modified and reproduced, with permission, from Simon RA: Management of severe asthma in relapse: Case discussion. In: *The Practical Management of Asthma.* Grune & Stratton, 1984.

11. Parenteral corticosteroids such as prednisolone are lifesaving in status asthmaticus. They probably act by reducing production of leukotrienes (see Chapter 18). The answer is **(G).**

12. Aminophylline is a salt of theophylline. Like the base theophylline, aminophylline can cause severe and potentially lethal overdose toxicity. The answer is **(A).**

13. Salmeterol is a long-acting β_2-selective sympathomimetic agent that is approved for prophylactic use in asthma. The answer is **(H).**

14. Zileuton is a selective inhibitor of 5-lipoxygenase. The answer is **(J).**

15. Zafirlukast inhibits LTD_4 at its receptors. The answer is **(I).**

16. The mediators probably most important in causing asthmatic bronchoconstriction are leukotrienes LTC_4 and LTD_4. Another leukotriene (LTB_4), prostaglandins, peptides, some enzymes, and histamine probably also play a role.

17. The most commonly used bronchodilators are the beta-adrenoceptor agonists. In some patients, a muscarinic blocking drug (eg, ipratropium) has a useful bronchodilating effect. Cromolyn and nedocromil inhibit the degranulation of mast cells and are useful as prophylactic agents in some patients. They are not useful in an acute attack. Systemic corticosteroids are reserved for patients with severe asthma who do not respond adequately to other agents, but inhaled steroids (eg, beclomethasone) are standard prophylactic therapy for all individuals with moderate or severe recurrent asthma.

18. The drug administered by the paramedics and by the personnel in the emergency room was epinephrine. This agent is extremely effective and has a rapid onset of action. However, it is probably no more effective than inhaled β_2-selective agonists (albuterol, metaproterenol, terbutaline). The drugs used in nebulizers include the β_2-selective agonists, epinephrine, and (rarely) isoproterenol. Note that nebulized drug is less efficacious than pressurized aerosols because the latter consist of smaller particles of drug-containing liquid that reach farther down into the airways.

Routine modern therapy of severe exacerbations of asthma includes oxygen in addition to frequent inhalation of β_2-selective bronchodilators and, frequently, systemic corticosteroids. Therapy of status asthmaticus is more complicated, requiring intubation and respiratory assistance, sedation, parenteral corticosteroids, and bronchodilators.

Skill Keeper Answer: Sympathomimetics in Asthma (see Chapter 9)

Direct-acting sympathomimetics are usually rapid in onset and short-acting (examples: epinephrine, albuterol; exception: salmeterol). Most direct-acting sympathomimetics have poor oral bioavailability. Indirect-acting sympathomimetics are usually longer-acting and have good bioavailability (example: ephedrine). An important disadvantage of the indirect-acting group is their CNS activity: most enter the CNS and produce undesirable stimulation. Even more important in asthma is the lack of receptor selectivity of the indirect-acting group. Because they release norepinephrine and epinephrine from stores, they produce all the α- and β_1-adrenoceptor-mediated effects of these catecholamines, which are undesirable in asthma. In contrast, the direct-acting agents can be tailored for selective β_2 activity. Furthermore, local application by aerosol administration is convenient and greatly reduces the systemic toxicity associated with oral or other systemic routes.

Part V. Drugs That Act in the Central Nervous System

Introduction to CNS Pharmacology 21

OBJECTIVES

You should be able to:

- Identify the major types of voltage-gated and ligand-gated ion channels in neuronal membranes.
- List the criteria for accepting a chemical as a neurotransmitter.
- Describe the mechanisms by which drugs modulate synaptic transmission.
- List the major excitatory central neurotransmitters.
- List the major inhibitory central neurotransmitters.
- Identify the major receptor subtypes of CNS neurotransmitters.

Learn the definitions that follow.

Table 21–1. Definitions.

Term	Definition
Voltage-gated ion channels	Transmembrane ion channels regulated by changes in membrane potential
Ligand-gated ion channels	Transmembrane ion channels that are regulated by interactions between neurotransmitters and their receptors; also called ionotropic receptors
Metabotropic receptors	G protein-coupled receptors that respond to neurotransmitters either by a direct action of G proteins on ion channels or by G protein enzyme activation that leads to formation of diffusible second messengers
EPSP	Excitatory postsynaptic potential; a depolarizing potential change
IPSP	Inhibitory postsynaptic potential; a hyperpolarizing potential change
Synaptic mimicry	Ability of an administered drug to mimic the actions of the natural synaptic transmitter; a criterion for identification of a putative neurotransmitter
Hierarchical systems	Neuronal pathways involved in sensory perception and motor control; relay or projection neurons and local circuit neurons; glutamate commonly the excitatory transmitter; GABA and glycine usually inhibitory transmitters
Diffuse systems	Neuronal pathways involved in global functions (sleep-wake, attention, appetite, affective state, etc); localized cell bodies but marked axonal branching and divergence; norepinephrine and serotonin commonly transmitters—excitatory or inhibitory depending on receptor subtypes

CONCEPTS

A. **Targets of CNS Drug Action:** Most drugs that act on the CNS appear to do so by changing ion flow through transmembrane channels of nerve cells.

1. **Types of ion channels:** Ion channels of neuronal membranes are of two major types: voltage-gated and ligand-gated (Figure 21–1). Voltage-gated ion channels respond to

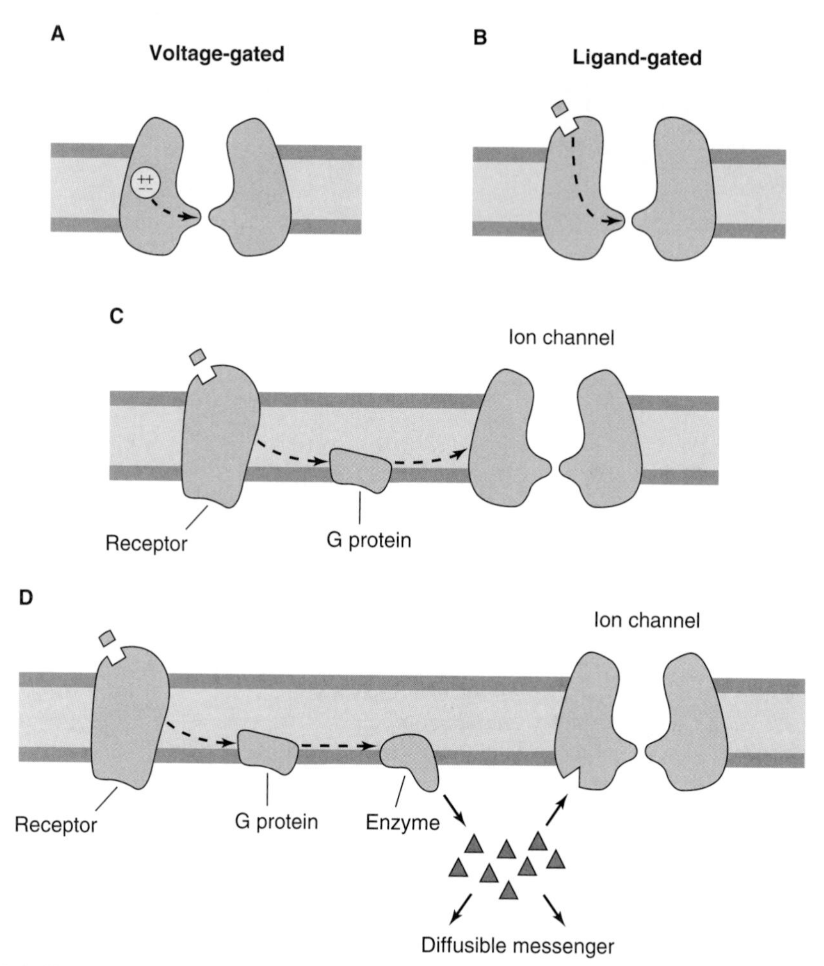

Figure 21–1. Types of ion channels and neurotransmitter receptors in the CNS. **A** shows a voltage-gated ion channel and **B** shows a ligand-gated ion channel. **C** shows a receptor coupled to a G protein that can interact directly with an ion channel. **D** shows a receptor coupled to a G protein that activates an enzyme; the activated enzyme generates a diffusible second messenger that can interact with an ion channel. (Reproduced, with permission, from Katzung BG [editor]: *Basic & Clinical Pharmacology,* 8th ed. McGraw-Hill, 2001.)

changes in membrane potential. They are concentrated on the axons of nerve cells and include the sodium channels responsible for action potential propagation. Cell bodies and dendrites also have voltage-sensitive ion channels for potassium and calcium. Ligand-gated ion channels (also called ionotropic receptors) respond to chemical neurotransmitters that bind to receptor subunits present in their macromolecular structure. Neurotransmitters also bind to G protein-coupled receptors (metabotropic receptors) that can modulate voltage-gated ion channels. Neurotransmitter-coupled ion channels are found on cell bodies and on both the presynaptic and the postsynaptic sides of synapses.

2. **Types of receptor-channel coupling:** In the case of ligand-gated ion channels, activation (or inactivation) is initiated by the interaction between chemical neurotransmitters and their receptors (see Figure 21–1). Coupling may be (1) through a receptor that acts directly on the channel protein (B), (2) through a receptor that is coupled to the ion channel through a G protein (C), or (3) through a receptor coupled to a G protein that modulates the formation of diffusible second messengers—including cAMP, inositol trisphosphate (IP_3), and diacylglycerol (DAG)—which secondarily modulate ion channels (D).
3. **Role of the ion current carried by the channel:** Excitatory postsynaptic potentials (EPSPs) are usually generated by the opening of sodium or calcium channels. In some

synapses, similar depolarizing potentials result from the *closing* of potassium channels. Inhibitory postsynaptic potentials (IPSPs) are generated by the opening of potassium or chloride channels. For example, activation of postsynaptic metabotropic receptors increases the efflux of potassium. Presynaptic inhibition can occur via a decrease in calcium influx elicited by activation of metabotropic receptors.

B. Sites and Mechanisms of Drug Action: A small number of neuropharmacologic agents exert their effects through direct interactions with molecular components of ion channels on axons. Examples include certain anticonvulsants (eg, carbamazepine, phenytoin), local anesthetics, and some drugs used in general anesthesia. However, the effects of most therapeutically important CNS drugs are exerted mainly at synapses. Possible mechanisms are indicated in Figure 21–2. Thus, drugs may act presynaptically to alter the synthesis, storage, release, reuptake, or metabolism of transmitter chemicals. Other drugs can activate or block both pre- and postsynaptic receptors for specific transmitters or can interfere with the actions of second messengers. The selectivity of CNS drug action is largely based on the fact that different groups of neurons utilize different neurotransmitters and that they are segregated into networks that subserve different CNS functions. A few neurotoxic substances damage or kill nerve cells. For example, 1-methyl-4-phenyl-1, 2, 3, 6-tetrahydropyridine (MPTP) is cytotoxic to neurons of the nigrostriatal dopaminergic pathway.

C. Role of CNS Organization: The CNS contains two types of neuronal systems: hierarchical and diffuse.

1. **Hierarchical systems:** These systems are clearly delimited in their anatomic distribution and generally contain large myelinated, rapidly conducting fibers. Hierarchical systems control major sensory and motor functions. The major excitatory transmitters in these systems are aspartate and glutamate. These systems also include numerous small inhibitory interneurons, which utilize γ-aminobutyric acid (GABA) or glycine as transmitters. Drugs

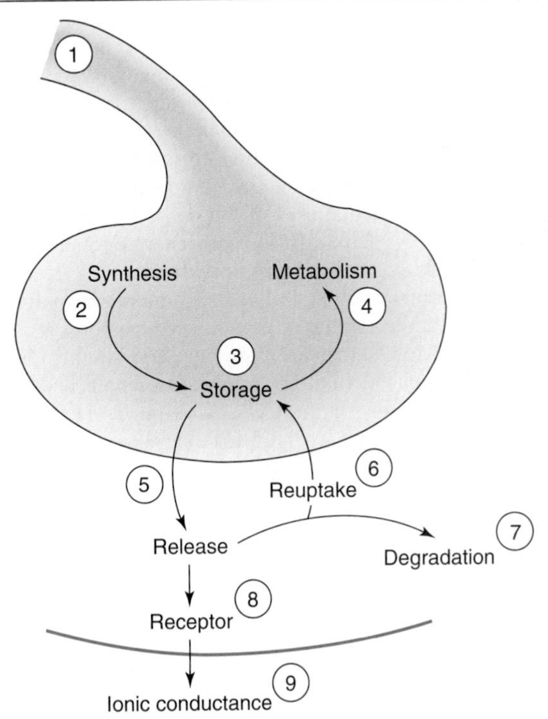

Figure 21–2. Sites of CNS drug action. Drugs may alter (1) the action potential in the presynaptic fiber; (2) the synthesis of transmitter; (3) the storage of transmitter; (4) the metabolism of transmitter within the nerve ending; (5) the release of transmitter; (6) the reuptake or (7) extracellular disposition of transmitter; (8) the postsynaptic receptor; or (9) the postsynaptic effects that follow receptor activation. (Reproduced, with permission, from Katzung BG [editor]: *Basic & Clinical Pharmacology,* 8th ed. McGraw-Hill, 2001.)

that affect hierarchical systems often have profound effects on the overall excitability of the CNS.

2. **Diffuse systems:** Diffuse systems are broadly distributed, with single cells frequently sending processes to many different areas. The axons are fine and branch repeatedly to form synapses with many cells. Axons commonly have periodic enlargements (varicosities) that contain transmitter vesicles. The transmitters in diffuse systems are often amines (norepinephrine, dopamine, serotonin) or peptides that commonly exert actions on metabotropic receptors. Drugs that affect these systems will often have marked effects on such CNS functions as attention, appetite, and emotional states.

D. Transmitters at Central Synapses:

1. **Criteria for transmitter status:** To be accepted as a neurotransmitter, a candidate chemical must be present in higher concentration in the synaptic area than in other areas (ie, must be localized in appropriate areas), must be released by electrical or chemical stimulation via a calcium-dependent mechanism, and must produce the same sort of postsynaptic response that is seen with physiologic activation of the synapse (ie, must exhibit synaptic mimicry). Table 21–2 lists the most important chemicals currently accepted as neurotransmitters in the CNS.
2. **Acetylcholine:** Approximately 5% of brain neurons have receptors for ACh. Most CNS responses to ACh are mediated by a large family of G protein-coupled muscarinic M_1 receptors that lead to slow excitation when activated. The ionic mechanism of slow excitation involves a *decrease* in membrane permeability to potassium. Of the nicotinic receptors present in the CNS (they are less common than muscarinic receptors), those on the Renshaw cells activated by motor axon collaterals in the spinal cord are the best-characterized. Drugs affecting the activity of cholinergic systems in the brain include the acetylcholinesterase inhibitors used in Alzheimer's disease (eg, tacrine) and the muscarinic blocking agents used in parkinsonism (eg, benztropine).
3. **Dopamine:** Dopamine exerts slow inhibitory actions at synapses in specific neuronal systems commonly via G protein-coupled activation of potassium channels. The D_2 receptor is the main dopamine subtype in basal ganglia neurons, and it is widely distributed at the supraspinal level. Dopaminergic pathways include the nigrostriatal, mesolimbic, and tuberoinfundibular tracts. In addition to the two receptors listed in Table 21–2, three other dopamine receptor subtypes have been identified (D_3, D_4, and D_5). Drugs affecting the activity of dopaminergic pathways include antipsychotics (eg, chlorpromazine), CNS stimulants (eg, amphetamine), and antiparkinsonism drugs (eg, levodopa).
4. **Norepinephrine:** Noradrenergic neuron cell bodies are mainly located in the brain stem and the lateral tegmental area of the pons. These neurons fan out broadly to provide most regions of the CNS with diffuse noradrenergic input. Excitatory effects are produced by activation of $alpha_1$ and $beta_1$ receptors. Inhibitory effects are caused by activation of $alpha_2$ and $beta_2$ receptors. CNS stimulants, monoamine oxidase inhibitors, and tricyclic antidepressants affect the activity of noradrenergic pathways.
5. **Serotonin:** Most serotonin (5-hydroxytryptamine; 5-HT) pathways originate from cell bodies in the raphe or midline regions of the pons and upper brain stem; these pathways innervate most regions of the CNS. Multiple 5-HT receptor subtypes have been identified and, with the exception of the $5\text{-}HT_3$ subtype, all are metabotropic. $5\text{-}HT_{1A}$ receptors and $GABA_B$ receptors share the same potassium channel. Serotonin is inhibitory at many CNS sites but can cause excitation of some neurons depending on the receptor subtype activated. Both excitatory and inhibitory actions can occur on the same neuron if appropriate receptors are present. Most of the agents used in the treatment of major depressive disorders affect serotonergic pathways (eg, tricyclic antidepressants, selective serotonin reuptake inhibitors). Reserpine, which may cause severe depression of mood, depletes vesicular stores of both serotonin and norepinephrine in CNS neurons.
6. **Glutamic acid:** Most neurons in the brain are excited by glutamic acid. Subtypes of glutamate receptors include the NMDA (*N*-methyl-D-aspartate) receptor, which is blocked by phencyclidine (PCP) and ketamine. NMDA receptors appear to play a role in synaptic plasticity related to learning and memory. Excessive activation of NMDA receptors following neuronal injury may be responsible for cell death. Glutamate metabotropic receptor activation can result in G-protein-coupled activation of phospholipase C or inhibition of adenylyl cyclase.

Table 21–2. Neurotransmitter pharmacology in the central nervous system.*

Transmitter	Anatomic Distribution	Receptor Subtypes	Receptor Mechanisms
Acetylcholine	Cell bodies at all levels, short and long axons	Muscarinic, M_1; blocked by pirenzepine and atropine	Excitatory; ↓ in K^+ conductance; ↑ IP_3 and DAG
		Muscarinic, M_2; blocked by atropine	Inhibitory; ↑ K^+ conductance; ↓ cAMP
	Motoneuron–Renshaw cell synapse	Nicotinic, N	Excitatory; ↑ cation conductance
Dopamine	Cell bodies at all levels, short, medium, and long axons	D_1; blocked by phenothiazines	Inhibitory; ↑ cAMP
		D_2; blocked by phenothiazines and haloperidol	Inhibitory (presynaptic); ↓ Ca^{2+} conductance; Inhibitory (postsynaptic); ↑ K^+ conductance; ↓ cAMP
Norepinephrine	Cell bodies in pons and brain stem project to all levels	$Alpha_1$; blocked by prazosin	Excitatory; ↓ K^+ conductance; ↑ IP_3 and DAG
		$Alpha_2$; activated by clonidine	Inhibitory (presynaptic); ↓ Ca^{2+} conductance Inhibitory (postsynaptic); ↑ K^+ conductance; ↓ cAMP
		$Beta_1$; blocked by propranolol	Excitatory; ↓ K^+ conductance; ↑ cAMP
		$Beta_2$; blocked by propranolol	Inhibitory; ? increase in electrogenic sodium pump; ↑ cAMP
Serotonin (5-hydroxy-tryptamine)	Cell bodies in midbrain and pons project to all levels	$5\text{-}HT_{1A}$; buspirone is a partial agonist	Inhibitory; ↑ K^+ conductance, ↓ cAMP
		$5\text{-}HT_{2A}$; blocked by clozapine, risperidone, and olanzapine	Excitatory; ↓ K^+ conductance; ↑ IP_3 and DAG
		$5\text{-}HT_3$; blocked by ondansetron	Excitatory; ↑ cation conductance
		$5\text{-}HT_4$	Excitatory; ↓ K^+ conductance
GABA	Supraspinal interneurons; spinal interneurons involved in presynaptic inhibition	$GABA_A$; facilitated by benzodiazepines and zolpidem	Inhibitory; ↑ Cl^- conductance
		$GABA_B$; activated by baclofen	Inhibitory (presynaptic); ↓ Ca^{2+} conductance Inhibitory (postsynaptic); ↑ K^+ conductance
Glutamate	Relay neurons at all levels	Four subtypes; NMDA subtype blocked by phencyclidine	Excitatory; ↑ Ca^{2+} or cation conductance
		Metabotropic subtypes	Inhibitory (presynaptic); ↓ Ca^{2+} conductance, ↓ cAMP Excitatory (postsynaptic); ↓ K^+ conductance, ↑ IP_3 and DAG
Glycine	Interneurons in spinal cord and brain stem	Single subtype; blocked by strychnine	Inhibitory; ↑ Cl^- conductance
Opioid peptides	Cell bodies at all levels	Three major subtypes: mu, delta, kappa	Inhibitory (presynaptic); ↓ Ca^{2+} conductance; ↓ cAMP
			Inhibitory (postsynaptic); ↑ K^+ conductance; ↓ cAMP

*Adapted, with permission, from Katzung BG (editor): *Basic & Clinical Pharmacology,* 8th ed. McGraw-Hill, 2001.

7. **GABA and glycine:** GABA is the primary neurotransmitter mediating IPSPs in neurons in the brain; it is also important in the spinal cord. $GABA_A$ receptor activation opens chloride ion channels. $GABA_B$ receptors (activated by baclofen) are coupled to G proteins that either open potassium channels or close calcium channels. Fast IPSPs are blocked by $GABA_A$ receptor antagonists, and slow IPSPs are blocked by $GABA_B$ receptor antagonists. Drugs that influence GABAergic systems include sedative-hypnotics (eg, barbiturates, benzodiazepines) and some anticonvulsants (eg, gabapentin). Glycine receptors, which are more numerous in the cord than in the brain, are blocked by strychnine, a spinal convulsant.
8. **Peptide transmitters:** Many peptides have been identified in the CNS, and some meet most or all of the criteria for acceptance as neurotransmitters. The best-defined ones are the opioid peptides (beta-endorphin, met- and leu-enkephalin, and dynorphin), which are distributed at all levels of the neuraxis. Some of the important therapeutic actions of opioid analgesics (eg, morphine) are mediated by receptors for these endogenous peptides. Substance P is localized in type C neurons involved in nociceptive sensory pathways in the spinal cord. Peptide transmitters differ from nonpeptide transmitters in that (1) the peptides are synthesized in the cell body and transported to the nerve ending via axonal transport, and (2) no reuptake or specific enzyme mechanisms have been identified for terminating their actions.

Skill Keeper: Biodisposition of CNS Drugs (see Chapter 1)

1. What characteristics of drug molecules afford access to the central nervous system?
2. What concerns do you have regarding CNS drug use in the pregnant patient?
3. How are CNS drugs eliminated from the body?

The Skill Keeper Answers appear at the end of the chapter.

QUESTIONS

DIRECTIONS: Each of the numbered items or incomplete statements in this section is followed by answers or by completions of the statement. Select the ONE lettered answer or completion that is BEST in each case.

1. Which one of the following chemicals does not satisfy the criteria for a neurotransmitter role in the CNS?
   (A) Acetylcholine
   (B) Dopamine
   (C) Glycine
   (D) Nitric oxide
   (E) Substance P
2. Many therapeutically useful drugs act via brain dopaminergic systems. Which one of the following mechanisms underlying their actions is LEAST likely to be useful in the management of Parkinson's disease?
   (A) Inhibition of dopamine reuptake
   (B) Increase in dopamine synthesis
   (C) Activation of dopamine receptors
   (D) Inhibition of dopamine metabolism
   (E) Blockade of dopamine receptors
3. Neurotransmitters may
   (A) Increase chloride conductance to cause inhibition
   (B) Increase potassium conductance to cause excitation
   (C) Increase sodium conductance to cause inhibition
   (D) Increase calcium conductance to cause inhibition
   (E) Exert all of the above actions

4. Which one of the following neurotransmitters does not change membrane excitability by decreasing K^+ conductance?
(A) Acetylcholine
(B) Dopamine
(C) Glutamic acid
(D) Norepinephrine
(E) Serotonin

5. Which one of the following receptors shares the same potassium channel as the 5-HT_{1A} receptor?
(A) Delta opioid receptor
(B) Dopamine D_2 receptor
(C) $GABA_B$ receptor
(D) Muscarinic M_1 receptor
(E) Substance P receptor

6. Which one of the following chemicals is most likely to function as a neurotransmitter in hierarchical systems?
(A) Dopamine
(B) Glutamate
(C) Met-enkephalin
(D) Norepinephrine
(E) Serotonin

7. Which one of the following statements about beta-endorphin is most accurate?
(A) It is exclusively located in the spinal cord
(B) Enzymes for its synthesis are located in nerve endings
(C) It selectively activates delta opioid receptors
(D) Its postsynaptic effects are terminated by active reuptake
(E) Its actions are mainly inhibitory

8. Activation of metabotropic receptors located presynaptically causes inhibition by decreasing the inward flux of
(A) Calcium
(B) Chloride
(C) Potassium
(D) Sodium
(E) None of the above

9. This compound is found in diffuse neuronal systems in the CNS, particularly in the raphe nuclei; it appears to play a major role in the expression of mood, since many antidepressant drugs are thought to increase its functional activity.
(A) Acetylcholine
(B) Dopamine
(C) Histamine
(D) Serotonin
(E) Substance P

10. In strychnine poisoning, convulsions occur due to antagonistic effects at receptors for
(A) Aspartate
(B) GABA
(C) Glutamate
(D) Glycine
(E) Norepinephrine

11. cAMP functions as a diffusible second messenger that can modify voltage-gated ion channels following activation of which of the following receptors?
(A) Acetylcholine M_1 receptors
(B) Beta-adrenoceptors
(C) 5-HT_3 receptors
(D) $GABA_A$ receptors
(E) Glycine receptors

12. One of the first neurotransmitter receptors to be identified in the CNS is located on the Renshaw cell in the spinal cord. Activation of this receptor results in excitation via an increase in cation conductance independently of G proteins. Which one of the following compounds is most likely to activate this receptor?

(A) Aspartate
(B) Baclofen
(C) Glutamate
(D) Nicotine
(E) Serotonin

13. This compound decreases the functional activities of several CNS neurotransmitters, including dopamine, norepinephrine, and serotonin. At high doses it may cause parkinsonism-like extrapyramidal system dysfunction.
(A) Amphetamine
(B) Baclofen
(C) Diazepam
(D) Ketamine
(E) Reserpine

14. This amine neurotransmitter is found in high concentrations in cell bodies in the pons and brain stem; at some sites, release of transmitter is autoregulated via presynaptic inhibition.
(A) Acetylcholine
(B) Dopamine
(C) Glutamate
(D) Norepinephrine
(E) Substance P

ANSWERS

1. Nitric oxide synthase (NOS), the enzyme that generates nitric oxide (NO), is found in some neurons in the CNS. While NO plays a significant physiologic function in relaxation of vascular smooth muscle, a role for nitric oxide in synaptic transmission in the CNS has not been clearly established. Substance P is a neurotransmitter released from unmyelinated sensory neurons in the spinal cord involved in nociception. The answer is **(D).**
2. The neuropathology of Parkinson's disease involves degeneration of dopaminergic neurons in the nigrostriatal pathway. Drugs that facilitate dopaminergic transmission have value in the management of parkinsonism. Levodopa increases dopamine synthesis; bromocriptine activates dopamine receptors; and selegiline inhibits dopamine metabolism. Drugs that act as inhibitors of brain dopamine *transporters* have not yet found a *therapeutic* niche. However, such drugs could have important therapeutic applications in Parkinson's disease and in the treatment of hyperprolactinemia. Antagonists of brain dopamine receptors are associated with extrapyramidal dysfunction, and such drugs are likely to exacerbate parkinsonism. The answer is **(E).**
3. Activation of chloride or potassium ion channels often generates inhibitory postsynaptic potentials (IPSPs) and inhibits nerve membranes. Activation of sodium and *inhibition* of potassium ion channels generate excitatory postsynaptic potentials (EPSPs). The answer is **(A).**
4. A decrease in K^+ conductance is associated with neuronal excitation. With the exception of dopamine, all of the neurotransmitters listed are able to cause excitation by this mechanism via their activation of specific receptors: acetylcholine (M_1), glutamate (metabotropic), norepinephrine ($alpha_1$ and $beta_1$), and serotonin ($5\text{-}HT_{2A}$). The answer is **(B).**
5. $GABA_B$ receptors and $5\text{-}HT_{1A}$ receptors share the same potassium ion channel, with a G protein involved in the coupling mechanism. The spasmolytic drug baclofen is an activator of $GABA_B$ receptors in the spinal cord. The anxiolytic drug buspirone may act as a partial agonist at brain $5\text{-}HT_{1A}$ receptors. The answer is **(C).**
6. Catecholamines (dopamine, norepinephrine), opioid peptides, and serotonin act as neurotransmitters in nonspecific or diffuse neuronal systems. Glutamate is the primary excitatory transmitter in hierarchical neuronal systems. The answer is **(B).**
7. The opioid peptides are widely distributed in the CNS at all levels of the neuraxis and are synthesized in the cell bodies. They activate several receptor subtypes and cause inhibition. No mechanism has been described for termination of the synaptic actions of endogenous peptides. The answer is **(E).**
8. Activation of metabotropic receptors located presynaptically results in the inhibition of calcium influx with a resultant decrease in the release of neurotransmitter from nerve endings. This type of presynaptic inhibition occurs following activation of dopamine D_2, norepinephrine $alpha_2$, glutamate, and mu opioid peptide receptors. The answer is **(A).**

9. Several amine transmitters may be involved in the control of mood states, especially norepinephrine and serotonin. Many of the cell bodies of serotonergic neurons are found in the raphe nuclei. Most of the drugs used for the treatment of major depressive disorders increase serotonergic activity in the CNS. The answer is **(D).**

10. Activation of both $GABA_A$ and glycine receptors present on neurons in the spinal cord leads to membrane hyperpolarization via increases in chloride ion conductance. In the case of glycine, its inhibitory action at the level of the spinal cord is opposed by strychnine, which acts as a glycine receptor antagonist. The answer is **(D).**

11. Metabotropic receptors can modulate voltage-gated ion channels directly (membrane-delimited action) and also by the formation of diffusible second messengers through G protein-mediated effects on enzymes involved in their synthesis. A classic example of the latter type of action is provided by the beta-adrenoceptor, which generates cAMP via the activation of adenylyl cyclase. The answer is **(B).**

12. Nicotinic receptors on the Renshaw cell are activated by the release of ACh from motoneuron collaterals. This results in the release of glycine, which, via interaction with its receptors on the motoneuron, causes membrane hyperpolarization—an example of feedback inhibition. The receptors were so-named because of their activation by nicotine. The answer is **(D).**

13. Reserpine is sometimes used in the treatment of hypertension. In addition to depleting vesicular stores of norepinephrine in sympathetic nerve endings, reserpine depletes brain dopamine and causes parkinsonism-like adverse effects. Reserpine also decreases vesicular stores of norepinephrine and serotonin in CNS neurons, which can result in depression of mood. The answer is **(E).**

14. Cell bodies of noradrenergic neurons located in the pons and brain stem project to all levels of the CNS. Agents that activate presynaptic $alpha_2$ receptors on such neurons (eg, clonidine, methyldopa) decrease central noradrenergic activity, an action thought to result in decreased vasomotor outflow. Glutamate and substance P are not amines. The answer is **(D).**

Skill Keeper Answers: Biodisposition of CNS Drugs (see Chapter 1)

1. Lipid solubility is an important characteristic of most CNS drugs in terms of their ability to cross the blood-brain barrier. Access to the CNS of water-soluble (polar) molecules is limited to those of low molecular weight such as lithium ion and alcohols such as ethanol.
2. CNS drugs readily cross the placental barrier and enter the fetal circulation. Concerns during pregnancy include possible effects on fetal development and the potential for drug effects on the neonate if CNS drugs are used near the time of delivery.
3. With the exception of lithium, almost all CNS drugs require metabolism to more water-soluble (polar) metabolites for their elimination. Thus, drugs that modify the activities of drug-metabolizing enzymes may impact on the clearance of CNS drugs, perhaps affecting the intensity or duration of their effects.

22 Sedative-Hypnotic Drugs

OBJECTIVES

You should be able to:

- Identify the major chemical classes of sedative-hypnotics.
- Describe the pharmacodynamics of benzodiazepines and barbiturates, including their mechanisms of action.
- Compare the pharmacokinetics of commonly used benzodiazepines and barbiturates and discuss how differences among them affect clinical use.
- Describe the clinical uses and the adverse effects of sedative-hypnotics.
- Identify the distinctive properties of buspirone, zolpidem, and zaleplon.

Learn the definitions that follow.

Table 22–1. Definitions.

Term	Definition
Sedation	Reduction of anxiety
Anxiolytic	A drug that reduces anxiety, a sedative
Hypnosis	Induction of sleep
REM sleep	Phase of sleep associated with rapid eye movements; most dreaming takes place during REM sleep
Tolerance	Reduction in drug effect requiring an increase in dosage to maintain the same response
Physiologic dependence	The state of response to a drug whereby removal of the drug evokes unpleasant symptoms, usually the opposite of the drug's effects
Psychologic dependence	The state of response to a drug whereby the drug taker feels compelled to use the drug and suffers anxiety when separated from the drug
Anesthesia	Loss of consciousness associated with absence of response to pain
Coma	Extremely deep anesthesia or depression of brain activity; precursor to respiratory and circulatory failure

CONCEPTS

A. Classification and Pharmacokinetics:

1. **Subgroups:** The sedative-hypnotics belong to a chemically heterogeneous class of drugs (Figure 22–1) almost all of which produce dose-dependent CNS depressant effects. The most important subgroup is the **benzodiazepines,** but representatives of other subgroups, including **barbiturates,** and miscellaneous agents (**carbamates, alcohols,** and **cyclic ethers**) are still in use. Newer drugs with distinctive characteristics include **buspirone, zolpidem,** and **zaleplon.**
2. **Absorption and distribution:** Most of these drugs are lipid-soluble and are absorbed well from the gastrointestinal tract, with good distribution to the brain. Drugs with the highest lipid solubility (eg, **thiopental**) enter the CNS rapidly and can be used as induction agents in anesthesia. The CNS effects of thiopental are terminated by rapid **redistribution** of the drug from brain to other tissues.
3. **Metabolism and excretion:** Sedative-hypnotics are metabolized prior to elimination from the body, mainly by hepatic enzymes. Metabolic rates and pathways vary among different drugs. Many benzodiazepines are converted initially to **active metabolites** with

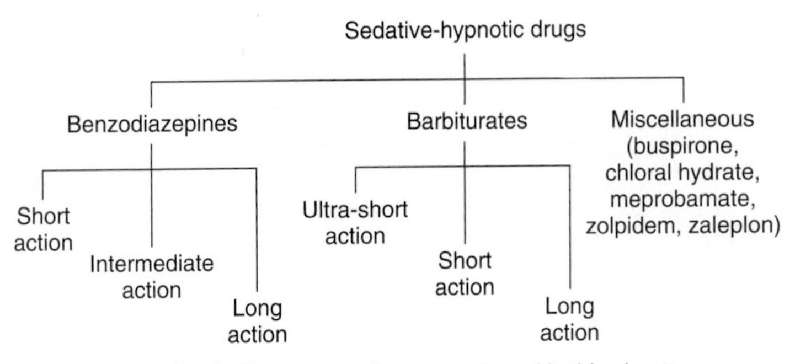

Figure 22–1. Subgroups of drugs reviewed in this chapter.

long half-lives. After several days of therapy with some drugs (eg, diazepam, flurazepam), accumulation of active metabolites can lead to excessive sedation. Lorazepam and oxazepam undergo extrahepatic conjugation and do not form active metabolites. With the exception of phenobarbital, which is excreted partly unchanged in the urine, the barbiturates are extensively metabolized via oxidation at the C5 position. Chloral hydrate is oxidized to trichloroethanol, an active metabolite. Rapid metabolism by liver enzymes is responsible for zolpidem's short duration of action. Zaleplon undergoes even more rapid hepatic metabolism by aldehyde oxidase and cytochrome P450. The duration of CNS actions of sedative-hypnotic drugs ranges from just a few hours (eg, zaleplon < zolpidem = triazolam < chloral hydrate) to more than 30 hours (eg, chlordiazepoxide, clorazepate, diazepam, phenobarbital).

B. Mechanism of Action: No single mechanism of action for sedative-hypnotics has been identified, and the different chemical subgroups may have different actions. Certain drugs (eg, benzodiazepines) facilitate neuronal membrane inhibition by actions at specific receptors.

1. **Benzodiazepines:** Receptors for benzodiazepines (BZ receptors) are present in many brain regions, including the thalamus, limbic structures, and the cerebral cortex. The BZ receptors form part of a $GABA_A$ receptor-chloride ion channel macromolecular complex. Binding of benzodiazepines to these receptors appears to facilitate the inhibitory actions of GABA, which are exerted through increased chloride ion conductance (Figure 22–2). Ben-

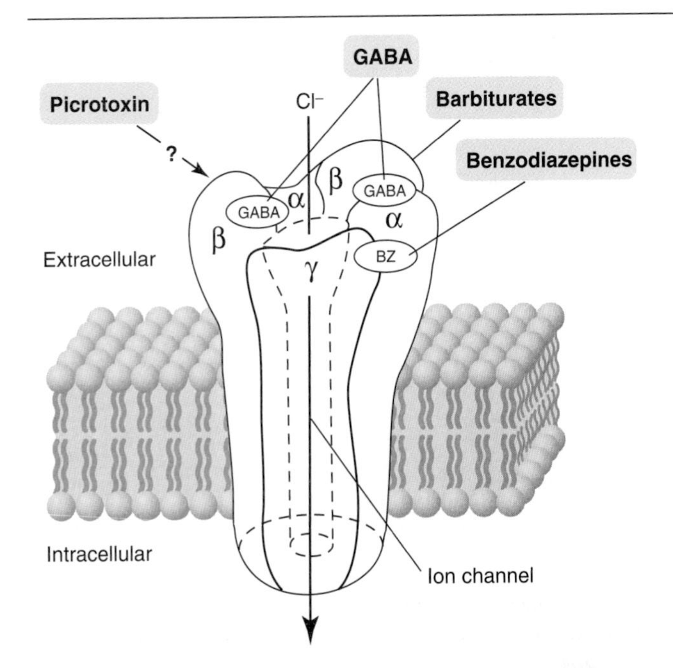

Figure 22–2. Mechanism of action of benzodiazepines. (Reproduced, with permission, from Zorumski CF, Isenberg KE: Insights into the structure and function of GABA-benzodiazepine receptors: ion channels and psychiatry. Am J Psychiatry 1991;148:162–173.)

zodiazepines increase the *frequency* of GABA-mediated chloride ion channel opening. **Flumazenil** reverses the CNS effects of benzodiazepines and is classified as an **antagonist** at BZ receptors. Certain beta-carbolines have a high affinity for BZ receptors and can elicit anxiogenic and convulsant effects. These drugs are classified as **inverse agonists.**

2. **Barbiturates:** Barbiturates depress neuronal activity in the midbrain reticular formation, facilitating and prolonging the inhibitory effects of GABA and glycine. They do not bind to BZ or GABA receptors but appear to interact with other sites on the chloride ion channel. Barbiturates increase the *duration* of GABA-mediated chloride ion channel opening. They may also block the excitatory transmitter glutamic acid, and, at high concentration, sodium channels.
3. **Other drugs:** The anxiolytic drug **buspirone** interacts with the 5-HT_{1A} subclass of brain serotonin receptors as a partial agonist, but the precise mechanism of its anxiolytic effect is unknown. The hypnotics **zolpidem** and **zaleplon** are not benzodiazepines but appear to exert their CNS effects via interaction with certain benzodiazepine receptors, classified as BZ_1 or $omega_1$ subtypes; their CNS depressant effects are antagonized by flumazenil.

C. **Pharmacodynamics:** The CNS effects of most sedative-hypnotics depend on dose, as shown in Figure 22–3. These effects range from sedation and relief of anxiety (anxiolysis), through hypnosis (facilitation of sleep), to anesthesia and coma. Depressant effects are additive when two or more drugs are given together. The steepness of the dose-response curve varies among drug groups; those with flatter curves, such as benzodiazepines, are safer for clinical use. Buspirone is a selective anxiolytic, with minimal depressant effects on the CNS.

1. **Sedation:** Sedative actions, with relief of anxiety, occur with all drugs in this class. Anxiolysis is usually accompanied by some impairment of psychomotor functions, and behavioral disinhibition may also occur. In animals, most sedative-hypnotics release punishment-suppressed behavior.
2. **Hypnosis:** Sedative-hypnotics promote sleep onset and increase the duration of the sleep state. Rapid eye movement (REM) sleep duration is usually decreased at high doses; a rebound increase in REM sleep may occur upon withdrawal from chronic drug use.
3. **Anesthesia:** At high doses loss of consciousness may occur, with amnesia and suppression of reflexes. Anterograde amnesia is more likely with benzodiazepines than with other sedative-hypnotics. Anesthesia can be produced by most barbiturates (eg, thiopental) and certain benzodiazepines (eg, midazolam).
4. **Anticonvulsant actions:** Suppression of seizure activity occurs with high doses of most

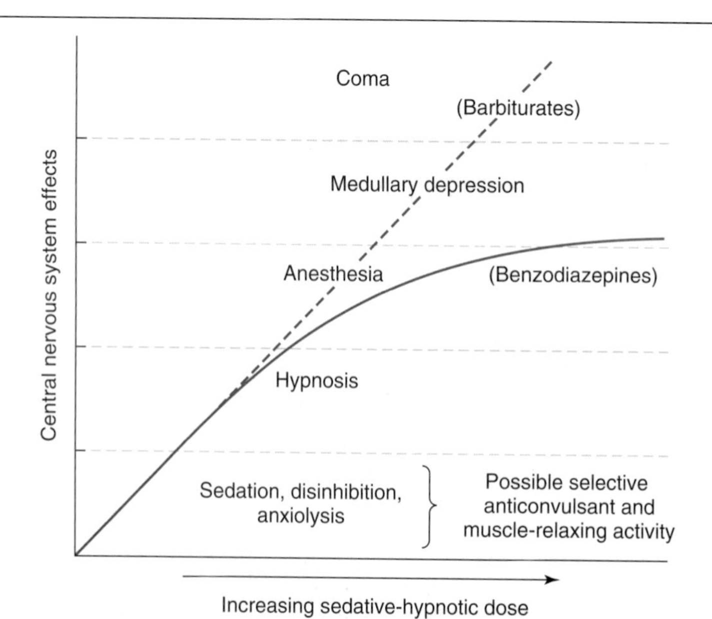

Figure 22–3. Relationships between dose of benzodiazepines and barbiturates and their CNS effects.

of the barbiturates and some of the benzodiazepines, but this is usually at the cost of marked sedation. Selective anticonvulsant action (ie, suppression of convulsions at doses that do not cause severe sedation) occurs with only a few of these drugs (eg, phenobarbital, clonazepam). High doses of intravenous diazepam, lorazepam, or phenobarbital are used in status epilepticus. In this condition, heavy sedation is desirable.

5. **Muscle relaxation:** Relaxation of skeletal muscle occurs at high doses of most sedative-hypnotics. Diazepam is effective at sedative dose levels for specific spasticity states, including cerebral palsy. Meprobamate also has some selectivity as a muscle relaxant.
6. **Medullary depression:** High doses can cause depression of medullary neurons, leading to respiratory arrest, hypotension, and cardiovascular collapse. These effects are the cause of death in suicidal overdose.

Skill Keeper: Loading Dose
(see Chapter 3)

Four hours after ingestion of an unknown quantity of phenobarbital, a patient was hospitalized and the drug concentration in the plasma was found to be 50 mg/L. Assume that in this patient pharmacokinetic parameters for phenobarbital are as follows: oral bioavailability = 100%; V_d = 40 L; CL = 6 L/d; half-life = 4 days. Estimate the dose of phenobarbital ingested. *The Skill Keeper Answer appears at the end of the chapter.*

7. **Tolerance and dependence:** Tolerance—a decrease in responsiveness—occurs when sedative-hypnotics are used chronically or in high dosage. Cross-tolerance may occur among different chemical subgroups. Psychologic dependence occurs frequently with most sedative-hypnotics and is manifested by the compulsive use of these drugs to reduce anxiety. Physiologic dependence constitutes an altered state that leads to an abstinence syndrome (withdrawal state) when the drug is discontinued. Withdrawal signs, which may include anxiety, tremors, hyperreflexia, and seizures, occur more commonly with shorter-acting drugs such as pentobarbital and secobarbital. Buspirone is not schedule-controlled because dependence is unlikely to occur with its use. The dependence liability of zolpidem and of zaleplon may be less than that of the benzodiazepines.

D. **Clinical Use:** Most of these uses can be predicted from the pharmacodynamic effects outlined above.

1. **Anxiety states:** Benzodiazepines with intermediate or long durations of action are favored in the drug treatment of most anxiety states. Alprazolam and clonazepam have greater efficacy than other benzodiazepines in panic and phobic disorders. The anxiolytic effects of buspirone occur without sedation or cognitive impairment but take a week or more to develop. Buspirone is commonly used for generalized anxiety disorders in patients with a past history of substance abuse.
2. **Sleep disorders:** Benzodiazepines, including estazolam, flurazepam, and triazolam, are widely used in primary insomnia and for the management of certain other sleep disorders. Zolpidem and zaleplon appear to cause less daytime cognitive impairment than most benzodiazepines and have minimal effects on sleep patterns.
3. **Other uses:** Thiopental is commonly used for the induction of anesthesia, and certain benzodiazepines (eg, diazepam, midazolam) are used as components of anesthesia protocols. Special uses include the management of seizure disorders (eg, clonazepam, phenobarbital) and muscle spasticity (diazepam). Longer-acting drugs (eg, chlordiazepoxide, diazepam) are used in the management of withdrawal states in persons physiologically dependent on ethanol and other sedative-hypnotics.

E. **Toxicity:**

1. **Psychomotor dysfunction:** This includes cognitive impairment, decreased psychomotor skills, and unwanted daytime sedation. These adverse effects are more common with benzodiazepines that have active metabolites with long half-lives (eg, diazepam, flurazepam). The dosage of a sedative-hypnotic should be reduced in elderly patients to avoid excessive

daytime sedation, which has been shown to increase the risk of falls and fractures. Short-acting hypnotics, especially triazolam, may cause daytime anxiety and amnesia. Anterograde amnesia may also occur with other benzodiazepines when used at high dosage, an action that forms the basis for their criminal use in cases of "date rape."

2. **Additive CNS depression:** This occurs when sedative-hypnotics are used with other drugs in the class as well as with alcoholic beverages, antihistamines, antipsychotic drugs, opioid analgesics, and tricyclic antidepressants. This is the most common type of drug interaction involving sedative-hypnotics. Additive CNS depression with buspirone is uncommon.
3. **Overdosage:** Overdosage causes severe respiratory and cardiovascular depression; these potentially lethal effects are more likely to occur with alcohols, barbiturates, and carbamates than with benzodiazepines. Management of intoxication requires maintenance of a patent airway and ventilatory support. Flumazenil may reverse CNS depressant effects of benzodiazepines, zolpidem, and zaleplon but has no beneficial actions in overdosage with other sedative-hypnotics.
4. **Other adverse effects:** Barbiturates and carbamates (but not benzodiazepines, buspirone, zolpidem, or zaleplon) induce the formation of the liver microsomal enzymes that metabolize drugs. This enzyme induction may lead to multiple drug interactions. Barbiturates may also precipitate acute intermittent porphyria in susceptible patients. Chloral hydrate may displace coumarins from plasma protein binding sites and increase anticoagulant effects.

DRUG LIST

The following drugs are important members of the group discussed in this chapter. Prototypes should be learned in detail; features of the major variants should be known well enough to distinguish the variants from prototypes and from each other; the other significant agents should be recognized as belonging to a specific subclass.

Subclass	Prototype	Major Variants	Other Significant Agents
Benzodiazepines	Chlordiazepoxide, diazepam, temazepam	Alprazolam, clonazepam	Flurazepam, lorazepam, nitrazepam, oxazepam, triazolam
Barbiturates	Phenobarbital, pentobarbital, thiopental		Secobarbital, methohexital
Carbamates	Meprobamate		
Alcohols	Ethanol	Chloral hydrate	
Others	Buspirone, zolpidem, zaleplon		

QUESTIONS

DIRECTIONS: Each of the numbered items or incomplete statements in this section is followed by answers or by completions of the sentence. Select the ONE lettered answer or completion that is BEST in each case.

1. Which one of the following is most likely to result from treatment with moderate doses of diazepam?
   (A) Alleviation of the symptoms of major depressive disorder
   (B) Agitation and possible hyperreflexia with abrupt discontinuance after chronic use
   (C) Increased porphyrin synthesis
   (D) Improved performance on tests of psychomotor function
   (E) Retrograde amnesia
2. A 56-year-old man, very overweight, complains of not sleeping well and feeling tired during the day. He tells his physician that his wife is the cause of the problem because she wakes him up several times during the night due to his loud snores. This appears to be a breathing-related sleep disorder, so you will probably write a prescription for

(A) Clorazepate
(B) Flurazepam
(C) Secobarbital
(D) Triazolam
(E) None of the above

3. Which one of the following statements concerning the barbiturates is accurate?
(A) Symptoms of the abstinence syndrome are more severe during withdrawal from phenobarbital than from secobarbital
(B) Compared with barbiturates, the benzodiazepines exhibit a steeper dose-response relationship
(C) Barbiturates may increase the half-lives of drugs metabolized by the liver
(D) An increase in urinary pH will accelerate the elimination of phenobarbital
(E) Respiratory depression caused by barbiturate overdosage can be reversed by flumazenil

4. Concerning the clinical uses of benzodiazepines and related drugs, which one of the following statements is accurate?
(A) Alprazolam is effective in the management of obsessive-compulsive disorders
(B) Clonazepam has effectiveness in patients who suffer from phobic anxiety states
(C) Diazepam is used for chronic management of bipolar affective disorder in patients who are unable to tolerate lithium
(D) Intravenous buspirone is useful in status epilepticus
(E) Symptoms of the alcohol withdrawal state may be alleviated by treatment with zaleplon

Items 5–6: The wife of a 24-year-old computer programmer considers him to be of a "nervous disposition." He is easily startled, worries about inconsequential matters, and sometimes complains of stomach cramps. At night he grinds his teeth in his sleep. There is no current history of drug abuse.

5. Assuming that the symptoms experienced by this young man are not related to a medical condition, the most appropriate drug treatment would be the judicious use of
(A) Buspirone
(B) Midazolam
(C) Phenobarbital
(D) Triazolam
(E) Zolpidem

6. Regarding the characteristic properties of the drug prescribed for this young man, the physician should inform the patient to anticipate
(A) Additive CNS depression with alcoholic beverages
(B) A significant effect on memory
(C) That the drug will take a week or so to begin working
(D) A need to gradually increase drug dosage because of tolerance
(E) That if he stops taking the drug abruptly he will experience withdrawal signs

7. Which one of the following statements best describes the mechanism of action of benzodiazepines?
(A) Benzodiazepines activate $GABA_B$ receptors in the spinal cord
(B) Their inhibition of GABA transaminase leads to increased levels of GABA
(C) Benzodiazepines block glutamate receptors in hierarchical neuronal pathways in the brain
(D) They increase the frequency of opening of chloride ion channels that are coupled to $GABA_A$ receptors
(E) They are direct-acting GABA receptor agonists in the CNS

Items 8–9: An 82-year-old woman, otherwise healthy for her age, has difficulty sleeping. Triazolam is prescribed for her at one-half of the conventional adult dose.

8. Which one of the following statements about the use of triazolam in this elderly patient is accurate?
(A) Ambulatory dysfunction does not occur in elderly patients taking one-half of the conventional adult dose
(B) Hypertension is a common adverse effect of benzodiazepines in patients over 70 years of age
(C) Over-the-counter cold medications may antagonize the hypnotic effects of the drug
(D) She may experience amnesia, especially if she also drinks alcoholic beverages
(E) Triazolam is distinctive in that it does not cause rebound insomnia on abrupt discontinuance

9. The most likely explanation for the increased sensitivity of elderly patients to a single dose of triazolam and other sedative-hypnotic drugs is
   (A) Changes in brain function that accompany the aging process
   (B) Decreased renal function
   (C) Increased cerebral blood flow
   (D) Decreased hepatic metabolism of lipid-soluble drugs
   (E) Changes in plasma protein binding
10. A 28-year-old woman has sporadic attacks of intense anxiety, with marked physical symptoms including hyperventilation, tachycardia, and sweating. If she is diagnosed as suffering from a panic disorder, the most appropriate drug to use is
   (A) Alprazolam
   (B) Chloral hydrate
   (C) Flurazepam
   (D) Meprobamate
   (E) Propranolol
11. Which one of the following drugs may increase anticoagulant effects by displacement of warfarin from plasma protein binding sites and is inactive until converted in the body to an active metabolite?
   (A) Buspirone
   (B) Chloral hydrate
   (C) Clorazepate
   (D) Secobarbital
   (E) Zaleplon
12. Which one of the following drugs has been used in the management of alcohol withdrawal states and in maintenance treatment of patients with tonic-clonic or partial seizure states? Its chronic use may lead to an increased metabolism of warfarin and phenytoin.
   (A) Chlordiazepoxide
   (B) Meprobamate
   (C) Phenobarbital
   (D) Triazolam
   (E) Zolpidem
13. A 40-year-old patient with liver dysfunction is scheduled for a surgical procedure. Lorazepam can be used for preanesthetic sedation in this patient without concern for excessive CNS depression because the drug is
   (A) A selective anxiolytic like buspirone
   (B) Actively secreted in the renal proximal tubule
   (C) Conjugated extrahepatically
   (D) Eliminated via the lungs
   (E) Reversible by administration of naloxone
14. This hypnotic drug facilitates the inhibitory actions of GABA, but it lacks anticonvulsant or muscle relaxing properties and has minimal effect on sleep architecture.
   (A) Buspirone
   (B) Diazepam
   (C) Flurazepam
   (D) Phenobarbital
   (E) Zaleplon
15. The most frequent type of drug interaction that occurs in patients using drugs of the sedative-hypnotic class is
   (A) Additive CNS depression
   (B) Antagonism of sedative or hypnotic actions
   (C) Competition for plasma protein binding
   (D) Induction of liver drug-metabolizing enzymes
   (E) Inhibition of liver drug-metabolizing enzymes

ANSWERS

1. Diazepam has no more effectiveness than placebo in the treatment of major depressions, but its use can cause a decrease in psychomotor function. Benzodiazepines do not increase activity of

liver drug-metabolizing enzymes or of enzymes involved in porphyrin synthesis. At high doses, benzodiazepines may cause anterograde, not retrograde, amnesia. With abrupt discontinuance following chronic use, anxiety and agitation may occur, sometimes with hyperreflexia and, rarely, seizures. The answer is **(B).**

2. Benzodiazepines and barbiturates are contraindicated in breathing-related sleep disorders because they will further compromise ventilation. In the obstructive sleep apnea syndrome (pickwickian syndrome), obesity is a major risk factor. The best prescription you can give this patient is to lose weight. The answer is **(E).**

3. Withdrawal symptoms from use of the shorter-acting barbiturate secobarbital are more severe than with phenobarbital. The dose-response curve for benzodiazepines is flatter than that for barbiturates. Induction of liver drug-metabolizing enzymes occurs with barbiturates and may lead to *decreases* in half-life of other drugs. Flumazenil is an antagonist at BZ receptors and is used to reverse CNS depressant effects of benzodiazepines. As a weak acid ($pK_a = 7$), phenobarbital will exist mainly in the ionized (nonprotonated) form in the urine at alkaline pH and will not be reabsorbed in the renal tubule. The answer is **(D).**

4. Benzodiazepines have no significant therapeutic benefit in the management of obsessive-compulsive disorders. Drugs effective for this condition increase the activity of serotonergic systems in the brain. Clonazepam has been used commonly as an anticonvulsant and also has efficacy in anxiety states, including agoraphobia. Clonazepam (not diazepam) has also been used as a back-up drug in bipolar affective disorder. The answer is **(B).**

5. The symptoms described suggest that this patient is suffering from a generalized anxiety disorder. Buspirone or longer-acting benzodiazepines are considered to be the drugs of choice for the management of such disorders. Midazolam and triazolam are short-acting benzodiazepines used in anesthesia protocols and for sleep disorders, respectively. The answer is **(A).**

6. Buspirone is a selective anxiolytic with pharmacologic characteristics quite different from those of most other drugs used in anxiety states. Buspirone has minimal effects on cognition or memory; it is not additive with ethanol in terms of CNS depression; tolerance is minimal; and it has no dependence liability. However, buspirone is not effective in *acute* anxiety because it has a slow onset of therapeutic action. The answer is **(C).**

7. Benzodiazepines are thought to exert most of their CNS effects by increasing the inhibitory effects of GABA. Benzodiazepines interact with specific receptors (BZ receptors) that are components of the $GABA_A$ receptor-chloride ion channel macromolecular complex to increase the frequency of chloride ion channel opening. Benzodiazepines are not GABA receptor agonists because they do not interact directly with this component of the complex. The answer is **(D).**

8. In elderly patients taking benzodiazepines, hypotension is far more likely than increased blood pressure. The elderly are more prone to CNS depressant effects of hypnotics; even a dose reduction of 50% may still cause excessive sedation with possible ambulatory impairment. Additive CNS depression occurs commonly with drugs used in OTC cold medications, and rebound insomnia occurs with the abrupt discontinuance of benzodiazepines used as sleeping pills. Amnestic effects of the benzodiazepines are enhanced by the concomitant use of alcoholic beverages. The answer is **(D).**

9. Decreased blood flow to vital organs, including the liver and kidney, occurs during the aging process. These changes may contribute to cumulative effects of sedative-hypnotic drugs. However, this does not explain the enhanced sensitivity of the elderly patient to a **single** dose of a central depressant, which appears to be due to changes in brain function that accompany aging. The answer is **(A).**

10. Alprazolam and clonazepam are the most effective of the benzodiazepines for the treatment of panic disorders. Propranolol has sometimes been used to attenuate excessive sympathomimetic activity in persons who suffer from performance anxiety ("stage fright"). The answer is **(A).**

11. Chloral hydrate is a prodrug and is metabolized to trichloroethanol, the active moiety. It displaces certain drugs from plasma protein binding sites and may cause bleeding when administered to patients given warfarin. The chronic use of chloral hydrate has been associated with an increased incidence of neoplastic disease. Clorazepate is also a prodrug hydrolyzed to form nordiazepam, the active metabolite. The benzodiazepines do not displace other drugs from plasma protein binding sites. The answer is **(B).**

12. Chronic administration of phenobarbital increases the activity of hepatic drug-metabolizing enzymes, including cytochrome P450 isozymes. This often increases the rate of metabolism of drugs administered concomitantly, with decreases in the intensity and duration of their effects. The answer is **(C).**

13. The elimination of most benzodiazepines involves their metabolism by liver enzymes, including cytochrome P450 isozymes. In a patient with liver dysfunction, lorazepam, which is metabolized extrahepatically, is less likely to cause excessive CNS depression. Benzodiazepines are not eliminated via the kidneys or lungs. Flumazenil is used to reverse excessive CNS depression caused by benzodiazepines. The answer is **(C).**
14. Zaleplon and zolpidem are related hypnotics which, though structurally different from benzodiazepines, appear to have a similar mechanism of action. However, neither drug is effective in the management of seizures nor in muscle spasticity states. Compared with benzodiazepines, zaleplon and zolpidem are less likely to alter sleep patterns. Remember—buspirone is not a hypnotic! The answer is **(E).**
15. While drug interactions based on pharmacokinetics do occur with sedative-hypnotics, the most common drug interaction is additive CNS depression. Additive effects can be predicted with concomitant use of alcoholic beverages, anticonvulsants, opioid analgesics and phenothiazines. Less obvious but equally important is enhanced CNS depression with many antihistamines, antihypertensives, and antidepressants of the tricyclic class. The answer is **(A).**

Skill Keeper Answer: Loading Dose
(see Chapter 3)

Since the half-life of phenobarbital is 4 days, one may assume that the plasma concentration 4 hours after drug ingestion is of an order of magnitude similar to that of the peak plasma level. If so, and assuming 100% bioavailability, then

$$\begin{aligned}\textbf{Dose ingested} &= \textbf{Plasma Conc.} \times \mathbf{V_d}\\ &= \textbf{50 mg/L} \times \textbf{40 L}\\ &= \textbf{2000 mg}\end{aligned}$$

23 Alcohols

OBJECTIVES

You should be able to:

- Describe the pharmacodynamics and pharmacokinetics of acute ethanol ingestion.
- List the toxic effects of chronic ethanol ingestion.
- Describe the fetal alcohol syndrome.
- Describe the treatment of ethanol overdosage.
- Outline the pharmacotherapy of (a) the alcohol withdrawal syndrome and (b) alcoholism.
- Describe the toxicity and treatment of acute poisoning with (a) methanol and (b) ethylene glycol.

Learn the definitions that follow.

Table 23–1. Definitions.

Term	Definition
Alcoholism	Compulsive use of ethanol
Psychologic and physiologic dependence	States wherein deprivation of the drug results in severe anxiety (psychologic dependence) and physical symptoms (physical dependence)
Tolerance, cross-tolerance	State of adaptation to a drug that results in reduced effects at a given dosage; cross-tolerance is tolerance to a second drug developed as a result of exposure to a first drug
Acute ethanol intoxication	The signs and symptoms of acute ingestion of a large quantity of ethanol (see text)
Alcohol withdrawal syndrome	The syndrome engendered by deprivation in an individual who has become physically dependent
Fetal alcohol syndrome	The syndrome of teratogenic effects of ethanol consumed by a pregnant woman (see text)
Wernicke-Korsakoff syndrome	Destruction of brain neurons that results from acute thiamine deficiency; most commonly occurs in alcoholics (see text)

CONCEPTS

Ethanol, a sedative-hypnotic drug, is the most important alcohol of pharmacologic interest. It has few medical applications, but its abuse as a recreational drug is responsible for major medical and socioeconomic problems. Other alcohols of toxicologic importance are methanol and ethylene glycol.

ETHANOL

A. **Pharmacokinetics:** After ingestion, ethanol is rapidly and completely absorbed; the drug is then distributed to most body tissues, and its volume of distribution is equivalent to that of total body water (0.5–0.7 L/kg). Two enzyme systems metabolize ethanol to acetaldehyde (Figure 23–1).

1. **Alcohol dehydrogenase (ADH):** This cytosolic, NAD-dependent enzyme, found mainly in the liver and gut, accounts for the metabolism of low to moderate doses of ethanol. Because of the limited supply of the coenzyme NAD, the reaction has *zero-order kinetics* that result in a fixed capacity for ethanol metabolism of 7–10 g/h. With chronic ethanol use, the requirement for NAD for its metabolism may lead to a deficiency of the coenzyme for its

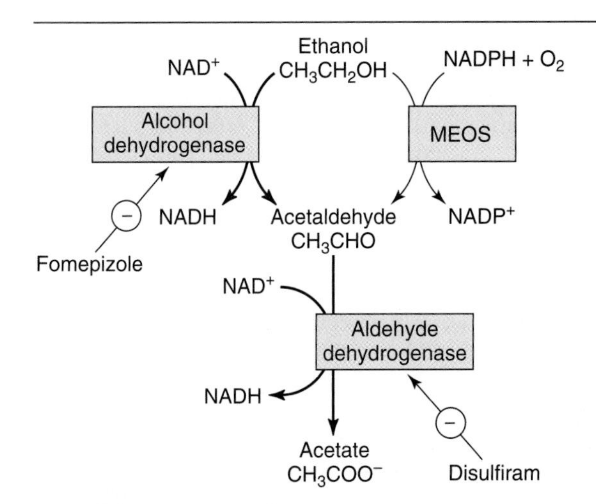

Figure 23–1. Metabolism of ethanol by alcohol dehydrogenase (ADH) and the microsomal ethanol-oxidizing system (MEOS). (Reproduced, with permission, from Katzung BG [editor]: *Basic & Clinical Pharmacology,* 8th ed. McGraw-Hill, 2001.)

normal metabolic functions. Gastrointestinal metabolism of ethanol is lower in women than in men.

2. **Microsomal ethanol-oxidizing system (MEOS):** At blood ethanol levels below 100 mg/dL, this liver microsomal mixed-function oxidase system contributes little to ethanol metabolism. However, the MEOS increases in activity with chronic exposure to ethanol or to inducing agents such as barbiturates, and this increase may be partially responsible for the development of tolerance.

   Acetaldehyde formed from the oxidation of ethanol is rapidly metabolized to acetate by aldehyde dehydrogenase, a mitochondrial enzyme found in the liver and many other tissues. Aldehyde dehydrogenase is inhibited by **disulfiram,** and by other drugs, including **metronidazole, oral hypoglycemics,** and some **cephalosporins.** Certain persons of Asian descent with a genetic deficiency of aldehyde dehydrogenase may experience a flushing reaction from accumulation of acetaldehyde after consumption of small quantities of ethanol.

B. Acute Effects:

1. **CNS:** The major acute effects of ethanol on the CNS include sedation, loss of inhibition, impaired judgment, slurred speech, and ataxia. Impairment of driving ability is thought to occur at ethanol blood levels between 60 mg/dL and 80 mg/dL. Blood levels of 120 to 160 mg/dL are usually associated with gross drunkenness. Levels greater than 300 mg/dL may lead to loss of consciousness, anesthesia, and coma with sometimes fatal respiratory and cardiovascular depression. Blood levels > 500 mg/dL are usually lethal. Chronic alcoholics function almost normally at much higher blood levels than occasional drinkers. Additive CNS depression occurs with concomitant administration of sedative-hypnotics, phenothiazines, and tricyclic antidepressants.

   The molecular mechanisms underlying the complex CNS effects of ethanol are not fully understood. Specific receptors for ethanol have not been identified, but ethanol appears to facilitate the action of GABA at $GABA_A$ receptors and inhibits the ability of glutamate to activate NMDA (*N*-methyl-D-aspartate) receptors. It has been suggested that alcohol "blackouts" may result from the latter action.

2. **Other organ systems:** Ethanol, even at relatively low blood concentrations, significantly depresses the heart. Vascular smooth muscle is relaxed, which leads to vasodilation, sometimes with marked hypothermia. Ethanol relaxes uterine smooth muscle. The drug also enhances the hypoglycemic effects of sulfonylureas and the antiplatelet actions of aspirin.

C. Chronic Effects:

1. **Tolerance and dependence:** Tolerance occurs mainly as a result of CNS adaptation but may be partly caused by an increased rate of ethanol metabolism. There is cross-tolerance to other sedative-hypnotic drugs. Both psychologic and physical dependence are marked, the latter demonstrated by an abstinence syndrome that occurs if a chronic user abruptly discontinues ethanol intake.
2. **Liver:** Gluconeogenesis is reduced and hypoglycemia and fat accumulation may occur as a result of NAD depletion; nutritional deficiencies may contribute to this process. Progressive loss of liver function occurs with hepatitis and cirrhosis. Hepatic dysfunction is often more severe in women than in men, perhaps because higher concentrations of alcohol reach the liver in women. Ethanol may induce an increase in the activity of hepatic microsomal drug-metabolizing enzymes. One form of cytochrome P450 that is inducible by ethanol converts acetaminophen to a hepatotoxic metabolite.
3. **Gastrointestinal system:** Irritation, inflammation, bleeding, and scarring of the gut wall occur after chronic heavy use of ethanol and may cause absorption defects and exacerbate nutritional deficiencies.
4. **CNS:** Peripheral neuropathies are the most common neurologic abnormalities in chronic alcoholics. More rarely, thiamine deficiency—along with ethanol use—leads to the **Wernicke-Korsakoff** syndrome, which is characterized by ataxia, confusion, and paralysis of the extraocular muscles. Prompt treatment with parenteral thiamine is essential to prevent permanent brain damage.
5. **Endocrine system:** Gynecomastia, testicular atrophy, and salt retention occur, partly because of altered steroid metabolism in the cirrhotic liver.

6. **Cardiovascular system:** Excessive ethanol use is associated with an increased incidence of hypertension, anemia, and myocardial infarction. However, the ingestion of modest quantities of ethanol (10–15 g/d) may *protect* against coronary heart disease.
7. **Fetal alcohol syndrome:** Ethanol use in pregnancy is associated with teratogenic effects that include mental retardation (most common), growth deficiencies, microcephaly, and a characteristic underdevelopment of the mid face region. Facial abnormalities are particularly associated with heavy consumption of alcohol in the first trimester of pregnancy.
8. **Neoplasia:** Ethanol is not a primary carcinogen, but its chronic use is associated with an increased incidence of neoplastic diseases, including breast carcinoma.

Skill Keeper: Elimination Half-Life (see Chapter 1)

Search "high and low" through drug information resources and you will *not* find data on the elimination half-life of ethanol! Can you explain why this is the case? *The Skill Keeper Answer appears at the end of the chapter.*

D. Treatment of Acute and Chronic Alcoholism:

1. **Excessive CNS depression:** Intoxication due to acute ingestion of ethanol is managed by maintenance of vital signs and prevention of aspiration after vomiting. Intravenous dextrose is standard. Thiamine administration is used to protect against the Wernicke-Korsakoff syndrome, and correction of electrolyte imbalance may also be required.
2. **Alcohol withdrawal syndrome:** In the chronic user of ethanol, discontinuance can lead to a withdrawal syndrome characterized by insomnia, tremor, anxiety, and, in severe cases, delirium tremens (DTs) and life-threatening seizures. Peripheral effects include nausea, vomiting, diarrhea, and arrhythmias. The abstinence syndrome is usually managed by administration of thiamine, correction of electrolyte imbalance, and the use of a long-acting sedative-hypnotic (eg, chlordiazepoxide, diazepam) with gradual dose-tapering. The intensity of the withdrawal syndrome may also be reduced by clonidine or propranolol.
3. **Treatment of alcoholism:** Alcoholism is a complex sociomedical problem, characterized by a high relapse rate. The aldehyde dehydrogenase inhibitor disulfiram is used adjunctively in some treatment programs. If ethanol is consumed by a patient who has taken disulfiram, acetaldehyde accumulation leads to nausea, headache, flushing, and hypotension (Figure 23–1). Several CNS neurotransmitter systems appear to be targets for drugs that may reduce the craving for alcohol. The opioid antagonist naltrexone has proved to be useful in this context, presumably through its ability to decrease the effects of endogenous opioid peptides in the brain. The selective serotonin reuptake inhibitors (eg, fluoxetine), which can increase serotonergic activity in the CNS, may also be helpful in some patients.

OTHER ALCOHOLS

A. Methanol: Methanol (wood alcohol) is sometimes used by alcoholics when they are unable to obtain ethanol and is a constituent of windshield cleaners and "canned heat." Intoxication from methanol alone may include visual dysfunction, gastrointestinal distress, shortness of breath, loss of consciousness, and coma. Methanol is metabolized to formaldehyde and formic acid, which can cause severe acidosis, retinal damage, and blindness. The formation of formaldehyde is retarded by prompt intravenous administration of ethanol, which acts as a preferred substrate for alcohol dehydrogenase and competitively inhibits the oxidation of methanol (Figure 23–2).

B. Ethylene Glycol: Industrial exposure to ethylene glycol (by inhalation or skin absorption) or self-administration (eg, by drinking antifreeze products) leads to severe acidosis and renal damage from the metabolism of ethylene glycol to oxalic acid. Prompt treatment with ethanol may slow or prevent formation of this toxic metabolite via competition for oxidation by alcohol dehydrogenase. Alcohol dehydrogenase is also inhibited by **fomepizole,** a drug used as an antidote in ethylene glycol toxicity, causing less CNS depression than ethanol.

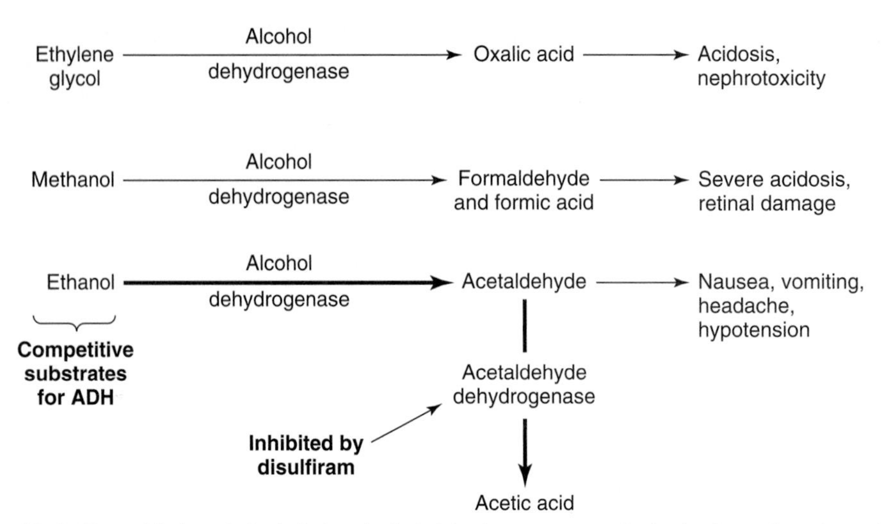

Figure 23–2. The oxidation of alcohols by alcohol dehydrogenase results in the formation of metabolites that cause serious toxicities. Ethanol, a preferred substrate for ADH, is used in methanol or ethylene glycol poisoning to slow the rate of formation of the toxic metabolites of these alcohols. Acetaldehyde formed from ethanol is oxidized rapidly by aldehyde dehydrogenase except in the presence of disulfiram.

QUESTIONS

DIRECTIONS: Each of the numbered items or incomplete statements in this section is followed by answers or by completions of the statement. Select the ONE lettered answer or completion that is BEST in each case.

1. Which one of the following effects is most likely after acute ingestion of ethanol resulting in a blood level of 80 mg/dL?
- **(A)** Cirrhosis
- **(B)** Hypertension
- **(C)** Increased activity of liver microsomal drug-metabolizing enzymes
- **(D)** Relaxation of uterine smooth muscle
- **(E)** Wernicke-Korsakoff syndrome

2. A 42-year-old man with a history of alcoholism is brought to the emergency room in a confused and delirious state. He has truncal ataxia and ophthalmoplegia. The most appropriate immediate course of action is to administer
- **(A)** Chlordiazepoxide
- **(B)** Disulfiram
- **(C)** Folic acid
- **(D)** Lorazepam
- **(E)** Thiamine

3. Which one of the following statements about the biodisposition of ethanol is accurate?
- **(A)** Ethanol is absorbed at all levels of the gastrointestinal tract
- **(B)** Acetic acid is the initial product of ethanol metabolism
- **(C)** After an intravenous dose, plasma levels of ethanol are lower in women than in men
- **(D)** The elimination of ethanol follows first-order kinetics
- **(E)** Alcohol dehydrogenase exhibits genetic variability

4. A freshman student (weight 70 kg) attends a college party where he rapidly consumes a quantity of an alcoholic beverage that results in a blood level of 5 mg/mL. Assuming that this young man has not had an opportunity to develop tolerance to ethanol, his present condition is BEST characterized as
- **(A)** Alert and competent to drive a car
- **(B)** Slightly inebriated
- **(C)** Sedated with increased reaction times
- **(D)** Able to walk, but not in a straight line
- **(E)** Comatose and near death

5. The regular consumption of a glass or two of wine each day with meals may decrease the risk of
(A) Cancer
(B) Coronary heart disease
(C) Gastritis
(D) Psychological dependence
(E) Viral hepatitis

Items 6–7: A homeless middle-aged male patient presents in the emergency room in a state of intoxication. You note that he is behaviorally disinhibited and rowdy. He tells you that he has recently consumed about a pint of a red-colored liquid that his friends were using to "get high." He complains that his vision is blurred and that it is "like being in a snowstorm." His breath smells a bit like formaldehyde.

6. The most likely cause of this patient's intoxicated state is the ingestion of
(A) Ethanol
(B) Ethylene glycol
(C) Isopropanol
(D) Hexane
(E) Methanol

7. Your management of this patient is LEAST likely to include
(A) Airway and respiratory support if needed
(B) Administration of activated charcoal
(C) Administration of bicarbonate to counteract metabolic acidosis
(D) Administration of ethanol before laboratory diagnosis is confirmed
(E) Initiation of dialysis procedures

8. Chronic use of ethanol is reported to increase
(A) Alcohol dehydrogenase
(B) Aldehyde dehydrogenase
(C) Microsomal ethanol-oxidizing system activity
(D) Monoamine oxidase
(E) NADH dehydrogenase

Items 9–10: A 40-year-old man who has consumed the equivalent of more than one-half pint of whisky a day for the last 5 years has in response to an "intervention" abruptly discontinued alcohol use. Within a few hours he became anxious and agitated, with signs of autonomic hyperexcitability. The following day he exhibited hand tremors and was delusional, with visual hallucinations. He was brought to the emergency room of a local hospital where his symptoms culminated in a seizure.

9. Which statement about the condition and management of this patient is accurate?
(A) Chlorpromazine should be given to sedate the patient
(B) Delirium tremens is an appropriate diagnosis of his condition
(C) Intravenous thiamine will reverse these symptoms
(D) Oral buspirone will alleviate withdrawal symptoms in alcohol dependency
(E) Naltrexone should be administered IV immediately

10. Which statement about the consequences and management of the chronic use of ethanol in this patient is accurate?
(A) Adequate nutrition would completely prevent organ system damage in alcohol abuse
(B) Because of his gender, he is more susceptible to hepatic dysfunction than a female in the same situation
(C) Following detoxication, the use of naltrexone may decrease the "craving" for alcohol
(D) The most important goal in alcohol withdrawal is to prevent respiratory depression
(E) Wernicke-Korsakoff syndrome that occurs in alcohol abuse is due to a deficiency of folic acid

11. The chronic abuse of alcohol predisposes to hepatic damage following overdose of acetaminophen because ethanol
(A) Blocks acetaminophen metabolism
(B) Causes thiamine deficiency
(C) Displaces acetaminophen from plasma proteins
(D) Induces liver drug-metabolizing enzymes
(E) Inhibits renal clearance of acetaminophen

12. The activity of this enzyme is specifically decreased in the Wernicke-Korsakoff syndrome
- **(A)** Alcohol dehydrogenase
- **(B)** Cytochrome P450
- **(C)** L-Aromatic amino acid decarboxylase
- **(D)** NADH dehydrogenase
- **(E)** Pyruvate dehydrogenase

ANSWERS

1. The emphasis in this question is on the word *acute.* An acute dose of ethanol relaxes both vascular and uterine smooth muscle. Vasodilation occurs and at high doses may lead to hypothermia. Blood pressure is not raised acutely, though chronic use of alcohol is a risk factor for hypertension. The effect of ethanol on the uterus is to prolong labor. The other effects listed are associated with *chronic* ethanol use. The answer is **(D).**

2. This patient has the symptoms of Wernicke's encephalopathy, including delirium, gait disturbances, and paralysis of the external eye muscles. The condition results from thiamine deficiency but is rarely seen in the absence of alcoholism. The answer is **(E).**

3. Ethanol is absorbed at all levels of the gastrointestinal tract. Acetaldehyde is the initial product of metabolism of ethanol. There are no differences between men and women in plasma levels of ethanol following its intravenous administration. Women have *higher* blood levels than men after *oral* ingestion, possibly because they have lower activity of gastric alcohol dehydrogenase. A characteristic feature of ethanol biodisposition is that its elimination via metabolism follows zero-order kinetics. Certain persons of Asian descent are deficient in *aldehyde dehydrogenase* and may experience a disulfiram-like reaction at low doses of ethanol. The answer is **(A).**

4. The blood level of ethanol achieved in this person is equivalent to 500 mg/dL and almost certainly was estimated postmortem. The quantity of ethanol ingested can be calculated from the product of plasma level and volume of distribution (0.5–0.7 L/kg). In this case, the young man ingested 200 g of ethanol, the equivalent of over 20 fluid ounces (550 mL) of distilled 80 proof spirits. The answer is **(E).**

5. Compared with those who abstain, individuals who regularly ingest modest quantities of ethanol (one or two drinks daily) are reported to have a *decreased* risk of coronary heart disease. The chronic use of ethanol is a risk factor for the other items listed. The answer is **(B).**

6. Behavioral disinhibition is a feature of early intoxication due to ethanol and most other alcohols but not ingestion of the solvent, hexane. Ocular dysfunction, including horizontal nystagmus and diplopia, is also a common finding in poisoning with alcohols, but the complaint of "flickering white spots before the eyes" or "being in a snowstorm" is highly suggestive of methanol intoxication. In some cases, the odor of formaldehyde may be present on the breath. In this patient, blood methanol levels should be determined as soon as possible. The answer is **(E).**

7. In all poisoning situations, it is important to establish adequate respiration. Bicarbonate may be needed to counteract metabolic acidosis. In patients with suspected methanol intoxication, ethanol (10% solution) is often given intravenously before laboratory diagnosis is confirmed to block the formation of toxic products of ADH-catalyzed metabolism of methanol. Blood levels of methanol in excess of 50 mg/dL are an absolute indication for hemodialysis. Activated charcoal does not bind alcohols. The answer is **(B).**

8. The microsomal ethanol-oxidizing system (MEOS) becomes significant in terms of ethanol metabolism only at blood levels in excess of 100 mg/dL. Chronic exposure to ethanol increases the activity of MEOS, and this effect may be contributory to "metabolic" tolerance. None of the other enzymes involved in ethanol metabolism change their activities with chronic use. Ethanol induces the formation of certain cytochrome P450 isozymes if used regularly. The answer is **(C).**

9. The patient is experiencing symptoms of the withdrawal syndrome from physical dependency on ethanol. Since seizures are possible, it would not be appropriate to attempt sedation with a phenothiazine such as chlorpromazine. Thiamine is usually administered to counteract the symptoms of Wernicke-Korsakoff syndrome but will not alleviate withdrawal symptoms. Neither buspirone nor naltrexone has value in the immediate management of alcohol withdrawal states. The patient is indeed suffering from delirium tremens. The answer is **(B).**

10. Attention to nutritional needs is not totally protective against organ system damage that occurs with chronic abuse of alcohol. Females are more susceptible to alcohol hepatotoxicity than males. Respiratory depression is a symptom of ethanol *overdose,* not withdrawal. Naltrexone, an opioid receptor antagonist, may have value in some patients to decrease the intensity of "craving." The answer is **(C).**

11. Chronic use of ethanol causes induction of a cytochrome P450 isozyme that converts acetaminophen to a cytotoxic metabolite. This appears to be the explanation for the increased susceptibility of alcoholics to hepatotoxicity with overdose of acetaminophen. The answer is **(D).**

12. Pyruvate dehydrogenase plays an important role in energy metabolism to provide ATP, utilizing thiamine pyrophosphate as a cofactor in the reaction. In thiamine deficiency, the activity of pyruvate dehydrogenase is decreased, impairing the formation of ATP. The answer is **(E).**

Skill Keeper Answer: Elimination Half-Life
(see Chapter 1)

Drug information resources will not provide data on the elimination half-life of ethanol because, in the case of this drug, it is not constant. The elimination of ethanol follows **zero-order kinetics** because the drug is metabolized at a constant rate irrespective of its concentration in the blood (see Chapter 3). The pharmacokinetic relationship between elimination half-life, volume of distribution, and clearance, given by

$$t_{1/2} = \frac{0.693 \times V_d}{CL}$$

is not applicable in the case of ethanol; its rate of metabolism is constant, but its clearance decreases with increase in blood level. The arithmetic plot of ethanol blood level versus time follows a straight line (not exponential decay).

Antiseizure Drugs 24

OBJECTIVES

You should be able to:

- List the major drugs used for partial seizures, generalized tonic-clonic seizures, absence and myoclonic seizures, and status epilepticus.
- Identify the mechanisms of antiseizure drug action.
- Describe the main pharmacokinetic features and adverse effects of major antiseizure drugs.

- Identify new antiseizure drugs and their important characteristics.
- Describe the factors that must be considered in designing a dosage regimen for an antiseizure drug.

Learn the definitions that follow.

Table 24–1. Definitions of seizure states.

Term	Definition
Seizures	Finite episodes of brain dysfunction resulting from abnormal discharge of cerebral neurons
Partial seizures, simple	Consciousness preserved; manifested variously as convulsive jerking, paresthesias, psychic symptoms (altered sensory perception, illusions, hallucinations, affect changes) and autonomic dysfunction
Partial seizures, complex	Impaired consciousness that is preceded, accompanied, or followed by psychologic symptoms
Tonic-clonic seizures, generalized	Tonic phase (less than 1 minute) involves abrupt loss of consciousness, muscle rigidity and respiration arrest; clonic phase (2–3 minutes) involves jerking of body muscles, with lip or tongue biting, and fecal and urinary incontinence; formerly called grand mal
Absence seizures, generalized	Impaired consciousness (often abrupt onset and brief), sometimes with automatisms, loss of postural tone, or enuresis; begin in childhood (formerly, petit mal) and usually cease by age 20 years
Myoclonic seizures	Single or multiple myoclonic muscle jerks
Status epilepticus	A series of seizures (usually tonic-clonic) without recovery of consciousness between attacks; it is a life-threatening emergency

CONCEPTS

A. Classification: Epilepsy comprises a group of chronic syndromes that involve the recurrence of seizures, ie, limited periods of abnormal discharge of cerebral neurons (see Table 24–1). Several chemical subgroups of antiseizure drugs are structurally related; these include **hydantoins** (eg, phenytoin), **barbiturates** (eg, phenobarbital), and **succinimides** (eg, ethosuximide). There are several unrelated subgroups, including two tricyclic compounds, **carbamazepine** and **oxcarbazepine; valproic acid,** a carboxylic acid; **benzodiazepines** (eg, diazepam, clonazepam); **felbamate,** a carbamate; **GABA derivatives** (eg, gabapentin, vigabatrin); **lamotrigine,** a phenyltriazine; and **topiramate,** a substituted monosaccharide. Subgroups of antiseizure drugs are selective in their therapeutic effects for specific types of seizures (Figure 24–1).

B. Pharmacokinetics: Antiseizure drugs are commonly used for long periods of time, and consideration of their pharmacokinetic properties is important for avoiding toxicity and drug interactions. For some of these drugs (eg, phenytoin), determination of plasma levels and

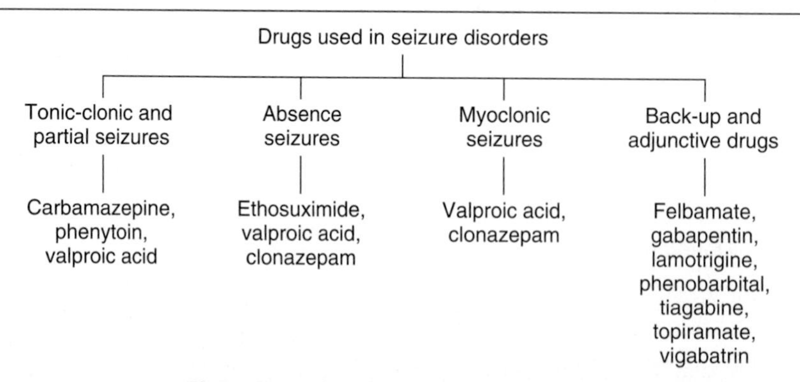

Figure 24–1. Subgroups of antiseizure drugs.

clearance in individual patients may be necessary for optimum therapy. In general, antiseizure drugs are well absorbed orally and have good bioavailability. Most are metabolized by hepatic enzymes, and in some cases (eg, primidone, trimethadione) active metabolites are formed.

Pharmacokinetic drug interactions are common in this drug group. In the presence of drugs that inhibit antiseizure drug metabolism or displace anticonvulsants from plasma protein binding sites, plasma concentrations of the antiseizure agents may reach toxic levels. On the other hand, drugs that induce hepatic drug-metabolizing enzymes (eg, rifampin) may result in plasma levels of the antiseizure agents that are inadequate for seizure control.

1. **Phenytoin:** The oral bioavailability of phenytoin is variable because of differences in first-pass metabolism. Phenytoin metabolism is nonlinear; elimination kinetics shift from first-order to zero-order at moderate to high dose levels. The drug binds extensively to plasma proteins (97–98%), and free (unbound) phenytoin levels in plasma are increased transiently by drugs that compete for binding (eg, sulfonamides, valproic acid). The metabolism of phenytoin is enhanced in the presence of inducers of liver metabolism (eg, phenobarbital, rifampin) and inhibited by other drugs (eg, cimetidine, isoniazid). **Fosphenytoin** is a water-soluble prodrug form of phenytoin that is used parenterally.
2. **Carbamazepine:** Carbamazepine induces formation of liver drug-metabolizing enzymes that increase metabolism of the drug itself and may increase the clearance of many other anticonvulsant drugs. Carbamazepine metabolism can be inhibited by other drugs (eg, propoxyphene, valproic acid).
3. **Valproic acid:** In addition to competing for phenytoin plasma protein binding sites, valproic acid inhibits the metabolism of phenytoin, phenobarbital, and lamotrigine. Hepatic biotransformation of valproic acid leads to formation of a toxic metabolite that has been implicated in the hepatotoxicity of the drug.
4. **Newer drugs:** Gabapentin and vigabatrin are unusual in that they are eliminated by the kidney, largely in unchanged form. Lamotrigine is eliminated via hepatic glucuronidation. Topiramate undergoes both hepatic metabolism and renal elimination of intact drug.

C. **Mechanisms of Action:** The general effect of antiseizure drugs is to suppress repetitive action potentials in epileptic foci in the brain. Different mechanisms are involved in achieving this effect. In the case of some drugs, multiple mechanisms may contribute to their antiseizure activities. Some of the recognized mechanisms are described below.

1. **Sodium channel blockade:** At therapeutic concentrations, phenytoin, carbamazepine, and lamotrigine block voltage-gated sodium channels in neuronal membranes. This action is rate-dependent (ie, dependent on the frequency of neuronal discharge) and results in prolongation of the inactivated state of the Na^+ channel and the refractory period of the neuron. Phenobarbital and valproic acid may exert similar effects at high doses.
2. **GABA-related targets:** As described in Chapter 22, benzodiazepines interact with specific receptors on the $GABA_A$ receptor-chloride ion channel macromolecular complex. In the presence of benzodiazepines, the *frequency* of chloride ion channel opening is increased; these drugs facilitate the inhibitory effects of GABA. Phenobarbital and other barbiturates also enhance the inhibitory actions of GABA but interact with a different receptor site on chloride ion channels that results in an increased *duration* of chloride ion channel opening.

   GABA transaminase is an important enzyme in the termination of action of GABA. The enzyme is irreversibly inactivated by vigabatrin at therapeutic plasma levels and can also be inhibited by valproic acid at very high concentrations. Inhibition of GABA transaminase is presumed to enhance the effects of GABA at synaptic sites. Tiagabine inhibits GABA transporters in neurons and glia. Gabapentin is a structural analog of GABA, but it does not activate GABA receptors directly and its mechanism of antiseizure action is unclear.
3. **Calcium channel blockade:** Ethosuximide inhibits low-threshold (T-type) Ca^{2+} currents, especially in thalamic neurons that act as pacemakers to generate rhythmic cortical discharge. A similar action is reported for valproic acid.
4. **Other mechanisms:** In addition to its action on calcium channels, valproic acid causes neuronal membrane hyperpolarization, possibly by enhancing K^+ channel permeability. In addition to its actions on sodium channels and GABA-chloride channels, phenobarbital also acts as an antagonist at some glutamate receptors. Topiramate appears to block sodium channels and potentiate the actions of GABA and may also block glutamate receptors.

Skill Keeper: Antiarrhythmic Drug Actions (see Chapter 14)

1. Which of the mechanisms of action of antiseizure drugs have theoretical implications regarding their activity in cardiac arrhythmias?
2. Can you recall any clinical uses of antiseizure drugs in the management of cardiac arrhythmias?

The Skill Keeper Answers appear at the end of the chapter.

D. **Clinical Use:** Diagnosis of a specific seizure type is important for prescribing the most appropriate antiseizure drug (or combination of drugs). Drug choice is usually made on the basis of established efficacy in the specific seizure state that has been diagnosed, the prior responsiveness of the patient, and the anticipated toxicity of the drug. Treatment may involve combinations of drugs, following the principle of adding known effective agents if the preceding drugs are not sufficient.

1. **Generalized tonic-clonic and partial seizures:** Valproic acid, carbamazepine, and phenytoin are the drugs of choice for generalized tonic-clonic (grand mal) seizures and for most cases of simple and complex partial seizures. Phenobarbital (or primidone) is now considered to be an alternative agent in adults but continues to be a primary drug in infants. Lamotrigine is also an alternative agent, but its usefulness is limited by its toxic potential (see below). Gabapentin may be used adjunctively in refractory cases. Topiramate is approved for adjunctive use with other agents in partial seizures, and vigabatrin may also be useful as a backup drug.
2. **Absence seizures:** Ethosuximide and valproic acid are the preferred drugs since they cause minimal sedation. Ethosuximide is often used in uncomplicated absence seizures if patients can tolerate its gastrointestinal side effects. Valproic acid is particularly useful in patients who have concomitant generalized tonic-clonic or myoclonic seizures. Clonazepam is effective as an alternative drug but has the disadvantages of causing sedation and tolerance.
3. **Myoclonic syndromes:** Myoclonic seizure syndromes are usually treated with valproic acid. Clonazepam can be effective, but the high doses required cause drowsiness. Lamotrigine is also reported to be effective in myoclonic syndromes in children. Felbamate has been used adjunctively with the primary drugs but has hematotoxic and hepatotoxic potential.
4. **Status epilepticus:** Intravenous diazepam or lorazepam is usually effective in terminating attacks and providing short-term control. For prolonged therapy, intravenous phenytoin is usually employed since it is highly effective and less sedating than benzodiazepines or barbiturates. However, phenytoin may cause cardiotoxicity (perhaps due to its solvent propylene glycol), and fosphenytoin (water-soluble) may prove to be safer. Phenobarbital has also been used in status epilepticus, especially in children. In very severe status epilepticus that does not respond to these measures, general anesthesia may be employed.
5. **Infantile spasms:** Corticotropin and corticosteroids are commonly used but cause characteristic cushingoid side effects. Benzodiazepines and other anticonvulsants may also be used, but their efficacy is limited.
6. **Other clinical uses:** Several antiseizure drugs are effective in the management of bipolar affective disorders, including valproic acid, carbamazepine, phenytoin, and gabapentin. Carbamazepine is the drug of choice for trigeminal neuralgia. Gabapentin has efficacy in pain of neuropathic origin and, like phenytoin, may have some value in migraine.

E. **Toxicity:** Chronic therapy with antiseizure drugs is associated with specific toxic effects, the most important of which are listed in Table 24–2.

1. **Teratogenicity:** Children born of mothers taking anticonvulsant drugs have an increased risk of congenital malformations. Neural tube defects (eg, spina bifida) are associated with the use of valproic acid; carbamazepine has been implicated as a cause of craniofacial anomalies and spina bifida; and fetal hydantoin syndrome has been described following phenytoin use by pregnant women.
2. **Overdosage toxicity:** Most of the commonly used anticonvulsants are CNS depressants, and respiratory depression may occur with overdosage. Management is primarily support-

Table 24–2. Adverse effects and complications of the use of antiseizure drugs.

Drug	Adverse Effects
Benzodiazepines	Sedation, tolerance, dependence
Carbamazepine	Diplopia, ataxia, enzyme induction, blood dyscrasias, teratogen
Ethosuximide	Gastrointestinal distress, lethargy, headache
Felbamate	Aplastic anemia, hepatotoxicity
Gabapentin	Sedation, behavioral changes in children, movement disorders, leukopenia
Lamotrigine	Sedation, ataxia, life-threatening skin disorders, hematotoxicity
Phenobarbital	Sedation, enzyme induction, tolerance, dependence
Phenytoin	Nystagmus, diplopia, ataxia, sedation, gingival hyperplasia, hirsutism, anemias, enzyme induction, teratogen
Tiagabine	Dizziness, tremor, difficulty in concentrating, psychosis (rare)
Topiramate	Sedation, mental dulling, renal stones, weight loss
Valproic acid	Gastrointestinal distress, hepatotoxicity (rare but possibly fatal), inhibition of drug metabolism, teratogen
Vigabatrin	Sedation, weight gain, agitation, confusion, psychosis, visual field defects with long-term use (possibly irreversible)

ive (airway management, mechanical ventilation), and flumazenil may be used in benzodiazepine overdose.

3. **Life-threatening toxicity:** Fatal hepatotoxicity has occurred with valproic acid, with greatest risk to children less than 2 years of age and patients taking multiple anticonvulsant drugs. Lamotrigine has caused skin rashes and life-threatening Stevens-Johnson syndrome or toxic epidermal necrolysis. Children are at higher risk (1–2% incidence), especially if they are also taking valproic acid. Reports of aplastic anemia and acute hepatic failure have limited the use of felbamate to severe, refractory seizure states.
4. **Withdrawal:** Withdrawal from antiseizure drugs should be accomplished gradually to avoid increased seizure frequency and severity. In general, withdrawal from anti-absence drugs is more easily accomplished than withdrawal from drugs used in partial or generalized tonic-clonic seizure states.

DRUG LIST

The following drugs are important members of the group discussed in this chapter. Prototypes should be learned in detail; features of the major variants should be known well enough to distinguish the variants from prototypes and from each other; the other significant agents should be recognized as belonging to a specific subclass.

Subclass	Prototype	Major Variant	Other Significant Agents
Barbiturates	Phenobarbital	Primidone	Metharbital
Benzodiazepines	Diazepam	Lorazepam, clorazepate	Clonazepam, nitrazepam
Carboxylic acids	Valproic acid	Sodium valproate	
Hydantoins	Phenytoin	Fosphenytoin	Mephenytoin
Succinimides	Ethosuximide	Phensuximide	
Tricyclics	Carbamazepine	Oxcarbazepine	
Newer agents	Felbamate, gabapentin, lamotrigine, tiagabine, topiramate, vigabatrin		

QUESTIONS

DIRECTIONS: Each of the numbered items or incomplete statements in this section is followed by answers or by completions of the statement. Select the ONE lettered answer or completion that is BEST in each case.

1. A 26-year-old woman develops a seizure disorder characterized by recurrent contractions of the muscles in the right hand which then spread to the right arm and to the right side of the face ("jacksonian march"). Consciousness is not impaired, and the attacks usually last for only a minute or two. Which one of the following drugs is LEAST likely to be useful in the treatment of this patient?
(A) Carbamazepine
(B) Ethosuximide
(C) Lamotrigine
(D) Phenytoin
(E) Primidone

2. A 9-year-old child is having learning difficulties at school. He has brief lapses of awareness with eyelid fluttering that occur every 5–10 minutes. EEG studies reveal brief 3-Hz spike and wave discharges appearing synchronously in all leads. Which one of the following drugs would be effective in this child but has the disadvantages of causing sedation and tolerance?
(A) Clonazepam
(B) Diazepam
(C) Ethosuximide
(D) Phenobarbital
(E) Valproic acid

3. Which one of the following statements concerning proposed mechanisms of action of anticonvulsant drugs is false?
(A) Diazepam facilitates GABA-mediated inhibitory actions
(B) Ethosuximide selectively blocks K^+ ion channels in thalamic neurons
(C) Phenobarbital has multiple actions, including enhancement of the effects of GABA, antagonism of glutamate receptors, and blockade of Na^+ ion channels
(D) Phenytoin prolongs the inactivated state of the Na^+ ion channel
(E) Vigabatrin elevates brain GABA levels

4. Which of the following antiseizure drugs is most likely to elevate the plasma concentration of other drugs administered concomitantly?
(A) Carbamazepine
(B) Diazepam
(C) Phenobarbital
(D) Phenytoin
(E) Valproic acid

Items 5–6: A young woman employed as a computer programmer suffers from myoclonic jerking with no overt signs of neurologic deficit. There is no history of generalized tonic-clonic seizures. You are considering drug therapy for this patient.

5. If the seizures are to be effectively controlled without excessive sedation, the most appropriate drug is
(A) Acetazolamide
(B) Carbamazepine
(C) Clonazepam
(D) Valproic acid
(E) Vigabatrin

6. In the management of this patient with the most appropriate drug, which one of the following considerations is LEAST important?
(A) Abdominal pain and heartburn are likely side effects
(B) Liver enzymes should be monitored
(C) She should be examined every 2 or 3 months for deep tendon reflex activity
(D) She should contact her physician immediately if she becomes pregnant
(E) The patient should avoid barbiturates

7. Which one of the following statements concerning the pharmacokinetics of antiseizure drugs is accurate?
(A) At high doses, phenytoin elimination follows first-order kinetics
(B) Valproic acid may increase the activity of hepatic ALA synthase and the synthesis of porphyrins
(C) The administration of phenytoin to patients in methadone maintenance programs has led to symptoms of opioid overdose, including respiratory depression
(D) Although ethosuximide has a half-life of approximately 40 hours, the drug is usually taken twice a day
(E) Treatment with vigabatrin may reduce the effectiveness of oral contraceptives

8. With chronic use in seizure states, the adverse effects of this drug include coarsening of facial features, hirsutism, gingival hyperplasia, and osteomalacia.
(A) Carbamazepine
(B) Ethosuximide
(C) Gabapentin
(D) Phenytoin
(E) Valproic acid

9. Which one of the following statements about vigabatrin is accurate?
(A) Blocks neuronal reuptake of GABA
(B) Drug of choice in absence seizures
(C) Is established to be teratogenic in humans
(D) Life-threatening skin disorders may occur
(E) Visual field defects occur in up to one-third of patients

10. Withdrawal of antiseizure drugs can cause increased seizure frequency and severity. Withdrawal is least likely to be a problem with
(A) Clonazepam
(B) Diazepam
(C) Ethosuximide
(D) Phenobarbital
(E) Phenytoin

11. A young female patient who suffers from bipolar affective disorder (BAD) has been managed with lithium. If she becomes pregnant, which one of the following drugs is likely to be effective in bipolar affective disorder with minimal risk of teratogenicity?
(A) Carbamazepine
(B) Clonazepam
(C) Phenytoin
(D) Valproic acid
(E) None of the above

12. The most likely mechanism involved in the antiseizure activity of carbamazepine is
(A) Block of sodium ion channels
(B) Block of calcium ion channels
(C) Facilitation of GABA actions on chloride ion channels
(D) Glutamate receptor antagonism
(E) Inhibition of GABA transaminase

13. Which one of the following statements about phenytoin is accurate?
(A) Displaces sulfonamides from plasma proteins
(B) Drug of choice in myoclonic seizures
(C) Half-life is increased if used with phenobarbital
(D) Isoniazid (INH) decreases steady state blood levels of phenytoin
(E) Toxicity may occur with only small increments in dose

14. A young male patient suffers from a seizure disorder characterized by tonic rigidity of the extremities followed in 15–30 seconds by tremor progressing to massive jerking of the body. This clonic phase lasts for a minute or two, leaving the patient in a stuporous state. The antiseizure drug of choice for chronic management of this patient is
(A) Clonazepam
(B) Ethosuximide
(C) Fosphenytoin
(D) Lamotrigine
(E) Valproic acid

DIRECTIONS (Items 15–18): The case history* below is followed by several short-answer questions. After reading the case history, write out brief answers (one to three sentences) to the questions based on your understanding of the material presented in this and preceding chapters. Then compare your answers with those given in the Answers section.

An 18-year-old woman was admitted for evaluation of therapy for frequent epileptic absence attacks associated with minor automatisms. The patient had a history of unsuccessful treatment with ethosuximide. The EEG showed generalized 3/s spike-and-wave complexes and intermittent left temporal discharges. Therapy was restarted using sodium valproate and carbamazepine. A 24-hour electroencephalographic study revealed 71 absence attacks. Increasing the valproate dosage from 1200 mg/d to 2400 mg/d was associated with a significant but transient decline in absence frequency. Mean serum levels of valproic acid at that time were 81 mg/L (109 mg/L peak, 36 mg/L trough) on a twice-daily dosage regimen. Slow withdrawal of carbamazepine resulted in a decrease in the number of clinical or electroencephalographic attacks. The addition of ethosuximide, 1000 mg/d, resulted in disappearance of all seizure activity. The mean serum ethosuximide level was 70 mg/L.

Six months later, an attempt was made to reduce the dosage of valproate. On a twice-daily dose of 300 mg (600 mg/d total), mean serum levels dropped to 34 mg/L. There was a prompt recurrence of seizures, but they declined again when valproate dosage was returned to 2400 mg/d. A follow-up study 8 months later demonstrated a continuing favorable response.

15. What was the rationale for the initial treatment with carbamazepine? Why was the drug subsequently withdrawn, and why did the frequency of the seizures decrease?
16. Why were blood levels of the drugs measured several times during the day?
17. What are the hazards of therapy with ethosuximide? With sodium valproate?
18. What alternative drugs are possible for the management of absence seizures? What are the side effects of such backup drugs?

ANSWERS

1. Simple partial seizures can have the characteristics described in this patient. The jacksonian march is due to progression of epileptiform discharges in the contralateral motor cortex. Phenytoin, carbamazepine, primidone, and lamotrigine are effective in partial seizures. The succinimides (ethosuximide, phensuximide) are not effective in partial seizures or in generalized tonic-clonic seizure states. The answer is **(B).**
2. Three of the drugs listed are effective in absence seizures. Ethosuximide and valproic acid are not sedating, and tolerance does not develop to their antiseizure activity. Clonazepam is effective but exerts troublesome CNS depressant effects, and tolerance develops with chronic use. At high doses, the drug has a dependence liability like most benzodiazepines. The answer is **(A).**
3. Though not completely understood, the mechanism of action of ethosuximide is thought to involve blockade of T-type Ca^{2+} ion channels in thalamic neurons. The drug does not block K^+ ion channels, which in any case would be likely to result in an increase (rather than a decrease) in neuronal excitability. The answer is **(B).**
4. With chronic use, the anticonvulsant barbiturates, carbamazepine, and phenytoin all induce the formation of hepatic drug-metabolizing enzymes. This action may lead to a *decrease* in the plasma concentration of other drugs used concomitantly. Valproic acid, an inhibitor of drug metabolism, can increase the plasma levels of many drugs, including carbamazepine, lamotrigine, phenobarbital, and phenytoin. Benzodiazepines have no major effects on the metabolism of other drugs. The answer is **(E).**
5. Valproic acid is highly effective in specific myoclonic syndromes and is usually considered to be the drug of choice since it is nonsedating. Clonazepam is a backup drug, since the high doses required cause excessive drowsiness. None of the other drugs listed are effective. Acetazolamide is rarely used in seizure states because tolerance develops rapidly; however, the drug may be useful in women who experience seizures at the time of menses. The answer is **(D).**

* Modified and reproduced, with permission, from Rowan AJ et al: Valproate-ethosuximide combination therapy for refractory absence seizures. Arch Neurol 1983;40:797.

6. Valproic acid often causes gastrointestinal distress and is potentially hepatotoxic. The use of this drug in pregnancy has been associated with teratogenicity (neural tube defects). Valproic acid inhibits the metabolism of barbiturates; marked CNS depression may result if such drugs are given concomitantly. Peripheral neuropathy, in the form of diminished deep tendon reflexes in the lower extremities, is associated with chronic use of phenytoin. The answer is **(C).**
7. Monitoring of plasma concentration of phenytoin may be critical in establishing an effective dosage, since the drug exhibits nonlinear elimination kinetics at high doses. Valproic acid has no effect on porphyrin synthesis. The enzyme-inducing activity of phenytoin has led to symptoms of opioid *withdrawal,* presumably due to an increase in the rate of metabolism of methadone. Vigabatrin does not affect the metabolism of oral contraceptives since it is not an inducer of liver drug-metabolizing enzymes. Twice-daily dosage of ethosuximide is common because it reduces the severity of adverse gastrointestinal effects. The answer is **(D).**
8. Common adverse effects of phenytoin include nystagmus, diplopia, and ataxia. With chronic use, abnormalities of vitamin D metabolism and coarsening of facial features may occur. Gingival overgrowth and hirsutism also occur to some degree in most patients. The answer is **(D).**
9. Vigabatrin inhibits the enzyme GABA transaminase and does not block the transporter mechanisms for GABA reuptake. The drug has been used in partial seizures, but long-term use is associated with visual field defects that may not be reversible in over 30% of patients. For this reason, the drug is a backup for treatment of patients refractory to the standard drugs. The answer is **(E).**
10. There are two problems with regard to withdrawal from antiseizure drugs: the effects of withdrawal itself and the need to continue suppression of seizures. Dose-tapering is an important principle in antiseizure drug withdrawal. As a rule, withdrawal from drugs used in absence seizures is easier than withdrawal from drugs used for partial and tonic-clonic seizures. Withdrawal is most difficult in patients who have been treated with barbiturates and benzodiazepines. The answer is **(C).**
11. Several antiseizure drugs have some effectiveness in bipolar affective disorder. Of the drugs listed, clonazepam does not appear to cause teratogenic effects and would be the "safest" during pregnancy. The answer is **(B).**
12. Carbamazepine's mechanism of action is similar to that of phenytoin, blocking sodium ion channels. Ethosuximide blocks calcium channels; benzodiazepines and barbiturates facilitate the inhibitory actions of GABA; topiramate may block glutamate receptors; and vigabatrin inhibits GABA metabolism. The answer is **(A).**
13. Sulfonamides have a very high binding affinity for plasma proteins and can displace phenytoin from its binding sites, increasing the plasma free fraction of the drug. Induction of liver drug-metabolizing enzymes by phenobarbital results in a *decreased* half-life of phenytoin, and isoniazid *increases* plasma levels of phenytoin by inhibiting its metabolism. Because of the dose-dependent elimination kinetics of phenytoin, some toxicity may occur with only small increments in dose. The answer is **(E).**
14. This patient is suffering from generalized tonic-clonic seizures. Several drugs have effectiveness in such seizure states, including carbamazepine, phenobarbital, phenytoin, and valproic acid. Clonazepam and ethosuximide are not effective. Lamotrigine is usually considered an "add-on" drug in the management of partial seizures. Fosphenytoin, more water-soluble than phenytoin, is available for parenteral use in the management of status epilepticus. The answer is **(E).**
15. Carbamazepine was probably used at the start of treatment to prevent the automatisms (complex partial seizures) that were reportedly part of the patient's seizure repertoire. Carbamazepine is considered a drug of choice for this seizure type. When it became apparent that such seizures were actually infrequent in this patient, the drug was withdrawn. Carbamazepine has been reported to make absence (or myoclonic) seizures worse.
16. Monitoring of blood levels can be important in the management of epilepsy because the therapeutic window of most antiepileptic drugs is narrow. The effective levels for valproate and ethosuximide are 50–100 mg/L. Thus, the levels measured in this patient while she was receiving the high dose of valproate were within the effective range for both agents. When the dose of valproate was reduced to 600 mg/d, the plasma levels dropped below the minimum effective range, and seizures recurred.
17. Ethosuximide is associated with a very low incidence of serious adverse effects. However, gastric irritation, lethargy, fatigue, and annoying CNS effects are quite common. In contrast, valproate carries with it a low but significant risk of serious hepatic injury; liver function

should be monitored. Valproic acid is contraindicated in pregnant women because it has been shown to cause spina bifida in infants born to mothers taking the drug. Valproic acid may inhibit the hepatic metabolism of other anticonvulsant drugs, including carbamazepine, lamotrigine, and phenytoin.

18. Alternative drugs for the management of absence seizures include clonazepam and lamotrigine. Clonazepam is less effective than ethosuximide or valproic acid; tolerance develops rapidly; and the doses used cause drowsiness, drooling, and ataxia. Lamotrigine has activity in absence seizures as well as in both generalized and partial seizures. Its most distinctive toxicity is life-threatening skin disorders, which can include Stevens-Johnson syndrome and toxic epidermal necrolysis.

Skill Keeper Answers: Antiarrhythmic Drug Actions (see Chapter 14)

1. Close similarities of structure and function exist between voltage-gated sodium channels in neurons and in cardiac cells. Drugs that exert antiseizure actions via their blockade of sodium channels in the CNS have the potential for a similar action in the heart. Delayed recovery of sodium channels from their inactivated state subsequently slows the rising phase of the action potential in Na+-dependent fibers and is characteristic of group I antiarrhythmic drugs. In theory, antiseizure drugs that block calcium ion channels might also have properties akin to those of group IV antiarrhythmic drugs.
2. In practice, the only antiseizure drug that has been used in cardiac arrhythmias is phenytoin, which has characteristics similar to group IB antiarrhythmic drugs. Phenytoin has been used for arrhythmias resulting from cardiac glycoside overdose and for ventricular arrhythmias unresponsive to lidocaine.

25 General Anesthetics

OBJECTIVES

You should be able to:

- Identify the main inhalation anesthetic agents and describe their pharmacodynamic properties.
- Describe the relationship of the blood:gas partition coefficient of an inhalation anesthetic with its speed of onset of anesthesia and its recovery time.
- List the factors that influence inhalation anesthetic biodisposition.
- Describe the main pharmacokinetic and pharmacodynamic characteristics of the intravenous anesthetics.

Learn the definitions that follow.

Table 25–1. Definitions.

Term	Definition
Balanced anesthesia	Anesthesia produced by a mixture of drugs, often including both inhaled and intravenous agents
Inhalation anesthesia	Anesthesia induced by inhalation of drug
Minimal alveolar anesthetic concentration (MAC)	The alveolar concentration of an anesthetic that is required to prevent a response to a standardized painful stimulus in 50% of patients
Analgesia	A state of decreased awareness of pain, sometimes with amnesia
General anesthesia	A state of unconsciousness, analgesia, and amnesia, with skeletal muscle relaxation and loss of reflexes

CONCEPTS

A. General Anesthesia: General anesthesia is a state characterized by unconsciousness, analgesia, amnesia, skeletal muscle relaxation, and loss of reflexes. General anesthetics are CNS depressants with actions that can be induced and terminated more rapidly than those of sedative-hypnotics. Modern anesthetics act very rapidly and achieve deep anesthesia quickly. With older and more slowly acting anesthetics, the progressively greater depth of central depression associated with increasing dose or time of exposure is traditionally described as **stages of anesthesia:**

1. **Analgesia:** In stage 1, the patient has decreased awareness of pain, sometimes with amnesia. Consciousness may be impaired but is not lost.
2. **Disinhibition:** In stage 2, the patient appears to be delirious and excited. Amnesia occurs, reflexes are enhanced, and respiration is typically irregular; retching and incontinence may occur.
3. **Surgical anesthesia:** In stage 3, the patient is unconscious and has no pain reflexes; respiration is very regular, and blood pressure is maintained.
4. **Medullary depression:** In stage 4, the patient experiences severe respiratory and cardiovascular depression that requires mechanical and pharmacologic support.

B. Anesthesia Protocols: For minor procedures, **conscious sedation** techniques that combine intravenous agents with local anesthetics are often used. For more extensive procedures, **balanced anesthesia** regimens are used that usually consist of short-acting intravenous agents with opioids and nitrous oxide. For major surgery, anesthesia protocols commonly include the use of intravenous drugs to induce the anesthetic state, inhaled anesthetics to maintain anesthesia, and neuromuscular blocking agents to effect muscle relaxation (Figure 25–1).

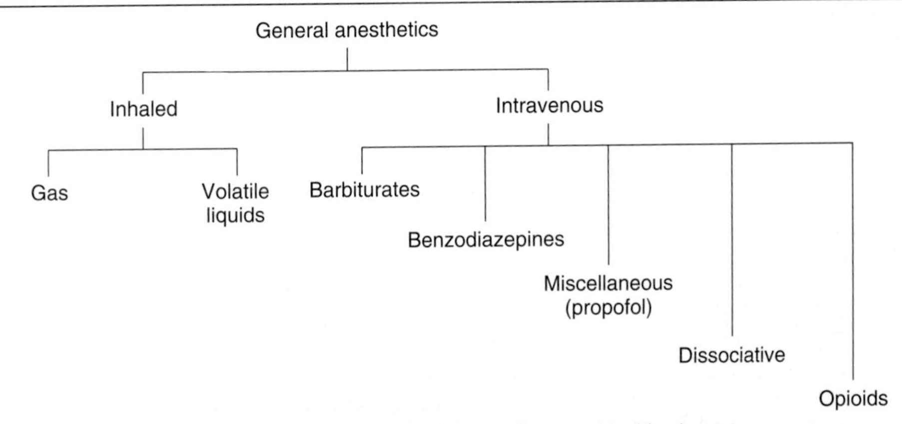

Figure 25–1. Subgroups of drugs discussed in this chapter.

C. Mechanisms of Action: The mechanisms of action of general anesthetics are unclear, but these drugs usually increase the threshold for firing of CNS neurons. The potency of most inhaled anesthetics is proportionate to their lipid solubility. Possible mechanisms of action include effects on ion channels by interactions with membrane lipids or proteins and effects on central neurotransmitter mechanisms. A potential "target" is the $GABA_A$ receptor, which is directly coupled to a chloride ion channel. Inhaled and intravenous anesthetics are reported to directly activate these receptors rather than just *facilitate* the actions of GABA (like sedative-hypnotics; see Chapter 22). CNS neurons in different regions of the brain have different sensitivities to general anesthetics; inhibition of neurons involved in pain pathways occurs before inhibition of neurons in the midbrain reticular formation.

INHALED ANESTHETICS

A. Classification and Pharmacokinetics: The agents currently used in inhalation anesthesia are nitrous oxide (a gas) and several easily vaporized liquid halogenated hydrocarbons, including halothane, desflurane, enflurane, isoflurane, sevoflurane, and methoxyflurane. They are administered as gases; their partial pressure, or "tension," in the inhaled air or in blood or other tissue is a measure of their concentration. Since the standard pressure of the total inhaled mixture is atmospheric pressure (760 mm Hg at sea level), the partial pressure may also be expressed as a percentage. Thus 50% nitrous oxide in the inhaled air would have a partial pressure of 380 mm Hg. The speed of induction of anesthetic effects depends on several factors:

1. **Solubility:** The more rapidly a drug equilibrates with the blood, the more quickly the drug passes into the brain to produce anesthetic effects. Drugs with a low blood:gas partition coefficient (eg, nitrous oxide) equilibrate more rapidly than do drugs with a higher blood solubility (eg, halothane), as illustrated in Figure 25–2. Partition coefficients for inhalation anesthetics are shown in Table 25–2.
2. **Inspired gas partial pressure:** A high partial pressure of the gas in the lungs results in more rapid achievement of anesthetic levels in the blood. Advantage is taken of this effect by the initial administration of gas concentrations higher than those required for maintenance of anesthesia.
3. **Ventilation rate:** The greater the ventilation, the more rapid the rise in alveolar and

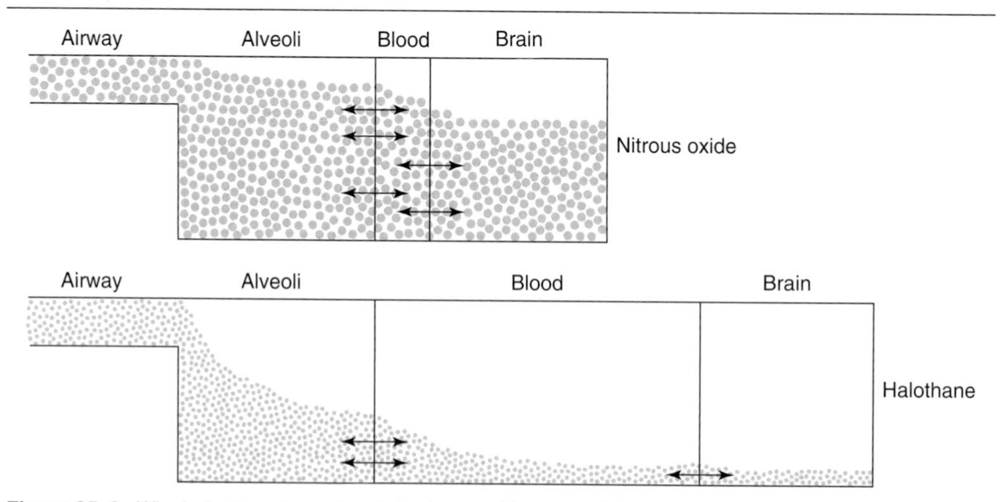

Figure 25–2. Why induction of anesthesia is slower with more soluble anesthetic gases and faster with less soluble ones. In this schematic diagram, solubility is represented by the size of the blood compartment (the more soluble the gas, the larger the compartment). For a given concentration or partial pressure of the two anesthetic gases in the inspired air, it will take much longer with halothane than with nitrous oxide for the blood partial pressure to rise to the same partial pressure as in the alveoli. Since the concentration in the brain can rise no faster than the concentration in the blood, the onset of anesthesia will be much slower with halothane than with nitrous oxide. (Reproduced, with permission, from Katzung BG [editor]: *Basic & Clinical Pharmacology,* 8th ed. McGraw-Hill, 2001.)

Table 25–2. Properties of inhalation anesthetics.*

Anesthetic	Blood:Gas Partition Coefficient	Minimum Alveolar Concentration (%)[1]	Metabolism
Nitrous oxide	0.47	> 100	None
Desflurane	0.42	6.5	< 0.1%
Sevoflurane	0.69	2.0	2–5% (fluoride)
Isoflurane	1.40	1.4	< 2%
Enflurane	1.80	1.7	8%
Halothane	2.30	0.75	> 40%
Methoxyflurane	12	0.16	> 70% (fluoride)

*Modified and reproduced, with permission, from Katzung BG (editor): *Basic & Clinical Pharmacology,* 8th ed. McGraw Hill, 2001.
[1]Minimum alveolar concentration (MAC) is the anesthetic concentration that eliminates the response in 50% of patients exposed to a standardized painful stimulus. In this table, MAC is expressed as a percentage of the inspired gas mixture.

blood partial pressure of the agent and the more rapid the onset of anesthesia (Figure 25–3). Advantage is taken of this effect in the induction of the anesthetic state.

4. **Pulmonary blood flow:** At high pulmonary blood flows, the gas partial pressure rises at a slower rate; thus, the speed of onset of anesthesia is reduced. At low flow rates, onset is faster. In circulatory shock, this effect may accelerate the rate of onset of anesthesia with agents of high blood solubility.
5. **Arteriovenous concentration gradient:** Uptake of soluble anesthetics into highly perfused tissues may decrease gas tension in mixed venous blood. This can influence the rate of onset of anesthesia, since achievement of equilibrium is dependent on the difference in anesthetic tension between arterial and venous blood.

B. Elimination: Anesthesia is terminated by redistribution of the drug from the brain to the blood and elimination of the drug through the lungs. The rate of recovery from anesthesia using agents with low blood:gas partition coefficients is faster than that of anesthetics with high blood solubility. This important property has led to the introduction of several newer inhaled anesthetics (eg, desflurane, sevoflurane) which, because of their low blood solubility, are characterized by recovery times that are considerably shorter than is the case with older agents.

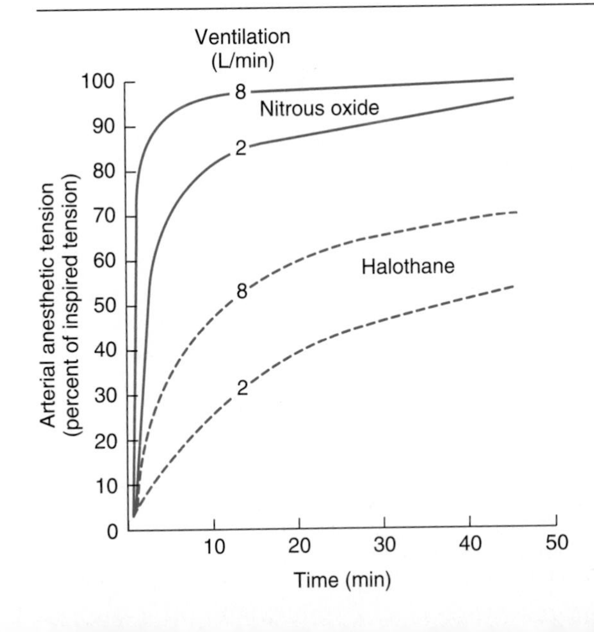

Figure 25–3. Ventilation rate and arterial anesthetic tensions. (Reproduced, with permission, from Katzung BG [editor]: *Basic & Clinical Pharmacology,* 8th ed. McGraw-Hill, 2001.)

Halothane and methoxyflurane are metabolized by liver enzymes to a significant extent (see Table 25–2). Metabolism of halothane and methoxyflurane has only a minor influence on the speed of recovery from their anesthetic effect but does play a role in potential toxicity of these anesthetics.

C. **Minimum Alveolar Anesthetic Concentration (MAC):** The potency of inhaled anesthetics is best measured by the minimum alveolar anesthetic concentration (MAC), defined as the alveolar concentration required to eliminate the response to a standardized painful stimulus in 50% of patients. Each anesthetic has a defined MAC (see Table 25–2), but this value may vary among different patients depending on age, cardiovascular status, and use of adjuvant drugs. Estimations of MAC value suggest a relatively "steep" dose-response relationship for inhaled anesthetics. MACs for infants and elderly patients are lower than those for adolescents and young adults. When several anesthetic agents are used simultaneously, their MAC values are additive.

D. **Effects of Inhaled Anesthetics:**
1. **CNS effects:** Inhaled anesthetics decrease brain metabolic rate. They reduce vascular resistance and thus increase cerebral blood flow. This may lead to an increase in intracranial pressure. High concentrations of enflurane may cause spike-and-wave activity and muscle twitching, but this effect is unique to this drug. Though nitrous oxide has low anesthetic potency (ie, a high MAC), it exerts marked analgesic and amnestic actions.
2. **Cardiovascular effects:** Most inhaled anesthetics decrease arterial blood pressure moderately. Enflurane and halothane are myocardial depressants that decrease cardiac output, while isoflurane causes peripheral vasodilation. Nitrous oxide is less likely to lower blood pressure than are other inhaled anesthetics. Blood flow to the liver and kidney is decreased by most inhaled agents. Halothane may sensitize the myocardium to the arrhythmogenic effects of catecholamines.
3. **Respiratory effects:** Rate of respiration may be increased by inhaled anesthetics, but tidal volume and minute ventilation are decreased, leading to an increase in arterial CO_2 tension. Inhaled anesthetics decrease ventilatory response to hypoxia even at subanesthetic concentrations (eg, during recovery). Nitrous oxide has the smallest effect on respiration.
4. **Toxicity:** Postoperative hepatitis has occurred (rarely) following halothane anesthesia in patients experiencing hypovolemic shock or other severe stress. Fluoride released by metabolism of methoxyflurane (and possibly enflurane) may cause renal insufficiency after prolonged anesthesia. Prolonged exposure to nitrous oxide decreases methionine synthase activity and may lead to megaloblastic anemia. Susceptible patients may develop **malignant hyperthermia** when exposed to halogenated anesthetics. This rare condition of uncontrolled release of calcium by the sarcoplasmic reticulum of skeletal muscle leads to muscle spasm, hyperthermia, and autonomic lability. Dantrolene is indicated for the treatment of this life-threatening condition, with supportive management of hyperthermia and cardiovascular instability.

Skill Keeper: Signaling Mechanisms
(see Chapter 2)

While receptors for inhaled anesthetics may exist, their molecular identities remain elusive. This is in contrast to most drugs that appear to act via interactions with specific receptor molecules involved in cell signaling. For review purposes, try to recall the major types of signaling mechanisms relevant to the actions of those drugs that act via receptors. *The Skill Keeper Answers appear at the end of the chapter.*

INTRAVENOUS ANESTHETICS

A. **Classification, Pharmacokinetics, and Pharmacodynamics:** Several chemical classes of drugs are used as intravenous agents in anesthesia.
1. **Barbiturates: Thiopental, thiamylal,** and **methohexital** have high lipid solubility, which promotes rapid entry into the brain and results in surgical anesthesia in one circula-

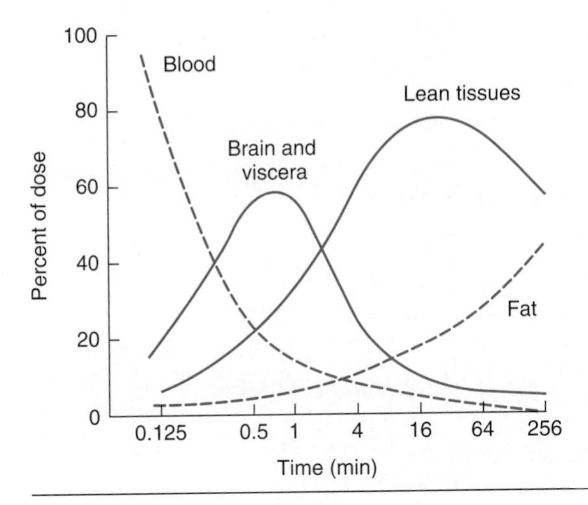

Figure 25–4. Redistribution of thiopental after intravenous bolus administration. (Reproduced, with permission, from Katzung BG [editor]: *Basic & Clinical Pharmacology,* 8th ed. McGraw-Hill, 2001.)

tion time (< 1 minute). These agents are used for induction of anesthesia and for short surgical procedures. Their anesthetic effects are terminated by redistribution from the brain to other tissues (Figure 25–4), but hepatic metabolism is required for their elimination from the body. They are respiratory and circulatory depressants; because they depress cerebral blood flow, they can also decrease intracranial pressure.

2. **Benzodiazepines: Midazolam** is widely used adjunctively with inhaled anesthetics and intravenous opioids. The onset of its CNS effects is slower than that of thiopental, and it has a longer duration of action. Cases of severe postoperative respiratory depression have occurred. The antagonist flumazenil accelerates recovery from midazolam and other benzodiazepines.
3. **Dissociative anesthetic: Ketamine** produces a state called "dissociative anesthesia" in which the patient remains conscious but has marked catatonia, analgesia, and amnesia. Ketamine is an antagonist of glutamic acid, blocking the actions of this excitatory transmitter at its NMDA receptor. The drug is a cardiovascular stimulant, and this action may lead to an increase in intracranial pressure. Emergence reactions, including disorientation, excitation, and hallucinations, which occur during recovery from ketamine anesthesia can be reduced by the preoperative use of benzodiazepines.
4. **Opioids: Morphine** and **fentanyl** are used with other CNS depressants (nitrous oxide, benzodiazepines) in anesthesia regimens and are especially valuable in high-risk patients who might not survive a full general anesthetic. Intravenous opioids may cause chest wall rigidity that can impair ventilation. Respiratory depression with these drugs may be reversed postoperatively with naloxone. **Neuroleptanesthesia** is a state of analgesia and amnesia produced when fentanyl is used with droperidol and nitrous oxide. Newer opioids related to fentanyl have been introduced for intravenous anesthesia. Alfentanil and remifentanil have been used for induction of anesthesia. Recovery from the actions of remifentanil is faster than recovery from other opioids used in anesthesia because of its rapid metabolism by blood and tissue esterases.
5. **Propofol:** Propofol produces anesthesia at a rate similar to that of the intravenous barbiturates, and recovery is more rapid. Propofol has antiemetic actions, and recovery is not delayed after prolonged infusion. The drug is commonly used as a component of balanced anesthesia and as an anesthetic in outpatient surgery. Propofol may cause marked hypotension during induction of anesthesia, primarily through decreased peripheral resistance. Total body clearance of propofol is greater than hepatic blood flow, suggesting that its elimination includes other mechanisms in addition to metabolism by liver enzymes.

DRUG LIST

The following drugs are important members of the group discussed in this chapter. Prototypes should be learned in detail; features of the major variants should be known well enough to distinguish the variants from the prototypes and from each other.

Subclass	Prototype	Major Variants
Inhaled anesthetics		
Volatile liquids	Halothane	Enflurane, desflurane, isoflurane, methoxyflurane, sevoflurane
Gas	Nitrous oxide	
Intravenous anesthetics		
Barbiturates	Thiopental	Thiamylal, methohexital
Opioids	Morphine	Fentanyl, alfentanil, remifentanil
Phenols	Propofol	
Benzodiazepines	Midazolam	
Dissociative agent	Ketamine	

QUESTIONS

DIRECTIONS: Each of the numbered items or incomplete statements in this section is followed by answers or by completions of the statement. Select the ONE lettered answer or completion that is BEST in each case.

1. A new halogenated gas anesthetic has a blood:gas partition coefficient of 0.5 and a MAC value of 1%. Which one of the following predictions about this agent is most accurate? (Refer to Table 25–2 for comparison of agents.)
- **(A)** The new agent will be more potent than halothane
- **(B)** It will be metabolized by the liver to release fluoride ions
- **(C)** It will be more soluble in the blood than isoflurane
- **(D)** Its speed of onset of action will be similar to that of nitrous oxide
- **(E)** Equilibrium between arterial and venous gas tensions will be achieved very slowly with this agent

2. Which one of the following statements concerning the effects of anesthetic agents is false?
- **(A)** Relaxation of bronchiolar smooth muscle occurs during halothane anesthesia
- **(B)** Mild generalized muscle twitching occurs at high doses of enflurane
- **(C)** Chest muscle rigidity often follows the administration of fentanyl
- **(D)** Intraoperative use of midazolam with inhalation anesthetics may prolong the postanesthesia recovery period
- **(E)** Severe hepatitis has been reported following the use of desflurane

3. A 23-year-old man has a pheochromocytoma, a blood pressure of 190/120 mm Hg, and a hematocrit of 50%. Pulmonary function and renal function are normal. His catecholamines are elevated, and he has a well-defined abdominal tumor on MRI. He has been scheduled for surgery. Of the agents listed below, which one should not be included in the anesthesia protocol?
- **(A)** Desflurane
- **(B)** Fentanyl
- **(C)** Halothane
- **(D)** Midazolam
- **(E)** Thiopental

4. Which one of the following statements concerning nitrous oxide is accurate?
- **(A)** It continues to be a useful component of anesthesia protocols because of its lack of cardiovascular depression
- **(B)** Megaloblastic anemia is a common adverse effect in patients exposed to nitrous oxide for periods longer than 2 hours
- **(C)** It is the most potent of the inhaled anesthetics
- **(D)** There is a direct association between the use of nitrous oxide and malignant hyperthermia
- **(E)** More than 30% of nitrous oxide is eliminated via hepatic metabolism

5. Which one of the following statements concerning anesthetic MAC values is most accurate?
- **(A)** Anesthetics with low MAC value have low potency
- **(B)** MACs give information about the slope of the dose-response curve
- **(C)** Nitrous oxide has an extremely low MAC value

(D) MAC values decrease in elderly patients
(E) Simultaneous use of opioid analgesics increases the MAC for inhaled anesthetics

6. Total intravenous anesthesia with fentanyl has been selected for a frail 72-year-old woman about to undergo cardiac surgery. Which one of the following statements about this anesthesia protocol is accurate?
(A) Intravenous opioids will provide useful cardiostimulatory effects
(B) Opioids control the hypertensive response to surgical stimulation
(C) Marked relaxation of skeletal muscles is anticipated
(D) Patient awareness may occur during surgery, with recall after recovery
(E) The patient is likely to experience pain during surgery

7. Which one of the following inhalation anesthetics has a low blood:gas partition coefficient but is not used for induction of anesthesia because of its pungency, which causes patients to hold their breath?
(A) Desflurane
(B) Enflurane
(C) Halothane
(D) Isoflurane
(E) Sevoflurane

Items 8–9: A 20-year-old male patient scheduled for hernia surgery was anesthetized with halothane and nitrous oxide, with tubocurarine provided for skeletal muscle relaxation. The patient rapidly developed tachycardia and became hypertensive. Generalized skeletal muscle rigidity was accompanied by marked hyperthermia. Laboratory values revealed hyperkalemia and acidosis.

8. This unusual complication of anesthesia is most probably due to
(A) Activation of brain dopamine receptors
(B) A genetically determined myopathy
(C) Block of autonomic ganglia
(D) Pheochromocytoma
(E) Release of acetylcholine from parasympathetic nerve endings

9. The patient should be treated immediately with
(A) Atropine
(B) Baclofen
(C) Dantrolene
(D) Edrophonium
(E) Succinylcholine

10. The inhalation anesthetic with the fastest onset of action is
(A) Enflurane
(B) Isoflurane
(C) Nitric oxide
(D) Nitrogen dioxide
(E) Nitrous oxide

11. If ketamine is used as the sole anesthetic in the attempted reduction of a dislocated shoulder joint, its actions will include
(A) Analgesia
(B) Bradycardia
(C) Hypotension
(D) Muscle rigidity
(E) Respiratory depression

12. An intravenous bolus dose of thiopental usually leads to loss of consciousness within 10–15 seconds. If no further drugs are administered, the patient will regain consciousness in just a few minutes. The reason for this is that thiopental is
(A) A good substrate for renal tubular secretion
(B) Exhaled rapidly
(C) Rapidly metabolized by hepatic enzymes
(D) Redistributed from brain to other body tissues
(E) Secreted in the bile

13. Respiratory depression following use of this agent may be reversed by administration of flumazenil
(A) Desflurane
(B) Fentanyl

(C) Ketamine
(D) Midazolam
(E) Propofol

14. Use of this agent is associated with a high incidence of disorientation, sensory and perceptual illusions, and vivid dreams during recovery from anesthesia
(A) Diazepam
(B) Fentanyl
(C) Ketamine
(D) Midazolam
(E) Thiopental

15. Postoperative vomiting is uncommon with this intravenous agent; patients are able to ambulate sooner than those who receive other anesthetics
(A) Enflurane
(B) Ketamine
(C) Morphine
(D) Propofol
(E) Remifentanil

ANSWERS

1. Inhaled anesthetics with low blood:gas solubility characteristically have a fast onset of action and a short duration of recovery. The new agent described here resembles nitrous oxide but is much more potent, as indicated by its low MAC value. Not all halogenated anesthetics undergo hepatic metabolism. The answer is **(D).**
2. Hepatitis following general anesthesia has been linked to use of *halothane,* though the incidence of severe hepatic necrosis is only about one out of 35,000 halothane administrations. The results of animal experiments suggest that halothane hepatotoxicity may be due to formation of a toxic metabolite produced under anoxic conditions. Hepatotoxicity has not been reported following desflurane administration; it may be relevant that this agent is the least metabolized of the fluorinated hydrocarbons. All of the other statements are correct. The answer is **(E).**
3. Halothane sensitizes the myocardium to catecholamines; arrhythmias may occur in patients with cardiac disease who have high circulating levels of epinephrine and norepinephrine (eg, patients with pheochromocytoma). Other modern anesthetics are considerably less arrhythmogenic. The answer is **(C).**
4. Bone marrow depression by nitrous oxide has **not** been reported in patients exposed to nitrous oxide anesthesia for periods as long as 6 hours. However, megaloblastic anemia may be an occupational hazard for staff working in poorly ventilated dental operating rooms. Nitrous oxide is the least potent of the inhaled anesthetics, and the compound has not been implicated in malignant hyperthermia. Over 98% of the gas is eliminated via exhalation. The answer is **(A).**
5. MAC value is inversely related to potency—a low MAC means that the anesthetic has a high potency. The MAC gives no information about the slope of the dose-response curve. Desflurane has the lowest blood:gas partition coefficient of the currently available inhaled anesthetics. Concomitant use of opioid analgesics with inhaled anesthetics lowers the MAC value. As is the case for most CNS depressants, the elderly patient is more sensitive, so MAC values are lower. The answer is **(D).**
6. High-dose intravenous opioids (eg, fentanyl, morphine) are widely used in anesthesia for cardiac surgery because they provide full analgesia and cause less cardiac depression than inhalation anesthetic agents. However, they are not cardiac stimulants, and fentanyl is more likely to cause skeletal muscle rigidity than relaxation. One disadvantage of this technique is patient recall, though the likelihood of patient awareness can be decreased by use of a benzodiazepine. Another disadvantage is the occurrence of hypertensive responses to surgical stimulation. The addition of vasodilators (eg, nitroprusside) or a beta-blocker (eg, esmolol) may be needed to prevent intraoperative hypertension. The answer is **(D).**
7. The pungency of desflurane leads to a high incidence of coughing and sometimes bronchospasm. Desflurane also causes a centrally mediated tachycardia and increase in blood pressure. Despite its low blood:gas partition coefficient, anesthesia with desflurane does not always lead to faster rates of recovery. The answer is **(A).**

8. Malignant hyperthermia is a rare but life-threatening reaction that may occur during general anesthesia with halogenated anesthetics and skeletal muscle relaxants, particularly succinylcholine and tubocurarine. Predisposing genetic factors include clinical myopathy associated with mutations in the gene loci for the skeletal muscle ryanodine receptor, the calcium release channel of the sarcoplasmic reticulum. The answer is **(B)**.
9. The drug of choice in malignant hyperthermia is dantrolene, which prevents release of calcium from the sarcoplasmic reticulum of skeletal muscle cells. Appropriate measures must be taken to lower body temperature, control hypertension, and restore acid-base and electrolyte balance. The answer is **(C)**.
10. The purpose of this easy question is to remind the reader that there are *three* medically important oxides of nitrogen. Nitric oxide (NO) is a powerful vasodilator (see Chapter 19). Nitrogen dioxide (NO_2) is a pulmonary irritant generated in fermenting silage; it may cause lethal pulmonary damage in farm workers. Nitrous oxide (N_2O) is the inhalation anesthetic agent discussed in this chapter. The answer is **(E)**.
11. Ketamine is a cardiovascular stimulant, increasing heart rate and blood pressure. This results in part from central sympathetic stimulation and possibly from inhibition of norepinephrine reuptake at sympathetic nerve endings. Analgesia and amnesia occur, with preservation of muscle tone and minimal depression of respiration. The answer is **(A)**.
12. The high lipophilicity of thiopental ensures rapid entry to the CNS following an intravenous bolus dose. As the blood level falls, thiopental exits the brain and is redistributed to other highly perfused tissues such as the liver and skeletal muscles. Thus, the brain level of thiopental rapidly declines to the point that consciousness is regained within a few minutes. Ultimately, the elimination of thiopental depends on its metabolism by the liver, but only 10–15% of thiopental is metabolized per hour. The answer is **(D)**.
13. Flumazenil is a benzodiazepine receptor antagonist (see Chapter 22). It accelerates recovery from postoperative depression of the CNS caused by midazolam and other benzodiazepines used in anesthesia. The short duration of action of flumazenil may necessitate multiple doses. The sedative actions of benzodiazepines are more reliably reversed by flumazenil than is respiratory depression. Use of flumazenil does not obviate the need for adequate monitoring of respiration and provision of ventilatory support when needed. The answer is **(D)**.
14. The emergence phenomena described are adverse effects of ketamine. Administration of diazepam immediately prior to ketamine anesthesia reduces the incidence of these effects. The answer is **(C)**.
15. Propofol is used extensively in balanced anesthesia protocols and is especially suitable for day surgery anesthesia. The favorable properties of the drug include an antiemetic effect and a rate of recovery more rapid than that following use of other intravenous drugs. Propofol does not cause cumulative effects, possibly because of its short half-life (2–8 minutes) in the body. The drug is also used for prolonged sedation in critical care settings. Opioids stimulate the chemoreceptor trigger zone causing emesis. The answer is **(D)**.

Skill Keeper Answer: Signaling Mechanisms (see Chapter 2)

1. Receptors that modify gene transcription: adrenal and gonadal steroids
2. Receptors on membrane-spanning enzymes: insulin
3. Receptors activating Janus kinases that modulate STAT molecules: cytokines
4. Receptors directly coupled to ion channels: nicotinic (ACh), GABA, glycine
5. Receptors coupled to enzymes via G proteins: many endogenous compounds (eg, ACh, NE, serotonin) and drugs
6. Receptors that are enzymes: acetylcholinesterase, angiotensin-converting enzyme, Na^+/K^+ ATPase, etc

26 Local Anesthetics

OBJECTIVES

You should be able to:

- Describe the mechanism of blockade of the nerve impulses by local anesthetics.
- Discuss the relation between pH, pK_a, and the speed of onset of local anesthesia.
- List the factors that determine the susceptibility of nerve fibers to blockade.
- List the major toxic effects of the local anesthetics.
- Explain use-dependent blockade by local anesthetics.

CONCEPTS

Local anesthesia is the condition that results when sensory transmission from a local area of the body to the CNS is blocked. The local anesthetics constitute a group of chemically similar agents that block the sodium channels of excitable membranes. Because these drugs can be administered locally by topical application or by injection in the target area, the anesthetic effect can be restricted to a localized area, eg, the cornea or an arm. When given intravenously, these drugs have effects on other tissues. Many drugs classified in other groups, eg, antihistamines and beta-blockers, have significant local anesthetic effects.

A. Chemistry and Subclasses: Most local anesthetic drugs are esters or amides of simple benzene derivatives. Subgroups within the local anesthetics are based on this chemical characteristic and on duration of action (Figure 26–1). All of the commonly used local anesthetics carry at least one amine function and are therefore weak bases that become charged through the gain of a proton (H^+). As discussed in Chapter 1, the degree of ionization is a function of the pK_a of the drug and the pH of the medium. Because the pH of tissue may differ from the physiologic 7.4 (for example, it may be as low as 6.4 in infected tissue), the degree of ionization of the drug will vary. Because the pK_a of most local anesthetics is between 8.0 and 9.0 (benzocaine is an exception), variations in pH associated with infection can have significant effects on the proportion of ionized to nonionized drug. The question of the active form of the drug (ionized versus nonionized) is discussed below.

B. Pharmacokinetics: Many shorter-acting local anesthetics are readily absorbed into the blood from the injection site after administration. The duration of local action is therefore limited unless blood flow to the area is reduced. This can be accomplished by administration of a vasoconstrictor (usually an α agonist sympathomimetic) with the local anesthetic agent. Cocaine is an important exception to this rule since it has intrinsic sympathomimetic action (because it in-

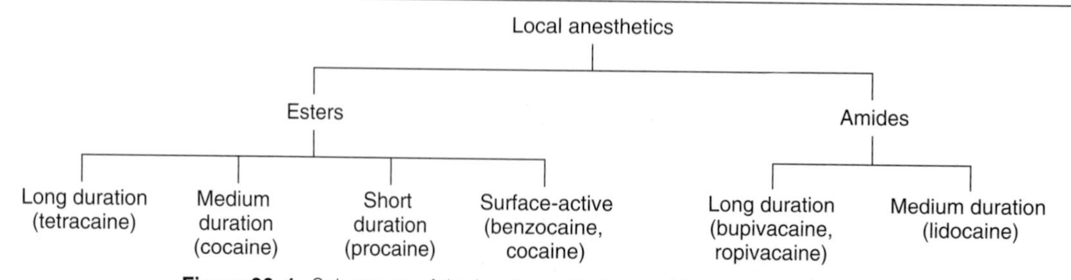

Figure 26–1. Subgroups of the local anesthetics and important examples.

hibits norepinephrine reuptake into nerve terminals); cocaine does not require any additional vasoconstrictor. The longer-acting agents, eg, tetracaine and bupivacaine, are also less dependent on the coadministration of vasoconstrictors. Surface activity (ability to reach superficial nerves when applied to the surface of mucous membranes) is a property of only a few local anesthetics, including cocaine and benzocaine.

Metabolism of ester local anesthetics is carried out by plasma cholinesterases and may be rapid. Procaine and chloroprocaine have half-lives of only 1–2 minutes. The amides are hydrolyzed in the liver and have half-lives from 1.8 hours to 6 hours. Bupivacaine and ropivacaine are very lipid-soluble and long-acting local anesthetics. Liver dysfunction may increase the elimination half-life of amide local anesthetics.

C. Mechanism of Action: Local anesthetics block voltage-dependent sodium channels and reduce the influx of sodium ions, thereby preventing depolarization of the membrane and blocking conduction of the action potential. Local anesthetics gain access to their receptors from the cytoplasm or the membrane (Figure 26–2). Since the drug molecule must cross the lipid membrane to reach the cytoplasm, the more lipid-soluble (nonionized, uncharged) form reaches effective intracellular concentrations more rapidly than does the ionized form. On the other hand, once inside the axon, the ionized (charged) form of the drug is the more effective blocking entity. Thus, both the nonionized and the ionized forms of the drug play important roles, the first in reaching the receptor site and the second in causing the effect. The affinity of the receptor site within the sodium channel for the local anesthetic is a function of the state of the channel—whether it is resting, open, or inactivated—and therefore follows the same rules of use-dependence and voltage-dependence that were described for the sodium channel-blocking antiarrhythmic drugs (see Chapter 14). In particular, if other factors are equal, rapidly firing fibers are usually blocked before slowly firing fibers.

D. Effects:

1. **Nerves:** Differential sensitivity of various types of nerve fibers to local anesthetics is associated with several factors, including fiber diameter, myelination, physiologic firing rate, and anatomic location (Table 26–1). In general, smaller fibers are blocked more easily than larger ones, and myelinated fibers are blocked more easily than unmyelinated ones. It is thought that activated pain fibers fire rapidly and that pain sensation may be selectively blocked by these drugs. Fibers located in the periphery of a thick nerve bundle are blocked sooner than those in the core because they are exposed earlier to higher concentrations of the anesthetic.

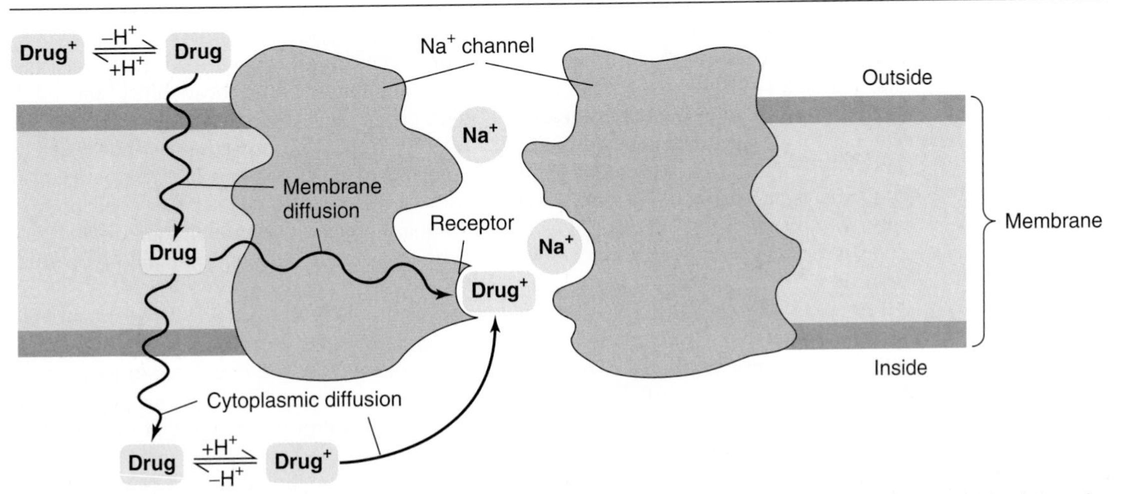

Figure 26–2. Schematic diagram of the sodium channel in an excitable membrane (eg, an axon) and the pathways by which a local anesthetic molecule *(Drug)* may reach its receptor. Sodium ions are not able to pass through the channel when the drug is bound to the receptor. The local anesthetic diffuses within the membrane in its uncharged form. In the aqueous extracellular and intracellular spaces, the charged form *(Drug⁺)* is also present.

Table 26–1. Susceptibility to block of types of nerve fibers.*

Fiber Type	Function	Diameter (μm)	Myelination	Conduction Velocity (m/s)	Sensitivity to Block
Type A					
Alpha	Proprioception, motor	12–20	Heavy	70–120	+
Beta	Touch, pressure	5–12	Heavy	30–70	++
Gamma	Muscle spindles	3–6	Heavy	15–30	++
Delta	Pain, temperature	2–5	Heavy	12–30	+++
Type B	Preganglionic autonomic	< 3	Light	3–15	++++
Type C					
Dorsal root	Pain	0.4–1.2	None	0.5–2.3	++++
Sympathetic	Postganglionic	0.3–1.3	None	0.7–2.3	++++

*Reproduced, with permission, from Katzung BG (editor): *Basic & Clinical Pharmacology,* 8th ed. McGraw-Hill, 2001.

2. **Other tissues:** The effects of these drugs on the heart are discussed in Chapter 14 (see class I antiarrhythmic agents). Most local anesthetics also have weak blocking effects on skeletal muscle neuromuscular transmission, but these actions have no clinical application. The mood elevation induced by cocaine probably reflects actions on dopamine or other amine-mediated synaptic transmission in the CNS rather than a local anesthetic action on membranes.

E. **Clinical Use:** The local anesthetics are most commonly used for minor surgical procedures. Local anesthetics are also used in spinal anesthesia and to produce autonomic blockade in ischemic conditions. Slow epidural infusion at low concentrations has been used successfully for postoperative analgesia (in the same way as epidural opioid infusion; Chapter 31). Repeated epidural injection in anesthetic doses may lead to tachyphylaxis, however.

F. **Interactions:** High concentrations of extracellular K^+ may enhance local anesthetic activity, while elevated extracellular Ca^{2+} may antagonize it.

G. **Toxicity:**

1. **CNS effects:** The important toxic effects of most local anesthetics are in the CNS. All local anesthetics are capable of producing a spectrum of central effects, including lightheadedness or sedation, restlessness, nystagmus, and tonic-clonic convulsions. Severe convulsions may be followed by coma with respiratory and cardiovascular depression.
2. **Cardiovascular effects:** With the exception of cocaine, all local anesthetics are vasodilators. Patients with preexisting cardiovascular disease may develop heart block and other disturbances of cardiac electrical function at high plasma levels of local anesthetics. Bupivacaine may produce severe cardiovascular toxicity, including arrhythmias and hypotension, if given intravenously. The ability of cocaine to block norepinephrine reuptake at sympathetic neuroeffector junctions and the drug's vasoconstricting actions contribute to cardiovascular toxicity. When used as a drug of abuse, cocaine's cardiovascular toxicity includes severe hypertension with cerebral hemorrhage, cardiac arrhythmias, and myocardial infarction.
3. **Other toxic effects:** Prilocaine is metabolized to products that include an agent capable of causing methemoglobinemia. The ester-type local anesthetics are metabolized to products that can cause antibody formation in some patients. Allergic responses to local anesthetics are rare and can usually be avoided by using an agent from the amide subclass. In high concentrations, local anesthetics may cause a local neurotoxic action that includes histologic damage and permanent impairment of function.
4. **Treatment of toxicity:** Severe toxicity is best treated symptomatically. Convulsions are often treated with intravenous diazepam or a short-acting barbiturate such as thiopental. Hyperventilation with oxygen is helpful. Occasionally, a neuromuscular blocking drug may be used to control violent convulsive activity. The cardiovascular toxicity of bupivacaine overdose is difficult to treat and has caused fatalities in healthy young adults.

Skill Keeper: Cardiac Toxicity of Local Anesthetics (see Chapter 14)

Explain how hyperkalemia facilitates the cardiac toxicity of local anesthetics. *The Skill Keeper Answer appears at the end of the chapter.*

DRUG LIST

The following drugs are important members of the group discussed in this chapter. Prototypes should be learned in detail; features of the major variants should be known well enough to distinguish the variants from prototypes and from each other; the other significant agents should be recognized as belonging to a specific subclass.

Subclass	Prototype	Major Variants	Other Significant Agents
Esters	Procaine	Cocaine, tetracaine	Benzocaine
Amides	Lidocaine	Bupivacaine	Etidocaine, prilocaine

QUESTIONS

DIRECTIONS: Each of the numbered items or incomplete statements in this section is followed by answers or by completions of the statement. Select the ONE lettered answer or completion that is BEST in each case.

1. Properties of local anesthetics include all of the following EXCEPT
   (A) Blockade of voltage-dependent sodium channels
   (B) Preferential binding to resting channels
   (C) Slowing of axonal impulse conduction
   (D) An increase in membrane refractory period
   (E) Effects on vascular tone
2. The pK_a of lidocaine is 7.9. In infected tissue at pH 6.9, the fraction in the ionized form will be
   (A) 1%
   (B) 10%
   (C) 50%
   (D) 90%
   (E) 99%
3. Which of the following statements about nerve blockade with local anesthetics is most correct?
   (A) Block is faster in onset in infected tissues
   (B) Block is faster in onset in unmyelinated fibers
   (C) Block is slower in onset in hypocalcemia
   (D) Block is faster in onset in hyperkalemia
   (E) Block is slower in onset in the periphery of a nerve bundle than in the center of a bundle
4. The most important effect of inadvertent IV administration of a large dose of an amide local anesthetic is
   (A) Bronchoconstriction
   (B) Hepatic damage
   (C) Nerve damage
   (D) Renal failure
   (E) Seizures
5. Factors that influence the action of local anesthetics include all of the following EXCEPT
   (A) Blood flow through the tissue in which the injection is made
   (B) Activity of acetylcholinesterase in the area
   (C) Use of vasoconstrictors

(D) Amount of local anesthetic injected
(E) Tissue pH

6. You have a vial containing 4 mL of a 2% solution of lidocaine. How much lidocaine is present in 1 mL?
(A) 2 mg
(B) 8 mg
(C) 20 mg
(D) 80 mg
(E) 200 mg

7. Which one of the following statements about the toxicity of local anesthetics is most correct?
(A) Serious cardiovascular reactions are more likely to occur with tetracaine than with bupivacaine
(B) Cyanosis may occur following injection of large doses of lidocaine, especially in patients with pulmonary disease
(C) Intravenous injection of local anesthetics may stimulate ectopic cardiac pacemaker activity
(D) In overdosage, hyperventilation (with oxygen) is helpful to correct acidosis and lower extracellular potassium
(E) Most local anesthetics cause vasoconstriction

8. Epinephrine added to a solution of lidocaine for a peripheral nerve block will
(A) Increase the risk of convulsions
(B) Increase the duration of anesthetic action of the local anesthetic
(C) Both **(A)** and **(B)**
(D) Neither **(A)** nor **(B)**

9. A child requires multiple minor surgical procedures in the nasopharynx. Which of the following drugs has high surface activity and vasoconstrictor actions that reduce bleeding in mucous membranes?
(A) Benzocaine
(B) Bupivacaine
(C) Cocaine
(D) Lidocaine
(E) Procaine
(F) Ropivacaine
(G) Tetracaine

10. A 24-year-old woman was given an epidural anesthetic for pain relief during labor. The drug selected had a slower onset and a longer duration of action than any of the other local anesthetics. Unfortunately, some of the drug was inadvertently injected intravenously and caused a marked drop in blood pressure and an arrhythmia. The drug was most likely
(A) Benzocaine
(B) Bupivacaine
(C) Cocaine
(D) Lidocaine
(E) Procaine
(F) Ropivacaine
(G) Tetracaine

DIRECTIONS (Items 11–12): The matching questions in this section consist of lettered options followed by two numbered items. For each numbered item, select the ONE lettered option that is most closely associated with it. Each lettered option may be selected once, more than once, or not at all.

(A) Benzocaine
(B) Bupivacaine
(C) Cocaine
(D) Lidocaine
(E) Procaine
(F) Ropivacaine

11. This drug is poorly soluble in aqueous fluids, remains at the site of its application, and is not absorbed into the systemic circulation. It has good surface activity and low toxic potential.
12. This drug has very poor surface activity, a short duration of action, and an ester structure.

ANSWERS

1. Local anesthetics bind preferentially to sodium channels in the open and inactivated states. Recovery from drug-induced block is 10–1000 times slower than recovery of channels from normal inactivation. Resting channels have a lower affinity for local anesthetics. The answer is **(B).**
2. Since the drug is a weak base, it will be more ionized (protonated) at pH values lower than its pK_a. Since the pH given is 1 log unit lower (more acid) than the pK_a, the ratio of ionized to nonionized drug will be approximately 90:10. The answer is **(D).** (Recall from Chapter 1 that at a pH equal to pK_a, the ratio is 1:1; at 1 log unit difference, the ratio is [approximately] 90:10; at 2 units difference, 99:1; etc.)
3. Smaller-diameter nerve fibers are more sensitive to local anesthetics and are blocked more rapidly than those of larger size. As the local concentration of drug declines during recovery from local anesthesia, smaller fibers continue to be blocked and are the last to recover. The answer is **(D).**
4. Of the effects listed, the most important in local anesthetic overdose (of both amide and ester types) concern the CNS. Such effects can include sedation or restlessness, nystagmus, convulsions, coma, and respiratory depression. Diazepam is used for seizures caused by local anesthetics, usually without significant effects on ventilation or circulation. The answer is **(E).**
5. The ester group of ester-type local anesthetics is hydrolyzed by plasma (and tissue) pseudocholinesterases. These drugs are poor substrates for acetylcholinesterase; the activity of this enzyme does not play a part in terminating the actions of local anesthetics. Individuals with genetically based defects in pseudocholinesterase activity are unusually sensitive to procaine and other esters. The answer is **(B).**
6. The fact that you have 4 mL of the solution of lidocaine is irrelevant. A 2% solution of any drug contains 2 g per 100 mL. The amount of lidocaine in 1 mL of a 2% solution is thus 0.02 g, or 20 mg. The answer is **(C).**
7. Acidosis due to tissue hypoxia favors local anesthetic toxicity because these drugs bind more avidly (or release less rapidly) from the sodium channel binding site when they are in the charged state. (Note that *onset* of therapeutic effect may be slower because charged local anesthetics penetrate the membrane less rapidly; see text.) Hyperkalemia depolarizes the membrane, which also favors local anesthetic binding. Oxygenation reduces both acidosis and hyperkalemia. The answer is **(D).**
8. Epinephrine will increase the duration of a nerve block when it is administered with short- and medium-duration local anesthetics. As a result of the vasoconstriction that prolongs the duration of this block, less local anesthetic is required, so the risk of toxicity, eg, a convulsion, is reduced. The answer is **(B).**
9. Cocaine is the only local anesthetic with intrinsic vasoconstrictor activity. It also has significant surface activity and is favored for head, neck, and pharyngeal surgery. Cocaine is an ester. The answer is **(C).**
10. You should be able to identify this drug as bupivacaine from its long duration of action. Unlike lidocaine, the actions of bupivacaine on cardiac cells occur in the normal heart. Accidental intravenous administration of bupivacaine may lead to arrhythmias and cardiovascular collapse. The answer is **(B).**
11. Benzocaine is an ester that is used for topical anesthesia. Because of its low toxic potential, it has been used for anesthesia of large surface areas, including those within the oral cavity. The answer is **(A).**
12. Procaine is an ester with short duration of action and negligible surface activity. The answer is **(E).**

Skill Keeper Answer: Cardiac Toxicity of Local Anesthetics (see Chapter 14)

Sodium channel blockers, eg, local anesthetics, bind more readily to open (activated) or inactivated sodium channels. Hyperkalemia depolarizes the resting membrane potential, so more sodium channels are in the inactivated state. (Conversely, hypercalcemia tends to hyperpolarize the resting potential and reduces the block of sodium channels.)

27 Skeletal Muscle Relaxants

OBJECTIVES

You should be able to:

- Describe the transmission process at the neuromuscular end plate and the points at which drugs can modify this process.
- Identify the major nondepolarizing neuromuscular blockers and one depolarizing neuromuscular blocker; compare their pharmacokinetics.
- Describe the differences between depolarizing and nondepolarizing blockers from the standpoint of tetanic and posttetanic twitch strength.
- Describe the method of reversal of nondepolarizing blockade.
- List the major drugs used in the treatment of acute and chronic skeletal muscle spasticity and describe their mechanisms.

Learn the definitions that follow.

Table 27–1. Definitions.

Term	Definition
Depolarizing blockade	Neuromuscular paralysis that results from persistent depolarization of the end plate, eg, by succinylcholine
Desensitization	A phase of blockade by a depolarizing blocker during which the end plate repolarizes but is less than normally responsive to agonists (acetylcholine or succinylcholine)
Malignant hyperthermia	Hyperthermia that results from massive release of calcium from the sarcoplasmic reticulum, leading to uncontrolled contraction and stimulation of metabolism in skeletal muscle
Nondepolarizing blockade	Neuromuscular paralysis that results from pharmacologic antagonism at the acetylcholine receptor of the end plate, eg, by tubocurarine
Spasmolytic	A drug that reduces abnormally elevated muscle tone (spasm) without paralysis, eg, baclofen, dantrolene
Stabilizing blockade	Synonym for nondepolarizing blockade

CONCEPTS

The drugs in this chapter are divided into two dissimilar groups (Figure 27–1). The **neuromuscular blocking drugs** are used to produce muscle paralysis in order to facilitate surgery or artificial ventilation. The **spasmolytic drugs** are used to reduce abnormally elevated tone caused by neurologic or muscle end plate disease.

NEUROMUSCULAR BLOCKING DRUGS

A. **Classification and Prototypes:** Skeletal muscle contraction is evoked by a nicotinic cholinergic transmission process. Blockade of transmission at the end plate (the postsynaptic structure bearing the nicotinic receptors) is clinically useful in producing relaxation of muscle, a requirement for surgery. The neuromuscular blockers are structurally related to acetylcholine. Most are antagonists (nondepolarizing type), and the prototype is **tubocurarine.** One neuromuscular blocker used clinically, **succinylcholine,** is an agonist at the nicotinic end plate receptor (depolarizing type).

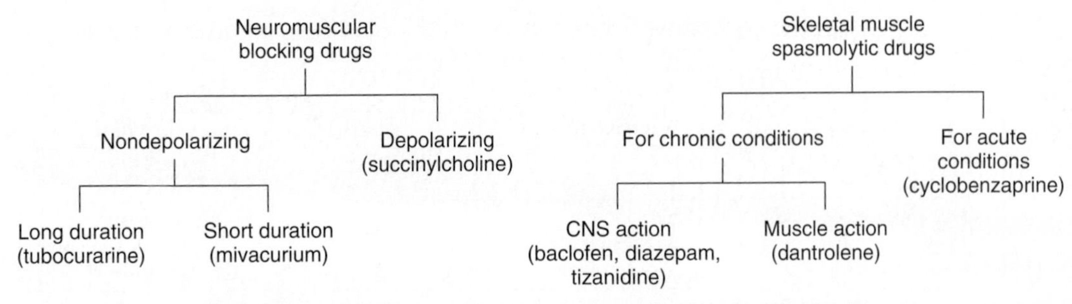

Figure 27–1. Subgroups and prototype drugs discussed in this chapter.

B. Nondepolarizing Neuromuscular Blocking Drugs:

1. **Pharmacokinetics:** All agents are given parenterally. Drugs that are metabolized (eg, mivacurium, by plasma cholinesterase) or eliminated in the bile (eg, vecuronium) usually have shorter durations of action than those eliminated by the kidney (eg, doxacurium, pancuronium, tubocurarine). Atracurium clearance involves spontaneous breakdown (Hofmann elimination) to form laudanosine and other products is largely independent of hepatic or renal function.
2. **Mechanism of action:** Nondepolarizing drugs prevent the action of ACh at the skeletal muscle end plate (Figure 27–2). They act as surmountable blockers, ie, the blockade can be overcome by increasing the amount of agonist (ACh) in the synaptic cleft. They behave as though they compete with acetylcholine at the receptor, and their effect is reversed by cholinesterase inhibitors. Some drugs in this group may also act directly to plug the ion channel operated by the acetylcholine receptor. Posttetanic potentiation is preserved in the presence of these agents, but tension during the tetanus fades rapidly. See Table 27–2 for additional details.

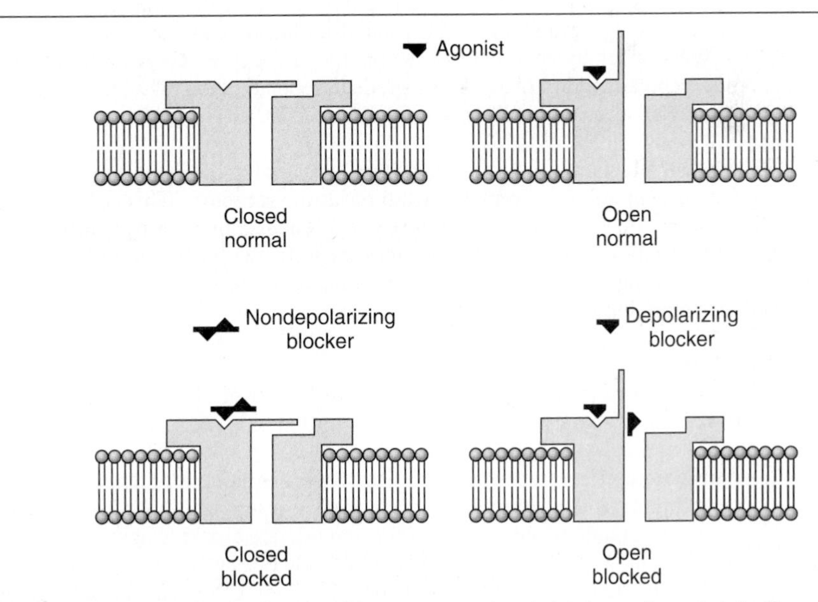

Figure 27–2. Drug interactions with the ACh receptor on the skeletal muscle end plate. **Top:** ACh, the normal agonist, opens the sodium channel. **Bottom left:** Nondepolarizing blockers bind to the receptor to prevent opening of the channel. **Bottom right:** Succinylcholine causes initial depolarization (fasciculation) and then persistent depolarization of the channel, which leads to muscle relaxation. (Reproduced, with permission, from Katzung BG [editor]: *Basic & Clinical Pharmacology,* 8th ed. McGraw-Hill, 2001.)

Table 27–2. Comparison of a typical nondepolarizing neuromuscular blocker (tubocurarine) and a depolarizing blocker (succinylcholine).*

Process	Tubocurarine	Succinylcholine	
		Phase I	Phase II
Administration of tubocurarine	Additive	Antagonistic	Augmented[1]
Administration of succinylcholine	Antagonistic	Additive	Augmented[1]
Effect of neostigmine	Antagonistic	Augmented[1]	Antagonistic
Initial excitatory effect on skeletal muscle	None	Fasciculations	None
Response to tetanic stimulus	Unsustained ("fade")	Sustained[2]	Unsustained
Posttetanic facilitation	Yes	No	Yes

*Reproduced, with permission, from Katzung BG (editor): *Basic & Clinical Pharmacology,* 8th ed. McGraw-Hill, 2001.
[1]It is not known whether this interaction is additive or synergistic (superadditive).
[2]The amplitude is decreased, but the response is sustained.

C. Depolarizing Neuromuscular Blocking Drugs:

1. **Pharmacokinetics:** Succinylcholine is composed of two acetylcholine molecules linked end to end. Succinylcholine is metabolized by plasma cholinesterase (butyrylcholinesterase or pseudocholinesterase), which determines the amount of drug reaching the end plate. It has a duration of action of only a few minutes if given as a single dose. Blockade may be prolonged in patients with genetic variants of plasma cholinesterase that metabolize succinylcholine very slowly. Succinylcholine is not rapidly hydrolyzed by acetylcholinesterase.
2. **Mechanism of action:** Depolarizing blockers act like nicotinic agonists and depolarize the neuromuscular end plate (Figure 27–2). The initial depolarization is often accompanied by twitching and fasciculations. Because tension cannot be maintained in skeletal muscle without periodic repolarization and depolarization of the end plate, continuous depolarization results in muscle relaxation and paralysis. As with the nondepolarizing blockers, some evidence suggests that these drugs can also plug the end plate channels.

   When given by continuous infusion, the effect of succinylcholine changes from continuous depolarization (phase I) to gradual repolarization with resistance to depolarization (phase II), ie, a curare-like block (see Table 27–2).

D. Reversal of Blockade: The action of nondepolarizing blockers is readily reversed by increasing the concentration of normal transmitter at the receptors. This is best accomplished by administration of cholinesterase inhibitors such as neostigmine or pyridostigmine. In contrast, the paralysis produced by depolarizing blockers is increased by cholinesterase inhibitors during phase I. During phase II, the block produced by succinylcholine is usually reversible by cholinesterase inhibitors.

E. Toxicity:

1. **Respiratory paralysis:** The action of full doses of neuromuscular blockers leads directly to respiratory paralysis. If mechanical ventilation is not provided, the patient will asphyxiate.
2. **Autonomic effects and histamine release:** Autonomic ganglia are stimulated by succinylcholine and blocked by tubocurarine. Succinylcholine also stimulates cardiac muscarinic receptors, while vecuronium is a moderate blocking agent. Tubocurarine is the most likely of these agents to cause histamine release, but it may also occur to a slight extent with atracurium, mivacurium, and succinylcholine. A summary of these autonomic effects is shown in Table 27–3.
3. **Specific effects of succinylcholine:** Muscle pain is a common postoperative complaint, and muscle damage has occurred. Succinylcholine may cause hyperkalemia, especially in patients with burn or spinal cord injury, peripheral nerve dysfunction, or muscular dystrophy. Increases in intragastric pressure may promote emesis.

Table 27–3. Autonomic effects of neuromuscular blocking drugs.*

Drug	Effect on Autonomic Ganglia	Effect on Cardiac Muscarinic Receptors	Ability to Release Histamine
Nondepolarizing			
Atracurium	None	None	Slight
Mivacurium	None	None	Slight
Pancuronium	None	Blocks moderately	None
Tubocurarine	Blocks	None	Moderate
Vecuronium, pipecuronium, rocuronium	None	None	None
Depolarizing			
Succinylcholine	Stimulates	Stimulates	Slight

*Modified and reproduced, with permission, from Katzung BG (editor): *Basic & Clinical Pharmacology,* 8th ed. McGraw-Hill, 2001.

4. **Interactions:** Inhaled anesthetics, especially isoflurane, strongly potentiate and prolong neuromuscular blockade. Aminoglycoside antibiotics and antiarrhythmic drugs potentiate and prolong the relaxant action of neuromuscular blockers to a lesser degree.

Skill Keeper: Autonomic Control of Heart Rate (see Chapter 6)

Tubocurarine can block bradycardia caused by phenylephrine but has no effect on bradycardia caused by neostigmine. Explain! *The Skill Keeper Answer appears at the end of the chapter.*

SPASMOLYTIC DRUGS

Certain chronic diseases of the CNS (eg, cerebral palsy, multiple sclerosis, stroke) are associated with abnormally high reflex activity in the neuronal pathways that control skeletal muscle; the result is painful spasm. Bladder and anal sphincter control are also affected in most cases and may require autonomic drugs for management. In other circumstances, acute injury or inflammation of muscle leads to spasm and pain. Such temporary spasm can sometimes be reduced with appropriate drug therapy.

The goal of spasmolytic therapy in both chronic and acute conditions is reduction of excessive skeletal muscle tone without reduction of strength. Reduced spasm results in reduction of pain and improved mobility.

A. **Drugs for Chronic Spasm:**

1. **Classification:** The spasmolytic drugs do not resemble acetylcholine in structure or effect. They act in the CNS or in the skeletal muscle cell rather than at the neuromuscular end plate. The spasmolytic drugs used in treatment of the chronic conditions mentioned above include **diazepam,** a benzodiazepine (see Chapter 22); **baclofen,** a GABA agonist; **tizanidine,** a congener of clonidine; and **dantrolene,** an agent that acts on the sarcoplasmic reticulum of skeletal muscle. These agents are usually used by the oral route. Refractory cases may respond to chronic intrathecal administration of baclofen. **Botulinum toxin** injected into selected muscles can reduce pain caused by severe spasm (see Chapter 6) and also has application in more generalized spastic disorders (eg, cerebral palsy). Gabapentin, an antiseizure drug, has been shown to be an effective spasmolytic in patients with multiple sclerosis.

2. **Mechanism of action:** The spasmolytic drugs act by several mechanisms. Three of the drugs act in the spinal cord. Diazepam facilitates GABA-mediated presynaptic inhibition, and baclofen acts as a $GABA_B$ agonist. Tizanidine, an imidazoline related to clonidine, reinforces both presynaptic and postsynaptic inhibition in the cord. All three drugs reduce the tonic output of the primary spinal motoneurons.

   Dantrolene acts in the skeletal muscle cell to reduce the release of activator calcium from the sarcoplasmic reticulum. Dantrolene is also effective in the treatment of malignant hyperthermia, a genetically determined disorder characterized by massive calcium release from the sarcoplasmic reticulum of skeletal muscle. Though rare, malignant hyperthermia can be triggered by general anesthesia protocols that include succinylcholine or tubocurarine (see Chapter 25). In this emergency condition, dantrolene is given intravenously.
3. **Toxicity:** The sedation produced by diazepam is significant but milder than that produced by other sedative-hypnotic drugs at doses that induce equivalent muscle relaxation. Baclofen produces less sedation than diazepam. Dantrolene causes significant muscle weakness but less sedation than either diazepam or baclofen. Tizanidine may cause drowsiness and hypotension.

B. **Drugs Used for Acute Muscle Spasm:** Many drugs are promoted for the treatment of acute spasm due to muscle injury. Most of these drugs are sedatives or act in the brain stem or spinal cord. **Cyclobenzaprine,** a typical member of this group, is believed to act in the brain stem, possibly by interfering with polysynaptic reflexes that maintain skeletal muscle tone. The drug is active by the oral route and has marked sedative and antimuscarinic actions. Cyclobenzaprine may cause confusion and visual hallucinations in some patients. It is not effective in muscle spasm due to cerebral palsy or spinal cord injury.

DRUG LIST

The following drugs are important members of the group discussed in this chapter. Prototypes should be learned in detail; features of the major variants should be known well enough to distinguish the variants from prototypes and from each other; the other significant agents should be recognized as belonging to a specific subclass.

Subclass	Prototype	Major Variants	Other Significant Agents
Nondepolarizing neuromuscular blockers			
Renal elimination, long duration	Tubocurarine		Pancuronium
Hepatic elimination, intermediate duration	Vecuronium		Rocuronium
Spontaneous or plasma ChE,[1] intermediate-short duration	Atracurium	Cisatracurium	Mivacurium
Depolarizing blockers	Succinylcholine		
Spasmolytic drugs	Diazepam, baclofen, dantrolene, tizanidine, botulinum toxin	Cyclobenzaprine	

[1]ChE: cholinesterase. (Atracurium breaks down spontaneously; mivacurium is metabolized by plasma ChE.)

QUESTIONS

DIRECTIONS: Each of the numbered items or incomplete statements in this section is followed by answers or by completions of the statement. Select the ONE lettered answer or completion that is BEST in each case.

1. Characteristics of phase I depolarizing neuromuscular blockade include
   (A) Easy reversibility with pharmacologic antagonists
   (B) Marked muscarinic blockade
   (C) Muscle fasciculations in the later stages of block

(D) Reversibility by pyridostigmine
(E) Well-sustained tension during a period of tetanic stimulation

Items 2–3: A patient underwent a surgical procedure of 2 hours. Anesthesia was provided by isoflurane, supplemented by intravenous midazolam and a nondepolarizing muscle relaxant. At the end of the procedure glycopyrrolate was administered followed by pyridostigmine.

2. The main reason for administering glycopyrrolate is to
(A) Prevent spasm of gastrointestinal smooth muscle
(B) Reverse the effects of the muscle relaxant
(C) Provide postoperative analgesia
(D) Prevent activation of cardiac muscarinic receptors
(E) Enhance the action of pyridostigmine

3. Glycopyrrolate would probably not be needed during reversal of the effects of a nondepolarizing relaxant if the agent used was
(A) Atracurium
(B) Mivacurium
(C) Pancuronium
(D) Tubocurarine
(E) Vecuronium

4. Characteristics of nondepolarizing neuromuscular blockade include which one of the following?
(A) Block of posttetanic potentiation
(B) Histamine blocking action
(C) Poorly sustained tetanic tension
(D) Significant muscle fasciculations during onset of block
(E) Stimulation of autonomic ganglia

5. Which of the following does not cause skeletal muscle contractions or twitching?
(A) Acetylcholine
(B) Nicotine
(C) Strychnine
(D) Succinylcholine
(E) Vecuronium

6. Which one of the following is most effective in the management of malignant hyperthermia?
(A) Baclofen
(B) Dantrolene
(C) Haloperidol
(D) Succinylcholine
(E) Vecuronium

7. Succinylcholine is associated with
(A) Antagonism by pyridostigmine during the early phase of blockade
(B) Blockade of autonomic ganglia
(C) Elevated serum enzymes indicative of muscle damage
(D) Histamine release in a genetically determined population
(E) Metabolism at the neuromuscular junction by acetylcholinesterase

8. A 22-year-old patient was given a bolus intravenous dose of a drug for muscle relaxation that should have lasted only 5–10 minutes. Instead, the patient required mechanical ventilation for over 8 hours. Which one of the following statements about this problem is false?
(A) The agent administered was succinylcholine
(B) This is an example of generic variation in drug metabolism
(C) Pseudocholinesterase in this patient is resistant to the inhibitory action of dibucaine
(D) The problem is not due to inadequate activity of acetylcholinesterase
(E) Neostigmine should be administered to establish the nature of the problem

9. Which one of the following drugs is most often associated with hypotension caused by histamine release?
(A) Diazepam
(B) Pancuronium
(C) Tizanidine
(D) Tubocurarine
(E) Vecuronium

10. Regarding the spasmolytic drugs, which one of the following statements is false?
 (A) Baclofen acts on neurons in the spinal cord to increase chloride ion conductance
 (B) Cyclobenzaprine is likely to dry oropharyngeal secretions and to decrease gut motility
 (C) Dantrolene has little effect on calcium release in cardiac muscle
 (D) Diazepam causes sedation at most doses required to reduce muscle spasms
 (E) Intrathecal use of baclofen is effective in some refractory cases of muscle spasticity

11. Which one of the following drugs has caused hyperkalemia leading to cardiac arrest in patients with neurologic disorders?
 (A) Baclofen
 (B) Dantrolene
 (C) Succinylcholine
 (D) Tubocurarine
 (E) Vecuronium

12. Which of the following phrases about atracurium is accurate?
 (A) Depolarizing blocker
 (B) Common ICU use for long-term immobilization
 (C) Inactivated by spontaneous breakdown
 (D) Prolonged action in pseudocholinesterase deficiency
 (E) Stimulates cardiac muscarinic receptors

13. Which one of the following drugs has spasmolytic activity and could also be used in the management of seizures caused by overdose of a local anesthetic?
 (A) Baclofen
 (B) Cyclobenzaprine
 (C) Dantrolene
 (D) Diazepam
 (E) Tizanidine

14. Which one of the following drugs given preoperatively will prevent postoperative pain caused by succinylcholine?
 (A) Baclofen
 (B) Dantrolene
 (C) Diazepam
 (D) Lidocaine
 (E) Tubocurarine

15. In anesthesia protocols that include succinylcholine, which one of the following is a premonitory sign of malignant hyperthermia?
 (A) Acidosis
 (B) Bradycardia
 (C) Hypotension
 (D) Transient hypothermia
 (E) Trismus

ANSWERS

1. Phase I depolarizing blockade is not associated with muscarinic blockade, nor is it reversible with cholinesterase inhibitors. Muscle fasciculations occur at the start of the action of succinylcholine. The answer is **(E).**

2. Acetylcholinesterase inhibitors used for reversing the effects of nondepolarizing muscle relaxants cause increases in ACh at all sites where it acts as a neurotransmitter. To offset the resulting side effects, including bradycardia, a muscarinic blocking agent is used concomitantly. The answer is **(D).**

3. One of the unusual characteristics of pancuronium is that it can block muscarinic receptors. It has sometimes caused tachycardia and hypertension and may cause dysrhythmias in predisposed individuals. The answer is **(C).**

4. Nondepolarizing blockers result in poorly sustained tetanic tension. They do not cause ganglionic stimulation or fasciculations at any time during their action. The answer is **(C).**

5. Nicotine, succinylcholine, and acetylcholine cause end plate depolarization and skeletal muscle contractions (they are nicotinic receptor agonists). Strychnine causes skeletal muscle contractions (convulsions) by blocking glycine receptors in the spinal cord. Vecuronium, a nondepolarizing blocker, does not cause contractions at any dose. The answer is **(E).**

6. Prompt treatment is essential in malignant hyperthermia to control body temperature, correct acidosis, and prevent calcium release. Dantrolene blocks the release of activator calcium from its stores in the sarcoplasmic reticulum, preventing the tension-generating interaction of actin with myosin. The answer is **(B).**
7. Succinylcholine use is associated with a rise in serum enzyme levels when muscle twitching and fasciculations are marked. Myoglobinuria may also occur. Histamine release due to succinylcholine is not genetically determined. The answer is **(C).**
8. Cholinesterase inhibitors (eg, neostigmine) markedly prolong the neuromuscular blockade caused by succinylcholine. They increase ACh at the end plate, which intensifies depolarization, and they also inhibit succinylcholine metabolism by pseudocholinesterase. About one in 500 persons have a single abnormal gene for pseudocholinesterase. Fewer than one in 3000 persons have two abnormal genes (homozygous atypical) that produce an enzyme with only 1% of the normal affinity for succinylcholine. The atypical enzyme is resistant to the inhibitory action of dibucaine. The answer is **(E).**
9. Hypotension may occur with tubocurarine and with the spasmolytic drug tizanidine. In the case of tubocurarine, the decrease in blood pressure may be due partly to histamine release and also to ganglionic blockade. Tizanidine causes hypotension via $alpha_2$ adrenoceptor activation like its congener clonidine. The answer is **(D).**
10. Baclofen does activate $GABA_B$ receptors in the spinal cord. However, these receptors are coupled to K^+ channels (see Chapter 21). The answer is **(A).**
11. Muscle depolarization by succinylcholine releases potassium, and the ensuing hyperkalemia can be life-threatening. Patients most susceptible include those with extensive burns, spinal cord injuries, neurologic dysfunction, or intra-abdominal infection. The answer is **(C).**
12. Atracurium (nondepolarizing) breaks down spontaneously in the plasma (Hofmann elimination) to form laudanosine, which has a long half-life. Since laudanosine enters the CNS and may cause seizures, prolonged administration of atracurium is usually avoided. The drug has no action on autonomic ganglia or muscarinic receptors. The answer is **(C).**
13. Diazepam is both an effective antiseizure drug and a spasmolytic. The spasmolytic action of diazepam is thought to be exerted partly in the spinal cord since it reduces spasm of skeletal muscle in patients with cord transection. Cyclobenzaprine is used for acute local spasm and has no antiseizure activity. The answer is **(D).**
14. The action of succinylcholine is antagonized by depolarizing blockers. To prevent fasciculations and postoperative pain caused by succinylcholine, a small nonparalyzing dose of a nondepolarizing drug is often given immediately before succinylcholine. The answer is **(E).**
15. Acidosis is a consequence of malignant hyperthermia. Bradycardia from activation of muscarinic receptors is characteristic of succinylcholine, and hypotension can result from histamine release. There is no transient phase of hypothermia, but severe contraction of the jaw muscles (trismus) is considered to be a premonitory sign of malignant hyperthermia. The answer is **(E).**

Skill Keeper Answer: Autonomic Control of Heart Rate (see Chapter 6)

Reflex changes in heart rate involve ganglionic transmission. Activation of $alpha_1$ receptors on blood vessels by phenylephrine elicits a reflex bradycardia since mean blood pressure is increased. One of the characteristic effects of tubocurarine is its block of autonomic ganglia—this action can interfere with reflex changes in heart rate. Tubocurarine would not prevent bradycardia due to neostigmine (an inhibitor of acetylcholinesterase) since this occurs via stimulation by acetylcholine of cardiac muscarinic receptors.

28 Drugs Used in Parkinsonism & Other Movement Disorders

OBJECTIVES

You should be able to:

- Describe the neurochemical imbalance underlying the symptoms of Parkinson's disease.
- Identify the mechanisms by which levodopa, dopamine receptor agonists, selegiline, and muscarinic blocking drugs alleviate parkinsonism.
- Describe the therapeutic and toxic effects of the major antiparkinsonism agents.
- Identify the compounds that inhibit dopa decarboxylase and catechol-*O*-methyltransferase and describe their use in parkinsonism.
- Identify the chemical agents and drugs that cause parkinsonism symptoms.
- Identify the drugs used in management of tremor, Huntington's disease, drug-induced dyskinesias, and Wilson's disease.

CONCEPTS

Movement disorders constitute a number of heterogeneous neurologic conditions with very different therapies (Figure 28–1).

PARKINSONISM

A. **Pathophysiology:** Parkinsonism is a common movement disorder that involves dysfunction in the basal ganglia and associated brain structures. Signs (mnemonic **RAFT**) include rigidity of skeletal muscles, akinesia (or bradykinesia), flat facies, and tremor at rest.

1. **Naturally occurring parkinsonism:** The naturally occurring disease is of uncertain origin and occurs with increasing frequency during aging from the fifth or sixth decade of life onward. Pathologic characteristics include a decrease in the levels of striatal dopamine and the degeneration of dopaminergic neurons in the nigrostriatal tract that normally *inhibit* the activity of striatal GABAergic neurons (Figure 28–2). Most of the postsynaptic dopamine

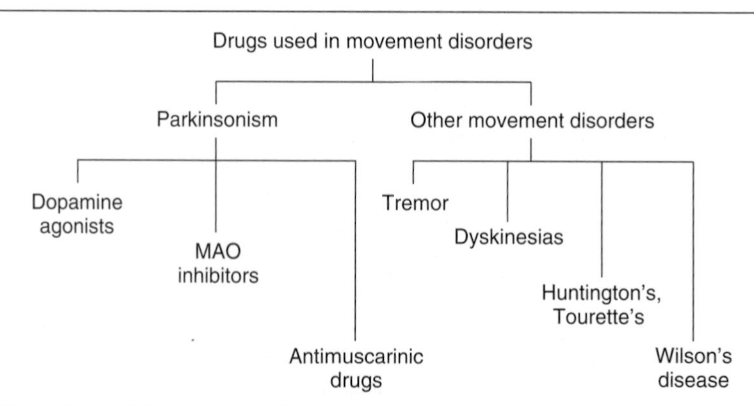

Figure 28–1. Some of the movement disorders and subgroups of drugs discussed in this chapter.

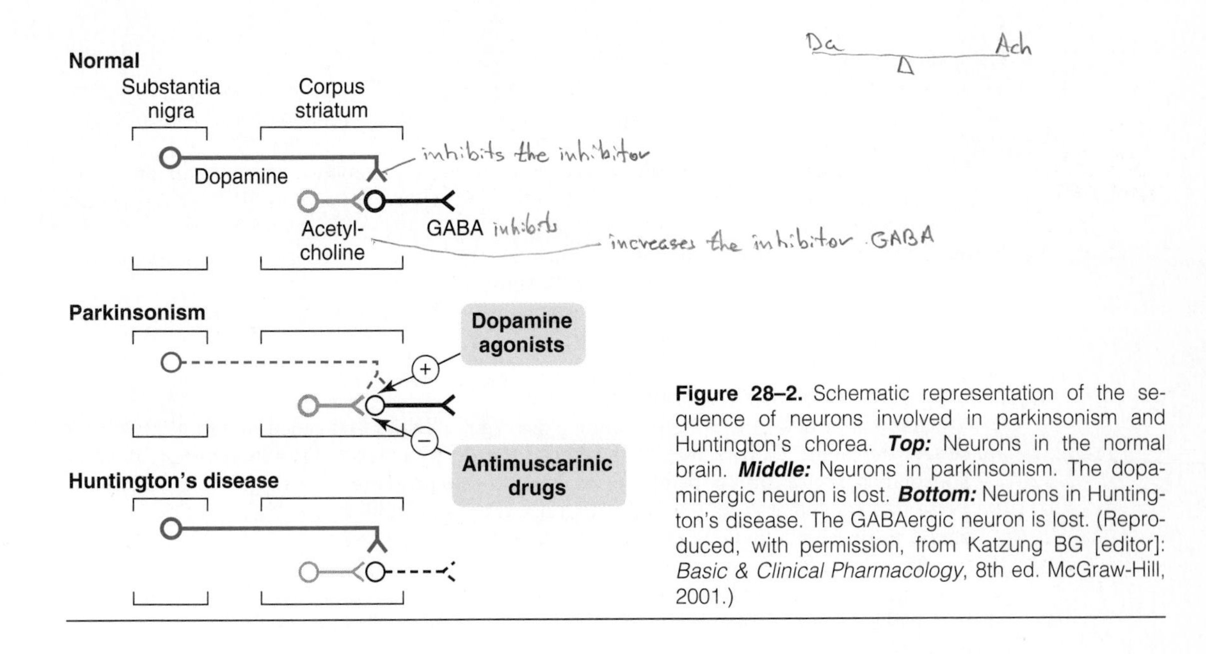

Figure 28–2. Schematic representation of the sequence of neurons involved in parkinsonism and Huntington's chorea. ***Top:*** Neurons in the normal brain. ***Middle:*** Neurons in parkinsonism. The dopaminergic neuron is lost. ***Bottom:*** Neurons in Huntington's disease. The GABAergic neuron is lost. (Reproduced, with permission, from Katzung BG [editor]: *Basic & Clinical Pharmacology*, 8th ed. McGraw-Hill, 2001.)

receptors on GABAergic neurons are of the D_2 subclass (negatively coupled to adenylyl cyclase). The reduction of normal dopaminergic neurotransmission leads to excessive *excitatory* actions of cholinergic neurons on striatal GABAergic neurons; thus, dopamine and acetylcholine activities are out of balance in parkinsonism (Figure 28–2).

2. **Drug-induced parkinsonism:** Many drugs can cause parkinsonian symptoms; these effects are usually reversible. The most important ones are the butyrophenone and phenothiazine **antipsychotic drugs,** which block brain dopamine receptors. At high doses, **reserpine** causes similar symptoms, presumably by depleting brain dopamine. MPTP (1-methyl-4-phenyl-1,2,3,6-tetrahydropyridine), a by-product of the attempted synthesis of an illicit meperidine analog, causes irreversible parkinsonism through destruction of dopaminergic neurons in the nigrostriatal tract. Treatment with inhibitors of monoamine oxidase (MAO) type B protects against MPTP neurotoxicity in animals.

DRUG THERAPY OF PARKINSONISM

Strategies of drug treatment of parkinsonism involve increasing dopamine activity in the brain or decreasing muscarinic cholinergic activity in the brain (or both).

A. Levodopa:

1. **Mechanisms:** Because dopamine has low bioavailability and does not readily cross the blood-brain barrier, its precursor, L-dopa (levodopa), is used. This amino acid is converted to dopamine by the enzyme aromatic L-amino acid decarboxylase (DOPA decarboxylase), which is present in many body tissues, including the brain. Levodopa is usually given with **carbidopa,** a drug that does not cross the blood-brain barrier but inhibits DOPA decarboxylase in peripheral tissues. With this combination, lower doses of levodopa are effective, and there are fewer peripheral side effects.
2. **Pharmacologic effects:** Levodopa ameliorates the signs of parkinsonism, particularly bradykinesia; moreover, the mortality rate is decreased. However, the drug does not cure parkinsonism, and responsiveness decreases with time, which may reflect progression of the disease. Clinical response to the drug may fluctuate quite rapidly, changing from akinesia to dyskinesia over a few hours. These so-called **on-off phenomena** may be related partly to changes in levodopa levels in plasma. Drug holidays sometimes reduce toxic effects but rarely affect response fluctuations. However, COMT inhibitors used adjunctively may improve levodopa responses (see below).

3. **Toxicity:** Most adverse effects are dose-dependent.
   a. **Gastrointestinal effects:** Anorexia, nausea, and emesis can be reduced by taking the drug in divided doses. Tolerance to the emetic action of levodopa usually occurs after several months.
   b. **Cardiovascular effects:** Postural hypotension is common, especially in the early stage of treatment. Other cardiac effects include tachycardia, asystole, and cardiac arrhythmias (rare).
   c. **Dyskinesias:** Choreoathetosis of the face and distal extremities occurs frequently. Some patients may exhibit chorea, ballismus, myoclonus, tics, and tremor.
   d. **Behavioral effects:** Behavioral effects may include anxiety, agitation, confusion, delusions, hallucinations, and depression.

B. Bromocriptine and Other Dopamine Agonists:

1. **Mechanism of action:** Bromocriptine is an ergot alkaloid that acts as a partial agonist at certain dopamine D_2 receptors in the brain; the drug increases the functional activity of dopamine neurotransmitter pathways, including those involved in extrapyramidal functions. **Pergolide** is another ergot derivative that activates dopamine receptors. Pergolide may decrease response fluctuations and prolong the effectiveness of levodopa, but the drug loses its efficacy with time.
2. **Clinical use:** Bromocriptine and pergolide have been used as individual drugs, in combinations with levodopa (and with anticholinergic drugs), and in patients who are refractory to or cannot tolerate levodopa.
3. **Toxicity:** **Gastrointestinal effects** include anorexia, nausea, and vomiting. **Cardiovascular effects** commonly include postural hypotension; cardiac arrhythmias may also occur. **Dyskinesias** may occur with abnormal movements similar to those caused by levodopa. **Behavioral effects** include confusion, hallucinations, and delusions; these occur more commonly with bromocriptine and pergolide than with levodopa. Like levodopa, bromocriptine and pergolide are contraindicated in patients with a history of psychosis. **Miscellaneous ergot-related effects** with bromocriptine include pulmonary infiltrates and erythromelalgia.
4. **Pramipexole and ropinirole:** Pramipexole and ropinirole are recently introduced dopamine receptor agonists; they are not ergot derivatives. These drugs are as effective as bromocriptine and do not cause the side effects typically associated with the use of ergots. They are presently considered to be first-line drugs in the initial management of Parkinson's disease. Dyskinesias, postural hypotension, lassitude, sleepiness, and fatigue have been reported.

C. Amantadine:

1. **Mechanism of action:** Amantadine enhances dopaminergic neurotransmission by unknown mechanisms that may involve increasing synthesis or release of dopamine or inhibition of reuptake of dopamine. The drug also has muscarinic blocking actions.
2. **Pharmacologic effects:** Amantadine may improve bradykinesia, rigidity, and tremor but is usually effective for only a few weeks. Amantadine also has antiviral effects.
3. **Toxicity:** **Behavioral effects** include restlessness, agitation, insomnia, confusion, hallucinations, and acute toxic psychosis. **Dermatologic reactions** include livedo reticularis. **Miscellaneous effects** may include gastrointestinal disturbances, urinary retention, and postural hypotension. Amantadine also causes peripheral edema that responds to diuretics.

D. Selegiline:

1. **Mechanism of action:** Selegiline is a selective inhibitor of MAO type B, the enzyme isoform that metabolizes dopamine in preference to norepinephrine and serotonin. Selegiline may increase brain dopamine levels.
2. **Pharmacologic effects:** The drug is used as an adjunct to levodopa in parkinsonism and has also been used as the sole agent in newly diagnosed patients. Hepatic metabolism of selegiline results in the formation of amphetamine.
3. **Toxicity:** Adverse effects include insomnia, mood changes, dyskinesias, gastrointestinal distress, and hypotension. Meperidine in combination with selegiline has caused agitation, delirium, and death. Selegiline has been implicated in the "serotonin syndrome" when used in patients taking selective serotonin reuptake inhibitors (see Chapter 30).

E. **Entacapone and Tolcapone:**
   1. **Mechanism of action:** Inhibitors of catechol-*O*-methyltransferase (COMT), the enzyme that converts levodopa to 3-*O*-methyldopa (3OMD). Increased plasma levels of 3OMD are associated with poor response to levodopa, partly because the compound competes with levodopa for active transport into the CNS.
   2. **Clinical uses:** The drugs are used as adjuncts to levodopa-carbidopa, improving response and prolonging "on-time."
   3. **Toxicity:** Adverse effects related to increased levels of levodopa include dyskinesias, gastrointestinal distress, and postural hypotension. Tolcapone has caused acute hepatic failure, necessitating routine monitoring of liver function tests.

F. **Acetylcholine-Blocking (Antimuscarinic) Drugs:**
   1. **Mechanism of action:** These drugs decrease the excitatory actions of cholinergic neurons on cells in the striatum by blocking muscarinic receptors.
   2. **Pharmacologic effects:** Drugs such as benztropine or trihexyphenidyl may improve the tremor and rigidity of parkinsonism but have little effect on bradykinesia. They are used adjunctively in parkinsonism and also alleviate the reversible extrapyramidal symptoms caused by antipsychotic drugs.
   3. **Toxicity:** CNS toxicity includes drowsiness, inattention, confusion, delusions, and hallucinations. Peripheral adverse effects are typical of atropine-like drugs. These agents exacerbate tardive dyskinesias that result from prolonged use of antipsychotic drugs.

Skill Keeper: Autonomic Drug Side Effects
(see Chapters 8 and 9)

Based on your understanding of the receptors affected by drugs used in Parkinson's disease, what types of autonomic side effects can you anticipate? *The Skill Keeper Answers appear at the end of the chapter.*

DRUG THERAPY OF OTHER MOVEMENT DISORDERS

A. **Tremor:** Physiologic and essential tremor are clinically similar conditions characterized by postural tremor. They may be alleviated by beta-blocking drugs such as **propranolol.** Beta-blockers should be used with caution in patients with congestive heart failure, asthma, diabetes, or hypoglycemia.

B. **Huntington's Disease and Gilles de la Tourette's Syndrome:** Huntington's disease, an inherited disorder, results from a brain neurotransmitter imbalance such that GABA functions are diminished and dopaminergic functions are enhanced (Figure 28–2). There may also be a cholinergic deficit, since choline acetyltransferase is decreased in the basal ganglia of patients with this disease. Drug therapy involves the use of amine-depleting drugs (eg, **tetrabenazine**) or antipsychotic agents (eg, **haloperidol** or a **phenothiazine**) that block dopamine receptors. Pharmacologic attempts to enhance brain GABA and acetylcholine activities have not been successful in patients with this disease.

   Tourette's syndrome is a disorder of unknown cause that responds to haloperidol and other dopamine D_2 receptor blockers including pimozide. Mecamylamine, a ganglion blocking drug that enters the CNS, may also have clinical value in Tourette's syndrome.

C. **Drug-Induced Dyskinesias:** Parkinsonism symptoms caused by antipsychotic agents are usually reversible by lowering drug dosage, changing the therapy to a drug that is less toxic to extrapyramidal function, or by adding muscarinic blockers. Levodopa and bromocriptine are not useful because dopamine receptors are blocked by the antipsychotic drugs. **Tardive dyskinesias** that develop from neuroleptic therapy are possibly a form of denervation supersensitivity. They are not readily reversed; no specific drug therapy is available.

D. **Wilson's Disease:** This recessively inherited disorder of copper metabolism results in deposition of copper salts in the liver and other tissues. Hepatic and neurologic damage may be severe or fatal. Treatment involves use of the chelating agent penicillamine (dimethylcysteine), which removes excess copper. Toxic effects of penicillamine include gastrointestinal distress, myasthenia, optic neuropathy, and blood dyscrasias.

DRUG LIST

The following drugs are important members of the group discussed in this chapter. Prototypes should be learned in detail; features of the major variants should be known well enough to distinguish the variants from prototypes and from each other.

Subclass	Prototype	Major Variants
Drugs used in parkinsonism		
Dopamine prodrug	Levodopa	
Levodopa adjunct		
DOPA decarboxylase inhibitor	Carbidopa	
COMT inhibitors	Tolcapone	Entacapone
Dopamine agonists	Bromocriptine	Pergolide, pramipexole, ropinirole
Indirect dopamine agonist	Amantadine	
MAO inhibitor	Selegiline	
Antimuscarinics	Benztropine	Biperiden, orphenadrine, trihexyphenidyl
Drugs used in tremor	Propranolol	
Drugs used in Huntington's disease	Haloperidol	
Drugs used in Tourette's syndrome	Haloperidol, pimozide, mecamylamine	Phenothiazines
Drugs used in Wilson's disease	Penicillamine	

QUESTIONS

DIRECTIONS: Each of the numbered items or incomplete statements in this section is followed by answers or by completions of the statement. Select the ONE lettered answer or completion that is BEST in each case.

Items 1–2: Bradykinesia has now made drug treatment necessary in a 60-year-old male patient with Parkinson's disease. You decide to initiate therapy with levodopa.

1. As the physician, you could tell the patient (and close family members) all of the following things about levodopa EXCEPT
- **(A)** Taking the drug in divided doses will decrease nausea and vomiting
- **(B)** He should be careful when he stands up because he may get dizzy
- **(C)** Uncontrollable muscle jerks may occur
- **(D)** A net-like reddish to blue discoloration of the skin is a likely side effect of the medication
- **(E)** The drug will probably improve his symptoms for a period of time but not indefinitely

2. As the physician who is prescribing levodopa, you will note that the drug
- **(A)** Causes less severe behavioral side effects if given with carbidopa
- **(B)** Fluctuates in its effectiveness with increasing frequency as treatment continues
- **(C)** Prevents extrapyramidal adverse effects of antipsychotic drugs
- **(D)** Protects against cancer in patients with melanoma
- **(E)** Has toxic effects that include pulmonary infiltrates

3. The major reason why carbidopa is of value in parkinsonism is that the compound
- **(A)** Crosses the blood-brain barrier
- **(B)** Inhibits monoamine oxidase type A
- **(C)** Inhibits aromatic L-amino acid decarboxylase

(D) Is converted to the false neurotransmitter carbidopamine
(E) Inhibits monoamine oxidase type B

4. Which one of the following statements about bromocriptine is accurate?
(A) It should not be administered to patients taking antimuscarinic drugs
(B) Effectiveness in Parkinson's disease requires its metabolic conversion to an active metabolite
(C) The drug is contraindicated in patients with a history of psychosis
(D) The drug should not be administered to patients already taking levodopa
(E) Mental disturbances occur more commonly with levodopa than with bromocriptine

5. A 72-year-old patient with parkinsonism presents with swollen feet. They are red, tender, and very painful. You could clear up these symptoms within a few days if you told the patient to stop taking
(A) Amantadine
(B) Benztropine
(C) Bromocriptine
(D) Levodopa
(E) Selegiline

6. A patient with parkinsonism is being treated with levodopa. He suffers from irregular, involuntary muscle jerks that affect the proximal muscles of the limbs. Which one of the following statements about these symptoms is accurate?
(A) The symptoms will usually be reduced if the dose of levodopa is increased
(B) Administration of other drugs that activate dopamine receptors will exacerbate dyskinesias
(C) The symptoms are likely to be alleviated by continued treatment with levodopa
(D) Dyskinesias are less likely to occur if levodopa is administered with carbidopa
(E) Coadministration of muscarinic blockers prevents the occurrence of dyskinesias during treatment with levodopa

7. A 51-year-old patient with parkinsonism is being maintained on levodopa-carbidopa with adjunctive use of selegiline. He presents with symptoms of severe depression, and treatment with antidepressants is appropriate. Which of the following is contraindicated?
(A) Amitriptyline
(B) Doxepin
(C) Imipramine
(D) Phenelzine
(E) Trazodone

8. Concerning the drugs used in parkinsonism, which of the following statements is accurate?
(A) Levodopa causes mydriasis and can precipitate an attack of acute glaucoma
(B) Useful therapeutic effects of amantadine continue for several years
(C) The primary therapeutic benefit of antimuscarinic drugs in parkinsonism is their ability to relieve bradykinesia
(D) Dopamine receptor agonists should not be used in Parkinson's disease prior to a trial of levodopa
(E) The concomitant use of selegiline may increase the peripheral adverse effects of levodopa

9. A previously healthy 50-year-old woman begins to suffer from slowed mentation and develops writhing movements of her tongue and hands. In addition, she has delusions of being persecuted. The woman has no past history of psychiatric or neurologic disorders. The most appropriate drug for treatment is
(A) Amantadine
(B) Bromocriptine
(C) Haloperidol
(D) Levodopa
(E) Trihexyphenidyl

10. Great caution must be exercised in the use of this drug (or drugs from the same class) in parkinsonian patients who have prostatic hypertrophy or obstructive gastrointestinal disease
(A) Benztropine
(B) Carbidopa
(C) Levodopa
(D) Ropinirole
(E) Selegiline

11. Which of the following statements about pramipexole is accurate?
    - **(A)** Activates dopamine D_2 receptors
    - **(B)** Commonly a first-line therapy for Parkinson's disease
    - **(C)** May cause postural hypotension
    - **(D)** Not an ergot derivative
    - **(E)** All of the above
12. This drug is protective against the selective neurotoxicity of MPTP, a chemical known to cause the destruction of dopaminergic neurons in the nigrostriatal tract
    - **(A)** Benztropine
    - **(B)** Entacapone
    - **(C)** Levodopa
    - **(D)** Ropinirole
    - **(E)** Selegiline
13. Tolcapone may be of value in patients being treated with levodopa-carbidopa because it
    - **(A)** Activates catechol-*O*-methyltransferase
    - **(B)** Decreases formation of 3-*O*-methyldopa
    - **(C)** Inhibits monoamine oxidase type B
    - **(D)** Inhibits dopamine reuptake
    - **(E)** Releases dopamine from nerve endings
14. Which one of the following drugs is most suitable for management of essential tremor in a patient who has pulmonary disease?
    - **(A)** Diazepam
    - **(B)** Levodopa
    - **(C)** Metoprolol
    - **(D)** Propranolol
    - **(E)** Terbutaline

ANSWERS

1. In prescribing levodopa, the patient should be informed about side effects, including gastrointestinal distress, postural hypotension, and dyskinesias. It would be reasonable to advise the patient that therapeutic benefits cannot be expected to continue indefinitely. Livedo reticularis (a net-like rash) is an adverse effect of treatment with amantadine. The answer is **(D).**
2. Levodopa causes less peripheral toxicity but more behavioral side effects when used with carbidopa. The drug is not effective in antagonizing the akinesia, rigidity, and tremor caused by treatment with antipsychotic agents. Levodopa is a precursor of melanin and may *activate* malignant melanoma. Use of levodopa is not associated with pulmonary dysfunction. The answer is **(B).**
3. Carbidopa is an inhibitor of aromatic L-amino acid decarboxylase, the enzyme that converts levodopa to dopamine. Since it does not enter the CNS, the drug acts only on the enzyme present in peripheral tissues (eg, liver). The use of carbidopa in combination with levodopa decreases the dose requirement and reduces peripheral side effects of levodopa. The answer is **(C).**
4. The use of dopaminergic agents in combination with antimuscarinic drugs is common in the treatment of parkinsonism. Bromocriptine does not complicate treatment with antimuscarinic drugs or amantadine. If combined with levodopa, bromocriptine should be used in reduced doses to avoid intolerable adverse effects. Confusion, delusions, and hallucinations occur more frequently with bromocriptine than with levodopa. Bromocriptine does not require bioactivation for its antiparkinson effects. The answer is **(C).**
5. The signs and symptoms described are those of *erythromelalgia,* an adverse effect of bromocriptine. The distal extremities (feet and hands) are usually involved. Arthralgia may occur along with the signs described. The answer is **(C).**
6. The form and severity of dyskinesias due to levodopa may vary widely in different patients. Dyskinesias occur in up to 80% of patients receiving levodopa for long periods. With continued treatment, dyskinesias may develop at a dose of levodopa that was previously well tolerated. They occur more commonly in patients treated with levodopa in combination with carbidopa or with other dopamine receptor agonists. Muscarinic receptor blockers do not prevent their occurrence. The answer is **(B).**

7. Remember that levodopa is a precursor of norepinephrine and epinephrine as well as dopamine and that norepinephrine and epinephrine are metabolized primarily by monoamine oxidase type A. In the presence of nonselective inhibitors of monoamine oxidases, levodopa may cause a hypertensive crisis. Though not contraindicated in Parkinson's disease, tricyclic antidepressants may interfere with the effectiveness of levodopa. The answer is **(D).**

8. The mydriatic action of levodopa may increase intraocular pressure, and the drug should be used cautiously in open-angle glaucoma and is contraindicated in angle-closure glaucoma. The effectiveness of amantadine is usually limited to just a few weeks. Antimuscarinic drugs may improve the tremor and rigidity of parkinsonism but have little effect on bradykinesia. Dopamine receptor agonists are commonly used as first-line agents in parkinsonism. As a selective inhibitor of MAO type B, selegiline does not exacerbate peripheral adverse effects of levodopa. The answer is **(A).**

9. Choreoathetosis with decreased mental abilities and psychosis (paranoia) suggest that this patient has Huntington's disease. Drugs that are partly ameliorative include agents that decrease dopaminergic activity such as the antipsychotic agents. The answer is **(C).**

10. Benztropine may cause urinary retention and gastrointestinal effects and should be used with caution in patients with prostatic hypertrophy or obstructive gastrointestinal disease and is contraindicated in those with angle-closure glaucoma. Relative contraindications regarding use of this class of drugs in Parkinson's disease are those for drugs that block acetylcholine at muscarinic receptors. The answer is **(A).**

11. Pramipexole is an agonist at dopamine receptors and may have greater selectivity for D_2 receptors in the striatum. It is not an ergot and appears to be less toxic than bromocriptine and pergolide. Pramipexole and ropinirole are often chosen for initial treatment of Parkinson's disease and sometimes have value in patients who have become refractory to levodopa. Side effects of these drugs include dyskinesias, postural hypotension, and somnolence. The answer is **(E).**

12. MPTP causes parkinson-like extrapyramidal dysfunction by destroying dopaminergic neurons in the nigrostriatal tract. This neurotoxic action requires the formation of toxic metabolites from the metabolism of MPTP by monoamine oxidase type B. Toxicity is prevented by selegiline, a selective inhibitor of MAO type B. MPTP is used as an experimental tool in animal models of parkinsonism. The answer is **(E).**

13. Tolcapone is an inhibitor of catechol-*O*-methyltransferase used adjunctively in patients treated with levodopa-carbidopa. The drug decreases the formation of 3-*O*-methyldopa (3OMD) from levodopa. This has the effect of improving patient response to levodopa, partly by increasing levodopa levels and also by decreasing competition between 3OMD and levodopa for active transport by carrier mechanisms involved in transport across the blood-brain barrier. The answer is **(B).**

14. Dysfunction of beta-adrenoceptors has been implicated in essential tremor, and management usually involves administration of propranolol. However, the more selective β_1 blocker metoprolol is equally effective and may be more suitable in a patient with pulmonary disease. The answer is **(C).**

Skill Keeper Answers: Autonomic Drug Side Effects (see Chapters 8 and 9)

Pharmacologic strategy in Parkinson's disease involves attempts to enhance dopamine functions or antagonize acetylcholine at muscarinic receptors. Thus, peripheral side effects must be anticipated.

1. Side effects referable to activation of peripheral dopamine (or adrenoceptors in the case of levodopa) include postural hypotension, tachycardia (possible arrhythmias), mydriasis, and emetic responses.
2. Side effects referable to antagonism of peripheral muscarinic receptors include dry mouth, mydriasis, urinary retention, and cardiac arrhythmias.

29 Antipsychotic Drugs & Lithium

OBJECTIVES

You should be able to:

- Describe the dopamine hypothesis of schizophrenia.
- List the major receptors blocked by antipsychotic drugs.
- Describe the pharmacodynamics of older antipsychotic drugs and relate these characteristics to their clinical uses.
- Identify the main characteristics and clinical uses of newer atypical antipsychotic drugs.
- List the major adverse effects of the antipsychotic drugs.
- Describe the pharmacokinetics and pharmacodynamics of lithium.

CONCEPTS

ANTIPSYCHOTIC DRUGS

The antipsychotic drugs **(neuroleptics)** are effective in controlling many manifestations of psychotic illness. Though the disease is not cured by drug therapy, the symptoms of schizophrenia, including thought disorder, emotional withdrawal, and hallucinations or delusions, may be attenuated by antipsychotic drugs. Unfortunately, protracted therapy (years) is often needed and can result in severe toxicity in some patients.

A. Classification: The major chemical subgroups of antipsychotic drugs are the **phenothiazines** (eg, chlorpromazine, thioridazine, fluphenazine); the **thioxanthenes** (eg, thiothixene); and the **butyrophenones** (eg, haloperidol).

Several newer drugs of varied **heterocyclic** structure are also effective in schizophrenia, including clozapine, loxapine, olanzapine, molindone, pimozide, risperidone, quetiapine, and sertindole. In some cases, these atypical antipsychotic drugs have proved to be more effective and less toxic than the older drugs. However, they are much more costly than standard drugs, most of which are prescribed generically.

B. Pharmacokinetics: The antipsychotic drugs are well absorbed when given orally and, because they are lipid-soluble, readily enter the CNS and most other body tissues. Many are bound extensively to plasma proteins. These drugs require metabolism by liver enzymes prior to elimination and have long plasma half-lives that permit once-daily dosing. Parenteral forms of several agents, including fluphenazine, thioridazine, and haloperidol, are available for rapid initiation of therapy.

C. Mechanism of Action:

1. **The dopamine hypothesis:** The dopamine hypothesis of schizophrenia proposes that the disorder is caused by a relative excess of functional activity of the neurotransmitter dopamine in specific neuronal tracts in the brain. This hypothesis is based on the following observations: (1) Many antipsychotic drugs block brain dopamine receptors (especially D_2 receptors). (2) Dopamine agonist drugs (eg, amphetamine, levodopa) exacerbate schizophrenia. (3) An increased density of dopamine receptors has been detected in certain brain regions of untreated schizophrenics. The dopamine hypothesis of schizophrenia is not fully satisfactory because antipsychotic drugs are only partly effective in most patients and because some effective drugs have a much higher affinity for other receptors than for D_2 receptors.

2. **Dopamine receptors:** Five different dopamine receptors (D_1–D_5) have been characterized. Each is G protein-coupled and contains seven transmembrane domains. The D_2 receptor, found in the caudate-putamen, nucleus accumbens, cerebral cortex, and hypothalamus, is negatively coupled to adenylyl cyclase. The therapeutic efficacy of most of the older antipsychotic drugs correlates with their relative affinity for the D_2 receptor. Unfortunately, there is also a correlation between blockade of D_2 receptors and extrapyramidal dysfunction.
3. **Other receptors:** Several newer antipsychotic agents have higher affinities for other receptors than for the D_2 receptor. For example, alpha adrenoceptor-blocking action correlates well with antipsychotic effect for many of the drugs (Table 29–1). Clozapine, a drug with significant D_4 and 5-HT_2 receptor-blocking actions, has low affinity for D_2 receptors. Most of the newer atypical drugs (olanzapine, quetiapine, risperidone, and sertindole) have high affinity for 5-HT_{2A} receptors, though they may also interact with D_2 and other receptors. Most of these atypical drugs cause less extrapyramidal dysfunction than standard drugs.

D. **Effects:** Dopamine receptor blockade is the major effect that correlates with therapeutic benefit for older antipsychotic drugs. Dopaminergic tracts in the brain include the mesocortical-mesolimbic pathways (regulating mentation and mood), the nigrostriatal tract (extrapyramidal function), the tuberoinfundibular pathways (control of prolactin release), and the chemoreceptor trigger zone (emesis). Mesocortical-mesolimbic dopamine receptor blockade presumably underlies antipsychotic effects, and a similar action on the chemoreceptor trigger zone leads to the useful antiemetic properties of some antipsychotic drugs. Adverse effects resulting from receptor blockade in the other dopaminergic tracts include extrapyramidal dysfunction and hyperprolactinemia (see below). The relative receptor blocking actions of different antipsychotic drugs are shown in Table 29–1.

E. **Clinical Use:**
1. **Treatment of schizophrenia:** Antipsychotic drugs reduce some of the positive symptoms of schizophrenia, including hyperactivity, bizarre ideation, hallucinations, and delusions. Consequently, they can facilitate functioning in both inpatient and outpatient environments. Beneficial effects may take several weeks to develop. Overall efficacy of the older antipsychotic drugs is equivalent, though individual patients may respond best to a specific drug. None of the traditional drugs have much effect on negative symptoms of schizophrenia. Among the newer atypical drugs, olanzapine and sertindole are reported to improve some of the negative symptoms of schizophrenia, including emotional blunting and social withdrawal, and clozapine and risperidone are often effective in patients refractory to standard drugs.
2. **Other psychiatric and neurologic indications:** Antipsychotic drugs may be useful in the initial treatment of mania, in the management of psychotic symptoms of schizoaffective disorders, in Tourette's syndrome, and for management of toxic psychoses caused by over-

Table 29–1. Relative receptor blocking actions of neuroleptic drugs.[1]

Drug	D_2 Block	D_4 Block	Alpha$_1$ Block	5-HT_2 Block	M Block	H_1 Block
Most phenothiazines and thioxanthenes	++	–	++	+	+	+
Thioridazine	++	–	++	+	+++	+
Haloperidol	+++	–	+	–	–	–
Clozapine	–	++	++	++	++	+
Molindone	++	–	+	–	+	+
Olanzapine	+	–	+	++	+	+
Quetiapine	+	–	+	++	+	+
Risperidone	++	–	+	++	+	+
Sertindole	++	–	+	+++	–	–

[1] **Key:** +, blockade; –, no effect. The number of plus signs indicates the intensity of receptor blockade.

dosage of certain CNS stimulants. Molindone is used mainly in Tourette's syndrome; it is rarely used in schizophrenia.

3. **Nonpsychiatric indications:** With the exception of thioridazine, most phenothiazines have antiemetic actions; prochlorperazine is promoted solely for this indication. H_1 receptor blockade, most often present in short side-chain phenothiazines, provides the basis for their use as antipruritics and sedatives and contributes to their antiemetic effects.

F. Toxicity:

1. **Reversible neurologic effects:** Dose-dependent extrapyramidal effects include a parkinson-like syndrome with bradykinesia, rigidity, and tremor. This toxicity may be reversed by a decrease in dose and may be antagonized by concomitant use of muscarinic blocking agents. Extrapyramidal toxicity occurs most frequently with haloperidol (Figure 29–1) and the more potent piperazine side-chain phenothiazines (eg, fluphenazine, trifluoperazine). Parkinsonism occurs infrequently with clozapine and is less common with several newer drugs, including olanzapine, risperidone, and sertindole. Other reversible neurologic dysfunctions include akathisia and dystonias; these usually respond to treatment with diphenhydramine or muscarinic blocking agents.
2. **Tardive dyskinesias:** This important toxicity includes choreoathetoid movements of the muscles of the lips and buccal cavity and may be irreversible. Tardive dyskinesias tend to develop after several years of antipsychotic drug therapy but have appeared as early as 6 months. Antimuscarinic drugs that usually ameliorate other extrapyramidal effects generally *increase* the severity of tardive dyskinesia symptoms. There is no effective drug treatment for tardive dyskinesia. Switching to clozapine does not exacerbate the condition. Tardive dyskinesia may be attenuated *temporarily* by increasing neuroleptic dosage; this suggests that tardive dyskinesia may be caused by dopamine receptor sensitization.
3. **Autonomic effects:** Autonomic effects result from blockade of peripheral muscarinic receptors and alpha adrenoceptors and are more difficult to manage in elderly patients. Tolerance to some of the autonomic effects occurs with continued therapy. As shown in Figure 29–1, thioridazine has the strongest autonomic effects and haloperidol the weakest. Clozapine and most of the atypical drugs have intermediate autonomic effects.
   a. **Muscarinic receptor blockade:** Atropine-like effects (dry mouth, constipation, urinary retention, and visual problems) are often pronounced during use of thioridazine and phenothiazines with aliphatic side chains (eg, chlorpromazine). These effects also occur with clozapine and most of the atypical drugs but not with sertindole. Antimuscarinic CNS effects may include a toxic confusional state similar to that produced by atropine and the tricyclic antidepressants.
   b. **Alpha receptor blockade:** Postural hypotension caused by alpha blockade is a common manifestation of many of these drugs, especially phenothiazines. In the elderly,

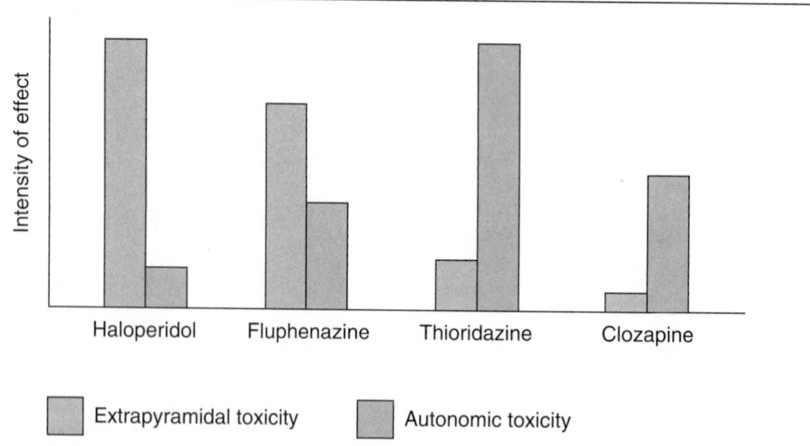

Figure 29–1. Relative extrapyramidal and autonomic toxicities of representative antipsychotic drugs. Extrapyramidal toxicities take the form of parkinsonism, akathisias, and dystonias. Autonomic toxicities are manifested as alpha-adrenoceptor blockade (orthostatic hypotension) or muscarinic blockade (dry mouth, blurred vision, urinary retention).

measures must be taken to avoid falls due to postural fainting. All of the atypical drugs can cause orthostatic hypotension. Failure to ejaculate is common in men treated with the phenothiazines.

4. **Endocrine and metabolic effects:** Endocrine and metabolic effects include hyperprolactinemia, weight gain, gynecomastia, the amenorrhea-galactorrhea syndrome, and infertility. These effects are predictable manifestations of dopamine receptor blockade in the pituitary; dopamine is the normal inhibitory regulator of prolactin secretion.
5. **Neuroleptic malignant syndrome:** Patients who are particularly sensitive to the extrapyramidal effects of antipsychotic drugs may develop a malignant hyperthermic syndrome. The symptoms include muscle rigidity, impairment of sweating, hyperpyrexia, and autonomic instability that may be life-threatening. Drug treatment involves the prompt use of dantrolene and perhaps dopamine agonists.

dantrolene

6. **Sedation:** Sedation is more marked with phenothiazines than with other antipsychotics; this effect is usually perceived as unpleasant by nonpsychotic individuals. With the exception of sertindole, the atypical drugs all block histamine receptors, an action that contributes to sedation.
7. **Miscellaneous toxicities:** Visual impairment caused by retinal deposits has occurred with **thioridazine;** at high doses, this drug may also cause severe conduction defects in the heart that result in fatal ventricular arrhythmias. **Sertindole** prolongs the QT interval of the ECG; the underlying myocardial effect may lead to cardiac arrhythmias. **Clozapine** causes a small but important (1–2%) incidence of agranulocytosis and at high doses has caused seizures.
8. **Overdosage toxicity:** Poisoning with antipsychotics other than thioridazine is not usually fatal. Hypotension often responds to fluid replacement. Neuroleptics lower the convulsive threshold and may cause seizures, which are usually managed with diazepam or phenytoin. Thioridazine overdose, because of cardiotoxicity, is more difficult to treat.

Skill Keeper: Receptor Mechanisms
(see Chapters 2, 6, and 21)

Antipsychotic drugs to varying degrees act as antagonists at several receptor types including those for acetylcholine, dopamine, norepinephrine, and serotonin. What are the second messenger systems for each of the following receptor subtypes that are blocked by antipsychotic drugs?

1. D_2
2. M_3
3. $Alpha_1$
4. $5\text{-}HT_{2A}$

The Skill Keeper Answers appear at the end of the chapter.

LITHIUM & OTHER DRUGS USED IN BIPOLAR (MANIC-DEPRESSIVE) DISORDER

A. **Pharmacokinetics:** Lithium is absorbed rapidly and completely from the gut. The drug is distributed throughout the body water and excreted by the kidneys with a half-life of about 20 hours. Plasma levels should be monitored, especially during the first weeks of therapy, to establish an effective and safe dosage regimen. The therapeutic plasma concentration is 0.6–1.4 meq/L. Plasma levels of the drug may be altered by changes in body water. Thus, dehydration or treatment with diuretics (thiazides), may result in an increase of lithium in the blood to toxic levels. Theophylline increases the renal clearance of lithium.

B. **Mechanism of Action:** The mechanism of action of lithium is not well defined. The drug inhibits the recycling of neuronal membrane phosphoinositides involved in the generation of inositol trisphosphate (IP_3) and diacylglycerol (DAG). These second messengers are important in amine neurotransmission, including that mediated by central adrenoceptors and muscarinic receptors (Figure 29–2).

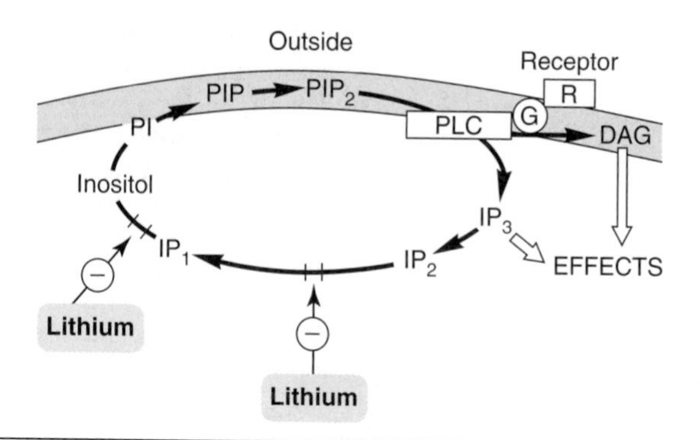

Figure 29–2. Postulated effect of lithium on the IP_3 and DAG second messenger system. The schematic diagram shows the synaptic membrane of a neuron in the brain. PLC, phospholipase-C; G, coupling protein; R, receptor; PI, PIP, PIP_2, IP_2, IP_1, intermediates in the production of IP_3. By interfering with this cycle, lithium may cause a use-dependent reduction of synaptic transmission. (Modified and reproduced, with permission, from Katzung BG [editor]: *Basic & Clinical Pharmacology,* 8th ed. McGraw-Hill, 2001.)

C. **Clinical Use:** Lithium carbonate is used in the treatment of bipolar affective disorder (manic-depressive disease). Maintenance therapy with lithium decreases manic behavior and reduces both the frequency and the magnitude of mood swings. Drug therapy with neuroleptics or benzodiazepines may also be required at the initiation of lithium treatment. Antidepressant drugs may be required adjunctively during maintenance. Alternative drugs of value in bipolar affective disorder include **carbamazepine, clonazepam, gabapentin,** and **valproic acid.**

D. **Toxicity:** Adverse neurologic effects of lithium include tremor, sedation, ataxia, and aphasia. Thyroid enlargement may occur, but thyroid dysfunction is rare. Reversible nephrogenic diabetes insipidus occurs commonly at therapeutic drug levels. Edema is a frequent adverse effect of lithium therapy; acneiform skin eruptions occur; and leukocytosis is always present. The use of lithium during pregnancy may increase the incidence of congenital cardiac anomalies (Ebstein's malformations). Lithium is contraindicated in nursing mothers.

DRUG LIST

The following drugs are important members of the drug groups discussed in this chapter. Prototypes should be learned in detail; the other significant agents should be recognized as belonging to a specific subclass.

Subclass	Prototype	Other Significant Agents
Phenothiazines		
Aliphatic	Chlorpromazine[1]	
Piperidine	Thioridazine	Mesoridazine
Piperazine	Trifluoperazine	Perphenazine, fluphenazine
Thioxanthenes	Thiothixene	
Butyrophenones	Haloperidol	
Heterocyclics	Clozapine, molindone, pimozide	Loxapine, olanzapine, quetiapine, risperidone, sertindole
Antimanic drugs	Lithium	Carbamazepine, clonazepam, gabapentin, valproic acid

[1]***Note:*** Some authorities consider chlorpromazine obsolete because of its high incidence of toxic effects.

QUESTIONS

DIRECTIONS: Each of the numbered items or incomplete statements in this section is followed by answers or by completions of the statement. Select the ONE lettered answer or completion that is BEST in each case.

1. Concerning hypotheses for the pathophysiologic basis of schizophrenia, which one of the following statements is accurate?
   (A) Positron emission tomography has shown decreased dopamine receptors in the brains of both untreated and drug-treated schizophrenics
   (B) Drugs that block dopamine receptors are useful for alleviating psychotic symptoms in parkinsonian patients
   (C) The clinical potency of many antipsychotic drugs correlates well with their beta adrenoceptor-blocking actions
   (D) Drug-induced psychosis can occur without activation of brain dopamine receptors
   (E) All effective antipsychotic drugs have high affinity for dopamine D_2 receptors
2. Fluphenazine has been prescribed for a 20-year-old male patient. His schizophrenic symptoms have improved enough for him to reside in a halfway house in the community. He visits his physician with a list of complaints about his medication. Which one of the following is not likely to be on his list?
   (A) Constipation
   (B) Dizziness if he stands up too quickly
   (C) He has become disinterested in sex
   (D) He salivates excessively
   (E) Newspaper print is hard to see
3. Which one of the following statements concerning adverse effects of antipsychotic drugs is accurate?
   (A) The late-occurring choreoathetoid movements caused by conventional antipsychotic drugs are reduced by antimuscarinic agents
   (B) Retinal pigmentation is a dose-dependent toxic effect of clozapine
   (C) Uncontrollable restlessness in a patient taking antipsychotic medications is usually alleviated by increasing the drug dose
   (D) Acute dystonic reactions occur very infrequently with olanzapine
   (E) Blurring of vision and urinary retention are common side effects of haloperidol
4. Chlorpromazine would not be an appropriate drug for management of
   (A) Acute mania
   (B) The amenorrhea-galactorrhea syndrome
   (C) Phencyclidine intoxication
   (D) Schizoaffective disorders
   (E) Tourette's syndrome
5. A schizophrenic patient developed bradykinesia, rigidity, and tremor during treatment with haloperidol. His drug therapy was changed to thioridazine, which was just as effective in reducing his psychiatric symptoms. However, thioridazine did not cause extrapyramidal dysfunction in this patient. The most likely explanation is that
   (A) Haloperidol has a low affinity for D_2 receptors
   (B) Thioridazine has greater alpha adrenoceptor-blocking actions
   (C) Haloperidol activates GABAergic neurons in the striatum
   (D) Thioridazine has greater blocking actions on brain muscarinic receptors
   (E) Haloperidol acts presynaptically to block dopamine release
6. Which one of the following statements concerning the treatment of bipolar affective disorder is accurate?
   (A) Lithium will alleviate the manic phase of bipolar disorder within 24 hours
   (B) Excessive intake of sodium chloride enhances the toxicity of lithium
   (C) Lithium dosage may need to be decreased in patients taking thiazides
   (D) The elimination rate of lithium is equivalent to that of creatinine
   (E) Lithium does not cross the placental barrier
7. A 30-year-old male patient is on drug therapy for a psychiatric problem. He complains that he feels "flat" and that he gets confused at times. He has been gaining weight and has lost his sex drive. As he moves his hands, you notice a slight tremor. He tells you that since he has been on medication he is always thirsty and frequently has to urinate. The drug he is most likely to be taking is
   (A) Clonazepam
   (B) Clozapine
   (C) Haloperidol

(D) Lithium
(E) Trifluoperazine

8. A young male patient diagnosed as schizophrenic develops severe muscle cramps with torticollis a short time after drug therapy is initiated with haloperidol. The best course of action would be to
(A) Add clozapine to the drug regimen
(B) Discontinue haloperidol and observe the patient
(C) Give oral diphenhydramine
(D) Switch the patient to fluphenazine
(E) Inject benztropine

9. The effective treatment of a bipolar patient has necessitated doses of lithium that result in plasma levels of 1.4 to 1.5 meq/L. Lately he has begun to suffer from increased motor activity, aphasia, mental confusion, and social withdrawal. The best course of action would be to
(A) Add amitriptyline to the drug regimen
(B) Continue lithium and add haloperidol
(C) Discontinue lithium and start valproic acid
(D) Discontinue lithium and start clozapine
(E) Increase the dose of lithium

10. Which one of the following statements about the actions of phenothiazines is accurate?
(A) They activate muscarinic receptors
(B) They are antiemetic
(C) They decrease serum prolactin levels
(D) They elevate the seizure threshold
(E) They raise blood pressure

11. A young patient who has been treated with an antipsychotic drug for a few weeks becomes easily fatigued and experiences periodic fevers. Petechiae are apparent on physical examination, and laboratory studies reveal leukopenia and thrombocytopenia. If a diagnosis is made that the patient is suffering from drug-induced agranulocytosis, he is most likely being treated with
(A) Chlorpromazine
(B) Clozapine
(C) Haloperidol
(D) Olanzapine
(E) Risperidone

12. In comparing the characteristics of thioridazine with other older antipsychotic drugs, which one of the following statements is accurate?
(A) Most likely to cause extrapyramidal dysfunction
(B) Least likely to cause urinary retention
(C) Most likely to be safe in patients with history of cardiac arrhythmias
(D) Least likely to cause dry mouth
(E) Most likely to cause ocular dysfunction

13. Within days of starting haloperidol treatment for a psychiatric disorder, a young male patient developed severe generalized muscle rigidity and a high fever. In the emergency room he was incoherent, with increased heart rate, hypotension, and diaphoresis. Laboratory studies indicated acidosis, leukocytosis, and increased creatine kinase. The most likely reason for these symptoms is that the patient was suffering from
(A) Agranulocytosis
(B) A severe bacterial infection
(C) Neuroleptic malignant syndrome
(D) Spastic retrocollis
(E) Tardive dyskinesia

14. This drug has a high affinity for 5-HT_2 receptors in the brain and does not cause extrapyramidal dysfunction or hematotoxicity; it is reported to improve both positive and negative symptoms of schizophrenia
(A) Chlorpromazine
(B) Clozapine
(C) Fluphenazine
(D) Olanzapine
(E) Risperidone

ANSWERS

1. PET scans of the brain of untreated schizophrenics have revealed small *increases* in dopamine receptors. Dopamine receptor blockers should be avoided in parkinsonism. While most conventional antipsychotic drugs block D_2 receptors, this action is not an absolute requirement for antipsychotic action, since clozapine and newer drugs have a very low affinity for such receptors. The clinical potency of antipsychotic drugs does not correlate well with their beta adrenoceptor-blocking actions. The effects of phencyclidine (PCP) closely parallel an acute schizophrenic episode, but PCP has no actions on brain dopamine receptors. The answer is **(D).**
2. Sedative effects occur with most of the phenothiazines; these drugs also act as antagonists at muscarinic and alpha adrenoceptors. Postural hypotension, blurring of vision, and constipation are common autonomic side effects, as is dry mouth. Effects on the male libido may result from increases in prolactin or from increased peripheral conversion of androgens to estrogens. The answer is **(D).**
3. Muscarinic blockers exacerbate tardive dyskinesias. Akathisias (uncontrollable restlessness) due to antipsychotic drugs may be relieved by a *reduction* in dosage. Ocular dysfunction does not occur with clozapine. Older antipsychotic drugs—especially those that are potent antagonists of dopamine receptors—may cause acute dystonic reactions early in treatment. Olanzapine has minimal dopamine receptor blocking action and is unlikely to cause this type of adverse effect. Haloperidol does not block muscarinic receptors. The answer is **(D).**
4. Hyperprolactinemia and the amenorrhea-galactorrhea syndrome may occur as an adverse effect during treatment with antipsychotic drugs that block dopamine receptors in the tuberoinfundibular tract. This prevents the normal inhibitory action of dopamine on release of prolactin from the anterior pituitary gland. The answer is **(B).**
5. Parkinsonian adverse effects occur more commonly with haloperidol than with thioridazine. One possible explanation is that thioridazine exerts more pronounced blocking actions at brain muscarinic receptors. This action partly compensates for dopamine receptor blockade in the nigrostriatal tract, so that extrapyramidal function is more effectively maintained. A second possibility (not listed) is that haloperidol has a higher affinity for dopamine D_2 receptors than does thioridazine. The answer is **(D).**
6. Clinical effects of lithium are slow in onset and may not be apparent before a week or two of daily treatment. Lithium is cleared exclusively by the kidney at a rate 20% of that of creatinine. Clearance is influenced by many factors, including renal function, serum sodium concentration, hydration state, pregnancy, and the presence of other drugs. High urinary levels of sodium inhibit renal tubular reabsorption of lithium, thus *decreasing* its plasma levels. By decreasing blood volume, thiazides may increase lithium plasma levels. Any drug that can cross the blood-brain barrier can cross the placental barrier! The answer is **(C).**
7. Confusion, mood changes, decreased sexual interest, and weight gain are symptoms that may be unrelated to drug administration. On the other hand, psychiatric drugs, including those used in the treatment of psychotic and affective disorders, may be responsible for such symptoms. Tremor and symptoms of nephrogenic diabetes insipidus are characteristic adverse effects of lithium that may occur at therapeutic blood levels of the drug. The answer is **(D).**
8. Acute dystonic reactions are usually very painful and should be treated immediately with parenteral administration of a muscarinic blocking agent. Adding clozapine will not be protective, and fluphenazine is as likely as haloperidol to cause acute dystonia. Oral administration of diphenhydramine is a possibility, but the patient may find it difficult to swallow and it would take a longer time to act. The answer is **(E).**
9. The symptoms described in this patient are toxic effects of lithium. The desired plasma level is usually in the range of 0.7–1.4 meq/L, but toxicity may occur at the top end of this range in some patients. Increasing the dose of lithium will increase blood levels and exacerbate these symptoms. Adding amitriptyline or haloperidol to the regimen would not alleviate the problem. A trial of an alternative drug (eg, carbamazepine, clonazepam, or valproic acid) is appropriate. Clozapine as a single agent has minimal efficacy in bipolar disorder. The answer is **(C).**
10. With the exception of thioridazine, phenothiazines exert strong antiemetic effects. Phenothiazines with short side chains have marked histamine H_1 receptor-blocking action and are used for relief of pruritus or, in the case of promethazine, as preoperative sedatives. All of the other actions listed are "opposites." The answer is **(B).**
11. Agranulocytosis occurs in a small percentage of patients taking clozapine. This potentially fatal abnormality can develop rapidly, usually between the 6th and 18th weeks of therapy.

Hematotoxicity is reversible if clozapine is discontinued immediately following a significant decrease in white count. The answer is **(B).**

12. Atropine-like side effects are more prominent with thioridazine than with other phenothiazines, but the drug is less likely to cause extrapyramidal dysfunction. At high doses, thioridazine causes retinal deposits which in advanced cases resemble retinitis pigmentosa. The patient may complain of browning of vision. The drug has quinidine-like actions on the heart and, in overdose, may cause arrhythmias and cardiac conduction block. The answer is **(E).**
13. The neuroleptic malignant syndrome is characterized by muscle rigidity, high fever, and autonomic instability. The syndrome may result from a too-rapid block of dopamine receptors in patients who are highly sensitive to the extrapyramidal effects of antipsychotic drugs. Management involves the physical control of fever, the use of muscle relaxants (eg, dantrolene or diazepam), and possibly administration of the dopamine receptor agonist bromocriptine. Like most drugs that increase brain dopaminergic activity, bromocriptine may exacerbate psychotic symptoms. The answer is **(C).**
14. Tricky? Many of the newer antipsychotic drugs have a greater affinity for 5-HT_2 receptors than dopamine receptors. However, since clozapine is hematotoxic, the choice comes down to olanzapine and risperidone, both of which block 5-HT receptors. Although the risk appears to be low, risperidone is reported to cause extrapyramidal dysfunction, including tardive dyskinesia. The answer is **(D).**

Skill Keeper Answers: Receptor Mechanisms (see Chapters 2, 6, and 21)

1. D_2: G_i linked, ↓ cAMP
2. M_3: G_q linked, ↑ IP_3 and DAG
3. $Alpha_1$: G_q linked, ↑ IP_3 and DAG
4. 5-HT_{2A}: G_q linked, ↑ IP_3 and DAG

30 Antidepressants

OBJECTIVES

You should be able to:

- Describe the probable mechanisms and the major properties of tricyclic antidepressants.
- List the toxic effects that occur during chronic therapy and with an acute overdose of tricyclic antidepressants.
- Identify the second- and third-generation heterocyclic antidepressants and their distinctive properties.
- Identify the selective serotonin reuptake inhibitors and list their major characteristics.
- Describe the therapeutic use and toxic effects of MAO inhibitors.
- Identify the major drug interactions associated with antidepressant drugs.

depression is low levels of norepinephrine and serotonin.

Learn the definitions that follow.

Table 30–1. Definitions.

Term	Definition
Amine hypothesis of mood	The hypothesis that major depressive disorders result from a functional deficiency of norepinephrine or serotonin at synapses in the central nervous system
Tricyclics	A group of structurally related drugs resembling phenothiazines chemically; block reuptake of both norepinephrine and serotonin
MAO inhibitors	Drugs that inhibit monoamine oxidase type A, which metabolizes norepinephrine and serotonin, or monoamine oxidase type B, which metabolizes dopamine
Selective serotonin reuptake inhibitors	A group of drugs that selectively inhibit the serotonin transporters of the nerve ending membrane
Heterocyclics (second- and third-generation antidepressants)	Drugs of varied chemical structures; several have actions different from those of tricyclic antidepressants or selective serotonin reuptake inhibitors

CONCEPTS

Depression is a common condition with both psychologic and physical manifestations. The three major types of depression are (1) **reactive depression,** a response to external events; (2) **bipolar affective (manic-depressive) disorder,** described in Chapter 29; and (3) **major depressive disorder,** or **endogenous depression,** a depression of mood without any obvious medical or situational causes. The drugs used in major depressive disorder are the subject of this chapter.

The **amine hypothesis of mood** postulates that brain amines, particularly norepinephrine (NE) and serotonin (5-HT), are neurotransmitters in pathways that function in the expression of mood. According to the amine hypothesis, a functional decrease in the activity of such amines would result in depression; a functional increase of activity would result in mood elevation. Difficulties with this hypothesis include the facts that (1) antidepressant drugs cause changes in amine activity within hours, but weeks may be required for them to achieve clinical effects; (2) most antidepressants ultimately cause a *down*-regulation of amine receptors; and (3) at least one antidepressant, bupropion, has minimal effects on brain NE or 5-HT.

A. Classification and Pharmacokinetics: The major classes of antidepressant drugs are shown in Figure 30–1: **tricyclic antidepressants, heterocyclic antidepressants, selective serotonin reuptake inhibitors,** and **monoamine oxidase inhibitors.**

1. **Tricyclics (TCAs):** Tricyclic antidepressant drugs (eg, **imipramine, amitriptyline**) are structurally related to the phenothiazine antipsychotics and share certain of their pharmacologic effects. The tricyclics are well-absorbed orally but may undergo first-pass metabolism. They have high volumes of distribution and are not readily dialyzable. Exten-

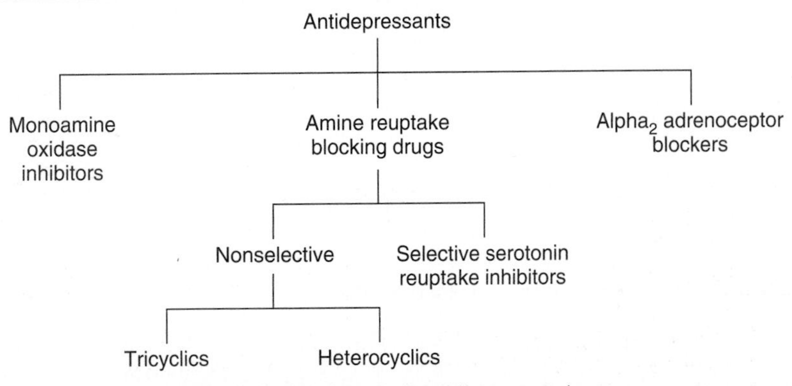

Figure 30–1. Major classes of antidepressant drugs.

sive hepatic metabolism is required prior to their elimination; plasma half-lives of 8–36 hours usually permit once-daily dosing. Some tricyclics form active metabolites.

2. **Heterocyclics:** These drugs have varied structures and include second-generation antidepressants (eg, **amoxapine, bupropion, maprotiline, trazodone**) and newer, third-generation drugs **(mirtazapine, nefazodone, venlafaxine).** The pharmacokinetics of most of these agents are similar to those of the tricyclic drugs. Nefazodone and trazodone are exceptions; their half-lives are quite short and usually require administration two or three times daily.
3. **Selective serotonin reuptake inhibitors (SSRIs): Fluoxetine** is the prototype of a group of drugs that selectively inhibit the reuptake of serotonin. All of them require hepatic metabolism and have half-lives of 18–24 hours. However, fluoxetine forms an active metabolite with a half-life of several days. Other members of this group (eg, **sertraline, citalopram, paroxetine**), do not form long-acting metabolites.
4. **MAO inhibitors (MAOIs):** These drugs (eg, **phenelzine, tranylcypromine, isocarboxazid**) are structurally related to amphetamines and are orally active. They inhibit both MAO-A (which metabolizes norepinephrine, serotonin, and tyramine) and MAO-B (which metabolizes dopamine). Tranylcypromine is the fastest in onset of effect but has a shorter duration of action (about a week) than do other MAO inhibitors (with durations of 2–3 weeks). In spite of these prolonged actions, the MAO inhibitors are given daily. These drugs are inhibitors of hepatic drug-metabolizing enzymes and cause many drug interactions.

B. Mechanisms of Antidepressant Action: Potential sites of action of antidepressants at central nervous system synapses are shown in Figure 30–2. By means of several mechanisms, almost all antidepressants result in a potentiation of the neurotransmitter actions of norepinephrine, serotonin, or both. The only exception is bupropion, which has an unknown mechanism of action. Long-term use of tricyclics and MAOIs, but not SSRIs, leads to down-regulation of beta receptors.

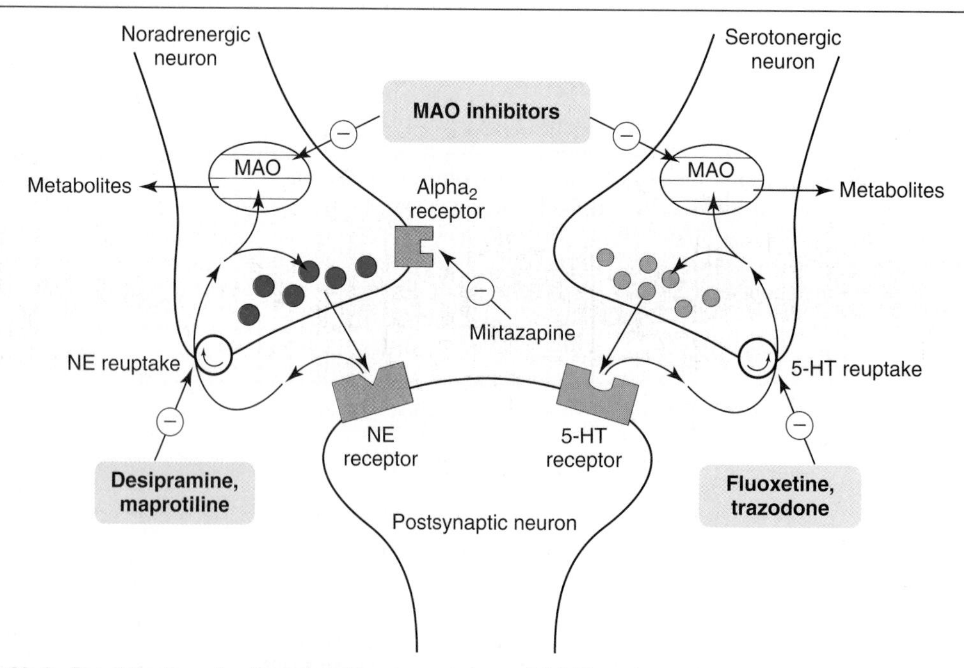

Figure 30–2. Possible sites of action of antidepressant drugs. Inhibition of neuronal reuptake of norepinephrine and serotonin increases the synaptic activities of these neurotransmitters. Inhibition of MAO increases the presynaptic stores of both norepinephrine and serotonin, which leads to increased neurotransmitter effects. Blockade of the presynaptic alpha$_2$ autoreceptor prevents feedback inhibition of the release of norepinephrine. ***Note:*** These are acute actions of antidepressants.

1. **Tricyclic antidepressants:** The acute effect of tricyclic drugs is to inhibit the reuptake mechanisms (transporters) responsible for the termination of the synaptic actions of both NE and 5-HT in the brain. This results in potentiation of their neurotransmitter actions at postsynaptic receptors.
2. **Heterocyclic antidepressants:** The acute actions of heterocyclics are varied. Some second-generation drugs inhibit the reuptake of NE (eg, maprotiline); others have more action on serotonin reuptake (eg, trazodone; see Table 30–2). The third-generation drug venlafaxine, though not a tricyclic, is a potent inhibitor of both NE and 5-HT transporters. Mirtazapine increases amine release from nerve endings by antagonism of presynaptic $alpha_2$ adrenoceptors involved in feedback inhibition.
3. **Selective serotonin reuptake inhibitors:** The acute effect of the selective serotonin reuptake inhibitors is a highly selective action on the 5-HT transporter.
4. **Monoamine oxidase inhibitors:** The MAO inhibitors increase brain amine levels by interfering with their metabolism in the nerve endings, resulting in an increase in the vesicular stores of norepinephrine and serotonin. When neuronal activity discharges the vesicles, increased amounts of the amines are released, enhancing the actions of these neurotransmitters.

C. Pharmacologic Effects:

1. **Amine uptake blockade:** The drugs that block norepinephrine transporters in the CNS (eg, tricyclics) also inhibit the reuptake of norepinephrine at nerve endings in the autonomic nervous system. Likewise, MAO inhibitors increase NE in sympathetic nerve terminals. In both cases, this can lead to peripheral autonomic sympathomimetic effects. However, long-term use of MAOIs can decrease blood pressure.
2. **Sedation:** Sedation is a common CNS effect of tricyclic drugs (although less so with protriptyline and desipramine) and of most heterocyclic agents (Table 30–2). MAO inhibitors, selective serotonin reuptake inhibitors, and bupropion are more likely to cause CNS-stimulating effects.
3. **Muscarinic receptor blockade:** Antagonism of muscarinic receptors occurs with all tricyclics and is particularly marked with amitriptyline and doxepin (Table 30–2). The newer

Table 30–2. Pharmacodynamics of common tricyclic antidepressants, heterocyclic agents, and selective serotonin reuptake inhibitors.[1,2]

Drug	Sedation	Muscarinic Receptor Block	NE Reuptake Block	5-HT Reuptake Block
Tricyclics				
Amitriptyline, doxepin	+++	+++	++	+++
Desipramine, protriptyline	+	+	+++	–
Imipramine, nortriptyline	++	++	++	+++
Heterocyclics (second generation)				
Amoxapine	++	++	++	+
Bupropion	–	–	–	–
Trazodone	+++	–	–	++
Maprotiline	++	++	+++	–
Heterocyclics (third generation)				
Mirtazapine	+++	–	–	–
Nefazodone	++	+++	–	+
Venlafaxine	–	–	+++	++
SSRIs				
Fluoxetine, citalopram, paroxetine, sertraline	–	+	–	+++

[1]Similar drugs have been grouped together for study purposes even though they may not be identical in their actions.
[2]**Key:** – = none; + = slight; ++ = moderate; +++ = marked.

agents appear to be less potent antimuscarinics; atropine-like effects are minimal with selective serotonin reuptake inhibitors, bupropion, and trazodone.

4. **Cardiovascular effects:** Cardiovascular effects occur most commonly with tricyclics and include hypotension—from alpha adrenoceptor blockade and depression of cardiac conduction. The latter effect may lead to arrhythmias.
5. **Seizures:** Because the convulsive threshold is lowered by tricyclic drugs and by MAO inhibitors, seizures may occur with overdoses of these agents. Overdoses of maprotiline and the SSRIs have also caused seizures.

D. Clinical Use:

1. **Major depressive disorders:** Endogenous depression is the major clinical indication for the antidepressant drugs. Patients typically vary in their responsiveness to individual agents. Because of more tolerable side effects and safety in overdose (see below), the newer drugs (SSRIs, certain heterocyclics) are now the most widely prescribed agents. They are sometimes effective in patients refractory to tricyclics or MAO inhibitors. As alternative agents, tricyclic drugs continue to be most useful in patients with psychomotor retardation, sleep disturbances, poor appetite, and weight loss. MAO inhibitors may be most useful in patients with significant anxiety, phobic features, and hypochondriasis. Selective serotonin reuptake inhibitors may decrease appetite; overweight patients often lose weight on these drugs, at least during the first 6–12 months of treatment.
2. **Other clinical uses:** Tricyclic drugs are also used in the treatment of bipolar affective disorders, acute panic attacks, phobic disorders (compare with alprazolam; Chapter 22), enuresis, and chronic pain states. Clomipramine and the selective serotonin reuptake inhibitors, including fluvoxamine, are effective in obsessive-compulsive disorders. SSRIs are also effective in patients who suffer from panic attacks, social phobias, bulimia, and premenstrual syndrome (PMS) and may also be useful in the treatment of alcohol dependence. Bupropion is used for management of patients attempting to withdraw from nicotine dependence.

E. Toxicity:

1. **Tricyclics:** The adverse effects of tricyclic antidepressants are largely predictable from their pharmacodynamic actions. These include (1) excessive sedation, lassitude, fatigue, and, occasionally, confusion; (2) sympathomimetic effects, including tachycardia, agitation, sweating, and insomnia; (3) atropine-like effects; (4) orthostatic hypotension, ECG abnormalities, and cardiomyopathies; (5) tremor and paresthesias; and (6) weight gain. Overdosage with tricyclics is extremely hazardous, and the ingestion of as little as a 2-week supply has been lethal. Manifestations include (1) agitation, delirium, neuromuscular irritability, convulsions, and coma; (2) respiratory depression and circulatory collapse; (3) hyperpyrexia; and (4) cardiac conduction defects and severe arrhythmias. The "three Cs" of coma, convulsions, and cardiotoxicity are characteristic.

   Tricyclic drug interactions (Table 30–3) include additive depression of the CNS with other central depressants, including ethanol, barbiturates, benzodiazepines, and opioids. Tricyclics may also cause reversal of the antihypertensive action of guanethidine by blocking its transport into sympathetic nerve endings. Less commonly, tricyclics may interfere with the antihypertensive actions of methylnorepinephrine (the active metabolite of methyldopa) and clonidine.
2. **Heterocyclic drug toxicity:** Mirtazapine and trazodone cause sedative effects. Amoxapine, maprotiline, mirtazapine, and trazodone cause some autonomic effects. Amoxapine is also a dopamine receptor blocker and may cause akathisia, parkinsonism, and the amenorrhea-galactorrhea syndrome. Adverse effects of bupropion include dizziness, dry mouth, aggravation of psychosis, and, at high doses, seizures. Seizures and cardiotoxicity are prominent features of overdosage with amoxapine and maprotiline. Venlafaxine has stimulant effects similar to those of the SSRIs. Both nefazodone and venlafaxine are inhibitors of cytochrome P450 isozymes. Through this action nefazodone inhibits the metabolism of alprazolam and triazolam, and venlafaxine inhibits the metabolism of haloperidol (see Table 30–3).
3. **SSRI toxicity:** Fluoxetine and the other SSRIs may cause nausea, headache, anxiety, agitation, insomnia, and sexual dysfunction. Jitteriness can be alleviated by starting with low doses or by adjunctive use of benzodiazepines. Extrapyramidal effects early in treatment

Table 30–3. Drug interactions observed with antidepressant medications.

Antidepressant	Taken With	Consequence
Fluoxetine	Lithium, tricyclics, warfarin	Increased blood levels of the second drug; doses may need to be decreased
Fluvoxamine	Alprazolam, theophylline, tricyclics, warfarin	Increased blood levels of the second drug; doses may need to be decreased
MAO inhibitors	Sympathomimetics, tyramine,	Hypertensive crisis
	SSRIs	Serotonin syndrome
Nefazodone	Alprazolam, triazolam	Increased blood levels of the second drug; doses may need to be decreased
Paroxetine	Procyclidine, theophylline, tricyclics, warfarin	Increased blood levels of the second drug; doses may need to be decreased
Sertraline	Tricyclics, warfarin	Increased effects; doses may need to be decreased
Tricyclics	CNS depressants (ethanol, sedative-hypnotics, etc)	Additive CNS depression[1]
	Clonidine, guanethidine, methyldopa	Decreased antihypertensive effects
	SSRIs	Serotonin syndrome

[1]Includes tricyclics and heterocyclics with sedative actions (eg, mirtazapine, nefazodone, and trazodone).

may include akathisia, dyskinesias, and dystonic reactions. Seizures are a consequence of gross overdosage. A withdrawal syndrome has been described for SSRIs that includes nausea, dizziness, anxiety, tremor, and palpitations.

4. **SSRI drug interactions:** The SSRIs are inhibitors of hepatic cytochrome P450 isozymes, an action that has led to increased activity of other drugs including tricyclic antidepressants and warfarin. Fluvoxamine inhibits the metabolism of cisapride, astemizole, and terfenadine, and the resultant cardiotoxicity has led to the withdrawal of the latter two drugs (see Table 30–3). Citalopram causes fewer drug interactions than other SSRIs.

   When SSRIs are used in combination with other drugs that enhance serotonergic functions, a dangerous interaction may occur. A **serotonin syndrome** was first described for an interaction between fluoxetine and an MAO inhibitor (see below). This life-threatening syndrome includes severe muscle rigidity, myoclonus, hyperthermia, cardiovascular instability, and marked CNS stimulatory effects, including seizures. Drugs implicated include MAO inhibitors, tricyclic antidepressants, meperidine, and possibly illicit recreational drugs such as MDMA ("ecstasy"). Antiseizure drugs, muscle relaxants, and blockers of 5-HT receptors (eg, cyproheptadine) have been used in management of the syndrome.

5. **MAO inhibitor toxicity:** Adverse effects of the MAO inhibitors include hypertensive reactions in response to indirectly acting sympathomimetics, hyperthermia, and CNS stimulation leading to agitation and convulsions. Hypertensive crisis may occur in patients taking MAO inhibitors who consume food that contains high concentrations of the indirect sympathomimetic tyramine (see Table 30–3). In the absence of indirect sympathomimetics, MAO inhibitors typically *lower* blood pressure; overdosage with these drugs may result in shock, hyperthermia, and seizures. MAO inhibitors should not be administered together with fluoxetine or other selective serotonin reuptake inhibitors because their combined use has caused a life-threatening **serotonin syndrome.**

DRUG LIST

The following drugs are important members of the group discussed in this chapter. Prototypes should be learned in detail; features of the major variants should be known well enough to distinguish the variants from prototypes and from each other; the other significant agents should be recognized as belonging to a specific subclass.

Subclass	Prototype	Major Variants	Other Significant Agents
Tricyclic drugs	Amitriptyline, imipramine	Desipramine, nortriptyline	Clomipramine, doxepin, protriptyline
Heterocyclics (second generation)	Amoxapine, bupropion, maprotiline, trazodone		
Heterocyclics (third generation)	Mirtazapine, nefazodone, venlafaxine		
Selective serotonin reuptake inhibitors	Fluoxetine	Fluvoxamine	Citalopram, paroxetine, sertraline
MAO inhibitors	Phenelzine	Tranylcypromine	Isocarboxazid

QUESTIONS

DIRECTIONS: Each of the numbered items or incomplete statements in this section is followed by answers or by completions of the statement. Select the ONE lettered answer or completion that is BEST in each case.

1. A 28-year-old woman presents with symptoms of major depression that are unrelated to a general medical condition, bereavement, or substance abuse. She is not currently taking any prescription or over-the-counter medications. Drug treatment is to be initiated with a selective serotonin reuptake inhibitor. In your information to the patient, you would NOT tell her that

(A) Divided doses may help to reduce nausea and gastrointestinal distress
(B) Muscle cramps and twitches sometimes occur
(C) She must inform you if she anticipates using other medications
(D) Taking the drug in the evening will ensure a good night's sleep
(E) The drug may require 2 weeks or more to become effective

2. Concerning the proposed mechanisms of action of antidepressant drugs, which one of the following statements is accurate?

(A) Bupropion is an effective inhibitor of NE and 5-HT transporters
(B) Chronic treatment with an antidepressant often leads to the up-regulation of adrenoceptors
(C) Elevation in amine metabolites in cerebrospinal fluid is characteristic of most depressed patients prior to drug therapy
(D) MAO inhibitors used as antidepressants selectively decrease the metabolism of norepinephrine
(E) The acute effect of most tricyclics is to block the neuronal reuptake of both norepinephrine and serotonin in the CNS

3. Which one of the following effects is unlikely to occur during treatment with amitriptyline?

(A) Alpha adrenoceptor blockade
(B) Elevation of the seizure threshold
(C) Mydriasis
(D) Sedation
(E) Urinary retention

4. A 54-year-old male patient was using fluoxetine for depression but decided to stop taking the drug. When questioned, he said that it affected his sexual performance and that "he wasn't getting any younger." You notice that he is a user of tobacco products. If you decide to reinstitute drug therapy in this patient, the best choice would be

(A) Amoxapine
(B) Bupropion
(C) Imipramine
(D) Sertraline
(E) Venlafaxine

5. Regarding the clinical use of antidepressant drugs, which one of the following statements is false?

(A) Patients should be advised not to abruptly discontinue antidepressant medications
(B) In selecting an appropriate drug for treatment of depression, the past history of patient response to specific drugs is a valuable guide

(C) In the treatment of major depressive disorders, sertraline is usually more effective than fluoxetine
(D) MAO inhibitors are sometimes effective in depressions with attendant anxiety, phobic features, and hypochondriasis
(E) Weight loss often occurs in patients taking SSRIs

Items 6–7: A patient under treatment for a major depressive disorder is brought to the emergency room after ingesting 30 times the normal daily therapeutic dose of amitriptyline.

6. Of the possible signs and symptoms in this patient, which one of the following is not likely to be observed?
(A) Acidosis
(B) Coma and shock
(C) Hot dry skin
(D) Hypotension
(E) Pinpoint pupils

7. In severe tricyclic antidepressant overdose, it would NOT be of value to
(A) Administer lidocaine (to control cardiac arrhythmias)
(B) Institute hemodialysis (to hasten drug elimination)
(C) Administer bicarbonate and potassium chloride (to correct acidosis and hypokalemia)
(D) Provide intravenous diazepam (to control seizures)
(E) Maintain the rhythm of the heart by electrical pacing

8. Drug interactions involving antidepressants do NOT include
(A) Additive impairment of driving ability in patients taking trazodone when ethanol is ingested
(B) Behavioral excitation and hypertension in patients taking MAO inhibitors with meperidine
(C) Elevated plasma levels of lithium if fluoxetine is administered
(D) Increased antihypertensive effects of methyldopa when tricyclics are administered
(E) Prolongation of tricyclic drug half-life in patients with cimetidine

9. A recently bereaved 74-year-old female patient was treated with a benzodiazepine for several weeks after the death of her husband, but she did not like the daytime sedation it caused. She has no major medical problems but appears rather infirm for her age and has poor eyesight. Because her depressive symptoms are not abating, you decide on a trial of an antidepressant medication. Which one of the following drugs would be the most appropriate choice for this patient?
(A) Amitriptyline
(B) Mirtazapine
(C) Paroxetine
(D) Phenelzine
(E) Trazodone

10. Regarding maprotiline, which one of the following statements is accurate?
(A) Blocks serotonin reuptake selectively
(B) Causes hypertension
(C) Raises the seizure threshold
(D) Sedation occurs commonly
(E) Has a tricyclic structure

11. Which one of the following drugs is most likely to be of value in obsessive-compulsive disorders (OCD)?
(A) Amitriptyline
(B) Bupropion
(C) Clomipramine
(D) Desipramine
(E) Mirtazapine

12. Compared with other antidepressant drugs, mirtazapine has the distinctive ability to act as an antagonist of
(A) $Alpha_2$ adrenoceptors
(B) Beta adrenoceptors
(C) D_2 receptors
(D) NE transporters
(E) 5-HT transporters

13. Established clinical uses of this drug include enuresis and chronic pain.
    (A) Bupropion
    (B) Fluvoxamine
    (C) Imipramine
    (D) Phenelzine
    (E) Selegiline
14. Which one of the following drugs is most likely to increase plasma levels of alprazolam, theophylline, and warfarin
    (A) Desipramine
    (B) Fluvoxamine
    (C) Imipramine
    (D) Nefazodone
    (E) Venlafaxine

DIRECTIONS (Items 15–18): This case history* is followed by discussion questions. Write out brief answers (two to five sentences) and then compare your answers with those given at the end of the Answers section.

A 47-year-old man visited an outpatient clinic with initial complaints of chronic tiredness, frequent bouts of stomach upset, and weight loss. Physical examination and laboratory studies were within normal limits. A psychiatric evaluation revealed that the patient had come to the clinic at the request of his wife, who thought that he was "depressed." He had been waking during the early morning hours and could not get back to sleep. The patient acknowledged that over the past year he had lost interest in his work and had started to worry about providing for his family. He admitted to having also lost interest in sex.

A diagnosis of major depression was made. Amitriptyline, 50 mg daily, was prescribed, to be taken at bedtime for 3 nights, and 100 mg daily thereafter, also taken at bedtime. Two weeks later, an interview indicated that the patient was sleeping better but that his appetite remained poor and his mood was unimproved. The dose of amitriptyline was increased to 200 mg/d.

Eight weeks after the initial visit, the patient had regained most of his lost weight and no longer had insomnia. However, he was not feeling much better. The side effects of the drug were bothersome, and he was becoming increasingly worried about his job and his family life. His feelings of inadequacy seemed to be increasing, and he had begun questioning what use he was to anybody. The psychiatrist initiated dose-tapering of amitriptyline and prescribed paroxetine (5 mg daily), with weekly increments of 5 mg up to a maximum dose of 20 mg/d.

Evaluation of the patient after 4 weeks of treatment with paroxetine revealed a major improvement in his mood. He had a renewed interest in his job and in the activities of his family. His sex life had improved overall, though he was occasionally anorgasmic. Dry mouth, constipation, and occasional "jitteriness" were his only complaints about the drug he was taking.

15. What drug groups are available for the treatment of major depression?
16. What reasons would support the initial choice of amitriptyline in this patient?
17. What reasons can you offer for the change in drug treatment to paroxetine?
18. What side effects and potential drug interactions are troublesome during treatment of depression with SSRIs?

ANSWERS

1. The SSRIs have CNS-stimulating effects. They may cause agitation, anxiety, "the jitters," and insomnia. The evening is not the best time to take such drugs. Anorexia and nausea, akathisia, dyskinesias, and dystonic reactions may occur. Because of the possibility of drug interactions, the physician needs to be informed of changes in drug regimens when maintaining a patient on antidepressants. The answer is **(D)**.
2. The mechanism of action of bupropion is unknown, but the drug does not inhibit amine trans-

---

* Modified and reproduced, with permission, from Coleman JH, Johnston JA: Affective disorders. Page 1021 in: *Applied Therapeutics*, 3rd ed. Katcher BS, Young LY, Koda-Kimble MA (editors). Applied Therapeutics, 1983.

porters. Levels of norepinephrine and serotonin metabolites in the cerebrospinal fluid of depressed patients prior to drug treatment are not higher than normal. Some studies have reported *decreased* levels of these metabolites. Down-regulation of adrenoceptors appears to be a common feature of all modes of chronic drug treatment of depression, including the use of drugs that have no direct actions on catecholamine receptors. MAO inhibitors used in depression are nonselective. The answer is **(E).**

3. Tricyclics modify peripheral sympathetic effects in two ways: through blockade of norepinephrine reuptake at neuroeffector junctions and through alpha adrenoceptor blockade. Sedation and atropine-like side effects are common with tricyclics, especially amitriptyline. In contrast to sedative-hypnotics, tricyclics lower the threshold to seizures. The answer is **(B).**
4. Selective serotonin reuptake inhibitors cause sexual dysfunction in some patients, with changes in libido, erectile dysfunction, and anorgasmia. Tricyclic antidepressants may also decrease libido or prevent ejaculation. Of the heterocyclic antidepressants bupropion is the least likely to affect sexual performance. The drug is also used in withdrawal from nicotine dependence. The answer is **(B).**
5. There is no evidence that any SSRI is more effective than another in its antidepressant efficacy. While an individual patient may respond more favorably to a specific drug, several controlled studies have shown equivalent effectiveness of these agents. However, SSRIs may be more effective than tricyclic antidepressants in some patients. The answer is **(C).**
6. Anticholinergic effects common in tricyclic drug overdosage include hot dry skin, decreased bowel sounds, tachycardia, and *dilated* pupils. Hypotension occurs frequently owing to marked blockade at alpha adrenoceptors. The answer is **(E).**
7. Tricyclic antidepressant overdose is a medical emergency. The "three Cs"—coma, convulsions, and cardiac problems—are the most common causes of death. Widening of the QRS complex on the ECG is a major diagnostic feature of cardiac toxicity. Arrhythmias resulting from cardiac toxicity are difficult to manage; they require the use of drugs with the least effect on cardiac conductivity (eg, lidocaine). There is no evidence that hemodialysis (or hemoperfusion) increases the rate of elimination of tricyclic antidepressants, presumably because of their large volume of distribution and their binding to tissue components. The answer is **(B).**
8. Tricyclic drugs block the uptake of guanethidine into sympathetic nerve endings, thus *reversing* its beneficial effects on blood pressure. While the precise mechanism is not defined, the tricyclics may also block the antihypertensive effects of clonidine and methyldopa. All of the other drug interactions have been reported. The answer is **(D).**
9. The elderly patient may be especially sensitive to antidepressant drugs that cause sedation, atropine-like side effects, or postural hypotension. Paroxetine (or another SSRI) is the best choice for this patient because it is the least likely of the drugs listed to exert such actions. The answer is **(C).**
10. Maprotiline is chemically similar to the tricyclic drug desipramine except that it has a tetracyclic structure. Maprotiline is almost equivalent to desipramine in terms of its sedative and muscarinic receptor blocking actions but has caused seizures at the top of its recommended dose range. Both drugs act selectively to block the reuptake of norepinephrine. The answer is **(D).**
11. Clomipramine, a tricyclic, is a more selective inhibitor of serotonin reuptake than other drugs in its class. This activity appears to be important in the treatment of obsessive-compulsive disorder (OCD). Patients with OCD are also responsive to sertraline and other selective serotonin reuptake inhibitors, and the SSRIs have now become the drugs of choice for this disorder since they are safer in overdose than tricyclics. The answer is **(C).**
12. Mirtazapine is the first of a new subclass of antidepressants—the alpha$_2$ antagonists. The drug also blocks histamine H_1 receptors (it is quite sedating), 5-HT_2 receptors, and 5-HT_3 receptors. It has minimal inhibitory activity on amine transporters. The answer is **(A).**
13. Enuresis is an established indication for tricyclics. Chronic pain states, which may be unresponsive to conventional analgesics, sometimes respond to tricyclic antidepressants. The answer is **(C).**
14. Fluvoxamine inhibits liver drug-metabolizing enzymes. Dosages of alprazolam, theophylline, and warfarin must be reduced if any of these drugs are given concomitantly with fluvoxamine. Nefazodone may also decrease the metabolism of benzodiazepines, and venlafaxine may inhibit haloperidol metabolism. The answer is **(B).**

15. Several drug groups are available for the treatment of major (endogenous) depression. These include the selective serotonin reuptake inhibitors (SSRIs), the tricyclic agents (TCAs), a group of heterocyclic antidepressants, and the monoamine oxidase inhibitors (MAOIs).
16. While the SSRIs are the most frequently used drugs for treatment of major depressions, the tricyclics remain valuable alternatives. In some patients a tricyclic may be the first choice, especially if the past history indicates a positive therapeutic response to such drugs. The sedative actions of tricyclics may be of value in depressed patients with insomnia or weight loss, since SSRIs tend to exacerbate such symptoms. *Generic* formulations of the tricyclics are much less costly than any of the other antidepressant drugs.
17. Limited effectiveness and toxicity are the major reasons for switching a patient from one antidepressant drug to another. SSRIs are sometimes superior to tricyclics in their clinical efficacy, and in this case amitriptyline had not proved effective after a reasonable trial (8 weeks). At that time, the depressive symptoms in this patient included feelings of worthlessness and possibly suicidal ideation. Tricyclic overdose is especially dangerous in depressed patients, who often use medications close at hand in attempting suicide. Ingestion of just a 2-week supply of amitriptyline can cause severe hypotension, cardiac arrhythmias, seizures, coma, and death ("one-prescription lethal").
18. The most common adverse effects associated with the SSRIs are nausea, headache, jitteriness, and insomnia. The SSRIs are less likely than tricyclics to cause weight gain, hypotension, and anticholinergic side effects. Sexual dysfunction may occur, including anorgasmia and decreased libido. SSRIs may cause seizures in overdose. Concomitant use of MAO inhibitors or tricyclics with SSRIs may cause a serotonin syndrome. The SSRIs are inhibitors of hepatic cytochrome P450 and may enhance the actions of other drugs, including tricyclic antidepressants and warfarin.

31 Opioid Analgesics & Antagonists

OBJECTIVES

You should be able to:

- Identify the endogenous opioid peptides.
- List the receptors activated by opioid analgesics and the endogenous opioid peptides.
- Given a list of major opioid agonists, rank them in analgesic efficacy.
- Identify opioid receptor antagonists and mixed agonist-antagonists.
- Describe the main pharmacodynamic and pharmacokinetic properties of agonist opioid analgesics and list their clinical uses.
- List the main adverse effects of acute and chronic use of opioid analgesics.
- Describe the clinical uses of the opioid receptor antagonists.
- List two opioids used for antitussive effects and one used for antidiarrheal effects.

Learn the definitions that follow.

Table 31–1. Definitions.

Term	Definition
Opiate	A drug derived from alkaloids of the opium poppy
Opioid	The class of drugs that includes opiates, opiopeptins, and all synthetic and semisynthetic drugs that mimic the actions of the opiates
Opioid peptides	Endogenous peptides that act on opioid receptors
Opioid agonist	A drug that activates some or all opioid receptor subtypes and does not block any
Partial agonist	A drug that can activate an opioid receptor to effect a submaximal response
Opioid antagonist	A drug that blocks some or all opioid receptor subtypes
Mixed agonist-antagonist	A drug that activates some opioid receptor subtypes and blocks other subtypes

CONCEPTS

A. Classification: Morphine and other natural derivatives of the opium poppy are **opiates.** Opiates, synthetic drugs, and the endogenous compounds that produce morphine-like effects comprise the **opioids.** The endogenous opiopeptins include pentapeptides (met-enkephalin, leu-enkephalin), dynorphins (17 amino acids), and beta-endorphins (31 amino acids). Opiopeptins are released from precursor proteins present in many regions of the CNS, including sites implicated in pain modulation. Precursor peptides are also found in the adrenal medulla and neural plexuses of the gut.

The opioids are derived from several chemical subgroups, including phenanthrenes, phenylheptylamines, phenylpiperidines, morphinans, and benzomorphans. A useful subdivision of the drugs is presented in Figure 31–1.

1. **Spectrum of clinical uses:** Opioid drugs can be subdivided on the basis of their major therapeutic uses (eg, as analgesics, antitussives, and antidiarrheal drugs).
2. **Strength of analgesia:** On the basis of their relative abilities to relieve pain, the analgesic opioids may be classified as strong, moderate, and weak agonists. Partial agonists are opioids that exert less analgesia than morphine, the prototype of a strong analgesic.
3. **Ratio of agonist to antagonist effects:** Opioid drugs may be classified as agonists (receptor activators), antagonists (receptor blockers), or mixed agonist-antagonists.

B. Pharmacokinetics: Most drugs in this class are well-absorbed, but morphine, hydromorphone, and oxymorphone undergo extensive first-pass metabolism when taken orally. Opioid drugs cross the placental barrier and exert effects on the fetus that can result in both respiratory depression and (with continuous exposure) physical dependence in neonates. Most opioids undergo metabolism by hepatic enzymes, usually to glucuronide conjugates, prior to their elimination by the kidney. Depending on the specific drug, the duration of their analgesic effects ranges from 1–2 hours (eg, fentanyl) to 6–8 hours (eg, buprenorphine); this may increase in patients with liver disease. One exception is remifentanil, a congener of fentanyl, which is metabolized by plasma and tissue esterases and has a very short half-life.

C. Mechanism of Action:

1. **Receptors:** Some of the effects of opioid analgesics have been interpreted in terms of

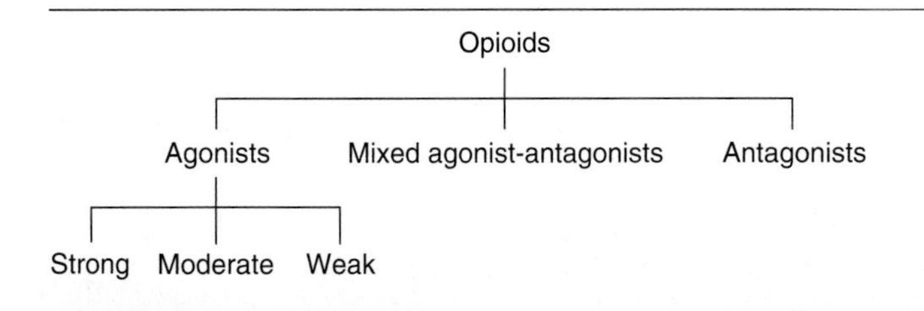

Figure 31–1. Subdivisions of drugs that act on opioid receptors.

their interactions with specific opioid receptors in the CNS and peripheral tissues. Certain opioid receptors are located on primary afferents and spinal cord pain *transmission* neurons (ascending pathways) and on neurons in the midbrain and medulla (descending pathways) that function in pain *modulation* (Figure 31–2). Other opioid receptors that may be involved in altering *reactivity* to pain are located on neurons in the basal ganglia, the hypothalamus, the limbic structures, and the cerebral cortex. Three opioid receptor types have been cloned and characterized pharmacologically.

a. **Mu (μ) and delta (δ) receptors:** Activation of mu and delta receptors contributes to analgesia at both spinal and supraspinal levels, to respiratory depression, and to physical dependence that can result from chronic use of some opioid analgesics.
b. **Kappa (κ) receptors:** Kappa receptor activation contributes to spinal analgesia and plays a role in the sedative effects of opioid drugs.

2. **Opioid peptides:** Opioid receptors are thought to be activated by endogenous peptides under physiologic conditions. These peptides (eg, enkephalins, dynorphin, beta-endorphin) bind to opioid receptors and can be displaced from binding by opioid antagonists. Although it remains unclear if these peptides function as classic neurotransmitters, they appear to modulate transmission at many sites in the brain and spinal cord, and in primary afferents.
3. **Ionic mechanisms:** Opioid analgesics *inhibit* synaptic activity, partly through direct activation of opioid receptors and partly through release of the endogenous opiopeptins, which are themselves inhibitory to neurons. All three major opioid receptors are coupled to their effectors by G proteins and activate phospholipase C or inhibit adenylyl cyclase. At the postsynaptic level, activation of these receptors opens K^+ ion channels to cause membrane

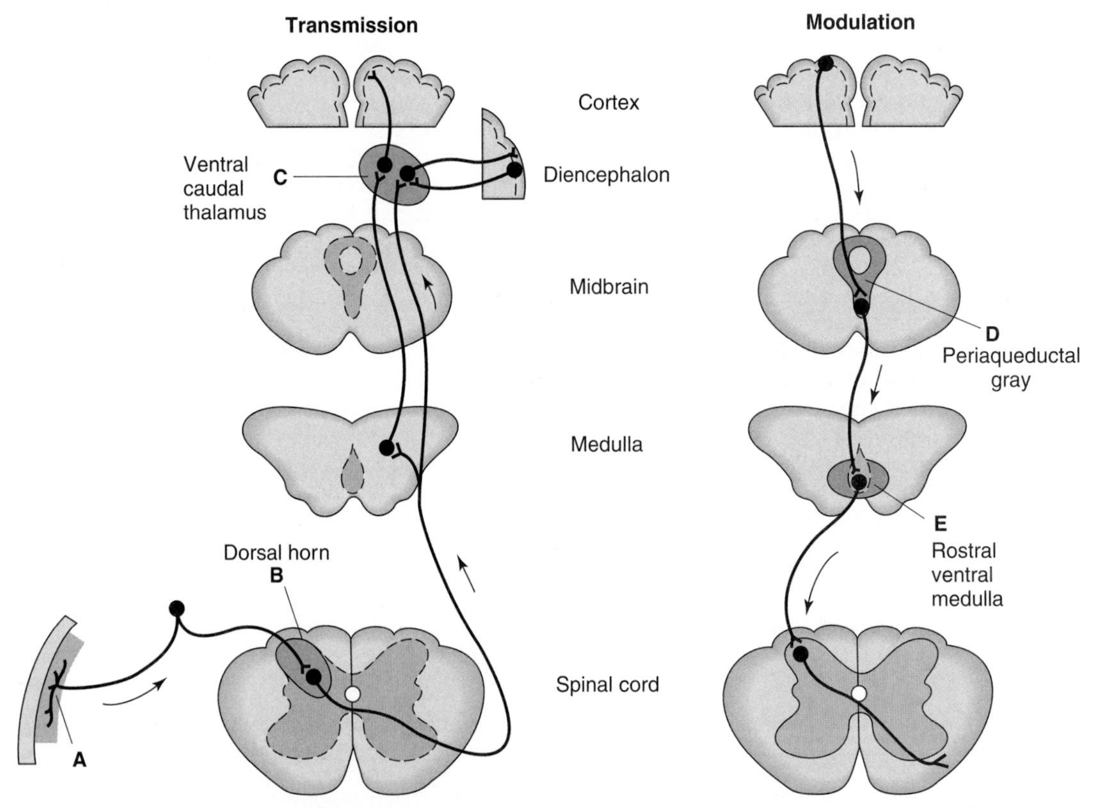

Figure 31–2. Putative sites of action (darker color) of opioid analgesics. On the left, sites of action on the pain transmission pathway from the periphery to the higher centers are shown. At ***A,*** possible direct action of opioids on painful peripheral tissues. ***B:*** Inhibition occurs in the spinal cord. ***C:*** Possible site of action in the thalamus. On the right, actions on pain-modulating neurons in the midbrain (site ***D***) and the medulla (site ***E***); these actions secondarily affect pain transmission pathways. (Reproduced, with permission, from Katzung BG [editor]: *Basic & Clinical Pharmacology,* 8th ed. McGraw-Hill, 2001.)

hyperpolarization (inhibitory postsynaptic potentials; IPSPs). At the presynaptic level, opioid receptor activation closes voltage-gated Ca^{2+} ion channels to inhibit neurotransmitter release (Figure 31–3). Presynaptic actions result in the inhibition of release of multiple neurotransmitters, including ACh, NE, 5-HT, glutamate, and substance P.

D. Acute Effects:

1. **Analgesia:** The opioids are the most powerful drugs available for the relief of pain. Strong agonists (ie, those with the highest analgesic efficacy) include morphine, methadone, meperidine, and fentanyl. Codeine, hydrocodone, and oxycodone are mild to moderate agonists. Propoxyphene is a very weak agonist drug.
2. **Sedation and euphoria:** These central effects may occur at doses below those required for maximum analgesia. Some patients experience dysphoria. At higher doses, the drugs may cause mental clouding and result in a stuporous state called narcosis.
3. **Respiratory depression:** Opioid actions in the medulla lead to inhibition of the respiratory center, with decreased response to carbon dioxide challenge. Increased Pco_2 may cause cerebrovascular dilation, resulting in increased blood flow and increased intracranial pressure.
4. **Antitussive actions:** Suppression of the cough reflex by unknown mechanisms is the basis for the clinical use of opioids as antitussives.
5. **Nausea and vomiting:** Nausea and vomiting are caused by activation of the chemoreceptor trigger zone and are increased by ambulation.
6. **Gastrointestinal effects:** Constipation occurs through decreased intestinal peristalsis, which is probably mediated by effects on opioid receptors in the enteric nervous system. This powerful action is the basis for the clinical use of these drugs as antidiarrheal agents.
7. **Smooth muscle:** Opioids cause contraction of biliary tract smooth muscle (which may cause biliary spasm), increased ureteral and bladder sphincter tone, and a reduction in uterine tone that may contribute to prolongation of labor.
8. **Miosis:** Pupillary constriction is a characteristic effect of all opioids except meperidine, which has a muscarinic blocking action.

Skill Keeper: Opiopeptins & Substance P (see Chapters 6 and 17)

These peptides are relevant to understanding the analgesic actions of opioid-analgesic drugs in terms of CNS function. What are the roles of these peptides in peripheral tissues? *The Skill Keeper Answer appears at the end of the chapter.*

E. Chronic Effects:

1. **Tolerance:** Marked tolerance develops to the above acute pharmacologic effects, with the exception of miosis and constipation. There is **cross-tolerance** between different opioid agonists.
2. **Dependence:** Psychologic and physical dependence is part of the basis for the abuse lia-

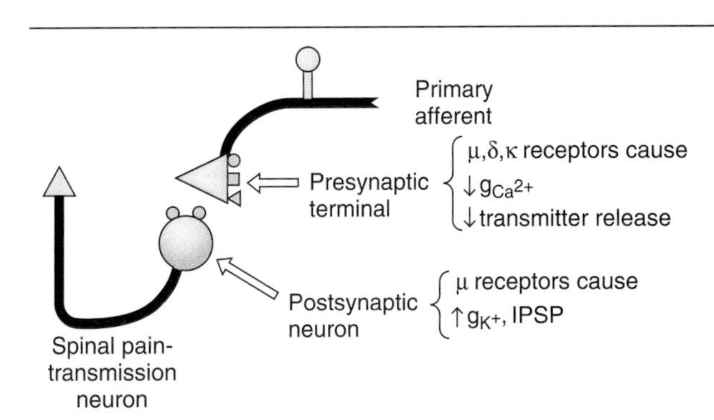

Figure 31–3. Spinal sites of opioid action. Mu, kappa, and delta agonists reduce transmitter release from presynaptic terminals of nociceptive primary afferents. Mu agonists also hyperpolarize second-order pain transmission neurons by increasing K^+ conductance, evoking an inhibitory postsynaptic potential. (Reproduced, with permission, from Katzung BG [editor]: *Basic & Clinical Pharmacology,* 8th ed. McGraw-Hill, 2001.)

bility of many drugs in this group, particularly the strong agonists. Physical dependence is revealed on abrupt discontinuance as an **abstinence syndrome,** which includes rhinorrhea, lacrimation, chills, gooseflesh, muscle aches, diarrhea, yawning, anxiety, and hostility. A more intense state of **precipitated withdrawal** results when an opioid antagonist is administered to a physically dependent individual.

F. Clinical Uses:

1. **Analgesia:** Treatment of relatively constant moderate to severe pain is the major indication. (See the Drug List for examples in each category.) In the acute setting, strong agonists are usually given parenterally. Prolonged analgesia, with some reduction in adverse effects, can be achieved with epidural administration of certain strong agonist drugs, eg, morphine. Fentanyl has been used by the transdermal route for analgesia. For more moderate pain and in the chronic setting, moderate agonists are given by the oral route.
2. **Cough suppression:** Useful antitussive drugs include codeine and dextromethorphan. They are given orally.
3. **Treatment of diarrhea:** Selective antidiarrheal opioids include diphenoxylate and loperamide. They are given orally.
4. **Management of acute pulmonary edema:** Morphine is useful in acute pulmonary edema because of its hemodynamic actions; its calming effects probably also contribute to relief of the pulmonary symptoms. It is given parenterally.
5. **Anesthesia:** Opioids are used as preoperative medications and as intraoperative adjunctive agents in balanced anesthesia protocols. High-dose intravenous opioids (eg, morphine, fentanyl) are often the major component of anesthesia for cardiac surgery.
6. **Opioid dependence:** Methadone, one of the longer-acting opioids, is used in the management of opioid withdrawal states and in maintenance programs for addicts. In withdrawal states, methadone permits a slow tapering of opioid effect that diminishes the intensity of abstinence symptoms. Buprenorphine (see below) has an even longer duration of action and is sometimes used in withdrawal states. In maintenance programs, the prolonged action of methadone blocks the euphoria-inducing effects of doses of shorter-acting opioids (eg, heroin, morphine).

G. Toxicity: Most of the adverse effects of the opioid analgesics (eg, constipation) are predictable extensions of their pharmacologic effects. In addition, overdose and drug interaction toxicities are very important.

1. **Overdose:** A triad of papillary constriction, comatose state, and respiratory depression is characteristic and may be fatal if not treated. Diagnosis of overdosage is confirmed if intravenous injection of naloxone, an antagonist drug, results in prompt signs of recovery. Treatment of overdose involves the use of antagonists such as naloxone and other therapeutic measures, especially ventilatory support.
2. **Drug interactions:** The most important drug interactions involving opioid analgesics are additive CNS depression with ethanol, sedative-hypnotics, anesthetics, antipsychotic drugs, tricyclic antidepressants, and antihistamines. Concomitant use of certain opioids (eg, meperidine) with MAO inhibitors increases the incidence of hyperpyrexic coma. Meperidine has also been implicated in the serotonin syndrome when used together with selective serotonin reuptake inhibitors.

H. Agonist-Antagonist and Partial Agonist Drugs:

1. **Analgesic activity:** The analgesic activity of some mixed agonist-antagonists (eg, butorphanol, nalbuphine) may be close to that of strong agonist drugs; others (eg, pentazocine) have only moderate efficacy. Buprenorphine, a partial agonist at mu receptors, is considered to be a strong analgesic.
2. **Receptors:** Butorphanol, nalbuphine, and pentazocine are kappa agonists, with weak mu receptor antagonist activity. This can lead to unpredictable results if these mixed agonist-antagonist drugs are used together with pure agonists. Buprenorphine has a long duration of effect since it binds strongly to mu receptors; this property renders its effects resistant to naloxone reversal.
3. **Effects:** The mixed agonist-antagonist drugs usually cause sedation at analgesic doses. Dizziness, sweating, and nausea may also occur, and anxiety, hallucinations, and nightmares are possible adverse effects. Respiratory depression may be less intense than with

pure agonists but is not as predictably reversed by naloxone. Tolerance develops with chronic use but is less than the tolerance that develops to the pure agonists; there is minimal cross-tolerance. Physical dependence occurs, but the abuse liability of mixed agonist-antagonist drugs is less than that of the full agonists (eg, fentanyl, morphine, meperidine).

I. Opioid Antagonists: Naloxone and naltrexone are pure opioid receptor antagonists that have few other effects at doses which produce marked antagonism of agonist effects. The major clinical use of the opioid antagonists is in the management of acute opioid overdose. Naloxone is given intravenously. Because it has a short duration of action (1–2 hours), multiple doses of naloxone may be required in opioid analgesic overdose. Naltrexone decreases the craving for ethanol and is approved for adjunctive use in alcohol dependency programs. It has a duration of action of 24–48 hours following oral use.

DRUG LIST

The following drugs are important members of the group discussed in this chapter. Prototypes should be learned in detail; features of the major variants should be known well enough to distinguish the variants from prototypes and from each other; the other significant agents should be recognized as belonging to a specific subclass.

Subclass	Prototypes	Major Variants	Other Significant Agents
Strong agonists	Morphine	Heroin, meperidine, methadone	Fentanyl, levorphanol
Moderate agonists	Codeine		Oxycodone, hydrocodone
Weak agonists	Propoxyphene		
Partial agonists	Buprenorphine		
Mixed agonist-antagonists	Pentazocine	Nalbuphine	Butorphanol
Antagonists	Naloxone	Naltrexone	
Antitussive	Dextromethorphan		Codeine
Antidiarrheal	Diphenoxylate		Loperamide

QUESTIONS

DIRECTIONS: Each of the numbered items or incomplete statements in this section is followed by answers or by completions of the statement. Select the ONE lettered answer or completion that is BEST in each case.

Items 1–2: Following surgery for prostatic carcinoma, a 63-year-old man is undergoing radiation treatment as an outpatient because the tumor has metastasized to bone. He has pain in his right hip that is exacerbated when he sits down and backache when he moves about. The pain has been managed with a fixed combination of oxycodone plus acetaminophen taken orally. Despite increasing doses of the analgesic combination, the pain is getting worse.

1. If you decide to continue oral medication for the increasing pain, the best choice of drug for this patient would be
(A) Butorphanol
(B) Codeine plus aspirin
(C) Levorphanol
(D) Pentazocine
(E) Propoxyphene

2. If the appropriate oral drug is prescribed, the patient will experience more pain relief (at least initially) and, possibly, some euphoria. However, he may have problems with nausea and sedation. Because of tolerance, it is possible that this patient will have to increase the dose of the analgesic as his condition progresses. Tolerance will not develop to a significant extent with respect to

(A) Constipation
(B) Euphoria
(C) Nausea and vomiting
(D) Sedation
(E) Urinary retention

3. Which one of the following actions of opioid analgesics is mediated via activation of kappa receptors?
(A) Cerebral vascular dilation
(B) Decreased uterine tone
(C) Euphoria
(D) Sedation
(E) Psychologic dependence

4. You are on your way to take an examination and you suddenly get an attack of diarrhea. If you stop at a nearby drugstore for an over-the-counter opioid with antidiarrheal action, you will be asking for
(A) Codeine
(B) Dextromethorphan
(C) Diphenoxylate
(D) Loperamide
(E) Nalbuphine

5. Fentanyl patches have been used to provide analgesia. The most dangerous adverse effect of this mode of administration is
(A) Cutaneous reactions
(B) Diarrhea
(C) Hypertension
(D) Relaxation of skeletal muscle
(E) Respiratory depression

6. A patient injured in an auto accident received 80 mg of meperidine. He subsequently developed a severe reaction characterized by tachycardia, hypertension, hyperpyrexia, and seizures. When questioned, the uninjured spouse revealed that the patient had been taking a drug for a psychiatric condition. Which of the following drugs is most likely to be responsible for this untoward interaction with meperidine?
(A) Alprazolam
(B) Amitriptyline
(C) Lithium
(D) Mirtazapine
(E) Phenelzine

7. A patient (weight 50 kg) with moderate pain was given a high dose (60 mg) of pentazocine intramuscularly at 10 AM. At 10:15 AM the pain intensified and continued to get worse. At 10:30 AM, 10 mg of morphine was given intramuscularly. Unfortunately, the addition of morphine provided very little additional analgesia for a further period of 90 minutes. The most plausible explanation for this type of drug interaction is that pentazocine is
(A) An agonist at kappa receptors
(B) An inhibitor of bioactivation of morphine
(C) An inducer of hepatic cytochrome P450
(D) An antagonist or partial agonist at mu and delta receptors
(E) Interfering with the systemic absorption of morphine

8. Opioid analgesics are either contraindicated or must be used with extreme caution in several clinical situations. For morphine, such situations do not include
(A) Adrenal insufficiency
(B) Biliary tract surgery
(C) Hypothyroidism
(D) Late stage of labor
(E) Pulmonary edema

Items 9–10: A heroin addict comes to the emergency room in an anxious and agitated state. He complains of chills, muscle aches, and diarrhea; he has also been vomiting. His symptoms include hyperventilation and hyperthermia. He claims to have had an intravenous "fix" approximately 12 hours ago. The attending physician notes that pupil size is greater than normal.

9. What is the most likely cause of these signs and symptoms?
(A) The patient has overdosed with an opioid
(B) These are early signs of the toxicity of MPTP, a contaminant in "street heroin"
(C) The signs and symptoms are those of the abstinence syndrome
(D) In addition to opioids, the patient has been taking barbiturates
(E) The patient has hepatitis B

10. Which one of the following will be most effective in alleviating the symptoms experienced by this patient?
(A) Acetaminophen
(B) Buprenorphine
(C) Codeine
(D) Diazepam
(E) Naltrexone

11. Which one of the following statements about nalbuphine is accurate?
(A) Activates mu receptors
(B) Does not cause respiratory depression
(C) Is nonsedating
(D) Pain-relieving action is not superior to that of codeine
(E) Response to naloxone in overdose may be unreliable

12. This drug, which does not activate opioid receptors, has been proposed as a maintenance drug in treatment programs for opioid addicts; a single oral dose will block the effects of injected heroin for up to 48 hours
(A) Amphetamine
(B) Buprenorphine
(C) Naloxone
(D) Naltrexone
(E) Propoxyphene

13. Which one of the following statements about dextromethorphan is accurate?
(A) Activates kappa receptors
(B) Analgesia equivalent to pentazocine
(C) Highly effective antiemetic
(D) Less constipation than codeine
(E) Use requires a prescription

14. This drug is a full agonist at opioid receptors. It has excellent oral bioavailability, analgesic activity equivalent to that of morphine, and a longer duration of action. Withdrawal signs on abrupt discontinuance are milder than those with morphine
(A) Fentanyl
(B) Hydromorphone
(C) Methadone
(D) Nalbuphine
(E) Oxycodone

15. Which one of the following statements about propoxyphene is accurate?
(A) Analgesia equivalent to oxycodone
(B) Antagonist at mu receptors
(C) Causes dose-limiting diarrhea
(D) Highly effective cough suppressant
(E) Seizures have occurred in overdose

ANSWERS

1. In most situations, pain associated with metastatic carcinoma will ultimately necessitate the use of an opioid analgesic that is equivalent in strength to morphine, so levorphanol would be indicated. Pentazocine or the combination of codeine plus salicylate are unlikely to be as effective as the original drug combination. Propoxyphene is less active than codeine alone. Butorphanol is a strong agent but is only available for parenteral injection. The answer is **(C).**

2. Chronic use of strong opioid analgesics leads to the development of tolerance to their analgesic, euphoric, and sedative actions. Tolerance also develops to their emetic effects and to effects on some smooth muscle, including the urethral sphincter muscle. However, tolerance does not develop to the constipating or miotic actions of the opioid analgesics. The answer is **(A)**.

3. Kappa receptor activation does not appear to be responsible for dependence, euphoria, or effects on smooth muscle. Increases in cerebral blood flow and (possibly) increased intracranial pressure result from the respiratory depressant actions of opioid analgesics. The latter effects are due to increased arterial P_{CO_2}, which results from mu receptor inhibition of the medullary respiratory center. However, the activation of kappa receptors contributes to analgesia at the spinal level and is probably responsible for sedative actions of the opioids. The answer is **(D)**.
4. Codeine and possibly nalbuphine could decrease gastrointestinal peristalsis but not without marked side effects (and a prescription). Dextromethorphan is a cough suppressant. The other two drugs listed are opioids with antidiarrheal actions. Diphenoxylate is not available over-the-counter since it is a constituent of a proprietary combination that includes atropine sulfate (Lomotil). Loperamide is available over-the-counter. The answer is **(D)**.
5. The fentanyl transdermal patch releases the drug over 72 hours. The blood levels achieved will often provide analgesia for postoperative pain but at the same time will increase arterial P_{CO_2} due to depression of the brain stem respiratory center. This effect has contributed to severe respiratory depression with occasional fatalities. The answer is **(E)**.
6. Concomitant administration of meperidine and MAO inhibitors has resulted in life-threatening hyperpyrexic reactions that may culminate in seizures or coma. Such reactions have even occurred when phenelzine was administered 14 days after a patient had been treated with meperidine! Note that concomitant use of SSRIs and meperidine has resulted in the serotonin syndrome, another life-threatening drug interaction (see Chapter 30). The answer is **(E)**.
7. Pentazocine is a weak agonist at mu and delta receptors. Its occupancy of these receptors can block the binding of pure agonists such as morphine. The result can be antagonism of morphine analgesia or a delay in its onset. The answer is **(D)**.
8. Intravenous morphine relieves the dyspnea of pulmonary edema associated with left ventricular failure. The mechanism may involve a decrease in perception of shortness of breath, relief of anxiety, and reductions in cardiac preload (decreased venous tone) and afterload (decreased peripheral resistance). Opioids cause exaggerated effects in Addison's disease and hypothyroidism, are contraindicated in head injury because they increase intracranial pressure, and may cause biliary muscle spasm. If given during labor, they may cause respiratory depression in the newborn. The answer is **(E)**.
9. The signs and symptoms are those of withdrawal in a patient physically dependent on an opioid agonist. Such signs and symptoms usually start within 6–10 hours after the last dose; their intensity depends on the degree of physical dependence that has developed. Peak effects usually occur at 36–48 hours. Mydriasis is a prominent feature of the abstinence syndrome; other symptoms include rhinorrhea, lacrimation, piloerection, muscle jerks, and yawning. The answer is **(C)**.
10. Prevention of signs and symptoms of withdrawal after chronic use of a strong opiate like heroin usually requires replacement with another strong opioid analgesic drug such as methadone. However, the partial agonist drug buprenorphine is also effective and has an even longer duration of action than methadone. Acetaminophen and codeine will not be effective. Beneficial effects of diazepam are restricted to relief of anxiety and agitation. The answer is **(B)**.
11. Mixed agonist-antagonist drugs may have analgesic efficacy almost equivalent to that of strong agonists. This is true for nalbuphine despite its antagonist action at mu receptors. Use of drugs in the agonist-antagonist subclass may lead to unpredictable results if combined with full agonists; agonist-antagonist drugs may precipitate an abstinence syndrome by blocking opioid receptors. While these drugs are less likely to cause respiratory depression, if depression does occur, reversal with opioid antagonists is unpredictable. The answer is **(E)**.
12. The opioid antagonist naltrexone has a much longer half-life than naloxone, and effects may last 2 days. A high degree of client compliance would be required for naltrexone to be of value in opioid dependence treatment programs. The same reservation is applicable to the use of naltrexone in alcoholism. The answer is **(D)**.
13. Dextromethorphan, an effective antitussive drug, is the dextrorotatory stereoisomer of a derivative of levorphanol. The drug is available without a prescription and is the active component in many over-the-counter cough suppressants. Dextromethorphan has no appreciable analgesic activity and minimal abuse liability. In comparison with codeine—also an effective antitussive—dextromethorphan causes less constipation. The answer is **(D)**.

14. Nalbuphine and oxycodone are not full agonists at opioid receptors, Fentanyl, hydromorphone, and methadone are full agonists with analgesic efficacy similar to that of morphine. Fentanyl, which is usually given intravenously, has a duration of action of just 60–90 minutes. Hydromorphone has poor oral bioavailability. Methadone has the greatest bioavailability of the drugs used orally, and its effects are more prolonged. Tolerance and physical dependence develop, and dissipate more slowly with methadone than with morphine. These properties underlie the use of methadone for detoxification and maintenance programs. The answer is **(C).**
15. Propoxyphene is chemically related to methadone but has very low analgesic activity. Propoxyphene causes a small additive analgesic effect when used in combination with aspirin or acetaminophen. Overdosage of propoxyphene results in severe toxicity, including respiratory depression, circulatory collapse, pulmonary edema, and seizures. The answer is **(E).**

Skill Keeper Answers: Opiopeptins & Substance P (see Chapters 6 and 17)

1. Precursor molecules that release opiopeptins are found at various peripheral sites, including the adrenal medulla and the pituitary gland and in some secretomotor neurons and interneurons in the enteric nervous system (ENS). In the gut these peptides appear to inhibit the release of ACh, presumably from parasympathetic nerve endings, and thereby inhibit peristalsis. In other tissues, opiopeptins may stimulate the release of transmitters or act as neurohormones.
2. Substance P, an undecapeptide, is a member of the tachykinin peptide group. It is an important sensory neuron transmitter in the ENS and, of course, in primary afferents involved in nociception. Substance P contracts intestinal and bronchiolar smooth muscle but is an arteriolar vasodilator (possibly via NO release). It may also play a role in renal and salivary gland functions.

Drugs of Abuse 32

OBJECTIVES

You should be able to:

- Describe the major actions of drugs that are commonly abused.
- Describe the major signs and symptoms of overdose with, and withdrawal from, CNS stimulants, opioid analgesics, and sedative-hypnotics, including ethanol.
- Describe the general principles of the management of overdose of commonly abused drugs.
- Identify the most likely causes of death from commonly abused agents.

Learn the definitions that follow.

Table 32–1. Definitions.

Term	Definition
Tolerance	A decreased response to a drug, necessitating larger doses to achieve the same effect. This can result from increased disposition of the drug (metabolic tolerance), an ability to compensate for the effects of a drug (behavioral tolerance), or changes in receptor or effector systems involved in drug actions (functional tolerance)
Psychologic dependence	Compulsive drug-using behavior in which the individual uses the drug for personal satisfaction, often despite known health risks
Physiologic dependence	A state characterized by signs and symptoms, frequently the opposite of those *caused* by a drug, when it is withdrawn from chronic use or when the dose is abruptly lowered. Psychologic dependence usually precedes physiologic dependence
Abstinence syndrome	A term used to describe the signs and symptoms that occur on withdrawal of a drug in a physiologically dependent person
Controlled substance	A drug deemed to have abuse liability that is listed on governmental Schedules of Controlled Drugs.[1] Such schedules categorize illicit drugs, control prescribing practices, and mandate penalties for illegal possession, manufacture, and sale of listed drugs. Controlled substance schedules are presumed to reflect current attitudes toward substance abuse; therefore, which drugs are regulated depends on a social judgment
Designer drug	A synthetic derivative of a drug, with slightly modified structure but no major change in pharmacodynamic action. Circumvention of the Schedules of Controlled Drugs is a motivation for the illicit synthesis of designer drugs

[1]An example of such a schedule promulgated by the United States Drug Enforcement Agency is shown in Table 32–2. Note that the criteria given by the agency do not always reflect the actual pharmacologic properties of the drugs.

CONCEPTS

Drug abuse is usually taken to mean the use of an illicit drug or the excessive or nonmedical use of a licit drug. It also denotes the deliberate use of chemicals that generally are not considered drugs by the lay public but may be harmful to the user. The motivation for drug abuse appears to be the anticipated feeling of pleasure derived from the CNS effects of the drug. If physiologic dependence is present, prevention of an abstinence syndrome acts as a reinforcement to continued drug abuse.

MAJOR CATEGORIES OF DRUGS OF ABUSE

A. **Sedative-Hypnotics:** The sedative-hypnotic drugs are responsible for many cases of drug abuse in the United States, Europe, and Japan. The group includes **ethanol, barbiturates,** and **benzodiazepines,** all of which are more readily available to the general public than are opioids, cocaine, or hallucinogens. Benzodiazepines are the most commonly prescribed drugs for anxiety and, as Schedule IV drugs, are judged by the United States government to have low abuse liability (Table 32–2). Ethanol is not listed in schedules of controlled substances with abuse liability.

Table 32–2. Schedules of Controlled Drugs.*

Schedule	Criteria	Examples
I	No medical use; high addiction potential	Flunitrazepam, heroin, LSD, marijuana, mescaline, methaqualone, PCP, DOM, MDMA
II	Medical use; high addiction potential	Strong opioid agonists, cocaine, short half-life barbiturates, amphetamines, methylphenidate
III	Medical use; moderate potential for dependence	Anabolic steroids, codeine and moderate opioid agonists, dronabinol, thiopental
IV	Medical use; low abuse potential	Benzodiazepines, chloral hydrate, meprobamate, weak opioid agonists, zolpidem, zaleplon

*Adapted, with permission, from Katzung BG (editor): *Basic & Clinical Pharmacology,* 8th ed. McGraw-Hill, 2001.

1. **Effects:** Sedative-hypnotics reduce inhibitions, suppress anxiety, and produce relaxation. All of these actions are thought to encourage repetitive use and the development of psychologic dependence. The drugs are CNS depressants, and their depressant effects are enhanced by concomitant use of opioid analgesics, antipsychotic agents, marijuana, and any other drug with sedative properties. Acute overdoses commonly result in death through depression of the medullary respiratory and cardiovascular centers (Table 32–3). Management of overdose includes maintenance of a patent airway plus ventilatory support. Flumazenil can be used to reverse the CNS depressant effects of benzodiazepines, but there is no antidote for the other sedative-hypnotics such as the barbiturates and ethanol.

   Flunitrazepam (Rohypnol), a potent rapid-onset benzodiazepine with marked amnestic properties, has been used in "date rape." Added to alcoholic beverages, chloral hydrate or gamma-hydroxybutyrate (GHB) will render the victim incapable of resisting rape.
2. **Withdrawal:** Physiologic dependence occurs with continued use of sedative-hypnotics; the signs and symptoms of the withdrawal (abstinence) syndrome are most pronounced with drugs that have a half-life of less than 24 hours (eg, ethanol, secobarbital, methaqualone). However, physiologic dependence may occur with any sedative-hypnotic, including the longer-acting benzodiazepines. The most important signs of withdrawal derive from excessive *CNS stimulation* and include anxiety, tremor, nausea and vomiting, delirium, and hallucinations (see Table 32–3). **Seizures** are not uncommon and may be life-threatening.

   Treatment of sedative-hypnotic withdrawal involves administration of a long-acting sedative-hypnotic (eg, chlordiazepoxide or diazepam) to suppress the acute withdrawal syndrome, followed by a gradual reduction of the dose. Clonidine or propranolol may also be of value to suppress sympathetic overactivity.

   A syndrome of **therapeutic withdrawal** has occurred on discontinuance of sedative-hypnotics after long-term therapeutic administration. In addition to the symptoms of classic withdrawal listed above, this syndrome includes weight loss, paresthesias, and headache. (See Chapters 22 and 23 for additional details.)

B. Opioid Analgesics:

1. **Effects:** The most commonly abused drugs in this group are **heroin, morphine, oxycodone,** and—among health professionals—**meperidine** and **fentanyl.** The effects of intravenous heroin are described by abusers as a "rush" or orgasmic feeling followed by euphoria and then sedation. Intravenous administration of opioids is associated with rapid development of tolerance and psychologic and physiologic dependence. Oral administration or smoking of opioids causes milder effects, with a slower onset of tolerance and dependence. Overdose of opioids leads to respiratory depression progressing to coma and death (see Table 32–3). Overdose is managed with intravenous naloxone and ventilatory support.
2. **Withdrawal:** Deprivation of opioids in physiologically dependent individuals leads to an abstinence syndrome that includes lacrimation, rhinorrhea, yawning, sweating, weakness, gooseflesh ("cold turkey"), nausea and vomiting, tremor, muscle jerks ("kicking the habit"), and hyperpnea. Although extremely unpleasant, withdrawal from opioids is rarely fatal (un-

Table 32–3. Signs and symptoms of overdose and withdrawal for selected drugs of abuse.

Drug	Overdose Effects	Withdrawal Symptoms
Amphetamines; methylphenidate; cocaine[1]	Agitation, hypertension, tachycardia, delusions, hallucinations, hyperthermia, seizures, death	Apathy, irritability, increased sleep time, disorientation, depression
Barbiturates; benzodiazepines; ethanol[2]	Slurred speech, "drunken" behavior, dilated pupils, weak and rapid pulse, clammy skin, shallow respiration, coma, death	Anxiety, insomnia, delirium, tremors, seizures, death
Heroin; other opioid analgesics	Constricted pupils, clammy skin, nausea, drowsiness, respiratory depression, coma, death	Nausea, chills, sweats, cramps, lacrimation, rhinorrhea, yawning, hyperpnea, tremor

[1]Cardiac arrhythmias, myocardial infarction, and stroke occur more frequently in cocaine overdose than with other CNS stimulants.
[2]Ethanol withdrawal includes the excited hallucinatory state of delirium tremens.

like withdrawal from sedative-hypnotics). Treatment involves replacement of the illicit drug with a pharmacologically equivalent agent (eg, methadone), followed by slow dose reduction. Clonidine and buprenorphine, a longer-acting opioid, have also been used to suppress withdrawal symptoms. The administration of naloxone to a person who is using strong opioids (but not overdosing) may cause more rapid and more intense symptoms of withdrawal ("precipitated withdrawal"). Neonates born to mothers physiologically dependent on opioids require special management of withdrawal symptoms.

C. **Stimulants:** A chemically heterogeneous subgroup, the stimulants include caffeine, nicotine, amphetamines, and cocaine.

1. **Caffeine and nicotine:**
   a. **Effects:** Caffeine (in beverages) and nicotine (in tobacco products) are legal in most Western cultures even though they have adverse medical effects. In the USA, cigarette smoking is now the major preventable cause of death; tobacco use is associated with a high incidence of cardiovascular, respiratory, and neoplastic disease. Psychologic dependence on caffeine and nicotine has been recognized for some time. More recently, demonstration of abstinence signs and symptoms has provided evidence for physiologic dependence.
   b. **Withdrawal:** Withdrawal from caffeine is accompanied by lethargy, irritability, and headache. The anxiety and mental discomfort experienced from discontinuing nicotine are major impediments to quitting the habit.
   c. **Toxicity:** Acute toxicity from overdosage of caffeine or nicotine includes excessive CNS stimulation with tremor, insomnia, and nervousness; cardiac stimulation and arrhythmias; and, in the case of nicotine, respiratory paralysis (Chapters 6 and 7). Severe toxicity has been reported in small children who ingest discarded gum or patches (containing nicotine) which are used as substitutes for tobacco products.
2. **Amphetamines:**
   a. **Effects:** Amphetamines cause a feeling of euphoria and self-confidence that contributes to the rapid development of psychologic dependence. Drugs in this class include **dextroamphetamine** and **methamphetamine** ("speed"), a crystal form of which ("ice") can be smoked. Chronic high-dose abuse leads to a psychotic state (with delusions and paranoia) that is difficult to differentiate from schizophrenia. Symptoms of overdose include agitation, restlessness, tachycardia, hyperthermia, hyperreflexia, and possibly seizures. There is no specific antidote, and supportive measures are directed toward control of body temperature and protection against seizures.
   b. **Tolerance and withdrawal:** Tolerance can be marked, and an abstinence syndrome, characterized by increased appetite, sleepiness, exhaustion, and mental depression, can occur upon withdrawal. Antidepressant drugs may be indicated.
   c. **Congeners of amphetamines:** Several chemical congeners of amphetamines have hallucinogenic properties. These include 2,5-dimethoxy-4-methylamphetamine **(DOM, STP),** methylene dioxyamphetamine **(MDA),** and methylene dioxymethamphetamine **(MDMA "ecstasy").** MDMA is purported to facilitate interpersonal communication and act as a sexual enhancer. Positron emission tomography (PET) studies of the brains of regular users of MDMA show a depletion of neurons in serotonergic tracts. Overdose toxicity includes the clinical features seen with overdose of amphetamine.
3. **Cocaine:** Cocaine has marked amphetamine-like effects ("super-speed"). Its abuse continues to be widespread in the USA, partly because of the availability of a free-base form ("crack") that can be smoked. The euphoria, self-confidence, and mental alertness produced by cocaine are short-lasting and positively reinforce its continued use.
   a. **Effects:** Overdoses with cocaine commonly result in fatalities from arrhythmias, seizures, or respiratory depression. Cardiac toxicity is due partly to blockade of norepinephrine reuptake by cocaine; its local anesthetic action contributes to the production of seizures. In addition, the powerful vasoconstrictive action of cocaine may lead to severe hypertensive episodes, resulting in myocardial infarcts and strokes. No specific antidote is available.
   b. **Withdrawal:** The abstinence syndrome following withdrawal from cocaine is similar to that following amphetamine discontinuance. Severe depression of mood is common and strongly reinforces the compulsion to use the drug. Antidepressant drugs may be indicated. Infants born to mothers who abuse cocaine (or amphetamines) have possible

teratogenic abnormalities (cystic cortical lesions), increased morbidity and mortality, and may be "cocaine-dependent." The signs and symptoms of CNS stimulant overdose and withdrawal are listed in Table 32–3.

D. Hallucinogens:

1. **Phencyclidine:** The arylcyclohexylamine drug **phencyclidine** (PCP; "angel dust") is probably the most dangerous of the currently popular hallucinogenic agents. Psychotic reactions are common with PCP, and impaired judgment often leads to reckless behavior. This drug should be classified as a **psychotomimetic.** Effects of overdosage with PCP include nystagmus, marked hypertension, and seizures, which may be fatal. Parenteral benzodiazepines (eg, diazepam, lorazepam) are used to curb excitation and protect against seizures.
2. **Miscellaneous hallucinogenic agents:** Several drugs with hallucinogenic effects have been classified as having abuse liability; these drugs include **lysergic acid diethylamide** (LSD), **mescaline,** and **psilocybin.** Hallucinogenic effects may also occur with scopolamine and other antimuscarinic agents. Terms that have been used to describe the CNS effects of such drugs include "psychedelic" and "mind-revealing." The perceptual and psychologic effects of such drugs are usually accompanied by marked somatic effects, particularly nausea, weakness, and paresthesias. Panic reactions ("bad trips") may also occur. There is little evidence that use of these agents leads to the development of physiologic dependence.

E. Marijuana:

1. **Classification:** Marijuana ("grass") is a collective term for the psychoactive constituents present in crude extracts of the plant *Cannabis sativa* (hemp), the active principles of which include the compounds **tetrahydrocannabinol (THC),** cannabidiol (CBD), and cannabinol (CBN). **Hashish** is a partially purified material that is more potent.
2. **Effects:** CNS effects of marijuana include a feeling of being "high," with euphoria, disinhibition, uncontrollable laughter, changes in perception, and achievement of a dreamlike state. Mental concentration may be difficult. Vasodilation occurs, and the pulse rate is characteristically increased. Habitual users show a reddened conjunctiva. A mild withdrawal state has been noted only in heavy long-term users of marijuana. The dangers of marijuana use concern its impairment of judgment and reflexes, effects that are potentiated by concomitant use of sedative-hypnotics, including ethanol. Potential therapeutic effects of marijuana include its ability to decrease intraocular pressure and its antiemetic actions. **Dronabinol** (a controlled-substance formulation of THC) is used to combat nausea in cancer chemotherapy.

F. Inhalants: Certain gases or volatile liquids are abused because they provide a feeling of euphoria or disinhibition. This class includes the following agents:

1. **Anesthetics:** This group includes nitrous oxide, chloroform, and diethylether. These agents are hazardous because they affect judgment and induce loss of consciousness. Inhalation of nitrous oxide as the pure gas (with no oxygen) has caused asphyxia and death. Ether is highly flammable.
2. **Industrial solvents:** Solvents and a wide range of volatile compounds are present in commercial products such as gasoline, paint thinners, aerosol propellants, glues, rubber cements, and shoe polish. Because of their ready availability, these substances are most frequently abused by children in early adolescence. Active ingredients that have been identified include benzene, hexane, methylethylketone, toluene, and trichloroethylene. Many of these are toxic to the liver, kidneys, lungs, bone marrow, and peripheral nerves and cause brain damage in animals.
3. **Organic nitrites:** Amyl nitrite, isobutyl nitrite, and other organic nitrites are referred to as "poppers" and are mainly used as sexual intercourse "enhancers." Inhalation of the nitrites causes dizziness, tachycardia, hypotension, and flushing. With the exception of methemoglobinemia, few serious adverse effects have been reported.

G. Steroids: In many countries, including the United States, anabolic steroids are controlled substances based on their potential for abuse. Effects sought by abusers are increases in muscle mass and strength rather than euphoria. However, excessive use can have adverse behavioral, cardiovascular, and musculoskeletal effects. Acne (sometimes severe), premature closure of the epiphyses, and masculinization in females are anticipated androgenic adverse effects. Hepatic dysfunction has been reported, and the anabolic steroids may pose an increased risk of myocardial infarct. Behavioral manifestations include increases in libido and aggression ("roid rage"). A withdrawal syndrome has been described with fatigue and depression of mood.

Skill Keeper: Drug of Abuse Overdose Signs & Symptoms (see Chapters 22 and 31)

In an emergency situation, behavioral manifestations of the toxicity of drugs of abuse can be of assistance in diagnosis. What other readily detectable markers will also be helpful? *The Skill Keeper Answer appears at the end of the chapter.*

DRUG LIST

The following drugs are important members of the group discussed in this chapter. Prototypes should be learned in detail; features of the major variants should be known well enough to distinguish the variants from prototypes and from each other; the other significant agents should be recognized as belonging to a specific subclass.

Subclass	Prototype	Major Variants	Other Significant Agents
Sedative-hypnotics	Secobarbital, benzodiazepines, ethanol	Pentobarbital, alprazolam, diazepam	Methaqualone, meprobamate
Opioids	Heroin	Fentanyl, meperidine	Strong agonist opioid analgesics
Stimulants	Amphetamine	Methamphetamine, phenmetrazine	DOM, MDA, MDMA
	Cocaine, caffeine, nicotine		
Hallucinogens	LSD, phencyclidine	Mescaline	Scopolamine
Marijuana	"Grass"	Hashish	Dronabinol
Inhalants	Nitrous oxide, toluene	Ether	Chloroform, benzene
	Amyl nitrite	Isobutyl nitrite	

QUESTIONS

DIRECTIONS: Each of the numbered items or incomplete statements in this section is followed by answers or by completions of the statement. Select the ONE lettered answer or completion that is BEST in each case.

Items 1–3: A 42-year-old homemaker with two school-age children suffers from anxiety with phobic symptoms and occasional panic attacks. No specific medical, financial, or domestic cause can be identified for her condition. Her prescription drugs include oral contraceptives and low-dose thyroxine. She also uses over-the-counter antihistamines for allergic rhinitis. She claims that ethanol use is restricted to a glass or two of wine with dinner. After several sessions with her psychiatrist, alprazolam is prescribed. The patient continues monthly sessions with her psychiatrist and is maintained on alprazolam for 3 years, with several dose increments over that time period. Her family notices that she does not seem to be improving, and that her speech is often slurred in the evenings. She is finally hospitalized with severe withdrawal signs one weekend while attempting to end her dependence on drugs.

1. Which one of the following statements about the use of alprazolam in this patient is false?

(A) Additive CNS depression will occur with ethanol and with over-the-counter antihistamines

(B) Alternative nondrug treatments should have been tried long before 3 years had elapsed

(C) Tolerance can be anticipated with chronic use of any benzodiazepine
(D) The anxiolytic effects of sedative-hypnotic drugs encourage dependence
(E) If she had discontinued alprazolam after 1 month, she would not have experienced any withdrawal signs at that time

2. The main reason for hospitalization of this patient was to be able to effectively control
(A) Anxiety
(B) Cardiac arrhythmias
(C) Respiratory depression
(D) Seizures
(E) Thyroid dysfunction

3. The symptoms being experienced by this hospitalized patient can best be ameliorated by the administration of
(A) Amphetamine
(B) Chlordiazepoxide
(C) Oxycodone
(D) Propranolol
(E) Secobarbital

4. Which one of the following statements about abuse of the opioid analgesics is false?
(A) A patient experiencing withdrawal from heroin is free of the symptoms of abstinence in 6–8 days
(B) In withdrawal from opioids, clonidine may be useful in reducing symptoms caused by sympathetic overactivity
(C) Lacrimation, rhinorrhea, yawning, and sweating are early signs of withdrawal from opioid analgesics
(D) Naloxone may precipitate a severe withdrawal state in abusers of opioid analgesics with symptoms starting in less than 15–30 minutes
(E) Methadone alleviates most of the symptoms of heroin withdrawal

5. A young male patient is brought to the emergency room of a hospital suffering from an overdose of cocaine following intravenous administration. His symptoms are unlikely to include
(A) Agitation
(B) Bradycardia
(C) Hyperthermia
(D) Myocardial infarct
(E) Seizures

6. Which one of the following statements about central nervous system stimulants is false?
(A) "Herbal ecstasy" causes amphetamine-like effects
(B) Withdrawal from caffeine may lead to severe headaches
(C) MDMA ("ecstasy," XTC) is reported to be neurotoxic to brain serotonergic systems
(D) While psychologic dependence to amphetamines is strong, physiologic dependence does not occur
(E) Treatment of cocaine overdose may include the use of diazepam and propranolol

7. Which one of the following statements about hallucinogens is accurate?
(A) Mescaline and related hallucinogens are thought to exert their CNS actions through dopaminergic systems in the brain
(B) Teratogenic effects are known to occur with the use of LSD during pregnancy
(C) Scopolamine is unique among hallucinogens in that animals will self-administer it
(D) Dilated pupils, tachycardia, tremor, and increased alertness are characteristic effects of psilocybin
(E) Phencyclidine can be anticipated to cause dry mouth and urinary retention

8. Which one of the following statements about inhalants is false?
(A) Solvent inhalation is mainly a drug abuse problem in boys age 8–12 years
(B) Euphoria, numbness, and tingling sensations with visual and auditory disturbances occur in most persons who inhale 35% nitrous oxide
(C) Methemoglobinemia is a common toxicologic problem following repetitive inhalation of industrial solvents
(D) Fluorocarbons may cause sudden death due to cardiac arrhythmias
(E) The use of isobutyl nitrite is likely to cause headache

9. Which one of the following signs or symptoms is likely to occur with marijuana?

(A) Bradycardia
(B) Conjunctival reddening
(C) Hypertension
(D) Increased psychomotor performance
(E) Mydriasis

Items 10–11: A college student is brought to the emergency room by friends. The physician is informed that the student had taken a drug and then "went crazy." The patient is agitated and delirious. Several persons are required to hold him down. His skin is warm and sweaty, and his pupils are dilated. Bowel sounds are normal. Signs and symptoms include tachycardia, marked hypertension, hyperthermia, increased muscle tone, and both horizontal and vertical nystagmus.

10. The most likely cause of these signs and symptoms is intoxication due to
(A) Hashish
(B) LSD
(C) Mescaline
(D) Phencyclidine
(E) Scopolamine

11. The management of this patient is unlikely to include
(A) Activated charcoal
(B) Benzodiazepine administration
(C) Haloperidol if psychosis ensues
(D) Nasogastric suction
(E) Urinary alkalinization to increase drug elimination

12. This agent has sedative and amnestic properties. Small doses added to alcoholic beverages are not readily detected by taste and have been used in "date rape" attacks. The drug is chemically related to a brain inhibitory neurotransmitter. Which one of the following most closely resembles the description given?
(A) Amyl nitrite
(B) Flunitrazepam
(C) Gamma-hydroxybutyrate
(D) Hashish
(E) Metcathinone

ANSWERS

1. Even normal therapeutic doses of benzodiazepines may lead to physiologic dependence with withdrawal symptoms. These can include increases in REM sleep (REM rebound), increased anxiety, agitation, and insomnia. The severity of withdrawal symptoms depends on the dose used and on the concomitant use of other sedative-hypnotics, including ethanol. In general, withdrawal symptoms are more severe with the use of shorter-acting sedative-hypnotics. The answer is **(E).**

2. In addition to the symptoms described above, abrupt withdrawal from sedative-hypnotic dependence may include hyperreflexia progressing to seizures, with ensuing coma and possibly death. The risk of a convulsion is increased if the patient abruptly withdraws from ethanol use at the same time. The answer is **(D).**

3. The standard approach to detoxification during withdrawal from physiologic dependence on barbiturates, benzodiazepines, or ethanol is the use of a long-acting sedative hypnotic with dose tapering. Chlordiazepoxide or diazepam is used most frequently. The answer is **(B).**

4. Symptoms of opioid withdrawal usually begin within 6–8 hours, and the acute course may last 6–8 days. However, a secondary phase of heroin withdrawal, characterized by bradycardia, hypotension, hypothermia, and mydriasis, may last 26–30 weeks. Methadone is commonly used in detoxification of the heroin addict because it is a strong agonist, has high oral bioavailability, and has a relatively long half-life. The answer is **(A).**

5. Overdoses with amphetamines or cocaine have many signs and symptoms in common. However, the ability of cocaine to block the reuptake of norepinephrine at sympathetic nerve terminals results in greater cardiotoxicity. Tachycardia is the rule, with the possibility of an arrhythmia, infarct, or stroke. The answer is **(B).**

6. Abuse of amphetamines results in marked tolerance and both psychologic and physiologic dependence. Withdrawal is manifested by signs and symptoms opposite to those produced by such drugs, including apathy and depression. "Herbal ecstasy" is a plant extract that causes CNS stimulation, decreased appetite, insomnia, and sympathomimetic effects; its primary ingredient is ephedrine, as is true of Ma-huang also. The answer is **(D).**

7. Psilocybin, mescaline, and LSD have similar central (via serotonergic systems) and peripheral (sympathomimetic) effects. None of these hallucinogenic drugs have been shown to have teratogenic potential. Contrast this with the established potential for teratogenicity or other fetal toxicity with abuse of ethanol, amphetamines, and cocaine. Unlike most hallucinogens, phencyclidine acts as a positive reinforcer of self-administration in animals. Scopolamine is not a positive reinforcer but does exert atropine-like effects. The answer is **(D).**
8. Male preteen children are most likely to "experiment" with solvent inhalation. Abuse of nitrous oxide is relatively common. Toxic inhalants such as heptane, hexane, methylethylketone, toluene, and trichloroethylene may result in central and peripheral neurotoxicity, liver and kidney damage, and pulmonary disease. Sudden death has occurred following inhalation of fluorocarbons. Industrial solvents rarely cause methemoglobinemia, but this (and headaches) may occur following excessive use of nitrites. The answer is **(C).**
9. Two of the most characteristic signs of marijuana use are increased pulse rate and reddening of the conjunctiva. Decreases in blood pressure and in psychomotor performance occur. Pupil size is *not* changed by marijuana. The answer is **(B).**
10. The signs and symptoms point to phencyclidine intoxication. The presence of both horizontal and vertical nystagmus is pathognomonic. The answer is **(D).**
11. Overdose with phencyclidine is dangerous. The basic principles of treatment are to maintain ventilation and to control seizures, blood pressure, and hyperthermia. Phencyclidine is secreted into the stomach, so removal of the drug may be hastened by activated charcoal or continual nasogastric suction. Phencyclidine is a weak base, and its renal elimination may be accelerated by urinary *acidification.* Treatment with antipsychotic drugs may be appropriate if psychotic symptoms follow the acute intoxication. The answer is **(E).**
12. Flunitrazepam fits part of the description of this "date rape" drug, but it is not chemically related to known neurotransmitters. Gamma-hydroxybutyrate (GHB; "Liquid ecstasy"), a popular street drug, is structurally related to GABA. GHB causes amnesia and in overdose has resulted in seizures, coma, and death. Metcathinone (khat, "Cat") is a natural plant alkaloid with CNS-stimulating properties similar to those of amphetamine. The answer is **(C).**

Skill Keeper Answer: Drug of Abuse Overdose Signs & Symptoms (see Chapters 22 and 31)

Readily detectable markers that may assist in diagnosis of the cause of drug overdose toxicity include changes in heart rate, blood pressure, respiration, body temperature, sweating, bowel signs, and pupillary responses. For example, in the case of drugs of abuse, tachycardia, hypertension, increased body temperature, decreased bowel signs, and mydriasis are common characteristics of overdose of CNS stimulants, including amphetamines, cocaine, and most hallucinogens.

Make a brief list of characteristics that would enable you to identify overdose with opioids and sedative-hypnotics.

Part VI: Drugs with Important Actions on Blood, Inflammation, & Gout

33 Agents Used in Anemias & Hematopoietic Growth Factors

OBJECTIVES

You should be able to:

- Describe the normal mechanism of regulation of iron absorption and storage in the body.
- List the anemias for which iron supplementation is indicated and those for which it is contraindicated.
- Describe the acute and chronic toxicity of iron.
- Sketch the dTMP cycle and show how folic acid and vitamin B_{12} affect the cycle.
- Describe the clinical applications of vitamin B_{12} and folic acid.
- Describe the major hazard involved in the use of folic acid as sole therapy for megaloblastic anemia.
- Name the major hematopoietic growth factors and discribe their clinical uses.

Learn the definitions that follow.

Table 33–1. Definitions.

Term	Definition
Cobalamin	Vitamin B_{12}
dTMP synthesis cycle	A set of biochemical reactions that produce deoxythymidylate (dTMP), an essential constituent of DNA synthesis. The cycle depends upon the conversion of dihydrofolate to tetrahydrofolate by the enzyme dihydrofolate reductase (Figure 33–2)
Folate trap	The accumulation of N^5-methyltetrahydrofolate and the resulting deficiency in tetrahydrofolate that is caused by vitamin B_{12} deficiency (Figure 33–2)
G-CSF	Granulocyte colony-stimulating factor, a hematopoietic growth factor that stimulates production and function of neutrophils
GM-CSF	Granulocyte-macrophage colony-stimulating factor, a hematopoietic growth factor that stimulates production of granulocytes (basophils, eosinophils, and neutrophils), and other myeloid cells
Megaloblastic anemia	A deficiency in serum hemoglobin and red blood cells (erythrocytes) in which the erythrocytes are abnormally large. This type of anemia is caused by folate or vitamin B_{12} deficiency.
Microcytic anemia	A deficiency in serum hemoglobin and red blood cells (erythrocytes) in which the erythrocytes are abnormally small. Often caused by iron deficiency
Neutropenia	An abnormal decrease in the number of neutrophils in the blood; patients with neutropenia are susceptible to serious infection
PBSCs	Peripheral blood stem cells; hematopoietic cells found in peripheral blood that have the capability to give rise to several different types of mature blood cells. PBSCs are used for autologous transplantation (transplantation with one's own cells) and allogeneic transplantation (transplantation with someone else's cells)
Pernicious anemia	A type of megaloblastic anemia that results from a lack of intrinsic factor, a protein that is produced by gastric mucosal cells and is required for intestinal absorption of vitamin B_{12}
Thrombocytopenia	An abnormal decrease in the number of platelets in the blood; patients with thrombocytopenia are susceptible to severe bleeding

CONCEPTS

BLOOD CELL DEFICIENCIES

A. Iron and Vitamin Deficiency Anemias: Microcytic hypochromic anemia, caused by iron deficiency, is the most common type of anemia. Megaloblastic anemias are caused by a deficiency of vitamin B_{12} or folic acid, cofactors required for the normal maturation of red blood cells. Pernicious anemia, the most common type of vitamin B_{12} deficiency anemia, is caused by a defect in the synthesis of intrinsic factor, a protein required for efficient absorption of dietary vitamin B_{12}, or by surgical removal of that part of the stomach that secretes intrinsic factor.

B. Other Blood Cell Deficiencies: Deficiency in the concentration of the various lineages of blood cells can be a manifestation of a disease or a side effect of radiation or cancer chemotherapy. Recombinant DNA-directed synthesis of hematopoietic growth factors now makes possible the treatment of more patients with deficiencies in erythrocytes, neutrophils, and platelets. Some of these growth factors also play an important role in stem cell transplantation.

C. Prototypes: Figure 33–1 illustrates the major drugs discussed in this chapter.

IRON

A. Role of Iron: Iron is the essential metallic component of heme, the molecule responsible for the bulk of oxygen transport in the blood. Although most of the iron in the body is present in hemoglobin, an important fraction is bound to transferrin, a transport protein, and to ferritin, a storage protein. Deficiency of iron occurs most often in women because of menstrual blood loss and in vegetarians or malnourished individuals because of inadequate dietary iron intake. Children and pregnant women have increased requirements for iron.

B. Regulation of Iron Stores: Regulation of body iron content occurs through modulation of intestinal absorption. There is no mechanism for the efficient excretion of iron. As a result, dysfunction of gastrointestinal regulation of iron absorption is one cause of diseases associated with excess iron stores, eg, hemochromatosis.

1. **Absorption:** Iron is absorbed as the ferrous ion (Fe^{2+}) and oxidized in the mucosal cell to the ferric (Fe^{3+}) form.
2. **Storage:** Trivalent ferric iron can be stored in the mucosa (bound to ferritin) or carried elsewhere in the body (bound to transferrin). Excess iron is stored in protein-bound form in the reticuloendothelial system and, in cases of gross overload, in parenchymal cells of the skin, liver, and other organs. An accumulation of storage iron occurs in hemolytic anemias (anemias caused by excess destruction of red blood cells) and in hemochromatosis.
3. **Elimination:** Minimal amounts of iron are lost from the body with sweat and saliva and in exfoliated skin and intestinal mucosal cells.

C. Clinical Use: Iron deficiency anemia is the only indication for the use of iron. Iron deficiency can be diagnosed from red blood cell changes (microcytic cell size, from diminished hemoglobin content of blood) and from measurements of serum and bone marrow iron stores. The disease is treated by dietary ferrous iron supplementation and, in special cases, by par-

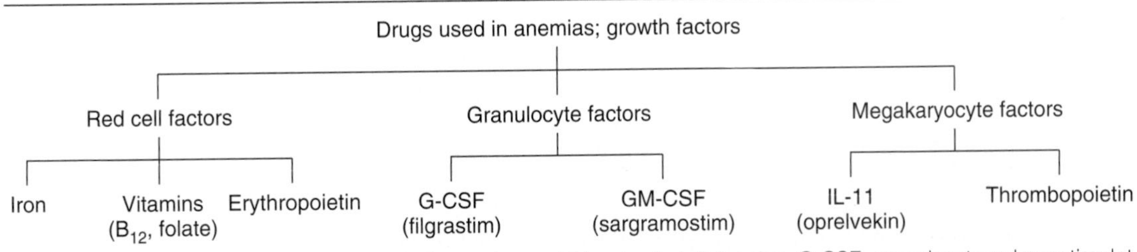

Figure 33–1. Drugs used in the treatment of anemias and blood cell deficiencies. G-CSF, granulocyte colony-stimulating factor; GM-CSF, granulocyte-macrophage colony-stimulating factor; IL-11, interleukin-11.

enteral administration of the metal (see Drug List). Iron should *not* be given in hemolytic anemia because iron stores are elevated, not depressed, in this type of anemia.

D. Toxicity of Iron: (See also Chapter 58.)

1. **Signs and symptoms:** Acute iron intoxication is most common in children and usually occurs as a result of accidental ingestion of iron supplementation tablets. Depending on the dose, necrotizing gastroenteritis, shock, metabolic acidosis, coma, and death may result. Chronic toxicity occurs most often in individuals who must receive frequent transfusions (eg, patients with sickle cell anemia) and in those with hemochromatosis, an inherited abnormality of iron absorption.
2. **Treatment of acute iron intoxication:** Immediate treatment is necessary and usually consists of removal of unabsorbed tablets from the gut, correction of acid-base and electrolyte abnormalities, and parenteral administration of deferoxamine, which chelates circulating iron.
3. **Treatment of chronic iron toxicity:** Treatment of hemochromatosis is usually by phlebotomy.

VITAMIN B_{12}

A. Role of Vitamin B_{12}: Vitamin B_{12} (cobalamin), a cobalt-containing molecule, is (along with folic acid) a cofactor in the transfer of one-carbon units, a step necessary for the synthesis of DNA. Impairment of DNA synthesis affects all cells, but because red blood cells must be produced continuously, deficiency of either B_{12} or folic acid usually manifests first as anemia. In addition, an important manifestation of vitamin B_{12} deficiency is the development of neurologic defects, which may become irreversible if not treated promptly.

B. Pharmacokinetics: Vitamin B_{12} is produced only by bacteria; this vitamin cannot be synthesized by multicellular organisms. It is absorbed from the gastrointestinal tract in the presence of intrinsic factor, a product of the parietal cells of the stomach. Vitamin B_{12} is stored in the liver in large amounts; a normal individual has enough to last 5 years. Plasma transport is accomplished by binding to transcobalamin II, a glycoprotein. When parenteral vitamin B_{12} is given, any in excess of the transport protein binding capacity is excreted. The two available forms of vitamin B_{12}, cyanocobalamin and hydroxocobalamin, have similar pharmacokinetics, but hydroxocobalamin is somewhat more firmly bound to plasma proteins and has a longer circulating half-life.

C. Pharmacodynamics: Vitamin B_{12} is essential in two reactions: conversion of methylmalonyl-CoA to succinyl-CoA and conversion of homocysteine to methionine. The second reaction is linked to folic acid metabolism and synthesis of deoxythymidylate (dTMP; Figure 33–2, reaction 2), a precursor required for DNA synthesis. In vitamin B_{12} deficiency, folates accumulate as N^5-methyltetrahydrofolate; the supply of tetrahydrofolate is depleted; and the production of red blood cells slows. Administration of folic acid to patients with vitamin B_{12} deficiency helps refill the tetrahydrofolate pool (Figure 33–2, reaction 3) and partially or fully corrects the anemia. However, the exogenous folic acid does not correct the neurologic defects of vitamin B_{12} deficiency.

D. Clinical Use and Toxicity: Vitamin B_{12} is available as hydroxocobalamin and cyanocobalamin, which have equivalent effects. The major application is in the treatment of naturally occurring pernicious anemia and anemia caused by gastric resection. Because B_{12} deficiency anemia is almost always caused by inadequate absorption, therapy should be by replacement of vitamin B_{12}, using parenteral therapy. Neither form of vitamin B_{12} has significant toxicity.

FOLIC ACID

A. Role of Folic Acid: Like vitamin B_{12}, folic acid is required for normal DNA synthesis, and its deficiency usually presents as megaloblastic anemia. In addition, deficiency of folic acid during pregnancy increases the risk of neural tube defects in the fetus.

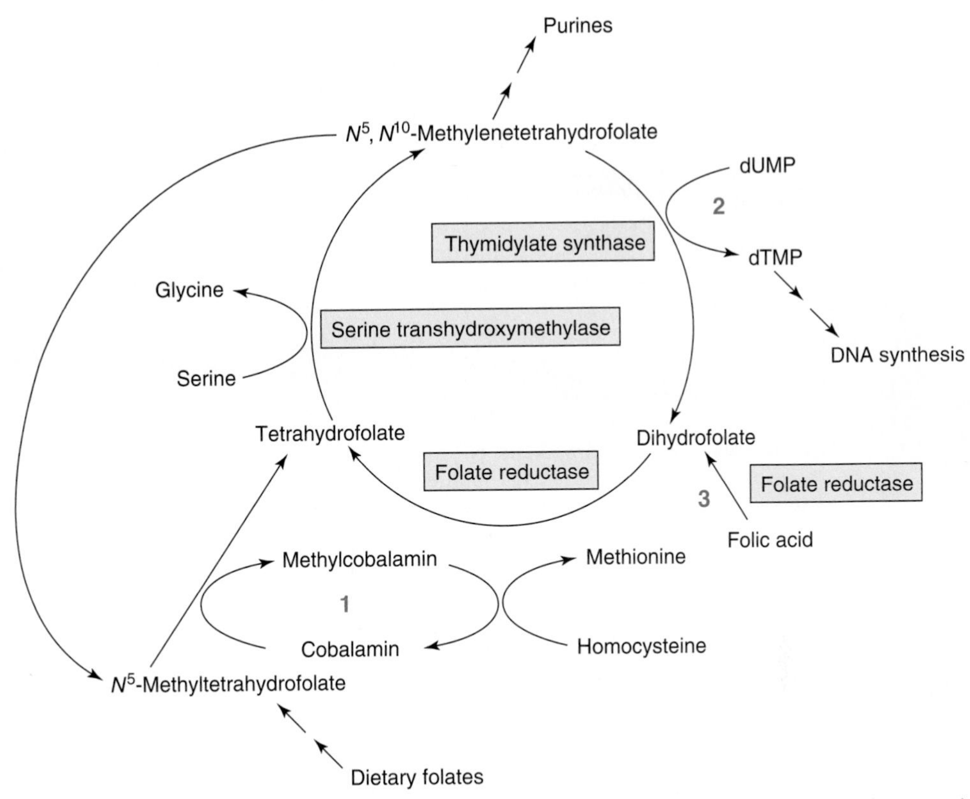

Figure 33–2. Enzymatic reactions that use folates. Section 1 shows the vitamin B_{12}-dependent reaction that allows most dietary folates to enter the tetrahydrofolate cofactor pool and becomes the "folate trap" in vitamin B_{12} deficiency. Section 2 shows the dTMP cycle. Section 3 shows the pathway by which folate enters the tetrahydrofolate cofactor pool. Double arrows indicate pathways with more than one intermediate step. (Reproduced, with permission, from Katzung BG [editor]: *Basic & Clinical Pharmacology,* 8th ed. McGraw-Hill, 2001.)

B. Pharmacokinetics: Folic acid is readily absorbed from the gastrointestinal tract. Only modest amounts are stored in the body, so a decrease in dietary intake is followed by anemia within a few months.

C. Pharmacodynamics: Folic acid is converted to tetrahydrofolate by the action of dihydrofolate reductase (Figure 33–2, reaction 3). One important set of reactions involving tetrahydrofolate and dihydrofolate constitutes the "dTMP cycle" (Figure 33–2, reaction 2), which supplies the dTMP required for DNA synthesis. Rapidly dividing cells, in which DNA must be rapidly synthesized, are highly sensitive to folic acid deficiency. For this reason, antifolate drugs are useful in the treatment of various infections and cancers.

D. Clinical Use and Toxicity: Folic acid deficiency is most often caused by dietary insufficiency or by malabsorption. Anemia due to folic acid deficiency is readily treated by oral folic acid supplementation. Folic acid supplements will also correct the anemia but not the neurologic deficits of vitamin B_{12} deficiency. Therefore, vitamin B_{12} deficiency must be ruled out before one selects folic acid as the sole therapeutic agent in the treatment of a patient with megaloblastic anemia. Folic acid has no recognized toxicity.

HEMATOPOIETIC GROWTH FACTORS

Almost a dozen glycoprotein hormones that regulate the differentiation and maturation of stem cells within the bone marrow have been discovered. Four growth factors, produced by recombinant DNA technology, have FDA approval for treatment of patients with blood cell deficiencies.

> **Skill Keeper: Routes of Administration**
> **(see Chapter 1)**
>
> All of the recombinant hematopoietic growth factors approved for clinical use are administered by injection.
>
> 1. Why can't the hematopoietic growth factors be given orally?
> 2. Which three routes of administration require drug injection? How do these three routes compare with regard to onset and duration of drug action and risk of adverse effects?
>
> *The Skill Keeper Answers appear at the end of the chapter.*

A. Erythropoietin: Erythropoietin is produced by the kidney; reduction in its synthesis is responsible for the anemia of renal failure. Through activation of specific receptors on erythroid progenitors in the bone marrow, erythropoietin stimulates the production of red cells and increases their release from the bone marrow.

Erythropoietin is routinely used for the anemias associated with renal failure and is sometimes effective for patients with other forms of anemia, eg, primary bone marrow disorders or anemias secondary to cancer chemotherapy or zidovudine treatment, bone marrow transplantation, AIDS, or cancer. Erythropoietin's toxicity is minimal and usually results from excessive increase in hematocrit.

B. Myeloid Growth Factors: Filgrastim (granulocyte colony-stimulating factor; G-CSF) and sargramostim (granulocyte-macrophage colony-stimulating factor; GM-CSF) stimulate the production and function of neutrophils. GM-CSF also stimulates the production of other myeloid and megakaryocyte progenitors. G-CSF and, to a lesser degree, GM-CSF mobilize hematopoietic stem cells, ie, increase their concentration in peripheral blood.

Both growth factors are used to accelerate the recovery of neutrophils after cancer chemotherapy and to treat other forms of secondary and primary neutropenia (eg, aplastic anemia, congenital neutropenia). When given to patients soon after autologous stem cell transplantation, G-CSF reduces the time to engraftment and the duration of neutropenia. G-CSF is used to mobilize peripheral blood stem cells (PBSCs) in preparation for autologous and allogeneic stem cell transplantation. The toxicity of G-CSF is minimal, though the drug sometimes causes bone pain. GM-CSF can cause more severe effects, including fever, arthralgias, and capillary damage with edema. Allergic reactions are rare.

C. Megakaryocyte Growth Factors: Oprelvekin (interleukin-11, IL-11) and thrombopoietin stimulate the growth of primitive megakaryocytic progenitors and increase the number of peripheral platelets. IL-11 is used for treatment of patients who have had a prior episode of thrombocytopenia after a cycle of cancer chemotherapy. In such patients, it reduces the need for platelet transfusions. The most common side effects of IL-11 are fatigue, headache, dizziness, and fluid retention. Thrombopoietin's effects appear to be similar to those of IL-11.

D. Other Hematopoietic Growth Factors: Other growth factors include monocyte colony stimulating factor (M-CSF), stem cell factor (SCF), and interleukins-3, -6, and -9. SCF and interleukin-3 have the broadest progenitor cell line effects, including red cell, granulocyte, monocyte-macrophage, megakaryocyte, eosinophil, and basophil cell lines.

DRUG LIST

The following drugs are important members of the group discussed in this chapter. Prototypes should be learned in detail; features of the major variants should be known well enough to distinguish the variants from prototypes and from each other; the other significant agents should be recognized as belonging to a specific subclass.

Subclass	Prototype	Major Variants	Other Significant Agents
Oral iron supplements	Ferrous sulfate		Ferrous gluconate, ferrous fumarate
Parenteral iron	Iron dextran		
Vitamin B_{12}	Cyanocobalamin	Hydroxocobalamin	
Folates	Folic acid		
Red cell factor	Erythropoietin (epoetin alfa)		
Myeloid growth factors	Filgrastim (G-CSF)	Sargramostim (GM-CSF)	
Megakaryocyte factors	Oprelvekin (interleukin-11, IL-11)	Thrombopoietin	

QUESTIONS

DIRECTIONS: Each of the numbered items or incomplete statements in this section is followed by answers or by completions of the statement. Select the ONE lettered answer or completion that is BEST in each case.

Items 1–4: A 23-year-old pregnant woman is referred by her obstetrician for evaluation of anemia. She is in her fourth month of pregnancy and has no previous history of anemia; her grandfather had pernicious anemia. Her hemoglobin is 10 g/dL (normal, 12–16 g/dL).

1. If this woman has macrocytic anemia, an increased serum concentration of transferrin, and a normal serum concentration of vitamin B_{12}, the most likely cause of her anemia is deficiency of
- **(A)** Cobalamin
- **(B)** Erythropoietin
- **(C)** Folic acid
- **(D)** Intrinsic factor
- **(E)** Iron

2. If the patient had the deficiency identified in Question 1, her infant would have a higher than normal risk of
- **(A)** A neural tube defect
- **(B)** Cardiac abnormality
- **(C)** Congential neutropenia
- **(D)** Kidney damage
- **(E)** Limb deformity

3. The laboratory data for your pregnant patient indicate that she does not have a macrocytic anemia but instead has a typical microcytic anemia of pregnancy. Optimal treatment of normocytic or mild microcytic anemia associated with pregnancy utilizes
- **(A)** A high-fiber diet
- **(B)** Erythropoietin injections
- **(C)** Ferrous sulfate tablets
- **(D)** Folic acid supplements
- **(E)** Hydroxocobalamin injections

4. If this patient has a young child at home and is taking iron-containing prenatal supplements, she should be warned that they are a common source of accidental poisoning in young children and advised to make a special effort to keep these pills out of her child's reach. Toxicity associated with acute iron poisoning usually includes
- **(A)** Dizziness, hypertension, and cerebral hemorrhage
- **(B)** Hyperthermia, delirium, and coma
- **(C)** Hypotension, cardiac arrhythmias, and seizures
- **(D)** Necrotizing gastroenteritis, shock, and metabolic acidosis
- **(E)** Severe hepatic injury, encephalitis, and coma

5. The iron stored in intestinal mucosal cells is complexed to

(A) Ferritin
(B) Intrinsic factor
(C) Oprelvekin
(D) Transcobalamin II
(E) Transferrin

6. Which of the following is most likely to be required by a 5-year-old boy with chronic renal insufficiency?
(A) Erythropoietin
(B) G-CSF
(C) Interleukin-11
(D) Stem cell factor
(E) Thrombopoietin

7. Relative to G-CSF, GM-CSF
(A) Has greater oral bioavailability
(B) Is more likely to cause thrombocytopenia
(C) Is more likely to elicit an allergic reaction
(D) Is more likely to prevent fevers in neutropenic patients
(E) Stimulates production of a wider variety of hematopoietic stem cells

8. An important biochemical consequence of vitamin B_{12} deficiency is accumulation of
(A) Dihydrofolate
(B) dTMP
(C) Folic acid
(D) N^5-methyltetrahydrofolate
(E) Tetrahydrofolate

Items 9–10: After undergoing surgery for breast cancer, a 53-year-old woman is scheduled to receive four cycles of cancer chemotherapy. The cycles are to be administered every 3–5 weeks. Her first cycle was complicated by severe chemotherapy-induced thrombocytopenia.

9. During the second cycle of chemotherapy, it would be appropriate to consider treating this patient with
(A) Erythropoietin
(B) G-CSF
(C) Interleukin-11
(D) Stem cell factor
(E) Vitamin B_{12}

10. Twenty months after finishing her chemotherapy, the woman had a relapse of breast cancer. The cancer was now unresponsive to standard doses of chemotherapy. The decision was made to treat the patient with high-dose chemotherapy followed by autologous stem cell transplantation. Which of the following drugs is most likely to be used to mobilize the peripheral blood stem cells needed for the patient's autologous stem cell transplantation?
(A) Erythropoietin
(B) G-CSF
(C) Interleukin-11
(D) Intrinsic factor
(E) Thrombopoietin

ANSWERS

1. Deficiencies of folic acid or vitamin B_{12} are the most common causes of megaloblastic anemia. If a patient with this type of anemia has a normal serum vitamin B_{12} concentration, folate deficiency is the most likely cause of the anemia. The answer is **(C).**
2. Deficiency of folic acid during early pregnancy is associated with increased risk of a neural tube defect in the newborn. In the USA, cereals and grains are supplemented with folic acid in an effort to decrease the incidence of neural tube defects. The answer is **(A).**
3. The anemia usually associated with pregnancy is a simple iron deficiency microcytic anemia. In this condition, only oral iron supplementation is indicated. The answer is **(C).**
4. Acute iron poisoning often causes severe gastrointestinal damage due to direct corrosive ef-

fects, shock due to fluid loss in the gastrointestinal tract, and metabolic acidosis due to cellular dysfunction. The answer is **(D).**

5. The iron stored in intestinal mucosal cells and cells of the reticuloendothelial system is complexed with ferritin. The answer is **(A).**
6. The kidney produces erythropoietin; patients with chronic renal insufficiency often require exogenous erythropoietin to avoid chronic anemia. The answer is **(A).**
7. GM-CSF has wider biologic activity than G-CSF; it stimulates early myeloid stem cells in addition to stimulating cells destined to become neutrophils. The answer is **(E).**
8. The conversion of N^5-methyltetrahydrofolate to methyltetrahydrofolate requires adequate supplies of cobalamin (vitamin B_{12}). In vitamin B_{12} deficiency, N^5-methyltetrahydrofolate accumulates, whereas supplies of dihydrofolate, tetrahydrofolate, and dTMP are depleted. The answer is **(D).**
9. Interleukin-11 stimulates platelet production and decreases the number of platelet transfusions required by patients undergoing bone marrow-suppressive therapy for cancer. The answer is **(C).**
10. The success of transplantation with peripheral blood stem cells depends upon infusion of adequate numbers of hematopoietic stem cells. Administration of G-CSF to the donor (in the case of autologous transplantation, the patient who also will be the recipient of the transplantation) greatly increases the number of hematopoietic stem cells harvested from the donor's blood and available for the transplantation procedure. The answer is **(B).**

Skill Keeper Answers: Routes of Administration (see Chapter 1)

1. All of the hematopoietic growth factors are proteins with molecular weights greater than 15,000. Like other proteinaceous drugs, the growth factors cannot be administered orally because they have such poor bioavailability. Their peptide bonds are destroyed by stomach acid and digestive enzymes.
2. Injections are required for the intravenous, intramuscular, and subcutaneous routes of administration. The intravenous route offers the fastest onset of drug action and shortest duration of drug action. Because the intravenous route can produce high blood levels, this route of administration has the most risk of producing concentration-dependent drug toxicity. Intramuscular injection has a quicker onset of action than subcutaneous injection, and larger volumes of injected fluid can be given. Because protective barriers may be breached by the needle or injection tubing used for drug injection, all three of these routes of administration carry a greater risk of infection than does oral drug administration.

34 Drugs Used in Coagulation Disorders

OBJECTIVES

You should be able to:

- List the three major classes of anticlotting drugs and compare their utility in venous and arterial thromboses.
- Name four types of anticoagulants and describe their mechanisms of action.
- Explain why the onset of warfarin's action is relatively slow.
- Compare the oral anticoagulants, standard heparin, and low-molecular-weight heparins in terms of their pharmacokinetics, mechanisms, and toxicities.
- Give several examples of warfarin's role in pharmacokinetic and pharmacodynamic drug interactions.
- Diagram the role of activated platelets at the site of a damaged blood vessel wall and show where the four major classes of antiplatelet drugs act.
- Compare the pharmacokinetics, clinical uses and toxicity of the major antiplatelet drugs.
- List three different drugs used to treat disorders of excessive bleeding.

Learn the definitions that follow.

Table 34–1. Definitions.

Term	Definition
Antithrombin III	An endogenous anticlotting protein that irreversibly inactivates thrombin and factor X. Its enzymatic action is markedly accelerated by heparin
Clotting cascade	System of serine proteases and substrates in the plasma and tissues that provides for very rapid generation of clotting factors to prevent loss of blood when damage occurs to a vessel
Extrinsic pathway	Factors in tissues that are important in triggering the clotting process
Glycoprotein IIb/IIIa	A large protein complex located on the surface of platelets. When activated by binding to fibrin or several other ligands, it triggers platelet aggregation
Intrinsic pathway	Factors in the plasma that are activated for clotting, eg, VII, IX, X, II
LMW heparins	Low molecular weight (LMW) heparins are preparations of heparin fractions of molecular weight 2000–6000. Regular heparin has a molecular weight range of 5000–30,000
Partial thromboplastin time (PTT)	Laboratory test used to monitor the anticoagulant effect of regular heparin; prolonged when drug effect is adequate
Prothrombin time test (PT)	Laboratory test used to monitor the anticoagulant effect of warfarin; prolonged when drug effect is adequate

CONCEPTS

The drugs used in clotting and bleeding disorders fall into two primary groups: (1) drugs used in patients at risk of vascular occlusion to decrease clotting or dissolve clots already present, and (2) drugs used to increase clotting in patients with clotting deficiencies (Figure 34–1). All of these drugs act at some point within the clotting process or cascade (as shown in Figure 34–2), a series of enzyme activation steps that originate within the blood itself (intrinsic system) or in tissues (extrinsic system).

The anticlotting drugs are used in the treatment of myocardial infarction and other acute coronary syndromes, atrial fibrillation, ischemic stroke, and deep vein thrombosis (DVT). The **anticoagulant** and **thrombolytic** drugs are effective in treatment of both venous and arterial thrombosis. **Antiplatelet** drugs are used primarily for treatment of arterial disease.

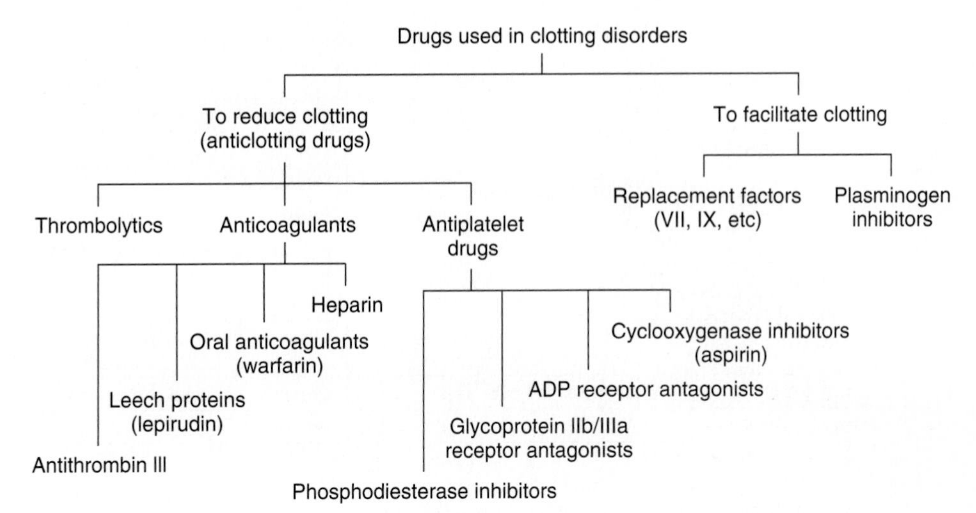

Figure 34–1. Classes of drugs used in the treatment of clotting disorders.

ANTICOAGULANTS

A. Classification and Prototypes: Anticoagulants reduce the formation of fibrin clots. Two major types of anticoagulants are available: heparin and its derivatives, which must be used parenterally; and the orally active coumarin derivatives (eg, warfarin). The two groups differ in their chemistry, pharmacokinetics, and pharmacodynamics (Table 34–2). Two other anticoagulant proteins are available: **lepirudin,** a recombinant form of hirudin, a protein found in leech saliva; and **human antithrombin III,** a commercial preparation of an endogenous human anticoagulant.

B. Heparin:

1. Chemistry: Heparin is a large sulfated polysaccharide polymer obtained from animal

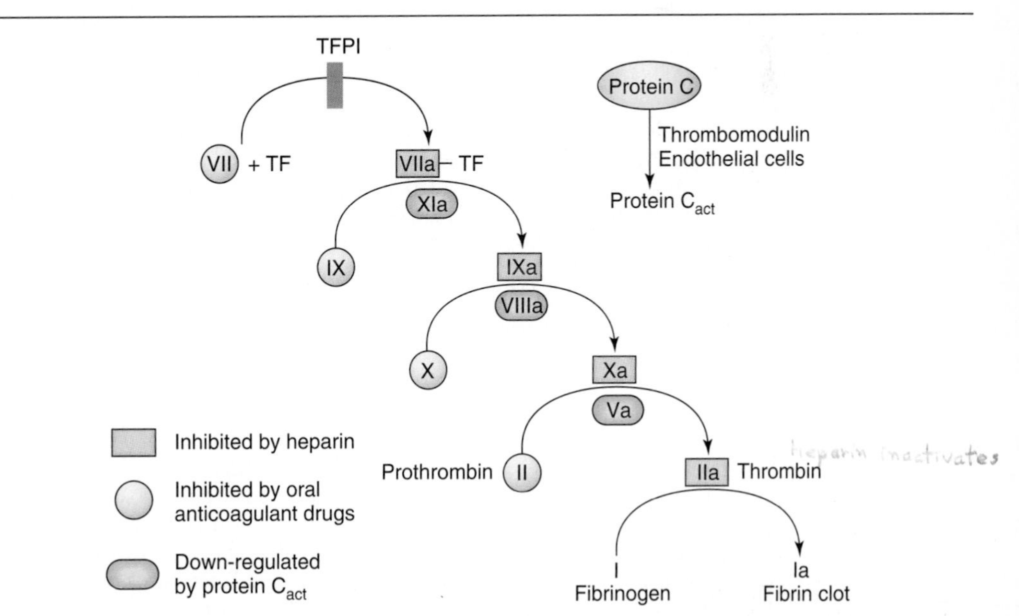

Figure 34–2. A model of drug coagulation showing the intrinsic system cascade. The extrinsic system generates tissue factor (TF), which is important in maintaining the velocity of the intrinsic system cascade. (Reproduced, with permission, from Katzung BG [editor]: *Basic & Clinical Pharmacology,* 8th ed. McGraw-Hill, 2001.)

Table 34–2. Properties of heparins and warfarin.

Property	Heparins	Warfarin
Structure	Large polymers, acidic	Small lipid-soluble molecule
Route of administration	Parenteral	Oral
Site of action	Blood	Liver
Onset of action	Rapid (seconds)	Slow, limited by half-lives of factors being replaced
Mechanism of action	Activates antithrombin III	Impairs synthesis of factors II, VII, IX, X
Monitoring	aPTT for regular heparin but not LMW heparins	PT
Antidote	Protamine (for regular heparin but not LMW heparins)	Vitamin K, plasma
Use	Mostly acute, over days	Chronic, over weeks to months
Use in pregnancy	Yes	No

sources. Each batch contains molecules of varying size with an average molecular weight of 15,000–20,000. Heparin is highly acidic and can be neutralized by basic molecules (eg, **protamine**). Heparin must be given parenterally (intravenously or subcutaneously). Intramuscular injection is avoided because of the risk of hematoma formation.

Low-molecular-weight (LMW) fractions of heparin have been developed. These (eg, enoxaparin) have molecular weights of 2000–6000. LMW heparins have greater bioavailability and longer durations of action than regular heparin; thus, doses can be given less frequently, eg, once or twice a day. They are given subcutaneously. Danaparoid, a heparan, is chemically distinct from heparin (no cross-hypersensitivity) and can be given intravenously or subcutaneously.

2. **Mechanism and effects:** Regular heparin binds to and activates endogenous antithrombin III (ATIII). The heparin-ATIII complex combines with and inactivates thrombin (activated factor II) and several other factors, especially factor X. In the presence of heparin, antithrombin III inhibits the coagulation factors approximately 1000-fold faster than in its absence. Low doses of heparin also coat the endothelial walls of vessels and reduce the activation of clotting elements by these cells. Because it acts on preformed blood components, heparin is also active in vitro—almost instantaneously. The action of heparin is monitored with the activated partial thromboplastin time laboratory test (aPTT or PTT).

   Low-molecular-weight heparins, like regular heparin, bind ATIII, and this complex has the same inhibitory effect on factor X as the regular heparin-ATIII complex. However, the short-chain heparin-ATIII complex has a smaller effect on thrombin. The aPTT test does not reliably measure the anticoagulant effect of the LMW heparins; this is a potential problem especially in renal failure, where their clearance may be decreased. Lepirudin is a powerful and selective thrombin inhibitor that can inactivate thrombin within a developing clot. This drug is relatively free of effects on platelets.
3. **Clinical use:** Because of its rapid effect, heparin is used when anticoagulation is needed immediately (eg, when starting therapy). Common uses include treatment of deep-vein thrombosis (DVT), pulmonary embolism, and acute myocardial infarction. Heparin is used in combination with thrombolytics for revascularization and in combination with glycoprotein IIb/IIIa inhibitors during angioplasty and placement of coronary stents. Because it does not cross the placental barrier, it is the drug of choice when an anticoagulant must be used in pregnancy. LMW heparins have similar clinical applications.

   Lepirudin is used for treatment of patients who have thrombosis and thrombocytopenia as a result of an antibody-mediated reaction to heparin (see below). Antithrombin III is used for treatment of patients who need anticoagulation but are resistant to heparin because of a genetic deficiency in antithrombin III and also in some cases of acquired antithrombin III deficiency (eg, disseminated intravascular coagulation).
4. **Toxicity:** Increased bleeding is the most common adverse effect of regular and LMW heparins and may result in hemorrhagic stroke. Additive interactions with other anticlotting drugs often occur. Regular heparin causes moderate transient thrombocytopenia in many patients and severe thrombocytopenia and thrombosis in a small percentage of patients who

produce an antibody that binds to a complex of heparin and platelet factor 4. LMW heparins and danaparoid are less likely to cause this immune-mediated thrombocytopenia. Prolonged use of regular heparin is associated with osteoporosis.

C. **Coumarin Anticoagulants:**

1. **Chemistry and pharmacokinetics:** The coumarin anticoagulants (eg, **warfarin**) are small, lipid-soluble molecules that are readily absorbed after oral administration. They cross the placental barrier readily and are potentially dangerous to the fetus. Warfarin is highly bound to plasma proteins (> 99%), and its elimination depends upon metabolism by hepatic cytochrome P450.
2. **Mechanism and effects:** Coumarins interfere with the normal posttranslational modification of clotting factors in the liver, a process that depends on vitamin K. The vitamin K-dependent factors include II (thrombin), VII, IX, and X. Because these factors have half-lives of 8–60 hours in the plasma, an anticoagulant effect is observed only after sufficient time has passed for the preformed normal factors to be eliminated. The action of warfarin can be reversed with vitamin K, but recovery requires the synthesis of new normal clotting factors and is therefore slow (6–24 hours). More rapid reversal can be achieved by transfusion with fresh or frozen plasma that contains normal clotting factors. The effect of warfarin is monitored by means of the prothrombin time (PT, or "pro time") test.
3. **Clinical use:** Warfarin is used for chronic anticoagulation in all of the clinical situations described above for heparin except in pregnant women.
4. **Toxicity:** Bleeding is the most important adverse effect of warfarin. Early in therapy, a period of hypercoagulability with subsequent dermal vascular necrosis can occur. This is due to deficiency of protein C, an endogenous vitamin K-dependent anticoagulant with a relatively short half-life. Warfarin can cause bone defects and hemorrhage in the developing fetus and therefore is contraindicated in pregnancy.

   Because warfarin has a narrow therapeutic window, its involvement in drug interactions is of major concern. Cytochrome P450-inducing drugs (eg, barbiturates, carbamazepine, phenytoin) increase warfarin's clearance and reduce the anticoagulant effect of a given dose. Cytochrome P450 inhibitors (eg, amiodarone, cimetidine, disulfiram) reduce warfarin's clearance and increase the anticoagulant effect of a given dose.

Skill Keeper: Treatment of Atrial Fibrillation (see Chapters 13 and 14)

Patients with chronic atrial fibrillation—a common supraventricular arrhythmia—routinely receive warfarin to prevent the development of blood clots in the poorly contracting atrium and to decrease the risk of embolism of such clots to the brain or other tissues. Such patients are also often treated with antiarrhythmic drugs. The primary goals of antiarrhythmic treatment are to slow the atrial rate and, most importantly, control the ventricular rate.

1. Which antiarrhythmic drugs are most appropriate for treating chronic atrial fibrillation?
2. Do any of these drugs have significant interactions with warfarin?

The Skill Keeper Answers appear at the end of the chapter.

ANTIPLATELET DRUGS

Platelet aggregation plays a central role in the clotting process and is especially important in clots that form in the arterial circulation. Platelets are believed to be especially important in coronary and cerebral artery occlusion. Platelet aggregation is facilitated by thromboxane, adenosine diphosphate (ADP), fibrin, serotonin, and other substances. Prostacyclin and increased intracellular cAMP inhibit aggregation.

A. **Classification and Prototypes:** Antiplatelet drugs include **aspirin** and other nonsteroidal anti-inflammatory drugs (NSAIDs), **dipyridamole** and inhibitors of ADP receptors (**ticlopidine** and **clopidogrel**), and glycoprotein IIb/IIIa receptor inhibitors (**abciximab, tirofiban,** and **eptifibatide**). These drugs increase bleeding time, a test used to monitor their effects.

B. **Mechanism of Action:** Aspirin and other NSAIDs inhibit thromboxane synthesis by blocking the enzyme cyclooxygenase. Thromboxane A_2 is a potent stimulator of platelet aggregation. Aspirin is particularly effective because it irreversibly inactivates the enzyme. Because the platelet lacks the machinery for synthesis of new protein, inhibition by aspirin persists until new platelets are formed (several days). Other NSAIDs cause a less persistent antiplatelet effect (hours).

Ticlopidine's and clopidogrel's mechanism of action involves irreversible inhibition of the ADP-receptor and thereby inhibition of ADP-mediated platelet aggregation.

Abciximab is a monoclonal antibody that reversibly inhibits the binding of fibrin and other ligands to the platelet glycoprotein IIb/IIIa receptor, a cell surface protein that is involved in platelet cross-linking. Eptifibatide and tirofiban also reversibly block the glycoprotein IIb/IIIa receptor.

The mechanism of dipyridamole is not well understood, but the drug may increase cAMP in platelets by inhibiting phosphodiesterases.

C. **Clinical Use:** Aspirin is used to prevent further infarcts in individuals who have had one or more myocardial infarcts and may also reduce the incidence of first infarcts. The drug is also used extensively to prevent transient ischemic attacks (TIAs), ischemic stroke, and other thrombotic events.

Clopidogrel and ticlopidine are effective in preventing transient ischemic attacks and ischemic strokes, especially in patients who cannot tolerate aspirin. These drugs prevent thrombosis in patients who have recently received a coronary artery stent.

The glycoprotein IIb/IIIa inhibitors prevent restenosis after coronary angioplasty and are used in acute coronary syndromes (eg, unstable angina and non-Q wave acute myocardial infarction).

D. **Toxicity:** Aspirin and other NSAIDs cause gastrointestinal and CNS effects (see Chapter 35). All antiplatelet drugs significantly enhance the effects of other anticlotting agents. Ticlopidine causes bleeding in up to 5% of patients and severe neutropenia in about 1%. Clopidogrel may be less hematotoxic. The major toxicities of the glycoprotein IIb/IIIa drugs are bleeding and, with chronic use, thrombocytopenia.

THROMBOLYTIC AGENTS

A. **Classification and Prototypes:** (Table 34–3) The thrombolytic drugs currently available are alteplase and reteplase (forms of tissue plasminogen activator, t-PA), anistreplase, urokinase, and streptokinase. All are given intravenously.

B. **Mechanism of Action:** Plasmin is the normal endogenous fibrinolytic enzyme. By splitting fibrin into fragments, plasmin promotes the breakdown and dissolution of clots (Figure 34–3). The thrombolytic enzymes catalyze the activation of the inactive precursor, plasminogen, to plasmin.

1. **Tissue plasminogen activator:** t-PA is a large human protein that directly converts fibrin-bound plasminogen to plasmin (Figure 34–3). In theory, this selectivity for plasminogen that has already bound to fibrin (ie, a clot) should result in greater selectivity and less danger of spontaneous bleeding. In fact, t-PA's selectivity appears to be quite limited. Alteplase is normal human plasminogen activator. Reteplase is a mutated form of human t-PA with similar effects but a slightly faster onset of action and longer duration of action.
2. **Urokinase:** Urokinase is extracted from cultured human kidney cells. Like t-PA, this human enzyme directly converts plasminogen to plasmin.
3. **Streptokinase:** Streptokinase is obtained from bacterial cultures. Though not itself an enzyme, it forms a complex with endogenous plasminogen. The complex catalyzes the rapid conversion of plasminogen to plasmin.
4. **Anistreplase:** This anisoylated plasminogen-streptokinase activator complex (APSAC) is a prodrug. As the anisoyl group is hydrolyzed in vivo (a slow, spontaneous process), the

Table 34–3. Properties of thrombolytic enzymes.

Agent	Source	Duration of Action	Comments
Alteplase, reteplase	Recombinant human protein	2–10 min	Active tissue plasminogen activator, (t-PA); converts plasminogen to plasmin; intravenous infusion (alteplase) or bolus doses (reteplase) required. Most expensive. Reteplase is somewhat longer-acting than alteplase
Anistreplase	Prodrug: streptokinase plus recombinant human plasminogen	1–2 hours	Slowly releases streptokinase-activated plasminogen; single bolus administration provides long duration of action
Streptokinase	Bacterial product	20–25 min	Streptokinase combines with plasminogen; the combination activates plasminogen to plasmin; intravenous infusion required. Least expensive
Urokinase	Human kidney cell culture	< 20 min	Active plasminogen activator

streptokinase-activated plasminogen is released and converts endogenous plasminogen to plasmin. This slow release provides for the relatively long half-life of this drug.

C. Clinical Use: The major application of the thrombolytic agents is in the emergency treatment of coronary artery thrombosis. Under ideal conditions (ie, treatment within 1–4 hours), these agents may cause prompt recanalization of the occluded vessel. Very prompt use (ie, within 3 hours of the first symptoms) of t-PA in patients with ischemic stroke appears to result in a significantly better clinical outcome. Cerebral hemorrhage must be positively ruled out before such use. The thrombolytic agents are also used in cases of multiple pulmonary emboli.

D. Toxicity: Bleeding is the most important hazard and has about the same frequency with all of these drugs. Cerebral hemorrhage is the most serious manifestation. Streptokinase, a bacterial protein, often evokes the production of antibodies and loses its effectiveness or even induces severe allergic reactions upon subsequent therapy. Patients who have had streptococcal infections may have preformed antibodies to the drug. Because they are human proteins, urokinase and t-PA are not subject to this problem. However, they (and anistreplase) are much more expensive than streptokinase and not much more effective.

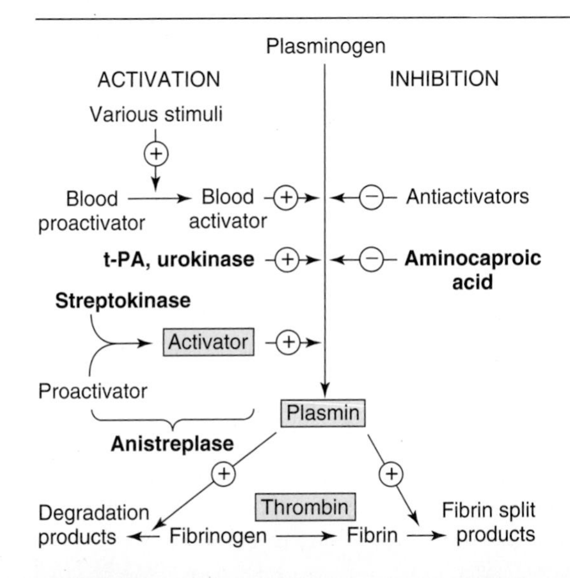

Figure 34–3. Diagram of the fibrinolytic system. The useful thrombolytic drugs are shown on the left in **bold** type. These drugs increase the formation of plasmin, the major fibrinolytic enzyme. The "activator" shown in the shaded box is a complex of streptokinase and plasminogen. Aminocaproic acid, a useful inhibitor of fibrinolysis, is shown on the right. (Reproduced, with permission, from Katzung BG [editor]: *Basic & Clinical Pharmacology,* 8th ed. McGraw-Hill, 2001.)

DRUGS USED IN BLEEDING DISORDERS

Inadequate blood clotting may result from vitamin K deficiency, genetically determined errors of clotting factor synthesis (eg, hemophilia), a variety of drug-induced conditions, and thrombocytopenia. Treatment, therefore, involves administration of vitamin K, preformed clotting factors, or antiplasmin drugs. Thrombocytopenia may be treated by administration of platelets.

A. **Vitamin K:** Deficiency of vitamin K, a fat-soluble vitamin, is particularly common in newborns and in older individuals with abnormalities of fat absorption. The deficiency is readily treated with oral or parenteral vitamin K supplements using phytonadione (K_1) or menadione (K_2). In the USA, all newborns receive an injection of phytonadione. Large doses of vitamin K_1 are used to reverse the anticoagulant effect of excess warfarin.

B. **Clotting Factors:** The most important agents used to treat hemophilia are fresh plasma and purified human blood clotting factors, especially **factor VIII** and **factor IX,** that are either purified from blood products or produced by recombinant DNA technology. These products are extremely expensive and carry a risk of infection (due to contamination by blood-borne pathogens) and immunologic reactions.

C. **Antiplasmin Agents:** Antiplasmin agents are valuable for the management of acute bleeding episodes in hemophiliacs and others with bleeding disorders. **Aminocaproic acid** and **tranexamic acid** are orally active agents that inhibit fibrinolysis by inhibiting plasminogen activation (Figure 34–3).

DRUG LIST

The following drugs are important members of the group discussed in this chapter. Prototypes should be learned in detail; features of the major variants should be known well enough to distinguish the variants from prototypes and from each other; the other significant agents should be recognized as belonging to a specific subclass.

Subclass	Prototype	Major Variants	Other Significant Agents
Anticoagulants			
Parenteral	Heparin	Enoxaparin	Dalteparin, danaparoid, antithombin III
Oral	Warfarin		
Antiplatelet drugs			
Cyclooxygenase inhibitors	Aspirin		
ADP receptor antagonists	Clopidogrel	Ticlopidine	
Glycoprotein IIb/IIIa inhibitors	Abciximab		Eptifibatide, tirofiban
Other	Dipyridamole		
Thrombolytic drugs	Streptokinase, alteplase	Reteplase	Anistreplase, urokinase
Clotting factors	Factor VIII	Factor IX	
Vitamin K	Phytonadione (K_1)		Menadione (K_2)
Antiplasmin drugs	Aminocaproic acid		Tranexamic acid

QUESTIONS

DIRECTIONS: Each of the numbered items or incomplete statements in this section is followed by answers or by completions of the statement. Select the ONE lettered answer or completion that is BEST in each case.

Items 1–3: A 58-year-old business executive is brought to the emergency room 2 hours after the onset of severe chest pain during a vigorous tennis game. She has a history of poorly controlled mild hypertension and elevated blood cholesterol but does not smoke. ECG changes confirm the diagnosis of myocardial infarction. The decision is made to attempt to open her occluded artery.

1. Conversion of plasminogen to plasmin is brought about by
   (A) Aminocaproic acid
   (B) Heparin
   (C) Lepirudin
   (D) Reteplase
   (E) Warfarin

2. If a fibrinolytic drug is used for treatment of this woman's acute myocardial infarction, the adverse drug effect that is most likely to occur is
   (A) Acute renal failure
   (B) Development of antiplatelet antibodies
   (C) Encephalitis secondary to liver dysfunction
   (D) Hemorrhagic stroke
   (E) Neutropenia

3. If this patient undergoes a percutaneous coronary procedure and placement of a stent in a coronary blood vessel, she may be given eptifibatide. The mechanism of eptifibatide's anticlotting action is
   (A) Activation of antithrombin III
   (B) Blockade of posttranslational modification of clotting factors
   (C) Inhibition of thromboxane production
   (D) Irreversible inhibition of platelet ADP receptors
   (E) Reversible inhibition of glycoprotein IIb/IIIa receptors

4. The following changes in plasma concentration of warfarin were observed in a patient when two other agents, drugs B and C, were given on a daily basis at constant dosage starting at the times shown. Which of the following statements most accurately describes what is shown in the graph below?
   (A) Drug B displaces warfarin from plasma proteins; drug C displaces warfarin from tissue binding sites
   (B) Drug B inhibits hepatic metabolism of warfarin; drug C displaces drug B from tissue binding sites
   (C) Drug B stimulates hepatic metabolism of warfarin; drug C displaces warfarin from plasma protein
   (D) Drug B increases renal clearance of warfarin; drug C inhibits hepatic metabolism of drug B

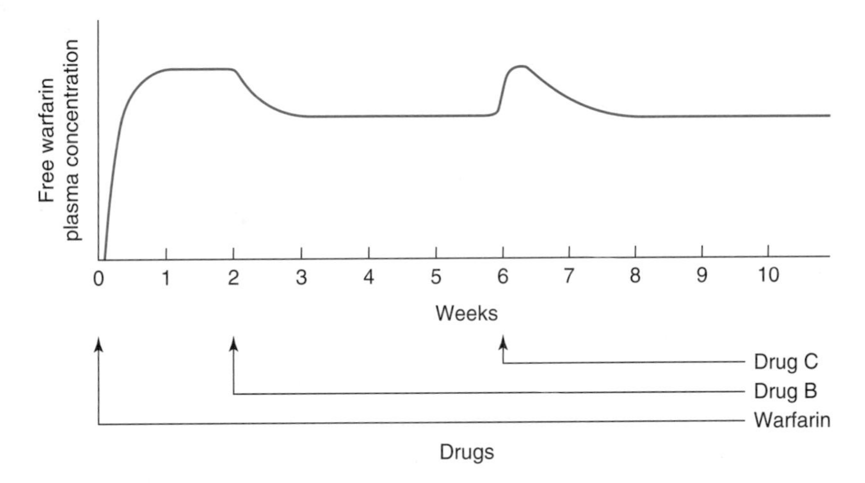

Items 5–7: A 65-year-old man is brought to the emergency room 30 minutes after the onset of right-sided weakness and aphasia (difficulty speaking). Imaging studies ruled out cerebral hemorrhage as the cause of his acute symptoms of stroke.

5. Prompt administration of which of the following drugs is most likely to improve this patient's clinical outcome?
   (A) Abciximab
   (B) Alteplase
   (C) Factor VIII
   (D) Streptokinase
   (E) Vitamin K
6. Over the next 2 days, the patient's symptoms resolved completely. To prevent a recurrence of this disease, the patient is most likely to be treated indefinitely with
   (A) Aminocaproic acid
   (B) Aspirin
   (C) Enoxaparin
   (D) Urokinase
   (E) Warfarin
7. If the patient is unable to tolerate the drug identified in Question 6, he may be treated with clopidogrel. Relative to ticlopidine, clopidogrel
   (A) Has a shorter duration of action
   (B) Is less likely to cause neutropenia
   (C) Is more likely to induce antiplatelet antibodies
   (D) Is more likely to precipitate serious bleeding
   (E) Will have a greater antiplatelet effect

Items 8–10: A 67-year-old woman presents with pain in her left thigh muscle. Duplex ultrasonography indicates the presence of deep vein thrombosis (DVT) in the affected limb.

8. The decision was made to treat this woman with enoxaparin. Relative to regular heparin, enoxaparin
   (A) Can be used without monitoring the patient's aPTT
   (B) Has a shorter duration of action
   (C) Is less likely to have a teratogenic effect
   (D) Is more likely to be given intravenously
   (E) Is more likely to cause thrombosis and thrombocytopenia
9. If this woman has marked resistance to heparin, she is most likely to be treated with
   (A) Abciximab
   (B) Antithrombin III
   (C) Plasminogen
   (D) Urokinase
   (E) Vitamin K_2
10. During the next week, the patient was started on warfarin and her heparin was discontinued. Two months later, she returned after a severe nosebleed. Laboratory analysis revealed an INR (international normalized ratio, the system now used for reporting results of the prothrombin time test) of 7.0 (INR value in such a warfarin-treated patient should be 2.5–3.5). In order to prevent severe hemorrhage, the warfarin should be discontinued and this patient should be treated immediately with
    (A) Alteplase
    (B) Aminocaproic acid
    (C) Factor VIII
    (D) Protamine
    (E) Vitamin K_1

ANSWERS

1. Heparin and warfarin are anticoagulants that affect activation or formation of proteins in the clotting cascade. Lepirudin is an inhibitor of thrombin, and aminocaproic acid is an inhibitor, not an activator, of fibrinolysis and the conversion of plasminogen to plasmin. Reteplase is the only thrombolytic drug listed. The answer is **(D).**
2. The most common serious adverse effect of the fibrolytics is bleeding, especially in the cerebral circulation. The fibrinolytics do not usually have serious effects upon the renal, hepatic, or hematologic systems. Unlike heparin, they do not induce antiplatelet antibodies. However,

streptokinase and anistreplase contain bacterial proteins and may induce formation of inactivating antibodies or even severe allergic reactions. The answer is **(D).**

3. Eptifibatide is a reversible inhibitor of the glycoprotein IIb/IIIa receptor, an integrin on the surface of platelets that serves as a key regulator of platelet aggregation. Glycoprotein IIb/IIIa receptor antagonists help to prevent platelet-induced occlusion of coronary stents. The answer is **(E).**
4. A drug that increases metabolism (clearance) of the anticoagulant will lower the steady state plasma concentration (both free and bound forms), whereas one that displaces the anticoagulant will increase the plasma level of the free form only until elimination of the drug has again lowered it to the steady state level. The answer is **(C).**
5. Controlled clinical trials have shown that alteplase improves the clinical outcome in patients with ischemic stroke if given within 3 hours after the onset of symptoms. Similar trials of streptokinase resulted in unacceptably high rates of bleeding. Glycoprotein IIb/IIIa receptor inhibitors like abciximab have not been tested in ischemic stroke. Vitamin K and factor VIII may actually worsen the patient's outcome. The answer is **(B).**
6. Aspirin, an irreversible inhibitor of platelet cyclooxygenase, has been shown to prevent recurrence of transient ischemic attacks and ischemic stroke. The answer is **(B).**
7. Ticlopidine and clopidogrel have similar mechanisms of action and therapeutic efficacy. The key difference between these two drugs is that clopidogrel is less likely to cause neutropenia and therefore does not require routine monitoring of blood cell counts during therapy. The answer is **(B).**
8. Enoxaparin is a low-molecular-weight (LMW) heparin. LMW heparins have a longer half-life than standard heparin and a more consistent relationship between dose and therapeutic effect. Enoxaparin is given subcutaneously, not intravenously. It is less—not more—likely to cause thrombosis and thrombocytopenia. Neither LMW heparins nor standard heparin are teratogenic. The aPTT is not useful for monitoring the effects of LMW heparins. The answer is **(A).**
9. Heparin's anticlotting effect is mediated by acceleration of the action of endogenous antithrombin III, a protease that inactivates clotting factors. Patients with genetic deficiencies in antithrombin III are resistant to heparin and prone to thrombosis. Antithrombin III isolated from pooled human plasma is available for use in such patients. The answer is **(B).**
10. The elevated INR indicates excessive anticoagulation with a high risk of hemorrhage. Warfarin should be discontinued and vitamin K_1 administered to accelerate formation of vitamin K-dependent factors. The answer is **(E).**

Skill Keeper Answers: Treatment of Atrial Fibrillation (see Chapters 13 and 14)

1. Beta adrenoceptor-blocking drugs (class II; eg, propranolol, acebutolol) and calcium channel-blocking drugs (class IV; eg, verapamil) are useful for treating atrial fibrillation because they slow AV nodal conduction and thereby help control ventricular rate. Drugs with class I or III antiarrhythmic action may be useful for maintaining sinus rhythm (eg, amiodarone). Through its vagotomimetic action, digoxin increases the effective refractory period in AV nodal tissue and decreases AV nodal conduction velocity.
2. With warfarin, one is always concerned about pharmacodynamic and pharmacokinetic drug interactions. None of the antiarrhythmic drugs mentioned above are likely to cause a pharmacodynamic interaction with warfarin. However, amiodarone is a cytochrome P450 enzyme inhibitor and increases warfarin's antithrombotic effects. Patients taking both drugs usually need to decrease their dose of warfarin.

35 Drugs Used in the Treatment of Hyperlipidemias

OBJECTIVES

You should be able to:

- Describe the proposed role of lipoproteins in the formation of atherosclerotic plaques.
- Describe the dietary management of hyperlipoproteinemia.
- List the four main classes of drugs used to treat hyperlipidemia and describe their mechanism of action, effects upon serum lipid concentrations, and adverse effects.
- Based on a set of baseline serum lipid values, propose a rational drug treatment regimen.
- Argue the merits of combined drug therapy for some diseases and list three rational drug combinations.

Learn the definitions that follow.

Table 35–1. Definitions.

Term	Definition
Apolipoproteins	Proteins located on the surface of lipoproteins; they play critical roles in the regulation of lipoprotein metabolism and uptake into cells
Chylomicrons	Largest of the lipoproteins; carry triglycerides and cholesteryl esters *from* the gut *to* the other tissues
FFA	Free fatty acids; products of triglyceride hydrolysis
HDL	High-density lipoproteins; transport cholesterol *from* the periphery *to* the liver
HMG-CoA reductase	3-Hydroxy-3-methylglutaryl-coenzyme A reductase; the enzyme that catalyzes the rate-limiting step in cholesterol biosynthesis
LDL	Low-density lipoproteins; major form in which lipid is recaptured by the liver; requires functional LDL receptors for normal endocytosis in hepatocytes
Lipoproteins	Macromolecular complexes in which lipids are transported in the blood
LPL	Lipoprotein lipase; an enzyme found in the peripheral tissue that hydrolyzes lipoproteins and depletes triglycerides in the lipoprotein complexes
PPAR-α	Peroxisome proliferator-activated receptor-alpha; one of a family of nuclear transcription regulators that participates in the regulation of metabolic processes
Triglyceride	Ester of three fatty acids with glycerol; a major form of fat storage
VLDL	Very low-density lipoproteins; secreted by the liver; the initial transporter of cholesterol and other lipids *from* the liver *to* the periphery

CONCEPTS

HYPERLIPOPROTEINEMIA

A. **Pathogenesis:** Premature or accelerated development of atherosclerosis is strongly associated with elevated levels of certain plasma lipoproteins, especially the lipoproteins associated with cholesterol transport. Elevations of low-density lipoproteins (LDL), intermediate-density lipoproteins (IDL), or very low-density lipoproteins (VLDL) constitute hyperlipoproteinemias. A *depressed* level of high-density lipoproteins (HDL) is also associated with increased risk of atherosclerosis. In some families, hypertriglyceridemia, an elevation of triglycerides, is similarly correlated with atherosclerosis. Chylomicronemia, the occurrence of chylomicrons in the serum while fasting, is a recessive trait that is correlated with a high incidence of acute pancreatitis and can be managed by restriction of total fat intake (Table 35–2).

Table 35–2. The primary hyperlipoproteinemias and their drug treatment.*

Condition	Single Drug	Drug Combination
Primary chylomicronemia (familial lipoprotein lipase or cofactor deficiency)	Dietary management	Niacin plus fibrate
Familial hypertriglyceridemia		
Severe	Niacin, fibrate	Niacin plus fibrate
Moderate	Niacin, fibrate	
Familial combined hyperlipidemia		
VLDL increased	Niacin, fibrate	
LDL increased	Niacin, reductase inhibitor, resin	Niacin plus resin or reductase inhibitor
VLDL, LDL increased	Niacin, reductase inhibitor	Niacin plus resin or reductase inhibitor
Familial dysbetalipoproteinemia	Fibrate, niacin	Fibrate plus niacin, or niacin plus reductase inhibitor
Familial hypercholesterolemia		
Heterozygous	Resin, reductase inhibitor, niacin	Two or three of the individual drugs
Homozygous	Niacin, atorvastatin	Resin plus niacin plus reductase inhibitor
LP(a) hyperlipoproteinemia	Niacin	

*Reproduced, with permission, from Katzung BG (editor): *Basic & Clinical Pharmacology,* 8th ed. McGraw-Hill, 2001.

Regulation of plasma lipoprotein levels involves a balance between dietary fat intake, hepatic processing, and utilization in peripheral tissues. Primary disturbances in regulation occur in various familial diseases. Secondary disturbances are associated with many endocrine conditions and diseases of the liver or kidneys.

The major enzymes involved in lipoprotein regulation are (1) acyl-CoA:cholesterol acyltransferase (ACAT), which esterifies some cholesterol in the core of chylomicrons; (2) lecithin:cholesterol acyltransferase (LCAT), which esterifies cholesterol and helps transfer it to LDL; (3) lipoprotein lipase (LPL), which hydrolyzes triglycerides to free fatty acids (FFA) and glycerol; and (4) 3-hydroxy-3-methylglutaryl-coenzyme A (HMG-CoA) reductase, which is essential in the synthesis of cholesterol and other steroids in the liver.

B. Treatment Strategies:

1. **Diet:** Dietary measures are the first method of management and may be sufficient to reduce lipoprotein levels to a safe range. Cholesterol and saturated fats are the primary dietary factors that contribute to elevated levels of plasma lipoproteins. Diets are designed to reduce the total intake of these substances. Alcohol intake raises triglyceride and VLDL levels.
2. **Drugs:** Drug therapy can reduce fat absorption from the intestine (resins), modify hepatic cholesterol synthesis (HMG-CoA reductase inhibitors), decrease secretion of lipoproteins (niacin), increase peripheral clearance of lipoproteins (fibrates), and can perhaps exert other effects. These drugs are all given orally (Figure 35–1).

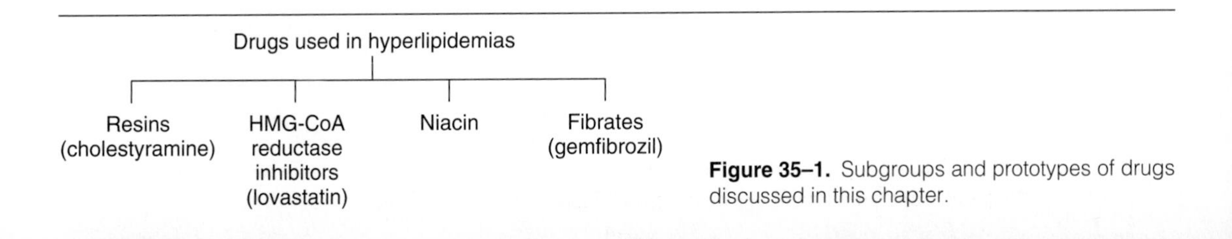

Figure 35–1. Subgroups and prototypes of drugs discussed in this chapter.

RESINS

A. Mechanism and Effects: Bile acid-binding resins (**cholestyramine** and **colestipol**) are large nonabsorbable polymers that bind bile acids and similar steroids in the intestine.

By preventing absorption of dietary cholesterol and reducing reabsorption of bile acids secreted by the liver, these agents divert hepatic cholesterol to synthesis of new bile acids, thereby reducing the availability of cholesterol for the production of plasma lipids (Figure 35–2). A compensatory increase in high-affinity LDL receptors, which increases the removal of LDL cholesterol from the blood, occurs in the liver.

The resins cause a modest reduction in LDL cholesterol (Table 35–3) but have little effect upon HDL cholesterol or triglycerides. In some patients with familial combined hyperlipidemia, resins can increase VLDL.

B. Clinical Use: The resins are used in patients with hypercholesterolemia (Table 35–2). They have also been used to reduce pruritus in patients with cholestasis and bile salt accumulation.

C. Toxicity: Adverse effects include bloating, constipation, and an unpleasant gritty taste. Absorption of vitamins (eg, vitamin K, dietary folates) and drugs (eg, digitalis, thiazides, warfarin, pravastatin, fluvastatin) may be impaired by the resins.

HMG-CoA REDUCTASE INHIBITORS

A. Mechanism and Effects: Lovastatin and simvastatin are prodrugs. The other HMG-CoA reductase inhibitors are active as given. In the body, the active drugs are structural analogs that

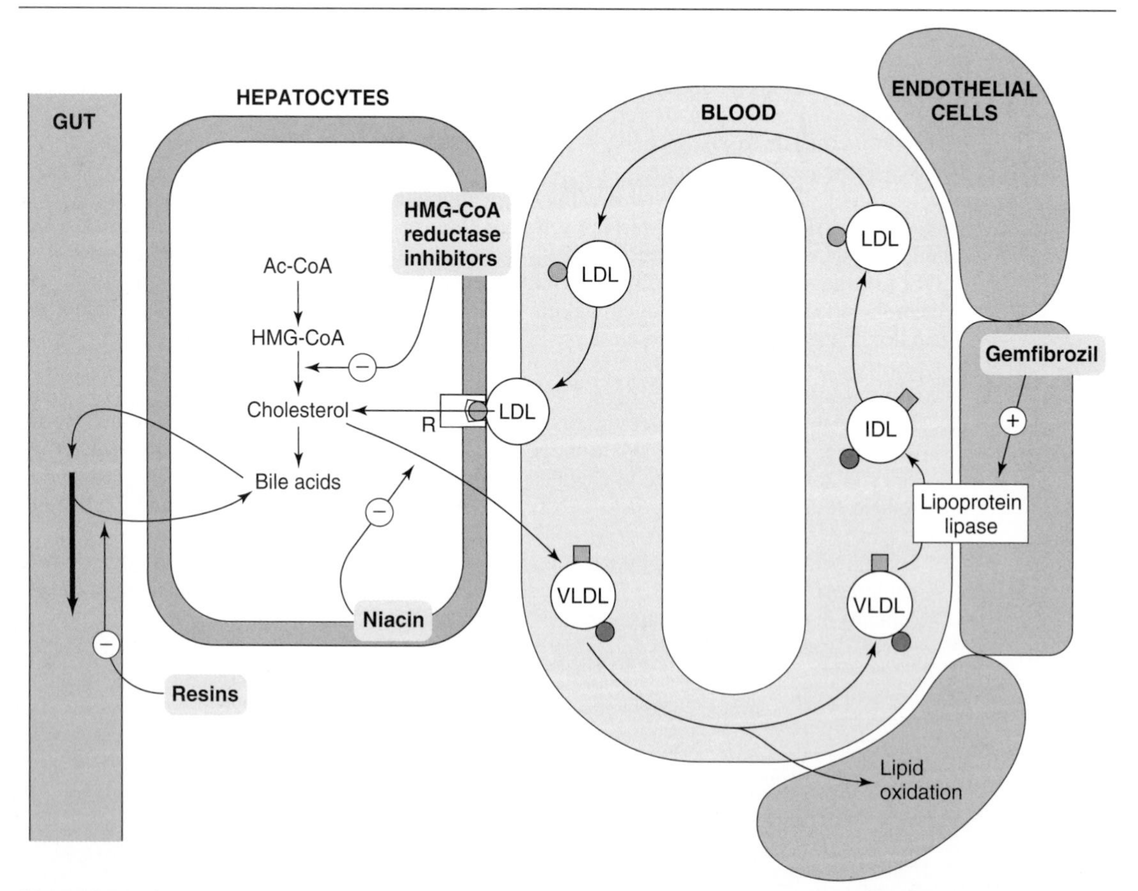

Figure 35–2. Schematic diagram of lipoprotein handling by hepatocytes and by vascular endothelial cells in vessels in peripheral tissues. The sites of action of the drugs are shown (+, stimulation; –, inhibition).

Table 35–3. Lipid-modifying effects of antihyperlipidemic drugs.*

Drug	LDL Cholesterol	HDL Cholesterol	Triglyceride
Atorvastatin	–25% to –40%	+5% to –10%	↓↓
Fluvastatin[1]	–20% to –30%	+5% to –10%	↓
Lovastatin[2]	–25% to –40%	+5% to –10%	↓
Cholestyramine, colestipol	–15% to –25%	+5%	±
Gemfibrozil	–10% to –15%	+15% to –20%	↓↓
Niacin	–15% to –40%	+25% to –35%	↓↓

*Modified, with permission, from Tierney LM, McPhee SJ, Papadakis MA (editors): *Current Medical Diagnosis & Treatment,* 40th ed. McGraw-Hill, 2001.

[1]Cerivastatin has effects similar to those of fluvastatin.

[2]Pravastatin and simvastatin have effects similar to those of lovastatin.

± = variable, if any.

competitively inhibit mevalonate synthesis by HMG-CoA reductase, a process essential for cholesterol biosynthesis in the liver (Figure 35–2). The liver compensates by increasing the number of high-affinity LDL receptors. This results in increased clearance of VLDL remnants (IDL) and LDL from the blood. Extrahepatic effects of HMG-CoA reductase inhibitors include decreases in endothelin-1 mRNA.

B. Clinical Use: "Statins" can reduce LDL cholesterol levels dramatically (see Table 35–3), especially when used in combination with other drugs (see Table 35–2). These drugs are used commonly because they are well tolerated and because large clinical trials have shown that they reduce the risk of coronary events and mortality in patients with ischemic heart disease.

Atorvastatin may have higher efficacy than the other reductase inhibitors, and it reduces triglycerides much more than the older drugs in this group. Cerivastatin and fluvastatin have less maximal efficacy than the other drugs in this group.

C. Toxicity: Mild elevations of serum aminotransferases are common but are not often associated with hepatic damage. Patients with preexisting liver disease may have more severe reactions. An increase in creatine kinase (released from skeletal muscle) is noted in about 10% of patients; in a few, severe muscle pain and even rhabdomyolysis may occur. HGM-CoA reductase inhibitors are metabolized by the cytochrome P450 system; drugs or foods (eg, grapefruit juice) that inhibit cytochrome P450 activity may increase the risk of hepatotoxicity and myopathy. Because of evidence that the HMG-CoA reductase inhibitors are teratogenic, these drugs should be avoided in pregnancy.

Skill Keeper: Angina (see Chapter 12)

The antihyperlipidemic drugs, especially the reductase inhibitors, are used very commonly to treat patients with various forms of ischemic heart disease. One of the most common manifestations of ischemic heart disease and coronary atherosclerosis is angina.

1. What are the three major forms of angina?
2. Name the three major drug groups used to treat angina and specify which form of angina each is useful for.

The Skill Keeper Answers appear at the end of the chapter.

NIACIN (NICOTINIC ACID)

A. Mechanism and Effects: Niacin (but not nicotinamide) directly reduces the secretion of VLDL from the liver (Figure 35–2) and inhibits hepatic synthesis of apolipoproteins or cholesterol. Consequently, LDL formation is reduced and there is a decrease in LDL cholesterol (Table 35–3). Increased clearance of VLDL by lipoprotein lipase in the periphery has also been demonstrated and probably accounts for the reduction in serum triglyceride concentrations. In addition, the levels of HDL may increase. Finally, niacin decreases circulating fibrinogen and increases tissue plasminogen activator.

B. Clinical Use: Because it lowers serum LDL cholesterol and triglyceride concentrations and increases HDL cholesterol concentrations, niacin has wide clinical utility (Table 35–2).

C. Toxicity: Cutaneous flushing is a common adverse effect. Pretreatment with aspirin or other NSAIDs reduces the intensity of this flushing, suggesting that it is mediated by prostaglandin release. Tolerance to the flushing reaction usually develops within a few days. Dose-dependent nausea and abdominal discomfort often occur. Pruritus and other skin conditions are reported. Moderate elevations of liver enzymes and even severe hepatotoxicity may occur. Hyperuricemia occurs in about 20% of patients, and carbohydrate tolerance may be moderately impaired.

FIBRIC ACID DERIVATIVES

A. Mechanism and Effects: Fibric acid derivatives (eg, gemfibrozil, fenofibrate, clofibrate) are ligands for the peroxisome proliferator-activated receptor-alpha (PPAR-α) protein, a receptor that regulates transcription of genes involved in lipid metabolism. This interaction with PPAR-α results in increased activity of lipoprotein lipase and enhanced clearance of triglyceride-rich lipoproteins (Figure 35–2). Cholesterol biosynthesis in the liver is secondarily reduced. The fibrates reduce serum triglyceride concentrations (Table 35–3). There may be a small reduction in LDL cholesterol and a small increase in HDL levels.

B. Clinical Use: Gemfibrozil and other fibrates are used to treat hypertriglyceridemia (Table 35–2). Because these drugs have only modest effects on LDL cholesterol, they often are combined with other cholesterol-lowering drugs for treatment of patients with elevated concentrations of both LDL and VLDL.

C. Toxicity: Nausea is the most common adverse effect with all members of this subgroup. Skin rashes are common with gemfibrozil. A few patients show decreases in white blood count or hematocrit, and these drugs can potentiate the action of anticoagulants. There is an increased risk of cholesterol gallstones; these drugs should be used with caution in patients with a history of cholelithiasis.

COMBINATION THERAPY

All patients with hyperlipidemia are treated first with dietary modification, but this is often insufficient and drugs must be added. Drug combinations are often required to achieve the maximum lowering possible with minimum toxicity and to achieve the desired effect upon the various lipoproteins (LDL, VLDL, and HDL). The most common combinations are listed in Table 35–2.

Certain drug combinations present challenges. Because resins interfere with the absorption of certain reductase inhibitors (pravastatin, cerivastatin, atorvastatin, and fluvastatin), these must be given at least 1 hour before or 4 hours after the resins. The combination of reductase inhibitors with either fibrates or niacin may increase the risk of myopathy.

DRUG LIST

The following drugs are important members of the group discussed in this chapter. Prototypes should be learned in detail; features of the major variants should be known well enough to distinguish the variants from prototypes and from each other; the other significant agents should be recognized as belonging to a specific subclass.

Subclass	Prototype	Major Variants	Other Significant Agents
Bile acid-binding resins	Cholestyramine		Colestipol
Cholesterol synthesis inhibitor	Lovastatin	Atorvastatin, pravastatin	Simvastatin, cerivastatin, fluvastatin
VLDL secretion inhibitor	Niacin		
Lipoprotein lipase stimulants	Gemfibrozil		Fenofibrate

QUESTIONS

DIRECTIONS: Each of the numbered items or incomplete statements in this section is followed by answers or by completions of the statement. Select the ONE lettered answer or completion that is BEST in each case.

1. Increased serum levels of which of the following may be associated with a *decreased* risk of atherosclerosis?
(A) Very low-density lipoproteins (VLDL)
(B) Low-density lipoproteins (LDL)
(C) Intermediate-density lipoproteins (IDL)
(D) High-density lipoproteins (HDL)
(E) Cholesterol

2. A 58-year-old man with a history of hyperlipidemia was treated with a drug. The chart below shows the results of the patient's fasting lipid panel before treatment and 6 months after initiating drug therapy. Normal values are also shown. Which of the following drugs is most likely to be the one that this man received? (All values represent mg/dL.)

Time of Lipid Measurement	Triglyceride	Total Cholesterol	LDL Cholesterol	VLDL Cholesterol	HDL Cholesterol
Before treatment	1000	640	120	500	20
Six months after starting treatment	300	275	90	150	40
Normal Values	< 150	< 200	< 130	< 30	> 35

(A) Atorvastatin
(B) Colestipol
(C) Gemfibrozil
(D) Lovastatin
(E) Niacin

Items 3–6: A 35-year-old woman appears to have familial combined hyperlipidemia. Her serum concentrations of total cholesterol, LDL cholesterol, and triglyceride are elevated. Her serum concentration of HDL cholesterol is somewhat reduced.

3. Which of the following drugs is most likely to cause an increase in this patient's triglyceride and VLDL cholesterol when used as monotherapy?
(A) Atorvastatin
(B) Cholestyramine
(C) Gemfibrozil
(D) Lovastatin
(E) Niacin

4. If this patient is pregnant, which of the following drugs should be avoided because of a risk of harming the fetus?
(A) Cholestyramine
(B) Fenofibrate

(C) Gemfibrozil
(D) Niacin
(E) Pravastatin

5. The patient is started on gemfibrozil. The major mechanism of action of gemfibrozil is
   (A) Increased excretion of bile acid salts
   (B) Increased expression of high-affinity LDL receptors
   (C) Increased lipid hydrolysis by lipoprotein lipase
   (D) Inhibition of secretion of VLDL by the liver
   (E) Reduction of secretion of HDL by the liver
6. When used as monotherapy, a major toxicity of gemfibrozil is increased risk of
   (A) Bloating and constipation
   (B) Cholelithiasis
   (C) Hyperuricemia
   (D) Liver damage
   (E) Severe cardiac arrhythmia

Items 7–10: A 43-year-old man has heterozygous familial hyperlipidemia. His serum concentrations of total cholesterol and LDL are markedly elevated. His serum concentration of HDL cholesterol, VLDL cholesterol, and triglyceride are normal or slightly elevated. This patient's mother and older brother died of myocardial infarctions before the age of 50. This patient has recently experienced mild chest pain when walking up stairs and has been diagnosed as having angina of effort. The patient is somewhat overweight. He drinks alcohol most evenings and smokes about one pack of cigarettes per week.

7. Alcohol drinking is associated with which of the following changes in serum lipid concentrations?
   (A) Decreased HDL cholesterol
   (B) Decreased IDL cholesterol
   (C) Decreased VLDL cholesterol
   (D) Increased LDL cholesterol
   (E) Increased triglyceride
8. If the patient has a history of gout, which of the following drugs is most likely to exacerbate this condition?
   (A) Colestipol
   (B) Gemfibrozil
   (C) Lovastatin
   (D) Niacin
   (E) Simvastatin
9. After being counseled about lifestyle and dietary changes, the patient was started on atorva-statin. During his treatment with atorvastatin, it is important to routinely monitor serum concentrations of
   (A) Blood urea nitrogen (BUN)
   (B) Alanine and aspartate aminotransferase
   (C) Platelets
   (D) Red blood cells
   (E) Uric acid
10. Six months after beginning atorvastatin, the patient's total and LDL cholesterol concentrations remained above normal and he continued to have anginal attacks despite good adherence to his antianginal medications. His physician decided to add niacin. The major recognized mechanism of action of niacin is
   (A) Decreased lipid synthesis in adipose tissue
   (B) Decreased oxidation of lipids in endothelial cells
   (C) Decreased secretion of VLDL by the liver
   (D) Increased endocytosis of HDL by the liver
   (E) Increased lipid hydrolysis by lipoprotein lipase

ANSWERS

1. Increased serum concentrations of most of the lipoproteins and total cholesterol is associated with increased risk of atherosclerosis. High serum concentrations of HDL cholesterol ("good cholesterol"), however, is associated with a decrease in the risk of atherosclerotic disease. The answer is **(D).**

2. This patient presents with striking hypertriglyceridemia, elevated VLDL cholesterol, and depressed HDL cholesterol. Six months after drug treatment was started, his triglyceride and VLDL cholesterols have dropped dramatically and his HDL cholesterol level had doubled. The drug that is most likely to have achieved all of these desirable changes, particularly the large increase in HDL cholesterol, is niacin. While gemfibrozil and atorvastatin lower triglyceride and VLDL concentrations, they do not cause such large increases in HDL cholesterol. The answer is **(E).**
3. In some patients with familial combined hyperlipidemia and elevated VLDL, the resins can increase VLDL and triglyceride concentrations even though they also lower LDL cholesterol. The answer is **(B).**
4. The HMG-CoA reductase inhibitors are contraindicated in pregnancy because of the risk of teratogenic effects. The answer is **(E).**
5. The major mechanism recognized for gemfibrozil is stimulation of lipoprotein lipase. The answer is **(C).**
6. A major toxicity of the fibrates is increased risk of gallstone formation, which may be due to enhanced biliary excretion of cholesterol. The answer is **(B).**
7. Chronic ethanol ingestion can increase serum concentrations of VLDL and triglyceride. This is one of the factors that puts patients with alcoholism at risk of pancreatitis. Chronic ethanol ingestion also has the possibly beneficial effect of raising, not decreasing, serum HDL concentrations. The answer is **(E).**
8. Niacin can exacerbate both hyperuricemia and glucose intolerance. The answer is **(D).**
9. The two primary adverse effects of the HMG-CoA reductase inhibitors are hepatotoxicity and myopathy. Patients taking these drugs should have liver function tests performed before starting therapy and then at regular intervals during therapy. Serum concentrations of alanine and aspartate aminotransferase are used as markers of hepatocellular toxicity. The answer is **(B).**
10. The major recognized effect of niacin is reduction of VLDL secretion by the liver (Figure 35–2). The answer is **(C).**

Skill Keeper Answers: Angina
(see Chapter 12)

1. The three major forms of angina are (a) angina of effort, which is associated with a fixed plaque that partially occludes one or more coronaries; (b) vasospastic angina, which involves unpredictably timed, reversible coronary spasm; and (c) unstable angina, which often immediately precedes a myocardial infarction and requires emergency treatment.
2. The three major drug groups used in angina are the nitrates, calcium channel blockers, and beta-blockers. Nitrates are used in all three types. Calcium channel blockers are useful for treatment of angina of effort and vasospastic angina. They can be added to beta-blockers and nitroglycerin in patients with refractory unstable angina. Beta-blockers are not useful in vasospastic angina or for an acute attack of angina of effort. They are primarily used for prophylaxis of angina of effort and also in emergency treatment of acute coronary syndromes.

36 Nonsteroidal Anti-inflammatory Drugs, Acetaminophen, & Drugs Used in Gout

OBJECTIVES

You should be able to:

- Contrast the functions of COX-1 and COX-2.
- Describe the effects of aspirin on prostaglandin synthesis.
- Contrast the actions and toxicity of aspirin, the older nonselective NSAIDs and the COX-2-selective drugs.
- List the toxic effects of aspirin.
- Name five DMARDs and compare their mechanisms of action and toxicity with those of the NSAIDs.
- Contrast the treatment of acute and chronic gout.
- Describe the mechanisms of action and toxicity of three different drug groups used in gout.
- Describe the effects and the major toxicity of acetaminophen.

CONCEPTS

ANTI-INFLAMMATORY DRUGS

Inflammation is a common nonspecific manifestation of many diseases. It may be acute or chronic, and the two forms may occur independently. The immune response is involved in most types of inflammation; thus, many of the treatment strategies applied to the reduction of inflammation are targeted at immune processes. The major drug groups used to treat inflammatory conditions are shown in Figure 36–1.

ASPIRIN & OTHER NONSTEROIDAL ANTI-INFLAMMATORY DRUGS (NSAIDs)

A. Classification and Prototypes: Aspirin (acetylsalicylic acid) is the prototype of the salicylates. The other older nonselective NSAIDs (ibuprofen, indomethacin, many others) vary primarily in their potency, analgesic and anti-inflammatory effectiveness, and duration of action. Ibu-

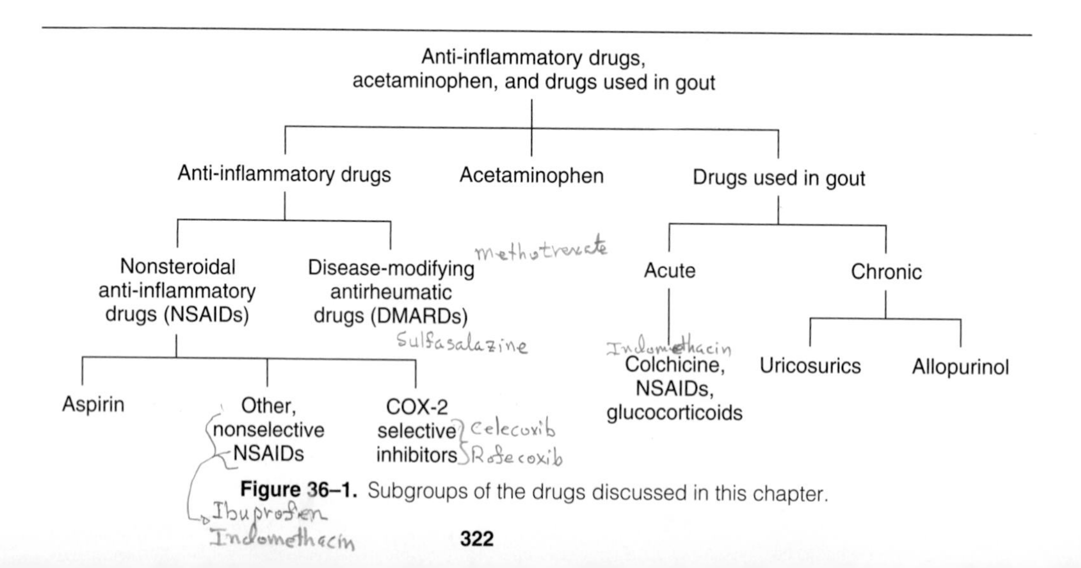

Figure 36–1. Subgroups of the drugs discussed in this chapter.

profen and naproxen have moderate effectiveness; indomethacin has greater anti-inflammatory effectiveness; and ketorolac has greater analgesic effectiveness. Celecoxib and rofecoxib are the first members of a new NSAID subgroup, the COX-2-selective inhibitors.

B. Mechanism of Action: As noted in Chapter 18, cyclooxygenase, the enzyme that converts arachidonic acid into the endoperoxide precursors of prostaglandin, has at least two different isoforms: COX-1 and COX-2 (Figure 18–1). COX-1 is primarily expressed in noninflammatory cells, whereas COX-2 is expressed in activated lymphocytes, polymorphonuclear cells, and other inflammatory cells.

Aspirin and the older nonselective NSAIDs inhibit both cyclooxygenase isoforms and thereby decrease prostaglandin and thromboxane synthesis throughout the body. Prostaglandins necessary for normal cell function are depleted, as well as prostaglandins involved in inflammation. Theoretically, the COX-2-selective inhibitors should have less effect upon the prostaglandins involved in normal cell function, particularly those in the gastrointestinal tract.

The major difference between the mechanisms of action of aspirin and other NSAIDs is that aspirin (but not its active metabolite, salicylate) acetylates and thereby irreversibly inhibits cyclooxygenase, whereas the inhibition produced by other NSAIDs is reversible. The irreversible action of aspirin results in a longer duration of its antiplatelet effect.

C. Effects: Arachidonic acid derivatives are important mediators of inflammation; cyclooxygenase inhibitors reduce the manifestations of inflammation, though they have no effect on underlying tissue damage or immunologic reactions. Prostaglandin synthesis in the CNS that is stimulated by pyrogens is suppressed by NSAIDs, resulting in reduction of fever (antipyretic action). The analgesic mechanism of these agents is less well understood. Activation of peripheral pain sensors may be diminished as a result of reduced production of prostaglandins in injured tissue; in addition, a central mechanism is operative. Cyclooxygenase inhibitors also interfere with the homeostatic function of prostaglandins. Most importantly, they reduce prostaglandin-mediated cytoprotection in the gastrointestinal tract and autoregulation of renal function.

D. Pharmacokinetics and Clinical Use:

1. **Aspirin:** Aspirin has three therapeutic dose ranges: the low range (< 300 mg/d) is effective in reducing platelet aggregation; intermediate doses (300–2400 mg/d) have antipyretic and analgesic effects; and high doses (2400–4000 mg/d) are used for their anti-inflammatory effect. Aspirin is readily absorbed and is hydrolyzed in blood and tissues to acetate and salicylic acid. Salicylate is a reversible nonselective inhibitor of cyclooxygenase. Elimination of salicylate is first-order at low doses, with a half-life of 3–5 hours. At high (anti-inflammatory) doses, half-life increases to 15 hours or more and elimination becomes zero-order. Excretion is via the kidney.
2. **Other NSAIDs:** The other NSAIDs are well absorbed after oral administration. Ibuprofen has a half-life of about 2 hours, is relatively safe, and is the least expensive of the older, nonselective NSAIDs. Indomethacin is a potent NSAID with increased toxicity. Naproxen and piroxicam are noteworthy because of their longer half-lives (12–24 hours), which permit less frequent dosing. These other NSAIDs are used for the treatment of mild to moderate pain—and especially the pain of inflammation such as that seen in rheumatoid arthritis and gout. COX-2 inhibitors are primarily used in inflammatory disorders. Selected NSAIDs are also used to treat other conditions, including dysmenorrhea, headache, and patent ductus arteriosus in premature infants. Ketorolac is notable as a drug used mainly as a systemic analgesic, not as an anti-inflammatory drug (though it has typical nonselective NSAID properties). It is the only NSAID available in a parenteral formulation.

E. Toxicity:

1. **Aspirin:** The most common adverse effect from therapeutic anti-inflammatory doses of aspirin is gastric upset. Chronic use can result in gastric ulceration, upper gastrointestinal bleeding, and renal effects, including acute failure and interstitial nephritis. Aspirin increases the bleeding time. When prostaglandin synthesis is inhibited by even small doses of aspirin, persons with aspirin hypersensitivity (especially associated with nasal polyps) may experience asthma from the increased synthesis of leukotrienes. This type of hypersensitivity to aspirin precludes treatment with any NSAID. At higher doses of aspirin, tinnitus, vertigo, hyperventilation, and respiratory alkalosis are observed. At very high doses, the drug

causes metabolic acidosis, dehydration, hyperthermia, collapse, coma, and death. Children with viral infections are at increased risk of developing Reye's syndrome (hepatic fatty degeneration and encephalopathy) if given aspirin.

2. **Nonselective NSAIDs:** Like aspirin, these agents may cause significant gastrointestinal disturbance, but the incidence is lower than with aspirin. There is a significant risk of renal damage with any of the NSAIDs, especially in patients with preexisting renal disease. Since these drugs are cleared by the kidney, renal damage results in higher, more toxic serum concentrations. Phenylbutazone, an older NSAID, should not be used chronically because it causes aplastic anemia and agranulocytosis. Serious hematologic reactions have also been noted with indomethacin.
3. **COX-2-selective inhibitors:** The COX-2-selective inhibitors may have a reduced risk of gastrointestinal effects, including gastric ulcers and serious gastrointestinal bleeding. Celecoxib is a sulfonamide and may cause a hypersensitivity reaction in patients who are allergic to other sulfonamides.

DISEASE-MODIFYING, SLOW-ACTING ANTIRHEUMATIC DRUGS (DMARDs, SAARDs)

A. **Classification and Prototypes:** This heterogeneous group of agents (Table 36–1) has anti-inflammatory actions in several connective tissue diseases. These agents are called disease-modifying because some evidence shows slowing or even reversal of joint damage—an effect never seen with NSAIDs. They are also called slow-acting because it may take 6 weeks to 6 months for their benefits to become apparent. **Corticosteroids** may be considered anti-inflammatory drugs with an intermediate rate of action, ie, slower than NSAIDs but faster than the other DMARDs. However, the corticosteroids are too toxic for chronic use (see Chapter 39) and are reserved for temporary control of severe exacerbations.

B. **Mechanisms of Action:** The mechanisms of action of these drugs are poorly understood. Cytotoxic drugs (eg, **methotrexate**) probably act by reducing the numbers of immune cells available to maintain the inflammatory response. The mechanism of action of **sulfasalazine** appears to differ from its mechanism in ulcerative colitis—sulfapyridine appears to be more important than the 5-aminosalicylic acid component. **Hydroxychloroquine** may interfere with the activity of T lymphocytes, decrease leukocyte chemotaxis, stabilize lysosomal membranes, interfere with DNA and RNA synthesis, and trap free radicals. Penicillamine appears to have anti-inflammatory effects similar to those of hydroxychloroquine. Organic gold compounds alter the activity of macrophages, cells that play a central role in inflammation, especially that of arthritis, and suppress phagocytic activity by polymorphonuclear leukocytes.

Several new DMARDs have been introduced recently. **Leflunomide** is a prodrug that is rapidly metabolized to a compound that inhibits dihydroorotate dehydrogenase, an enzyme required by

Table 36–1. Some slow-acting antirheumatic drugs.

Drug	Other Clinical Uses	Toxicity When Used for Rheumatoid Arthritis
Sulfasalazine	Inflammatory bowel disease	Rash, gastrointestinal disturbance, dizziness, headache, leukopenia
Hydroxychloroquine	Antimalarial	Rash, gastrointestinal disturbance, ototoxicity, myopathy, peripheral neuropathy
Methotrexate	Anticancer	Nausea, mucosal ulcers, hematotoxicity, teratogenicity
Cyclosporine	Tissue transplantation	Nephrotoxicity, hypertension, peripheral neuropathy
Infliximab	Crohn's disease	Upper respiratory infection
Etanercept		Injection site reactions
Leflunomide		Teratogen, hepatotoxicity, gastrointestinal disturbance, skin reactions
Gold compounds		Many adverse effects, including diarrhea, dermatitis, hematologic abnormalities (including aplastic anemia)
Penicillamine	Chelating agent	Many adverse effects, including proteinuria, dermatitis, gastrointestinal disturbance, hematologic abnormalities (including aplastic anemia)

activated lymphocytes for synthesis of the pyrimidines that are needed for RNA synthesis. In lymphocytes, inhibition of this enzyme results in cell cycle arrest. Other cell types are not affected to the same degree because they can use other biochemical pathways to synthesize pyrimidines. **Infliximab** and **etanercept** are recombinant proteins that bind to and prevent the action of tumor necrosis factor-alpha (TNF-α), a cytokine that appears to play a key role in chronic inflammation.

C. Effects: DMARDs are used in patients with rheumatoid arthritis not responsive to other agents. Some of these drugs are also used in other rheumatic diseases such as lupus erythematosus, arthritis associated with Sjögren's syndrome, and juvenile rheumatoid arthritis.

D. Pharmacokinetics and Clinical Use: Sulfasalazine, hydroxychloroquine, methotrexate, cyclosporine, penicillamine and leflunomide are given orally. Infliximab and etanercept are given by injection. Gold compounds are available for parenteral use (gold sodium thiomalate and aurothioglucose) and for oral administration (auranofin).

E. Toxicity: All disease-modifying agents can cause severe or fatal toxicities. Careful monitoring of patients who take these drugs is mandatory. Their major adverse effects are listed in Table 36–1.

ACETAMINOPHEN

A. Classification and Prototype: Acetaminophen is the only over-the-counter non-anti-inflammatory analgesic commonly available in the USA. Phenacetin, a toxic prodrug that is metabolized to acetaminophen, is still available in some other countries.

B. Mechanism of Action: The mechanism of analgesic action of acetaminophen is unclear. The drug is a weak cyclooxygenase inhibitor in peripheral tissues, which accounts for its lack of anti-inflammatory effect. Acetaminophen may be a more effective inhibitor of prostaglandin synthesis in the CNS, and this CNS activity may account for its analgesic and antipyretic action.

C. Effects: Acetaminophen is an analgesic and antipyretic agent lacking anti-inflammatory or antiplatelet effects.

D. Pharmacokinetics and Clinical Use: Acetaminophen is effective for the same indications as intermediate-dose aspirin. Acetaminophen is therefore useful as an aspirin substitute, especially in children with viral infections and in individuals with any type of aspirin intolerance. Acetaminophen is well absorbed orally and metabolized in the liver. Its half-life, which is 2–3 hours in persons with normal hepatic function, is unaffected by renal disease.

E. Toxicity: In therapeutic dosages, acetaminophen has negligible toxicity in most individuals. However, when taken in overdose or by patients with severe liver impairment, the drug is a very dangerous hepatotoxin. The mechanism of toxicity requires oxidation to cytotoxic intermediates by phase I P450 enzymes. This occurs if substrates for phase II conjugation reactions (acetate and glucuronide) are lacking (see Chapter 4). People who regularly consume three or more alcoholic drinks per day are at increased risk of acetaminophen-induced hepatotoxicity (see also Chapters 4 and 23).

Skill Keeper: Opioid Analgesics & Antagonists (see Chapter 31)

While the NSAIDs and acetaminophen are extremely useful for the treatment of mild to moderate pain, adequate control of more intense pain usually requires treatment with an opioid.

1. Name one strong, one moderate, and one weak opioid drug.
2. Briefly describe the most common adverse effects of strong and moderate opioids.
3. What drug should be administered in the event of an opioid overdose?

The Skill Keeper Answers appear at the end of the chapter.

DRUGS USED IN GOUT

A. Classification and Prototypes: Gout is associated with increased body stores of uric acid. Acute attacks involve joint inflammation caused by precipitation of uric acid crystals. Treatment strategies include (1) reducing inflammation during acute attacks (with colchicine, NSAIDs, or glucocorticoids; Figure 36–2); (2) accelerating renal excretion of uric acid with uricosuric drugs (probenecid or sulfinpyrazone); and (3) reducing (with allopurinol) the conversion of purines to uric acid by xanthine oxidase.

B. Anti-inflammatory Drugs Used for Gout:

1. **Mechanisms:** Potent NSAIDs such as **indomethacin** are effective in inhibiting the inflammation of acute gouty arthritis. These agents act through the reduction of prostaglandin formation and through the inhibition of crystal phagocytosis by macrophages (Figure 36–2). **Colchicine,** a selective inhibitor of microtubule assembly, reduces leukocyte migration and phagocytosis; the drug may also reduce production of leukotriene B_4, and it decreases free radical formation as well.
2. **Effects:** NSAIDs and glucocorticoids reduce the synthesis of mediators of inflammation by inflammatory cells in the gouty joint. Because it reacts with tubulin and interferes with microtubule assembly, colchicine is a general mitotic poison. Tubulin is necessary for normal cell division, motility, and many other processes.
3. **Pharmacokinetics and clinical use:** Indomethacin or a glucocorticoid is preferred for the treatment of acute gouty arthritis. While colchicine can be used, the doses required cause significant gastrointestinal disturbance, particularly diarrhea. Lower doses of colchicine are used to prevent attacks of gout in patients with a history of multiple acute attacks. Colchicine is also of value in the management of Mediterranean fever, a disease of unknown cause characterized by fever, hepatitis, peritonitis, pleuritis, arthritis, and, occasionally, amyloidosis. Indomethacin, some glucocorticoids, and colchicine are used orally; parenteral preparations of glucocorticoids and colchicine are also available.
4. **Toxicity:** Indomethacin may cause renal damage or bone marrow depression. Short courses of glucocorticoids can cause behavioral changes and impaired glucose control. Because colchicine can severely damage the liver and kidney, dosage must be carefully limited and monitored. Overdose is often fatal.

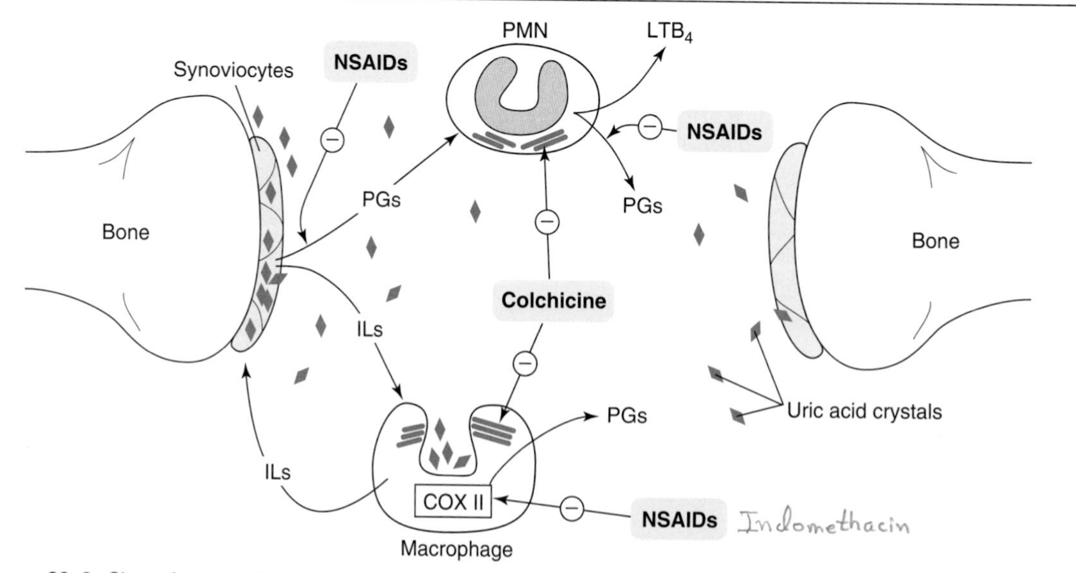

Figure 36–2. Sites of action of some anti-inflammatory drugs in a gouty joint. Synoviocytes damaged by uric acid crystals release prostaglandins (PGs), interleukins (ILs), and other mediators of inflammation. Polymorphonuclear leukocytes (PMNs), macrophages, and other inflammatory cells enter the joint and also release inflammatory substances, including leukotrienes (eg, LTB_4), that attract additional inflammatory cells. Colchicine acts on microtubules in the inflammatory cells. NSAIDs act on cyclooxygenase-2 in all of the cells of the joint.

C. Uricosuric Agents:

1. **Mechanism:** Uricosuric agents **(probenecid, sulfinpyrazone)** are weak acids that compete with uric acid for reabsorption by the weak acid transport mechanism in the S_2 segment of the proximal renal tubule. At low doses, these agents may also compete with uric acid for secretion by the tubule and (occasionally) can even elevate serum uric acid concentration. Elevation of uric acid levels by this mechanism occurs with aspirin (another weak acid) over much of its dose range.
2. **Effects:** Uricosuric drugs act primarily in the kidney and inhibit the secretion of a large number of other weak acids (eg, penicillin, methotrexate) in addition to inhibiting the reabsorption of uric acid.
3. **Pharmacokinetics and clinical use:** Chronic gout is treated orally with a uricosuric or allopurinol. These drugs are of no value in acute gouty arthritis and are best withheld for 1–2 weeks after an acute episode.
4. **Toxicity:** Uricosuric drugs may precipitate an attack of acute gouty arthritis during the early phase of their action. This can be avoided by simultaneously administering colchicine or indomethacin. Because they are sulfonamides, the uricosuric drugs may share allergenicity with other classes of sulfonamide drugs (diuretics, antimicrobials, oral hypoglycemic drugs).

D. Allopurinol:

1. **Mechanism:** Allopurinol is converted to oxipurinol (alloxanthine) by xanthine oxidase, the enzyme that converts hypoxanthine to xanthine and xanthine to uric acid. Allopurinol and oxipurinol are irreversible suicide inhibitors of this enzyme.
2. **Effects:** Inhibition of conversion to uric acid increases the concentrations of the more soluble hypoxanthine and xanthine and decreases the concentration of the less soluble uric acid. As a result, there is less likelihood of precipitation of uric acid crystals in joints and tissues.
3. **Pharmacokinetics and clinical use:** Allopurinol is given orally in the management of chronic gout. It is usually withheld for 1–2 weeks after an acute episode of gouty arthritis. Allopurinol may also be used in cancer chemotherapy to slow the formation of uric acid from purines released by the death of large numbers of neoplastic cells.
4. **Toxicity and drug interactions:** Like uricosuric drugs, allopurinol can precipitate acute attacks of gout during the early phase of treatment. Allopurinol causes gastrointestinal upset and, rarely, peripheral neuritis and vasculitis. Allopurinol inhibits the metabolism of mercaptopurine and azathioprine, drugs that depend upon xanthine oxidase for elimination.

DRUG LIST

The following drugs are important members of the groups discussed in this chapter. Prototypes should be learned in detail; features of the major variants should be known well enough to distinguish the variants from the prototypes and from each other; the other significant agents should be recognized as belonging to a specific subclass.

Subclass	Prototype	Major Variants	Other Significant Agents
Anti-inflammatory drugs Salicylates	Aspirin		Sodium salicylate
Nonselective NSAIDs	Ibuprofen	Indomethacin, ketorolac	Naproxen, many others
COX-2-selective inhibitors	Celecoxib	Rofecoxib	
Slow-acting antirheumatic drugs	Methotrexate	Hydroxychloroquine, sulfasalazine	Infliximab, etanercept, leflunomide, penicillamine, gold
Acetaminophen class	Acetaminophen		Phenacetin
Drugs used in gout Anti-inflammatory drugs	Colchicine		NSAIDs, eg, indomethacin, glucocorticoids
Uricosurics	Probenecid		Sulfinpyrazone
Xanthine oxidase inhibitors	Allopurinol		

QUESTIONS

DIRECTIONS: Each of the numbered items or incomplete statements in this section is followed by answers or by completions of the statement. Select the ONE lettered answer or completion that is BEST in each case.

1. The effects of aspirin do not include
(A) Reduction of fever
(B) Reduction of prostaglandin synthesis in inflamed tissues
(C) Impaired autoregulation of kidney function
(D) Reduction of bleeding tendency
(E) Tinnitus and vertigo

2. Which one of the following pairs of a drug effect and mechanism of action is false?
(A) Allopurinol action in gout: Inhibits oxidation of hypoxanthine
(B) Aspirin antiplatelet action: Inhibits cyclooxygenase
(C) Hydroxychloroquine antirheumatic action: Interferes with T lymphocyte action
(D) Probenecid uricosuric action: Increases secretion of uric acid by the loop of Henle
(E) Indomethacin closure of patent ductus arteriosus: Blocks PGE production in the ductus of the newborn

3. Which one of the following effects does not occur in salicylate intoxication?
(A) Hyperventilation
(B) Hypothermia
(C) Metabolic acidosis
(D) Respiratory alkalosis
(E) Tinnitus

4. Which one of the following drugs is not useful in dysmenorrhea?
(A) Aspirin
(B) Colchicine
(C) Ibuprofen
(D) Rofecoxib
(D) Naproxen

5. Which of the following drugs is MOST likely to increase serum concentrations of conventional doses of methotrexate, a weak acid that is primarily cleared in the urine?
(A) Acetaminophen
(B) Allopurinol
(C) Colchicine
(D) Hydroxychloroquine
(E) Probenecid

6. The main advantage of ketorolac over aspirin is that ketorolac
(A) Can be combined more safely with an opioid such as codeine
(B) Can be obtained as an over-the-counter agent
(C) Does not prolong the bleeding time
(D) Is available in a parenteral formulation that can be injected intramuscularly or intravenously
(E) Is less likely to cause acute renal failure in patients with some preexisting degree of renal impairment

Items 7–8: A 52-year-old woman presented with intense pain, warmth, and redness in the first toe on her left foot. Examination of fluid withdrawn from the inflamed joint revealed crystals of uric acid.

7. In the treatment of this woman's acute attack of gout, the advantage of using indomethacin instead of colchicine is that indomethacin is
(A) Less likely to cause acute renal failure
(B) Less likely to cause severe diarrhea
(C) Less likely to precipitate sudden gastrointestinal bleeding
(D) More likely to prevent another acute attack
(E) More likely to reduce the symptoms of inflammation

8. Over the next 7 months, the patient had two more attacks of acute gout. Her serum concentration of uric acid was elevated. The decision was made to put her on chronic drug therapy to try to prevent subsequent attacks. Which of the following drugs could be used to decrease this woman's rate of production of uric acid?

(A) Allopurinol
(B) Aspirin
(C) Colchicine
(D) Hydroxychloroquine
(E) Probenecid

Items 9–10: A 54-year-old woman presented with signs and symptoms consistent with an early stage of rheumatoid arthritis. The decision was made to initiate NSAID therapy.

9. Which of the following patient characteristics is a possible reason for the use of celecoxib in the treatment of her arthritis?
(A) A history of a severe rash after treatment with a sulfonamide antibiotic
(B) A history of gout
(C) A history of peptic ulcer disease
(D) A history of sudden onset of bronchospasm after treatment with aspirin
(E) A history of type 2 diabetes

10. Although the patient's disease was adequately controlled with an NSAID and methotrexate for some time, her symptoms began to worsen and radiologic studies of her hands indicated progressive destruction in the joints of several fingers. Treatment with a new second-line agent for rheumatoid arthritis was considered. This drug is available only in a parenteral formulation; its mechanism of anti-inflammatory action is antagonism of tumor necrosis factor. The drug being considered is
(A) Cyclosporine
(B) Etanercept
(C) Penicillamine
(D) Phenylbutazone
(E) Sulfasalazine

ANSWERS

1. Aspirin clearly *increases* bleeding tendency (by its antiplatelet effects). The answer is **(D).**

2. Probenecid inhibits the reabsorption of uric acid in the proximal tubule. (Both secretion and reabsorption of weak acids occur in the proximal tubule, not the loop of Henle.) The answer is **(D).**

3. Salicylate intoxication is associated with *hyperthermia,* not hypothermia, because the drug causes uncoupling of oxidative phosphorylation, resulting in increased metabolism. The answer is **(B).**

4. Primary dysmenorrhea is caused by excessive production of prostaglandin $F_{2\alpha}$. NSAIDs that inhibit cyclooxygenase are far more effective in relieving symptoms than other analgesics. Colchicine, which is not analgesic and is anti-inflammatory only in gout and Mediterranean fever, would never be used in this condition. The answer is **(B).**

5. Methotrexate, a weak acid, depends upon active tubular excretion in the proximal tubule for efficient elimination. Probenecid competes with methotrexate for binding to the proximal tubule transporter and thereby decreases the rate of clearance of methotrexate. The answer is **(E).**

6. Ketorolac exerts typical NSAID effects. It prolongs the bleeding time and can impair renal function, especially in a patient with preexisting renal disease. Ketorolac is not available over-the-counter. Its primary use is as a parenteral agent for pain management, especially for treatment of postoperative patients. The answer is **(D).**

7. Indomethacin and colchicine have equivalent efficacy in the treatment of acute gout. Colchicine is now more likely to be used chronically to prevent other attacks. Indomethacin is more—not less—likely to precipitate sudden gastrointestinal bleeding and acute renal failure. In the dose used to treat acute gout, colchicine frequently causes significant diarrhea. The answer is **(B).**

8. Allopurinol is the only drug listed that decreases production of uric acid. Probenecid increases uric acid excretion. Colchicine and hydroxychloroquine do not affect uric acid metabolism. Aspirin actually slows renal secretion of uric acid and raises uric acid blood levels. It should not be used in gout. The answer is **(A).**

9. Celecoxib is a COX-2-selective inhibitor. Its advantage over nonselective NSAIDs may be reduced gastrointestinal toxicity. Celecoxib is being used in patients who need NSAIDs but who also have a high risk of gastrointestinal toxicity, such as patients with a history of ulcer disease. Celecoxib is a sulfonamide, so it should be avoided in patients with sulfonamide allergy. Like all NSAIDs, it should not be used in patients with hypersensitivity to aspirin. It does not offer any advantages over other NSAIDs in patients with gout or diabetes. The answer is **(C).**

10. Etanercept is a recombinant protein that binds to tumor necrosis factor and prevents its inflammatory effects. The answer is **(B).**

Skill Keeper Answers: Opioids (see Chapter 31)

1. Morphine is the prototype of the strong opioids. Meperidine is a variant used commonly for analgesia. Methadone is a strong agonist used in maintenance programs for patients addicted to opioids. Codeine, oxycodone, and hydrocodone are moderate agonists, whereas propoxyphene is a weak agonist.
2. Constipation and sedation occur with therapeutic doses; constipation should be managed with stool softeners. In overdose, opioids cause a triad of pinpoint pupils, coma, and respiratory depression.
3. Naloxone, a nonselective opioid receptor antagonist, is the antidote for opioid overdose.

Part VII. Endocrine Drugs

Hypothalamic & Pituitary Hormones 37

OBJECTIVES

You should be able to:

- List the major hypothalamic releasing hormones.
- Describe the major anterior pituitary hormones and their effects.
- Describe the major posterior pituitary hormones and their effects.
- Describe the major drugs used as substitutes for the natural hypothalamic and pituitary hormones.
- Name the drugs that are used for treatment of acromegaly and hyperprolactinemia.

CONCEPTS

The hypothalamus and pituitary gland synthesize several hormones that regulate other glands and tissues throughout the body. One group of hypothalamic hormones (releasing hormones) regulates the release of anterior pituitary hormones. The other hypothalamic hormones (oxytocin and vasopressin) are transported to the posterior pituitary where they are released into the general circulation. The hormones currently recognized as most important (and their targets) are listed in Table 37–1. Except for prolactin-inhibiting hormone (dopamine), all of these endocrine agents are peptides.

Table 37–1. Links between hypothalamic, pituitary, and target gland hormones.

Hypothalamic Hormone	Pituitary Hormone	Target Organ	Target Organ Hormone
Growth hormone-releasing hormone (GHRH)	Growth hormone (GH)	Liver	Somatomedins
Somatostatin[1]	Growth hormone (GH)	Liver	Somatomedins
Thyrotropin-releasing hormone (TRH)	Thyroid-stimulating hormone (TSH)	Thyroid	Thyroxine, triiodothyronine
Corticotropin-releasing hormone (CRH)	Adrenocorticotropic hormone (ACTH)	Adrenal cortex	Glucocorticoids, mineralocorticoids, androgens
Gonadotropin-releasing hormone (GnRH or LHRH)	Follicle-stimulating hormone (FSH) Luteinizing hormone (LH)	Gonads	Estrogen, progesterone, testosterone
Prolactin-releasing hormone (PRH)	Prolactin (PRL)	Lymphocytes	Lymphokines
Prolactin-inhibiting hormone (PIH, dopamine)		Breast	
Oxytocin	None	Smooth muscle, especially uterus	
Vasopressin	None	Renal tubule, smooth muscle	

[1]Inhibits GH and TSH release. Also found in gastrointestinal tissues; inhibits release of gastrin, glucagon, and insulin.

HYPOTHALAMIC HORMONES

A. Growth Hormone-Releasing Hormone (GHRH): GHRH consists of several large peptides with GHRH activity; two shorter synthetic peptides with similar activity are available for clinical use. In normal individuals, they produce a rapid increase in plasma growth hormone levels; their primary use is to determine the cause of growth hormone deficiency.

B. Somatostatin (Somatotropin Release-Inhibiting Hormone; SRIF): Somatostatin, a 14-amino-acid peptide, is found in the pancreas and other parts of the gastrointestinal system as well as in the CNS. In addition to inhibiting the release of growth hormone, somatostatin inhibits the release of thyrotropin, glucagon, insulin, and gastrin. Somatostatin is of no clinical value because of its short duration of action. **Octreotide,** a synthetic octapeptide somatostatin analog with a longer duration of action, has been found useful in the management of acromegaly, carcinoid, gastrinoma, glucagonoma, and other endocrine tumors. Regular octreotide must be administered subcutaneously two to four times daily. Once a brief course of regular octreotide has been demonstrated to be effective and tolerated, a slow-release intramuscular formulation is administered every 4 weeks for long-term therapy.

C. Thyrotropin-Releasing Hormone (TRH): TRH is a tripeptide that stimulates release of thyrotropin from the anterior pituitary. TRH also increases prolactin production but has no effect on the release of growth hormone or ACTH.

D. Corticotropin-Releasing Hormone (CRH): This 41-amino-acid peptide stimulates secretion of both ACTH and beta-endorphin (a closely related peptide) from the pituitary. CRH can be used in the diagnosis of abnormalities of ACTH secretion because ACTH secretion by nonpituitary tumors (eg, of the lung) rarely increases in response to stimulation by CRH, whereas secretion by the pituitary in Cushing's disease consistently increases after CRH stimulation.

E. Gonadotropin-Releasing Hormone (GnRH or LHRH): GnRH is a decapeptide; **leuprolide** is a synthetic nonapeptide with similar activity. When given in pulsatile doses (resembling physiologic cycling), these agents stimulate gonadotropin release. In contrast, steady dosing causes a marked inhibition of gonadotropin release—in effect, a medical castration. GnRH is used in the diagnosis and treatment (by pulsatile administration) of hypogonadal states in female and male patients. Leuprolide and several analogs (nafarelin, gosarelin, buserelin) are used to suppress gonadotropin secretion (by administration in steady dosage) in patients with prostatic carcinoma or other gonadal steroid-sensitive tumors, endometriosis, or precocious puberty. GnRH agonists are also used to suppress endogenous gonadotropin release in women who are undergoing controlled ovarian hyperstimulation and in assisted reproduction technology (eg, in vitro fertilization). **Ganirelix,** a new GnRH *antagonist,* is used to prevent premature surges of luteinizing hormone during controlled ovarian hyperstimulation.

F. Prolactin-Inhibiting Hormone (PIH, Dopamine): Dopamine is the physiologic inhibitor of prolactin release. Because of its peripheral effects and the need for parenteral administration, dopamine is not useful in the control of hyperprolactinemia, but **bromocriptine** and other orally active ergot derivatives (eg, cabergoline, pergolide) are effective in reducing prolactin secretion from the normal gland as well as from pituitary tumors.

Skill Keeper: Drugs That Cause Hyperprolactinemia (see Chapter 29)

As many as 25% of infertile women have hyperprolactinemia. In women, hyperprolactinemia causes galactorrhea, oligomenorrhea, or amenorrhea as well as infertility (the amenorrhea-galactorrhea syndrome). While prolactin-secreting tumors are the most common cause of hyperprolactinemia, the condition can also be precipitated by treatment with drugs that interfere with the control of prolactin release.

1. What types of pharmacologic actions are most likely to cause hyperprolactinemia?
2. Name several drugs with this type of pharmacologic action.

The Skill Keeper Answers appear at the end of the chapter.

ANTERIOR PITUITARY HORMONES

A. Growth Hormone (Somatotropin): Human growth hormone is available in two forms through recombinant DNA technology: somatropin and somatrem (somatotropin with an extra methionine). These products are useful in the treatment of GH deficiency in children and adults. Treatment with GH of girls with Turner's syndrome frequently leads to increased final adult height. Growth hormone treatment also improves growth in children with failure to thrive because of chronic renal failure or HIV infection and has efficacy in treatment of adults with AIDS-associated wasting. Recombinant bovine GH is used in dairy cattle to increase milk production.

B. Thyroid-Stimulating Hormone (TSH): In thyroid cells, this peptide increases iodine uptake and production of thyroid hormones. TSH has been used as a diagnostic tool to distinguish primary from secondary hypothyroidism.

C. Adrenocorticotropin (ACTH): This peptide is formed from a large precursor peptide, pro-opiomelanocortin. This precursor is also the source of melanocyte-stimulating hormone, beta-endorphin, and met-enkephalin. **Cosyntropin,** a synthetic analog, is used for diagnostic purposes in patients with abnormal corticosteroid production.

D. Follicle-Stimulating Hormone (FSH): FSH is a glycoprotein that stimulates gametogenesis and follicle development in women and spermatogenesis in men. The preparation usually used is urofollitropin, a product extracted from the urine of postmenopausal women.

E. Luteinizing Hormone (LH): LH is the major stimulant of gonadal steroid production. In women, LH also regulates follicular development and ovulation. No pure preparation of LH is currently in use. **Human chorionic gonadotropin (hCG),** which has an almost identical structure, is used in place of LH for treatment of hypogonadism in men and women and as part of controlled ovarian hyperstimulation and assisted reproductive technology programs.

F. Menotropins: Menotropins are human menopausal gonadotropins that consist of FSH and LH from the urine of postmenopausal women. The product is often used in combination with human chorionic gonadotropin in the treatment of hypogonadal states and as part of controlled ovarian hyperstimulation and assisted reproductive technology programs.

G. Prolactin: Prolactin, a glycoprotein hormone responsible for lactation, is not used in therapy.

POSTERIOR PITUITARY HORMONES

A. Oxytocin: Oxytocin is a nonapeptide synthesized in cell bodies in the paraventricular nuclei of the hypothalamus and transported through the axons of these cells to the posterior pituitary, where the peptide is released into the circulation. Oxytocin is an effective stimulant of uterine contraction and is often used intravenously to induce or reinforce labor. Because it causes contraction of smooth muscle in the myoepithelial cells of the mammary gland, oxytocin also can be used by lactating women as a nasal spray to stimulate milk let-down.

B. Vasopressin (Antidiuretic Hormone, ADH): Vasopressin is synthesized in the supraoptic nuclei of the hypothalamus and released from the posterior pituitary. As discussed in Chapter 15, vasopressin acts on V_2 receptors and increases the synthesis or insertion of water channels by a cAMP-dependent mechanism, resulting in an increase in water permeability in the collecting tubules of the kidney. The increased water permeability permits water reabsorption into the hypertonic renal papilla, thus causing the antidiuretic effect. Vasopressin also causes smooth muscle contraction (a V_1 effect). **Desmopressin,** a selective agonist of V_2 receptors, is used in the treatment of pituitary diabetes insipidus.

DRUG LIST

The drugs listed in Table 37–2 are pituitary hormone analogs or agents used for their effects on pituitary-related endocrine function. Many of the natural hormones described in Table 37–1 are also used as drugs.

Table 37–2. Pituitary hormone analogs or agents used for their effects on pituitary-related endocrine function.

Drug	Actions	Clinical Use	Comment
Somatropin, somatrem	Growth hormone	Pituitary deficiency	Proteins from recombinant synthesis; somatrem has one additional methionine
Octreotide	Somatostatin analog	Multiple uses to inhibit glandular secretion	Longer-acting than natural somatostatin
Cosyntropin	ACTH analog, stimulates adrenal cortex	Corticosteroid substitute; diagnosis; infantile spasms (seizures)	Cosyntropin is a 1–24 amino acid active fragment of ACTH
Leuprolide, goserelin, nafarelin	GnRH receptor agonists	Infertility, cancer	Stimulates gonads if given in pulses; inhibits if given continuously
Ganirelix	GnRH antagonist	Infertility	Inhibits LH release immediately
Urofollitropin	FSH-like activity	Infertility	Isolated from human urine
Human chorionic gonadotropin (hCG)	LH-like activity	Infertility	Isolated from human urine
Menotropins	FSH plus LH activity	Infertility	Isolated from human urine
Bromocriptine, pergolide, cabergoline	Inhibit prolactin release	Stop lactation; inhibit growth of pituitary tumors	Ergot alkaloid derivatives with potent dopamine agonist activity
Desmopressin	Antidiuretic hormone analog	Pituitary diabetes insipidus	A V_2 receptor agonist; longer-acting than vasopressin (ADH)

QUESTIONS

DIRECTIONS: Each of the numbered items or incomplete statements in this section is followed by answers or by completions of the statement. Select the ONE lettered answer or completion that is BEST in each case.

1. Which one of the following compounds is not a hormone?
(A) Bromocriptine
(B) Somatomedin
(C) Somatotropin
(D) Thyroxine
(E) Vasopressin

2. A 29-year-old woman who was in her 41st week of gestation had been in labor for 12 hours. Although her uterine contractions had been strong and regular initially, they had diminished in force during the past hour. Which of the following drugs would be administered to facilitate this woman's labor and delivery?
(A) Dopamine
(B) Leuprolide
(C) Oxytocin
(D) Prolactin
(E) Vasopressin

3. Which one of the following hormones is not synthesized in the hypothalamus?
(A) Corticotropin-releasing hormone
(B) Luteinizing hormone
(C) Oxytocin
(D) Thyrotropin-releasing hormone
(E) Vasopressin

4. An important difference between leuprolide and the new drug ganirelix is that ganirelix
(A) Can be administered as an oral formulation
(B) Can be used alone to restore fertility to hypogonadal men and women
(C) Immediately reduces gonadotropin secretion

(D) Initially stimulates pituitary production of LH and FSH
(E) Must be administered in a pulsatile fashion

5. A 27-year-old woman with amenorrhea, infertility, and galactorrhea was treated with a drug that successfully restored ovulation and menstruation. Before being given the drug, the woman was carefully questioned about previous mental health problems, which she did not have. She was advised to take the drug orally. The drug used to treat this patient was probably
(A) Bromocriptine
(B) Desmopressin
(C) Human gonadotropin hormone
(D) Leuprolide
(E) Octreotide

6. Who is LEAST likely to be treated with somatropin?
(A) A 3-year-old cow on a dairy farm
(B) A 4-year-old girl with an XO genetic genotype
(C) A 4-year-old boy with chronic renal failure and growth deficiency
(D) A 10-year-old boy with polydipsia and polyuria
(E) A 37-year-old AIDS patient who is 180 cm tall and weighs 52 kg

7. Hormones that are useful in the diagnosis of endocrine insufficiency include
(A) Corticotropin-releasing hormone
(B) Cosyntropin
(C) Gonadotropin-releasing hormone
(D) Thyrotropin-releasing hormone
(E) All of the above

8. A 47-year-old man exhibited signs and symptoms of acromegaly. Radiologic studies showed the presence of a large pituitary tumor. Surgical treatment of the tumor was only partially effective in controlling his disease. At this point, which of the following drugs is most likely to be used as pharmacologic therapy?
(A) Cosyntropin
(B) Desmopressin
(C) Leuprolide
(D) Octreotide
(E) Somatropin

9. Which of the following drugs is LEAST likely to be used as part of a controlled ovarian hyperstimulation protocol?
(A) Human chorionic gonadotropin
(B) Leuprolide
(C) Menotropins
(D) Pergolide
(E) Urofollitropin

ANSWERS

1. Bromocriptine, an ergot alkaloid, is not produced in the body. The answer is **(A).**
2. Oxytocin is the only drug listed that is an effective stimulant of uterine contraction. The answer is **(C).**
3. Luteinizing hormone is synthesized in the anterior pituitary. The answer is **(B).**
4. Leuprolide is an agonist of GnRH receptors, whereas ganirelix is an antagonist. While both drugs can be used to inhibit gonadotropin release, ganirelix does so immediately whereas leuprolide does so only after about a week of sustained activity. The answer is **(C).**
5. Bromocriptine, a dopamine receptor agonist, is used to treat the amenorrhea-galactorrhea syndrome, which is a consequence of hyperprolactinemia. Because of its central dopaminergic effects, the drug should not be used in patients with a history of schizophrenia or other forms of psychotic illness. The answer is **(A).**
6. Somatropin, recombinant human GH, promotes growth in children with Turner's syndrome (an XO genetic genotype) or chronic renal failure. It also helps combat the AIDS-associated wasting syndrome. Bovine GH promotes milk production in cows. Growth hormone would not be appropriate for the boy with polydipsia and polyuria, which is probably symptomatic of a form of diabetes. The answer is **(D).**

7. All are correct. The answer is **(E).**
8. Octreotide, a somatostatin analog, has some efficacy in reducing the excess GH production that causes acromegaly. The answer is **(D).**
9. In controlled ovarian hyperstimulation, the strategy is to suppress a woman's endogenous ovarian regulation with a GnRH agonist, to hyperstimulate follicle production by administration of drugs with LH and FSH activity, and then to induce ovulation with human chorionic gonadotropin. The only drug listed that does not have a role in this process is the dopamine receptor agonist pergolide. The answer is **(D).**

Skill Keeper Answers: Drugs That Cause Hyperprolactinemia (see Chapter 29)

1. Drugs that block $dopamine_2$ receptors can cause hyperprolactinemia by blocking the inhibitory effects of endogenous dopamine upon the pituitary cells that release prolactin. Drugs that deplete central neurons of amine neurotransmitters and drugs with an inhibiting action on dopaminergic mechanisms in the hypothalamus may also cause hyperprolactinemia.
2. The older **antipsychotic drugs** (eg, phenothiazines, haloperidol), with their strong $dopamine_2$ receptor-blocking activity, are most likely to be the pharmacologic cause of hyperprolactinemia (see Chapter 29). This adverse effect is less likely with the newer antipsychotic drugs (eg, olanzapine). **Reserpine** can cause hyperprolactinemia by depleting stores of dopamine in central neurons. Drugs or drug groups that cause hyperprolactinemia through mechanisms that are not well characterized include methyldopa (an antihypertensive), amphetamines, tricyclic and other types of antidepressants, and opioids.

38 Thyroid & Antithyroid Drugs

OBJECTIVES

You should be able to:

- List the principal drugs used in the treatment of hypothyroidism.
- List the principal drugs used in the treatment of hyperthyroidism and compare the onset and duration of their action.
- Sketch the biochemical pathway for thyroid hormone synthesis and release and indicate the sites of action of antithyroid drugs.
- Describe the major toxicities of thyroxine and the antithyroid drugs.

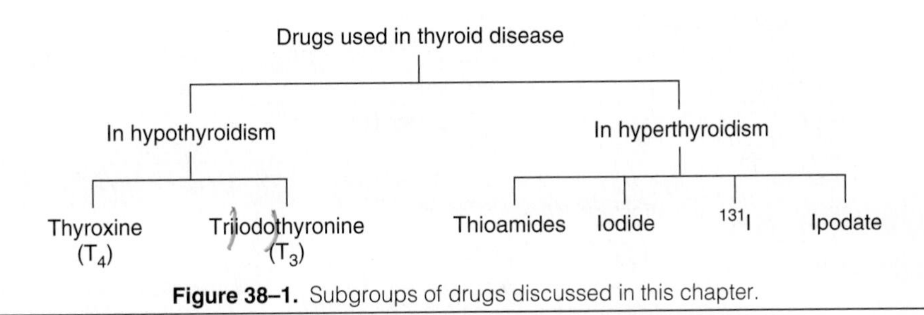

Figure 38–1. Subgroups of drugs discussed in this chapter.

CONCEPTS

The thyroid secretes two types of hormones: iodine-containing amino acids (thyroxine and triiodothyronine) and a peptide (calcitonin). Thyroxine and triiodothyronine have very general effects on growth, development, and metabolism. Calcitonin is important in calcium metabolism and is discussed in Chapter 41. This chapter describes the drugs used in the treatment of hypothyroidism and hyperthyroidism (Figure 38–1).

THYROID HORMONES

A. Synthesis and Transport of Thyroid Hormones: The thyroid secretes two iodine-containing hormones: triiodothyronine (T_3) and thyroxine (T_4). The iodine necessary for the synthesis of these molecules is derived from food or iodine supplements. Iodine uptake is an active process, and the iodide ion is highly concentrated in the thyroid gland. The tyrosine residues of a protein, thyroglobulin, are iodinated in the gland to form monoiodotyrosine (MIT) or diiodotyrosine (DIT). Thyroxine (T_4) is formed from the combination of two molecules of DIT, while triiodothyronine (T_3) contains one molecule of MIT and one of DIT. Some T_3 is released from the thyroid, but much of the circulating T_3 is formed by the deiodination of T_4 in the tissues. After release from the gland, both T_3 and T_4 are bound to thyroxine-binding globulin, a transport protein in the blood.

Thyroid function is controlled by the pituitary through the release of thyrotropin (TSH) and by the availability of iodide. High levels of thyroid hormones inhibit the release of TSH, providing an effective negative feedback control mechanism. In Graves' disease, lymphocytes release a thyroid-stimulating immunoglobulin (TSI; also called TSH receptor-stimulating antibody) that causes thyrotoxicosis. Since these lymphocytes are not susceptible to negative feedback, blood concentrations of thyroid hormone may become very high.

Iodide concentrations higher than normal inhibit iodination of tyrosine, an effect that is useful in the treatment of thyroid disease. Inadequate iodine intake results in diffuse enlargement of the thyroid (goiter).

B. Mechanisms of Action of Thyroxine and Triiodothyronine: T_3 is about ten times more potent than T_4; since T_4 is converted to T_3 in target cells, the liver, and the kidneys, most of the effect of circulating T_4 is probably due to T_3.

Thyroid hormone binds to receptors in the nucleus that control the expression of genes responsible for many metabolic processes. The T_3 receptor exists in two monomeric forms: alpha and beta. When activated by T_3, the α and β monomers combine to form $\alpha\alpha$, $\beta\beta$, or $\alpha\beta$ dimers. These T_3-activated dimers bind to DNA response elements and control the synthesis of RNA, which codes for specific proteins that mediate the actions of thyroid hormones.

The proteins synthesized under T_3 control differ depending upon the tissue involved; these proteins include Na^+/K^+ ATPase, specific contractile proteins in smooth muscle and the heart, enzymes involved in lipid metabolism, important developmental components in the brain, etc. T_3 may also have a separate membrane receptor-mediated effect in some tissues.

1. **Effects of thyroid hormone:** The organ level actions of the thyroid drugs include normal growth and development of the nervous, skeletal, and reproductive systems and control of metabolism of fats, carbohydrates, proteins, and vitamins. The results of excess thyroid activity (thyrotoxicosis) and hypothyroidism (myxedema) are summarized in Table 38–1.

Table 38–1. Summary of thyroid hormone effects.*

System	Thyrotoxicosis	Hypothyroidism
Skin and appendages	Warm, moist skin; sweating; heat intolerance; fine, thin hair	Pale, cool, puffy skin; dry and brittle hair; brittle nails
Eyes, face	Retraction of upper lid with wide stare; periorbital edema; exophthalmos (Graves' disease)	Drooping of eyelids; periorbital edema; puffy, nonpitting facies; large tongue
Cardiovascular system	Decreased peripheral vascular resistance, increased heart rate, stroke volume, cardiac output, pulse pressure; high-output congestive heart failure; increased inotropic/chronotropic effects; arrhythmias; angina	Increased peripheral vascular resistance, decreased heart rate, stroke volume, cardiac output, pulse pressure; low-output congestive heart failure; ECG: bradycardia, prolonged PR interval; pericardial effusion
Respiratory system	Dyspnea; decreased vital capacity	Pleural effusions; hypoventilation and CO_2 retention
Gastrointestinal system	Increased appetite; increased frequency of bowel movements; hypoproteinemia	Decreased appetite; decreased frequency of bowel movements; ascites
Central nervous system	Nervousness; hyperkinesia; emotional lability	Lethargy; general slowing of mental processes; neuropathies
Musculoskeletal system	Weakness and muscle fatigue; increased deep tendon reflexes; hypercalcemia; osteoporosis	Stiffness and muscle fatigue; decreased deep tendon reflexes; increased alkaline phosphatase, LDH, AST
Renal system	Mild polyuria; increased renal blood flow; increased glomerular filtration rate	Impaired water excretion; decreased renal blood flow; decreased glomerular filtration rate
Hematopoietic system	Increased erythropoiesis; anemia[1]	Decreased erythropoiesis; anemia[1]
Reproductive system	Menstrual irregularities; decreased fertility; increased gonadal steroid metabolism	Hypermenorrhea; infertility; decreased libido; impotence; oligospermia; decreased gonadal steroid metabolism
Metabolic system	Increased basal metabolic rate; hyperglycemia; increased free fatty acids; decreased cholesterol and triglycerides; increased hormone degradation; increased requirements for fat- and water-soluble vitamins; increased drug detoxification	Decreased basal metabolic rate; delayed degradation of insulin, with increased sensitivity; increased cholesterol and triglycerides; decreased hormone degradation; decreased requirements for fat- and water-soluble vitamins; decreased drug detoxification

*Modified, with permission, from Katzung BG (editor): *Basic & Clinical Pharmacology,* 8th ed. McGraw-Hill, 2001.
[1]The anemia of hyperthyroidism is usually normochromic and caused by increased red blood cell turnover. The anemia of hypothyroidism may be normochromic, hyperchromic, or hypochromic and may be due to decreased production rate, decreased iron absorption, or decreased folic acid absorption, or may represent autoimmune pernicious anemia.

2. **Clinical use:** Thyroid hormone therapy can be accomplished with either thyroxine or triiodothyronine. Synthetic levothyroxine (T_4) is the form of choice for most cases. T_3 (liothyronine) is faster-acting but has a shorter half-life and is more expensive.
3. **Toxicity:** Toxicity is that of thyrotoxicosis (Table 38–1). Older patients, those with cardiovascular disease, and those with long-standing hypothyroidism are highly sensitive to the stimulatory effects of T_4 on the heart. Such patients should receive lower initial doses of T_4.

ANTITHYROID DRUGS

A. Thioamides: Propylthiouracil (PTU) and methimazole are small sulfur-containing molecules that inhibit thyroid hormone production by several mechanisms. The most important effect is to block iodination of the tyrosine residues of thyroglobulin (Figure 38–2). In addition, these drugs may block coupling of DIT and MIT. The thioamides can be used by the oral route and are effective in most patients with uncomplicated hyperthyroidism. Since synthesis of thyroid hormone rather than release is inhibited, the onset of activity of these drugs is usually slow, of-

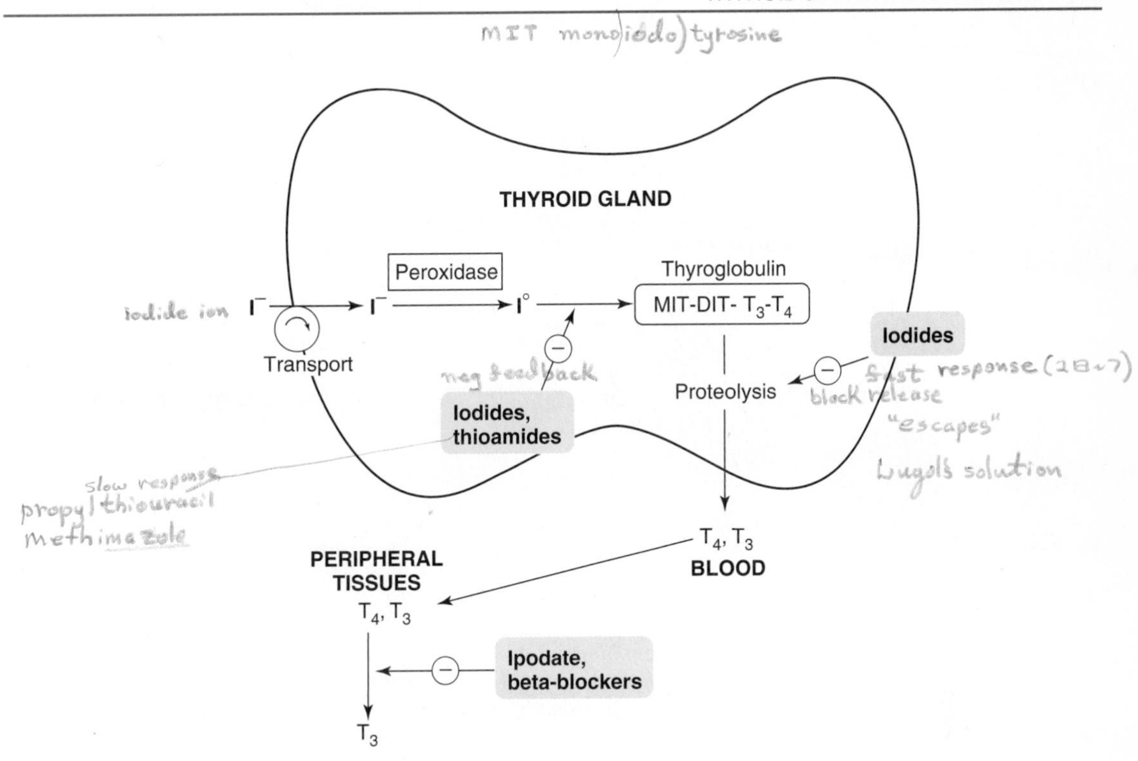

Figure 38–2. Sites of action of some antithyroid drugs. I^-, iodide ion; I°, elemental iodine. Not shown: radioactive iodine (^{131}I), which destroys the gland through radiation.

ten requiring 3–4 weeks for full effect. However, high-dose PTU inhibits the conversion of T_4 to T_3. PTU is less likely than methimazole to cross the placenta and enter breast milk, but it should be used cautiously in pregnant and nursing women. Toxic effects include skin rash (common) and severe immune reactions (rare) such as vasculitis, hypoprothrombinemia, and agranulocytosis. These effects are usually reversible.

B. Iodide Salts and Iodine: Iodide salts inhibit organification (iodination of tyrosine) and thyroid hormone release (Figure 38–2); these salts also decrease the size and vascularity of the hyperplastic thyroid gland. Since iodide salts inhibit release as well as synthesis of the hormones, their onset of action occurs rapidly—within 2–7 days. However, the effects are transient; the thyroid gland "escapes" from the iodide block after several weeks of treatment. Iodide salts are used in management of "thyroid storm," severe thyrotoxicosis, and to prepare patients for surgical resection of a hyperactive thyroid. The usual forms of this drug are Lugol's solution (iodine and potassium iodide) and saturated solution of potassium iodide.

C. Radioactive Iodine: Radioactive iodine (^{131}I) is taken up and concentrated in the thyroid gland so avidly that a dose large enough to severely damage the gland can be given without endangering other tissues. Unlike the thioamides and iodide salts, an effective dose of ^{131}I can produce a permanent cure of thyrotoxicosis without surgery. ^{131}I should not be used in pregnant or nursing women.

D. Iodinated Radiocontrast Media: Certain iodinated radiocontrast media (eg, ipodate) effectively suppress the conversion of T_4 to T_3 via 5′-deiodinase in the liver, kidney, and other peripheral tissues (Figure 38–2). Inhibition of hormone release from the thyroid may also play a part. Ipodate has proved to be very useful in rapidly reducing T_3 concentrations in thyrotoxicosis.

E. Other Drugs: Other agents used in the treatment of thyrotoxicosis include the beta-blockers. Propranolol also inhibits 5′-deiodinase. These agents are particularly useful in controlling the tachycardia and other cardiac abnormalities of severe thyrotoxicosis.

DRUG LIST

The following drugs are important members of the group discussed in this chapter. Prototypes should be learned in detail; the other significant agents should be recognized as belonging to a specific subclass.

Subclass	Prototype	Other Significant Agents
Thyroid hormones	Thyroxine (T_4), triiodothyronine (T_3)	
Antithyroid drugs	Propylthiouracil, iodide salts, ^{131}I, ipodate	Methimazole
Miscellaneous	Propranolol	

QUESTIONS

DIRECTIONS: Each of the numbered items or incomplete statements in this section is followed by answers or by completions of the sentence. Select the ONE lettered answer or completion that is BEST in each case.

Items 1–3: A 24-year-old woman is found to have thyrotoxicosis. She appears to be in good health otherwise. It is decided to place her on antithyroid drug therapy.

1. Agents that could be used to treat this woman's thyrotoxicosis do not include
- **(A)** Methimazole
- **(B)** Potassium iodide
- **(C)** Propylthiouracil
- **(D)** Radioactive iodine
- **(E)** Thyroglobulin

2. Potential drug toxicities that might be considered in this case are LEAST likely to include
- **(A)** Iodide ion: Acne-like rash
- **(B)** Ipodate: Skin rash
- **(C)** Methimazole: Agranulocytosis
- **(D)** Propylthiouracil: Lupus erythematosus-like syndrome
- **(E)** Radioactive iodine: Radiation damage to the ovaries

3. The patient is lost to follow-up before therapy is begun, but she returns 6 months later for a prenatal workup. Although 3 months pregnant, she has lost weight, has a marked tremor, and her resting heart rate is 120/min. Her thyrotoxicosis is obviously worse, and the gland is larger and more vascular. It is decided to correct her thyroid abnormality surgically. Before surgery can be done, however, her gland should be reduced in size and vascularity by administering
- **(A)** Iodide ion
- **(B)** Ipodate
- **(C)** Propranolol
- **(D)** Propylthiouracil
- **(E)** Radioactive iodine

4. Actions of thyroxine do not include
- **(A)** Acceleration of cardiac rate
- **(B)** Decreased glomerular filtration rate
- **(C)** Fine tremor of skeletal muscles
- **(D)** Increased appetite
- **(E)** Stimulation of oxygen consumption

5. Effects of iodide salts given in large doses do not include
- **(A)** Decreased size of the thyroid gland
- **(B)** Decreased vascularity of the thyroid gland
- **(C)** Decreased hormone release
- **(D)** Decreased iodination of tyrosine
- **(E)** Increased ^{131}I uptake

6. Symptoms of hypothyroidism (myxedema) do not include
- **(A)** Dry, puffy skin
- **(B)** Increased appetite

(C) Large tongue and drooping of the eyelids
(D) Lethargy, sleepiness
(E) Slow heart rate

7. When initiating thyroxine therapy for an elderly patient with long-standing hypothyroidism, it is important to begin with small doses to avoid
(A) A flare of exophthalmos
(B) Acute renal failure
(C) Hemolysis
(D) Overstimulation of the heart
(E) Seizures

DIRECTIONS (Items 8–10): The matching questions in this section consist of a list of five lettered options followed by several numbered items. For each numbered item, select the ONE lettered option that is most closely associated with it. Each lettered option may be selected once, more than once, or not at all.

(A) ^{131}I
(B) Ipodate
(C) Propranolol
(D) Propylthiouracil
(E) Triiodothyronine

8. Produced in the peripheral tissues when thyroxine is administered
9. Radiocontrast medium that is also useful in thyrotoxicosis
10. Produces a permanent reduction in thyroid activity

DIRECTIONS (Items 11–13): This case history* is followed by discussion questions. Write out brief answers (two to five sentences) and then compare your answers with those given at the end of the Answers section.

A 27-year-old woman was referred for evaluation of thyroid disease. She had a 3-month history of intermittent heat intolerance, sweats, tremor, tachycardia, and muscle weakness. She had lost weight in spite of a marked increase in appetite. She denied taking any medications before seeing her family physician. She had been taking iodide drops since seeing her doctor and initially noted a decrease in symptoms. For the past month, however, they had worsened.

Physical examination revealed blood pressure 180/90 mm Hg, heart rate 110/min, minimal proptosis, and an enlarged thyroid gland. Laboratory tests showed elevated thyroxine, resin T_3 uptake, radioactive iodine uptake, and antimicrosomal antibodies. A diagnosis of hyperimmune hyperthyroidism (Graves' disease) was made.

11. What therapeutic measures should be considered in this case? Why did the iodide drops the patient was taking reduce symptoms at first and then lose their effectiveness?
12. What are the benefits and hazards of pharmacologic therapy in hyperthyroidism?
13. What therapy should be considered if thyrotoxic crisis (thyroid storm) occurs?

ANSWERS

1. Thyroglobulin contains thyroxine in its protein-bound form. This compound would never be used in thyrotoxicosis. The answer is **(E).**
2. The toxicities listed are all possible except radiation damage to the ovaries. Iodine is so avidly taken up by the thyroid that large doses of radioactive iodide can be given without damage to other tissues. The answer is **(E).**
3. Surgical treatment is often preferred in hyperthyroidism that occurs during pregnancy because this offers minimal risk to the fetus and the fetal thyroid. Before surgical removal, a large, highly vascular thyroid gland should be prepared by administration of a short course of iodide ion. This treatment reduces the gland's size and vascularity and makes surgery much safer.

* Modified and reproduced, with permission, from Dong BJ: Thyroid diseases. In: *Applied Therapeutics,* 3rd ed. Katcher BS, Young LY, Koda-Kimble MA (editors). Applied Therapeutics, 1983.

Short-term administration of iodide will not harm the fetus. Propylthiouracil may be considered for less severe thyrotoxicosis occurring during pregnancy. The answer is **(A).**

4. Thyroid hormone *increases* glomerular filtration rate. The answer is **(B).**

5. Iodide has a negative feedback effect on the thyroid and decreases the rate of iodine uptake. The answer is **(E).**

6. Appetite decreases in myxedema as the metabolic rate decreases. The answer is **(B).**

7. Patients with long-standing hypothyroidism, especially elderly ones, are highly sensitive to the stimulatory effects of thyroxine upon cardiac function. Administration of regular doses can cause overstimulation of the heart and cardiac collapse. The answer is **(D).**

8. T_4 is converted into T_3 in the periphery. The answer is **(E).**

9. Ipodate is a radiocontrast agent. The answer is **(B).**

10. Radioactive iodine is the only medical therapy that produces a permanent reduction of thyroid activity. The answer is **(A).**

11. The major therapies available for Graves' disease are surgery, thyroid-suppressant drugs, and radioactive iodine in sufficient dosage to destroy the gland. Ipodate—an iodine-containing x-ray contrast material—and beta-blockers are of value in severe thyrotoxicosis.

Iodide therapy (usually saturated solution of potassium iodide) is useful in reducing thyroid hormone release and in decreasing the vascularity of the gland prior to surgery. However, escape from the inhibitory effect of iodide often occurs in Graves' disease, and the increased iodine substrate made available by the therapy may actually accentuate the disease.

12. Radioactive iodine is often the treatment of choice for young adult patients. This treatment provides a permanent cure. (In fact, hypothyroidism is common after treatment and is managed with levothyroxine replacement therapy.) There is no evidence—even after 35 years of follow-up—that this exposure to radioactivity causes increased incidence of neoplastic disease.

Antithyroid drugs include iodide (discussed above) and the thioamides. The principal thioamides are propylthiouracil and methimazole. Almost all patients respond to these agents. However, immunologic complications are not rare. Skin rashes are the most common. Agranulocytosis, cholestatic jaundice, hepatocellular damage, and exfoliative dermatitis are uncommon.

Surgical thyroidectomy is the treatment of choice for patients with very large or multinodular glands. Patients are treated preoperatively with antithyroid drugs until they are euthyroid, and they then receive iodine for 2 weeks prior to surgery to reduce vascularity of the gland.

13. Patients in thyrotoxic crisis usually have multiple system involvement. The cardiovascular system is particularly susceptible, and severe tachycardia, arrhythmias, and heart failure are common. The sympathetic nervous system is hyperactive, and this is one of the major causes of the cardiovascular effects. The CNS is also affected, and signs may include severe agitation, delirium, and coma.

Ipodate, which inhibits the conversion of thyroxine to triiodothyronine, is useful in reducing the intensity of thyroid storm. Sympathoplegic drugs are also useful, and propranolol is the most commonly used agent. Further release of hormone from the gland is blocked by intravenous administration of sodium iodide supplemented by oral potassium iodide. Synthesis is inhibited by oral or, if necessary, parenteral antithyroid drugs. Corticosteroids are sometimes used.

Corticosteroids & Antagonists 39

OBJECTIVES

You should be able to:

- Describe the major naturally occurring glucocorticosteroid and its actions.
- List several synthetic glucocorticoids and the differences between these agents and the naturally occurring hormone.
- Describe the actions of the naturally occurring mineralocorticoid and one synthetic agent in this subgroup.
- List the indications for the use of corticosteroids in adrenal and nonadrenal disorders.

CONCEPTS

The corticosteroids are those steroid hormones produced by the adrenal cortex. They consist of two major physiologic and pharmacologic groups: (1) glucocorticoids, which have important effects on intermediary metabolism, catabolism, immune responses, and inflammation; and (2) mineralocorticoids, which regulate sodium and potassium reabsorption in the collecting tubules of the kidney. This chapter reviews the glucocorticoids, the mineralocorticoids, and the adrenocorticosteroid antagonists (Figure 39–1).

GLUCOCORTICOIDS

A. Mechanism of Action: Corticosteroids enter the cell and bind to cytosolic receptors that transport the steroid into the nucleus. The steroid-receptor complex alters gene expression by binding to glucocorticoid response elements (GREs) or mineralocorticoid-specific elements (Figure 39–2). Tissue-specific responses to steroids are made possible by the presence in each tissue of different protein regulators that control the interaction between the hormone-receptor complex and particular response elements.

B. Organ and Tissue Effects:

1. Metabolic effects: Glucocorticoids stimulate gluconeogenesis. As a result, blood sugar

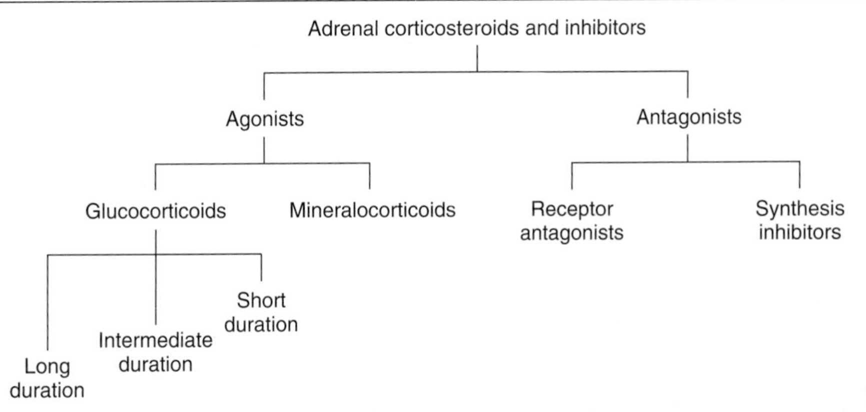

Figure 39–1. Subgroups of drugs discussed in this chapter.

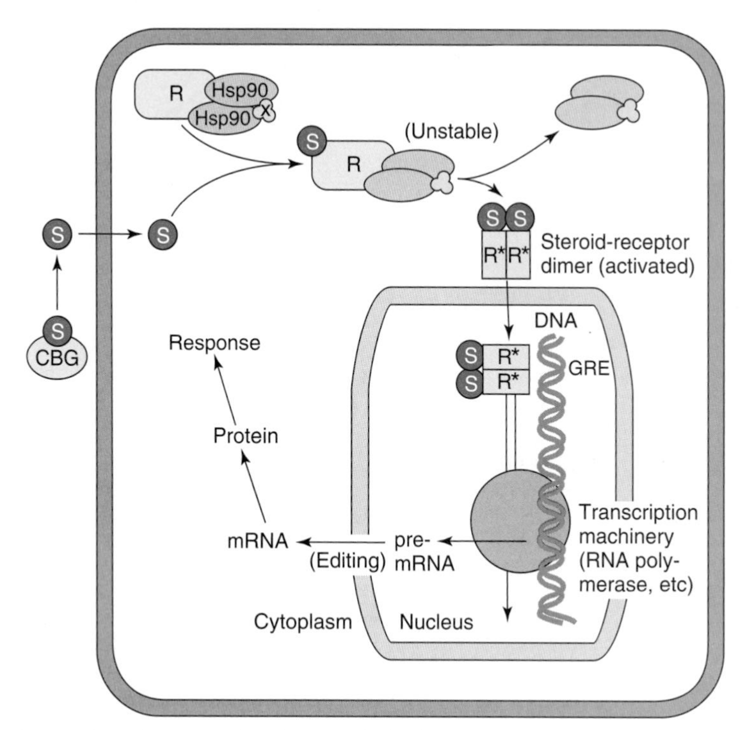

Figure 39–2. Mechanism of glucocorticoid action. This figure models the interaction of a steroid, S (eg, cortisol), with its receptor, R, and the subsequent events in a target cell. The steroid is present in the blood bound to the corticosteroid-binding globulin, CBG, but enters the cell as the free molecule. The intracellular receptor is bound to stabilizing proteins, including heat shock protein 90 (Hsp90) and several others, represented as "X" in the figure. When the complex binds a molecule of steroid, the Hsp90 and associated molecules are released. The steroid-receptor complex enters the nucleus as a dimer, binds to the glucocorticoid response element (GRE) on the gene, and regulates gene transcription by RNA polymerase II and associated transcription factors. The resulting mRNA is edited and exported to the cytoplasm for the production of protein that brings about the final hormone response. (Reproduced, with permission, from Katzung BG [editor]: *Basic & Clinical Pharmacology,* 8th ed. McGraw-Hill, 2001.)

rises, muscle protein is catabolized, and insulin secretion is stimulated. Both lipolysis and lipogenesis are stimulated, with a net increase of fat deposition in certain areas, eg, the face (moon facies) and the shoulders and back (buffalo hump).

2. **Catabolic effects:** As noted above, glucocorticoids cause muscle protein catabolism. In addition, lymphoid and connective tissue, fat, and skin undergo wasting under the influence of high concentrations of these steroids. Catabolic effects on bone can lead to osteoporosis. In children, growth is inhibited.
3. **Immunosuppressive effects:** Glucocorticoids inhibit some of the mechanisms involved in cell-mediated immunologic functions, especially those dependent on lymphocytes. These agents are actively lymphotoxic and are important in the treatment of hematologic cancers. The drugs do not interfere with the development of normal acquired immunity but delay rejection reactions in patients with organ transplants.
4. **Anti-inflammatory effects:** Glucocorticoids have a dramatic effect on the distribution and function of leukocytes. These drugs increase neutrophils and decrease lymphocytes, eosinophils, basophils, and monocytes. The migration of leukocytes is also inhibited. The biochemical mechanisms underlying these cellular effects include the induced synthesis of an inhibitor of phospholipase A_2 (see Chapter 18), decreased mRNA for COX-2, decreases in IL2 and IL3, and decreases in platelet activating factor (PAF), an inflammatory cytokine.
5. **Other effects:** Glucocorticoids such as cortisol are required for normal renal excretion of water loads. The glucocorticoids also have effects on the CNS. When given in large doses (especially if given for long periods), these drugs may cause profound behavioral disturbances. Large doses stimulate gastric acid secretion and decrease resistance to ulcer formation.

C. Important Glucocorticoids:

1. **Cortisol:** The major natural glucocorticoid is cortisol (hydrocortisone). The physiologic secretion of cortisol is regulated by ACTH and varies during the day (circadian rhythm), with the peak occurring in the morning and the trough around midnight. In the plasma, cortisol is 95% bound to corticosteroid-binding globulin. Given as a drug, cortisol is well absorbed from the gastrointestinal tract, is cleared by the liver, and has a short duration of action compared with its synthetic congeners (Table 39–1). Although it diffuses poorly across normal skin, cortisol is readily absorbed across inflamed skin and mucous membranes.

   The cortisol molecule also has a small but significant salt-retaining (mineralocorticoid) effect. This is an important cause of hypertension in patients with a cortisol-secreting adrenal tumor or a pituitary ACTH-secreting tumor (Cushing's syndrome).

2. **Synthetic glucocorticoids:** The mechanism of action of these agents is identical to that of cortisol. A large number are available for use; prednisone and its active metabolite, prednisolone, dexamethasone, and triamcinolone are representative. Their properties (when compared to cortisol) include longer half-life and duration of action, reduced salt-retaining effect, and better penetration of lipid barriers for topical activity (Table 39–1).

   Special glucocorticoids have been developed for use in asthma and other conditions in which good surface activity on mucous membranes or skin is needed and systemic effects are to be avoided. **Beclomethasone** and **budesonide** readily penetrate the airway mucosa but have very short half-lives after they enter the blood, so that systemic effects and toxicity are greatly reduced.

D. Clinical Uses:

1. **Adrenal disorders:** Glucocorticoids are essential to preserve life in patients with chronic adrenal cortical insufficiency (Addison's disease) and are necessary in acute adrenal insufficiency associated with life-threatening shock, infection, or trauma. Glucocorticoids are also used in certain types of congenital adrenal hyperplasia, in which synthesis of abnormal forms of corticosteroids are stimulated by ACTH. In these conditions, administration of a potent synthetic glucocorticoid suppresses ACTH secretion sufficiently to reduce the synthesis of the abnormal steroids.
2. **Nonadrenal disorders:** Many disorders respond to corticosteroid therapy. Some of these are inflammatory or immunologic in nature (eg, asthma, organ transplant rejection, collagen diseases, exophthalmos). Other applications include the treatment of hematopoietic cancers, neurologic disorders, chemotherapy-induced vomiting, hypercalcemia, and mountain sickness. Betamethasone, a glucocorticoid with a low degree of protein binding, is given to pregnant women in premature labor to hasten maturation of the fetal lungs. The degree of benefit differs considerably in different disorders, and the toxicity of corticosteroids given chronically limits their use.

E. Toxicity: Most of the toxic effects of the glucocorticoids are predictable from the effects already described. Some are life-threatening and include adrenal suppression (from suppression of ACTH secretion), metabolic effects (growth inhibition, diabetes, muscle wasting, osteoporosis), salt retention, and psychosis. Methods for minimizing these toxicities include local appli-

Table 39–1. Properties of representative corticosteroids.

Agent	Duration of Action (hours)	Anti-inflammatory Potency[1]	Salt-Retaining Potency[1]	Topical Activity
Primarily glucocorticoid				
Cortisol	8–12	1	1	0
Prednisone	12–24	4	0.3	(+)
Triamcinolone	15–24	5	0	+++
Dexamethasone	24–36	30	0	+++++
Primarily mineralocorticoid				
Aldosterone	1–2	0.3	3000	0
Fludrocortisone	8–12	10	125–250	0

[1]Relative to cortisol.

cation (eg, aerosols for asthma), alternate-day therapy (to reduce pituitary suppression), and tapering the dose soon after achieving a therapeutic response. To avoid adrenal insufficiency in patients who have had long-term therapy, additional "stress doses" may need to be given during serious illness or before major surgery. Patients who are being withdrawn from glucocorticoids after protracted use should have their doses tapered slowly, over the course of several months, to allow recovery of normal adrenal function.

MINERALOCORTICOIDS

A. Aldosterone: The major natural mineralocorticoid in humans is aldosterone, which has already been mentioned in connection with hypertension (see Chapter 11) and control of its secretion by angiotensin II (see Chapter 17). The secretion of aldosterone is regulated by ACTH and by the renin-angiotensin system and is very important in the regulation of blood volume and blood pressure (see Figure 6–4). Aldosterone has a short half-life and little glucocorticoid activity (Table 39–1). Its mechanism of action is the same as that of the glucocorticoids.

B. Other Mineralocorticoids: Other mineralocorticoids include deoxycorticosterone, the naturally occurring precursor of aldosterone, and **fludrocortisone.** The latter has significant glucocorticoid activity. Because of its long duration of action (Table 39–1), fludrocortisone is favored for replacement therapy after adrenalectomy and in other conditions in which mineralocorticoid therapy is needed.

CORTICOSTEROID ANTAGONISTS

A. Receptor Antagonists: Spironolactone, an antagonist of aldosterone at its receptor, has been discussed in connection with the diuretics (see Chapter 15). **Mifepristone (RU 486)** is an inhibitor at glucocorticoid receptors as well as progesterone receptors (see Chapter 40) and has been used in the treatment of Cushing's syndrome.

B. Synthesis Inhibitors: Several drugs are used in the treatment of adrenal cancer when surgical therapy is impractical or unsuccessful because of metastases. The most important of these drugs are **aminoglutethimide, metyrapone,** and **ketoconazole.**

Ketoconazole (an antifungal drug) inhibits the P450 enzymes necessary for the synthesis of all steroids and is used in a number of conditions in which reduced steroid levels are desirable, eg, adrenal carcinoma, hirsutism, breast cancer. Aminoglutethimide blocks the conversion of cholesterol to pregnenolone and also inhibits synthesis of all hormonally active steroids. It can be used in conjunction with other drugs for treatment of steroid-producing adrenocortical cancer. Metyrapone inhibits the normal synthesis of cortisol but not that of cortisol precursors; the drug can be used in diagnostic tests of adrenal function.

DRUG LIST

The following drugs are important members of the group discussed in this chapter. Prototypes should be learned in detail; features of the major variants should be known well enough to distinguish the variants from prototypes and from each other; the other significant agents should be recognized as belonging to a specific subclass.

Subclass	Prototype	Major Variants	Other Significant Agents
Agonists			
Glucocorticoids	Cortisol (hydrocortisone), prednisone	Dexamethasone, triamcinolone, beclomethasone	Triamcinolone acetonide
Mineralocorticoids	Aldosterone	Fludrocortisone	
Antagonists			
Receptor antagonists	Spironolactone	Mifepristone	
Synthesis inhibitors	Aminoglutethimide, metyrapone	Ketoconazole	

QUESTIONS

DIRECTIONS: Each of the numbered items or incomplete statements in this section is followed by answers or by completions of the statement. Select the ONE lettered answer or completion that is BEST in each case.

1. Effects of the glucocorticoids do not include
(A) Altered fat deposition
(B) Increased blood glucose
(C) Increased skin protein synthesis
(D) Inhibition of leukotriene synthesis
(E) Reduction in circulating lymphocytes

2. Toxic effects of the corticosteroids do not include
(A) Growth inhibition
(B) Hypertension
(C) Hypoglycemia
(D) Psychosis
(E) Salt retention

3. A 46-year-old male patient has Cushing's syndrome that is due to the presence of an adrenal tumor. Which of the following drugs would be expected to reduce the signs and symptoms of this man's disease?
(A) Betamethasone
(B) Cortisol
(C) Fludrocortisone
(D) Ketoconazole
(E) Triamcinolone

4. In the treatment of congenital adrenal hyperplasia in which there is excess production of cortisol precursors due to a lack of 21β-hydroxylase activity, the purpose of administration of a synthetic glucocorticoid is
(A) Inhibition of aldosterone synthesis
(B) Normalization of renal function
(C) Prevention of hypoglycemia
(D) Recovery of normal immune function
(E) Suppression of ACTH secretion

5. A glucocorticoid response element is
(A) A protein regulator that controls the interaction between an activated steroid receptor and DNA
(B) A short DNA sequence that binds tightly to RNA polymerase
(C) A small protein that binds to an unoccupied steroid receptor protein and prevents it from becoming denatured
(D) A specific nucleotide sequence that is recognized by a steroid hormone receptor-hormone complex
(E) The portion of the steroid receptor that binds to DNA

6. Glucocorticoids have not been proved to be effective in the treatment of
(A) Acute lymphocytic leukemia
(B) Addison's disease
(C) Asthma
(D) Chemotherapy-induced vomiting
(E) Osteoporosis

7. For patients who have been on long-term therapy with a glucocorticoid and who now wish to discontinue the drug, gradual tapering of the glucocorticoid is needed to allow recovery of
(A) Depressed release of insulin from pancreatic B cells
(B) Hematopoiesis in the bone marrow
(C) Normal osteoblast function
(D) The control by vasopressin of water excretion
(E) The hypothalamic-pituitary-adrenal system

Items 8–9: A 54-year-old man with miliary tuberculosis has developed signs of severe acute adrenal insufficiency.

8. This patient is not likely to develop
(A) Hypoglycemia if food is withheld
(B) Moon face

(C) Reduced ability to combat infection
(D) Reduced ability to excrete a water load
(E) Reduced blood volume

9. The patient should be treated immediately. Which of the following combinations is most rational?
   (A) Aldosterone and fludrocortisone
   (B) Cortisol and fludrocortisone
   (C) Dexamethasone and metyrapone
   (D) Fludrocortisone and metyrapone
   (E) Triamcinolone and dexamethasone

DIRECTIONS (Items 10–14): This case history* is followed by discussion questions. Write out brief answers (two to five sentences) and then compare your answers with those given at the end of the Answers section.

A 60-year-old woman was referred for management of severe rheumatoid arthritis. She had had the disease for 15 years and had been treated until age 55 with aspirin. She was then switched to ibuprofen, which diminished the gastrointestinal adverse effects she had developed from aspirin. One year before referral, she started to complain of increased joint pain and stiffness, and laboratory studies confirmed that the disease had become more active. Several attempts to control her symptoms with increased dosage of ibuprofen and with a trial of another NSAID were not successful, and the decision was made to add corticosteroids to the regimen.

Prednisone was started in a dosage of 5 mg daily, given in the morning. After a period of evaluation, the dose was increased to 10 mg and then to 15 mg daily. At this dosage, the patient's symptoms were tolerable.

10. What are the relative advantages and disadvantages of corticosteroids versus NSAIDs in the treatment of inflammatory disease?
11. Why was prednisone given to this patient in the morning?
12. What is the advantage of alternate-day therapy with corticosteroids? Which steroids are unsuitable for alternate-day therapy?
13. What other well-established disease-modifying antirheumatic drugs (DMARDs) may also be useful in a patient with rheumatoid arthritis?
14. What new drugs have recently become available for the treatment of rheumatoid arthritis?

ANSWERS

1. Glucocorticoids stimulate protein breakdown, not synthesis (except in the liver). The answer is **(C).**
2. Corticosteroids may induce hyperglycemia of sufficient magnitude to require insulin therapy. The answer is **(C).**
3. Ketoconazole inhibits many types of cytochrome P450 enzymes. It can be used to reduce the unregulated overproduction of corticosteroids by adrenal tumors. The answer is **(D).**
4. 21β-Hydroxylase deficiency prevents normal synthesis of cortisol and causes accumulation of cortisol precursors. The hypothalamic-pituitary system responds to the low levels of cortisol by increasing ACTH release. High levels of ACTH induce adrenal hyperplasia and excess production of steroids, which are diverted to the androgen pathway to cause virilization. A high dose of glucocorticoid is administered to suppress release of ACTH. The answer is **(E).**
5. Activated steroid hormone receptors mediate their effects upon gene expression by binding to hormone response elements, which are short sequences of DNA located near steroid-regulated genes. The answer is **(D).**
6. Chronic treatment with glucocorticoids *increases* the risk of osteoporosis. The answer is **(E).**
7. Exogenous glucocorticoids act at the hypothalamus and pituitary to suppress the production of CRF and ACTH. As a result, adrenal production of endogenous corticosteroids is suppressed. On discontinuance, the recovery of normal hypothalamic-pituitary-adrenal function occurs

* Modified and reproduced, with permission, from Kishi DT: Disorders of the adrenals. In: *Applied Therapeutics,* 3rd ed. Katcher BS, Young LY, Koda-Kimble MA (editors). Applied Therapeutics, 1983.

slowly. Glucocorticoid doses must be tapered slowly, over several months, in order to prevent adrenal insufficiency. The answer is **(E).**

8. Moon face is a manifestation of hypercortisolism, not adrenal insufficiency. The answer is **(B).**

9. A rational combination of drugs should include agents with complementary effects, ie, a glucocorticoid and a mineralocorticoid. The combination with these characteristics is cortisol and fludrocortisone. (Note that while fludrocortisone may have sufficient glucocorticoid activity for a patient with mild disease, a patient in severe acute adrenal insufficiency needs a full glucocorticoid such as cortisol.) The answer is **(B).**

10. Corticosteroids are more effective than NSAIDs in controlling acute severe flare-ups of joint inflammation. However, the severe toxicities of corticosteroids (adrenocortical suppression, weight gain, buffalo hump, striae, osteoporosis, diabetes, peptic ulcers, cataracts, glaucoma, and psychoses) preclude their use for chronic therapy in most patients.

11. The normal diurnal variation of glucocorticoid release includes a peak in the morning hours and a trough late at night. Therefore, a single morning dose of an intermediate-acting (12–24 hours) agent such as prednisone mimics the normal variation and reduces the degree of suppression of the pituitary.

12. Alternate-day therapy permits maintenance of a greater degree of pituitary-adrenal interaction and also allows temporary recovery of peripheral tissues from stimulation by high levels of glucocorticoid. This is particularly valuable in growing children. The longest-acting corticosteroids are not suitable for alternate-day regimens because the duration of pituitary suppression extends over 48 hours, and nothing is gained. Such long-acting agents include dexamethasone and betamethasone.

13. Older disease-modifying antirheumatic drugs (DMARDs) used frequently in rheumatoid arthritis include hydroxychloroquine, methotrexate, steroids, and sulfasalazine. Gold salts and penicillamine may be effective but cause severe toxicity (see Chapter 36).

14. Newer drugs that have become available for the treatment of rheumatoid arthritis include the COX-2 inhibitors, etanercept, infliximab, and leflunomide (see Chapter 36).

Gonadal Hormones & Inhibitors — 40

OBJECTIVES

You should be able to:

- Describe the hormonal changes that occur during the menstrual cycle.
- Name three estrogens and four progestins. Describe their pharmacologic effects, clinical uses, and toxicity.
- List the benefits and hazards of oral contraceptives.
- List the benefits and hazards of postmenopausal estrogen therapy.
- Describe the use of sex hormones and their antagonists in the treatment of cancer in women and men.
- List or describe the toxic effects of anabolic steroids used to build muscle mass.
- Define the terms "SERM" and "mixed agonists." Name two SERMs and describe their unique properties.

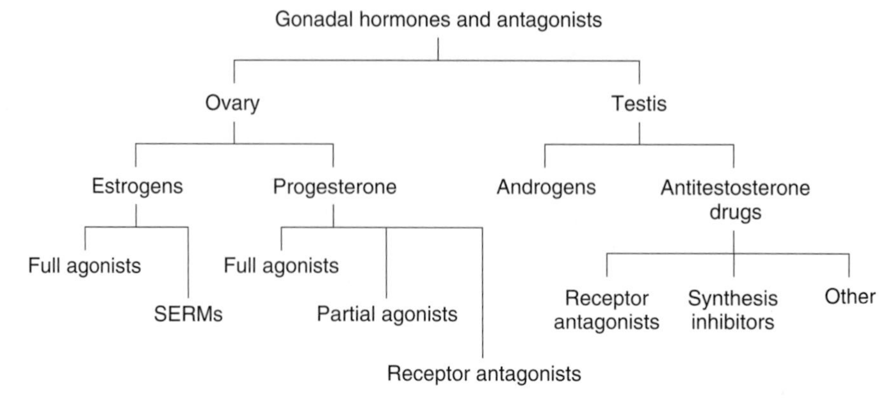

Figure 40–1. Subgroups of drugs discussed in this chapter.

CONCEPTS

The gonadal hormones include the steroids of the ovary (estrogens and progestins) and testis (chiefly testosterone). Because of their importance as contraceptives, many synthetic estrogens and progestins have been produced. These include partial agonists, receptor antagonists, and some drugs with mixed effects, ie, agonist effects in some tissues and antagonist effects in other tissues. Mixed agonists with estrogenic effects are called **selective estrogen receptor modulators (SERMs).** Synthetic androgens, including those with anabolic activity, are also available for clinical use. A diverse group of drugs with antiandrogenic effects are used in treatment of prostate cancer, benign prostatic hyperplasia in men, and hirsutism in women. The drug group is outlined in Figure 40–1.

OVARIAN HORMONES

The ovary is the primary source of sex hormones in women during the child-bearing years, ie, between puberty and menopause. When properly regulated by FSH and LH from the pituitary, each menstrual cycle consists of the following events: A follicle in the ovary matures, secretes increasing amounts of estrogen, releases an ovum, and is transformed into a progesterone-secreting corpus luteum. If the ovum is not fertilized and implanted, the corpus luteum degenerates; the uterine endometrium (which has proliferated under the stimulation of estrogen and progesterone) is shed as part of the menstrual flow, and the cycle repeats. The mechanism of action of both estrogen and progesterone involves entry into cells, binding to cytosolic receptors, and translocation of the receptor-hormone complex into the nucleus, where it modulates gene expression (see Figure 39–2).

A. Estrogens: The major ovarian estrogen in women is estradiol. The steroid has low oral bioavailability but is available in a micronized form for oral use. Estradiol can also be administered via transdermal patch, vaginal cream, or intramuscular injection. Mixtures of conjugated estrogens from biologic sources (eg, Premarin) are used orally, especially in hormone replacement therapy (HRT). Synthetic estrogens with high bioavailability (eg, ethinyl estradiol, mestranol) are used in oral contraceptives.

1. **Effects:** Estrogen is essential for normal female sexual development. It is responsible for the growth of the genital structures (vagina, uterus, and uterine tubes) during childhood and for the appearance of secondary sexual characteristics and the growth spurt associated with puberty. Estrogen has many metabolic effects: It modifies serum protein levels and reduces bone resorption. It enhances the coagulability of blood and increases plasma triglyceride levels while reducing LDL cholesterol. Estrogen is also an effective feedback suppressant of pituitary FSH (Figure 40–2).
2. **Clinical use:** An important therapeutic use of estrogens is in the treatment of primary hypogonadism in young females (Table 40–1). Another use is as hormone replacement therapy in women with estrogen deficiency due to premature ovarian failure, menopause, or surgical removal of the ovaries. HRT ameliorates hot flushes and atrophic changes in the urogenital tract. It is effective also in preventing bone loss and development of osteoporosis

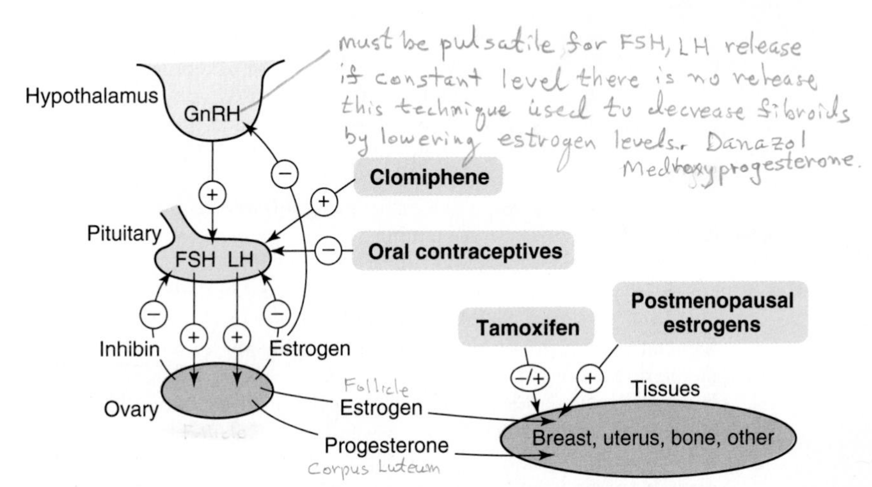

Figure 40–2. Sites of action of several ovarian hormones and their analogs. Clomiphene, a partial agonist, is mainly an antagonist at pituitary estrogen receptors; this prevents negative feedback and increases the output of the pituitary gonadotropic hormones. Tamoxifen, a SERM, is mainly an antagonist at estrogen receptors in the breast but acts as an agonist in bone. Contraceptives reduce FSH and LH output from the pituitary by activating feedback receptors.

and may reduce the risk of coronary artery disease, memory loss, and Alzheimer's disease. The estrogens are very important as a component of oral contraceptives (see below).

3. **Toxicity:** In hypogonadal girls, the dose of estrogen must be adjusted carefully to prevent premature closure of the epiphyses. When used as HRT, estrogen increases the risk of en-

Table 40–1. Representative applications for the gonadal hormones and hormone antagonists.

Clinical Application	Drugs
Hypogonadism in girls, women	Conjugated estrogens, ethinyl estradiol, estradiol esters
Hormone replacement therapy	Estrogen component: Conjugated estrogens, estradiol, estrone, estriol Progestin component: Progesterone, medroxyprogesterone acetate
Oral contraception	Combined: ethinyl estradiol or mestranol plus a progestin Progestin only: norethindrone or norgestrel
Implanted or depot injection contraception	Norgestrel (implant); medroxyprogesterone (intramuscular depot injection)
Postcoital contraception	Oral contraceptive, norgestrel, mifepristone, conjugated estrogens
Intractable dysmenorrhea or uterine bleeding	Conjugated estrogens, ethinyl estradiol, oral contraceptive, GnRH agonist, depot injection of medroxyprogesterone acetate
Infertility	Clomiphene; hMG and hCG; GnRH analogs; bromocriptine
Abortifacient	Mifepristone (RU 486) and prostaglandin; methotrexate and prostaglandin
Endometriosis	Oral contraceptive, depot injection of medroxyprogesterone acetate, GnRH agonist, danazol
Breast cancer	Tamoxifen
Osteoporosis in postmenopausal women	Conjugated estrogens, estradiol, raloxifene
Hypogonadism in boys, men; replacement therapy	Testosterone enanthate or cypionate; methyltestosterone; fluoxymesterone, testosterone (patch)
Anabolic protein synthesis	Oxandrolone, stanozolol
Prostate hypertrophy (benign)	Finasteride
Prostate carcinoma	GnRH agonist, flutamide, cyproterone
Hirsutism	Combined oral contraceptive, GnRH agonist, cyproterone, spironolactone, flutamide

dometrial cancer; this effect is prevented by use of a progestin. Dose-dependent toxicity includes nausea and breast tenderness and increased risk of migraine headache, thromboembolic events (eg, deep vein thrombosis), gallbladder disease, hypertriglyceridemia, and hypertension. A significant number of women using HRT experience uterine bleeding.

B. Progestins: Progesterone is the major progestin in humans. A micronized form is used orally for HRT, and progesterone-containing vaginal creams are also available. Synthetic progestins (eg, medroxyprogesterone) have improved oral bioavailability. The 19-nortestosterone compounds differ primarily in their degree of androgenic effects. Older drugs (eg, L-norgestrel and norethindrone) are more androgenic than the newer progestins (eg, norgestimate, desogestrel).

1. **Effects:** Progestins cause development of secretory tissue in the breast and maturation of the uterine endometrium. They have much less effect than the estrogens on plasma proteins but significantly affect carbohydrate metabolism and stimulate the deposition of fat. High doses inhibit the production of FSH and thereby suppress ovarian function.
2. **Clinical use:** A major therapeutic use of the progestins is as a component of oral or implantable contraceptives. They are used in HRT to prevent estrogen-induced endometrial cancer. Large doses of medroxyprogesterone can be used to produce anovulation and amenorrhea in women with dysmenorrhea, endometriosis, or bleeding disorders.
3. **Toxicity:** The toxicity of progestins is low. However, they may increase blood pressure and decrease high-density plasma lipoproteins (HDL). Long-term use of high doses is associated with reversible decrease in bone density and delayed resumption of ovulation after termination of therapy.

C. Hormonal Contraceptives: Three different types of **oral contraceptives** for women are in use in the USA: combination estrogen-progestin tablets that are taken in constant dosage throughout the menstrual cycle (monophasic preparations); combination preparations (biphasic and triphasic) in which the progestin dosage rises during the month (to mimic the natural cycle); and progestin-only preparations. Two parenteral progestin preparations are used: norgestrel implants that prevent conception for up to 5 years and medroxyprogesterone acetate depot injections that provide contraceptive action for approximately 3 months. Progestisert is an intrauterine device (IUD) that slowly releases progesterone over the course of 1 year; the steroid suppresses endometrial growth and thereby reduces menstrual bleeding, which can be heavy with regular IUDs.

The **postcoital contraceptives** will prevent pregnancy if administered within 72 hours after unprotected intercourse. Several types are available, including conjugated estrogens, combined contraceptives, L-norgestrel, and mifepristone (RU 486), a progesterone antagonist that is described below.

1. **Mechanism of action:** The combination oral contraceptives have several actions, including inhibition of ovulation (the primary action) and effects on the uterine tubes and endometrium that decrease the likelihood of fertilization and implantation. Oral progestin-only agents do not always inhibit ovulation and may act through the other mechanisms listed. However, implantable and injected progestin-only contraceptives appear to act mainly through inhibition of ovulation. The mechanisms of action of postcoital contraceptives are not well understood. When administered before the LH surge, they inhibit ovulation. They also affect implantation and possibly fertilization.
2. **Other clinical uses and beneficial effects:** Combination oral contraceptives are used in young women with primary hypogonadism after their growth has been achieved to prevent estrogen deficiency. Combinations of oral contraceptives and progestins are used to treat acne, hirsutism, dysmenorrhea, and endometriosis. Users of combination oral contraceptives have reduced risks of ovarian cysts, ovarian and endometrial cancer, benign breast disease, and pelvic inflammatory disease as well as a lower incidence of ectopic pregnancy, iron deficiency anemia, and rheumatoid arthritis.
3. **Toxicity:** The incidence of dose-dependent toxicity has fallen since the introduction of the low-dose combined oral contraceptives.
   a. **Thromboembolism:** The major toxic effects of the oral contraceptives relate to their actions on blood coagulation. There is a well-documented increase in the risk of thromboembolic events (myocardial infarction, stroke, deep vein thrombosis, pulmonary embolism) in older women, in smokers, in women with a personal or family history of such problems, and in women with genetic defects that affect the production or func-

tion of clotting factors. However, the risk of thromboembolism incurred by the use of these drugs is usually less than the risk imposed by pregnancy.

b. **Breast cancer:** Despite extensive study, evidence regarding the effects of combined oral contraceptives on breast cancer is still confusing. Evidence suggests that lifetime risk of breast cancer is not changed but that there may be an earlier onset of breast cancer.

c. **Other toxicities:** The low-dose combined oral and progestin-only contraceptives cause significant breakthrough bleeding, especially during the first few months of therapy. Other toxicities of the oral contraceptives include nausea, breast tenderness, headache, skin pigmentation, and depression. Preparations containing older, more androgenic progestins can cause weight gain, acne, and hirsutism. The high dose of estrogen in the estrogen-containing postcoital contraceptives is associated with significant nausea.

> **Skill Keeper: Cytochrome P450 & Oral Contraceptives**
> **(see Chapters 4 and 61)**
>
> Oral contraceptives usually contain the lowest doses of the estrogen and progestin components that prevent pregnancy. The margin between effective and ineffective serum concentrations of the steroids is narrow, which presents a risk of unintended pregnancy resulting from drug-drug interactions. Most steroidal contraceptives are metabolized by cytochrome P450 isozymes.
>
> 1. How many drugs can you identify that decrease the efficacy of hormonal contraceptives by increasing their metabolism?
> 2. When one of these drugs is prescribed for a woman who already is using a combined oral contraceptive, what should be done to prevent pregnancy?
>
> *The Skill Keeper Answers appear at the end of the chapter.*

D. **Selective Estrogen Receptor Modulators (SERMs):** SERMs are mixed estrogen agonists that have estrogen agonist effects in some tissues and act as partial agonists or antagonists of estrogen in other tissues.

1. **Tamoxifen:** Tamoxifen is a SERM effective in the treatment of hormone-responsive breast cancers, where it acts as an *antagonist* to prevent receptor activation by endogenous estrogens (Figure 40–2). Prophylactic use of tamoxifen reduces the incidence of breast cancer in women who are at very high risk. Tamoxifen acts as an *agonist* at endometrial receptors, causing hyperplasia and increasing the risk of endometrial cancer. The drug also causes hot flushes and increases the risk of venous thrombosis. Tamoxifen has more agonist than antagonist action on bone, and thus prevents osteoporosis in women who are taking the drug for breast cancer. **Toremifene** is structurally related to tamoxifen and has similar properties, indications, and toxicity.
2. **Raloxifene:** Raloxifene is used for prevention of osteoporosis in postmenopausal women. It has partial agonist effects on bone and increases serum HDL. Like tamoxifen, raloxifene has antagonist effects in breast tissue and reduces the incidence of breast cancer in women who are at very high risk. Unlike tamoxifen, the drug has no estrogenic effects on endometrial tissue. Adverse effects include hot flushes and increased risk of venous thrombosis.

E. **Estrogen and Progesterone Agonists, Antagonists, and Synthesis Inhibitors:**

1. **Clomiphene:** Clomiphene is used to induce ovulation in anovulatory women who wish to become pregnant. It is a nonsteroidal compound with tissue-selective actions. By selectively blocking estrogen receptors in the pituitary, clomiphene reduces negative feedback and increases FSH and LH output. The increase in gonadotropins stimulates ovulation.
2. **Diethylstilbestrol:** Diethylstilbestrol (DES) is a nonsteroidal compound with estrogen agonist activity. It is no longer used commonly because of its association with the development of infertility, ectopic pregnancy, and vaginal adenocarcinoma in the daughters of women who were treated with large doses of DES during pregnancy.

3. **Mifepristone (RU 486):** Mifepristone is an orally active steroid antagonist of progesterone and glucocorticoids. Its major use is as an abortifacient in early pregnancy (up to 49 days after the last menstrual period). When given as a single oral dose followed by administration of a prostaglandin E or prostaglandin F analog, a very high percentage of complete abortion is achieved with a low incidence of serious toxicity.
4. **Danazol:** Danazol is a weak partial agonist that binds to progestin, androgen, and glucocorticoid receptors in cells and to steroid transport proteins in the blood. Danazol also inhibits several P450 enzymes involved in gonadal steroid synthesis. The drug is sometimes used in the treatment of endometriosis and fibrocystic disease of the breast.
5. **Aromatase inhibitors: Anastrozole** and related compounds (eg, letrozole) are nonsteroidal inhibitors of aromatase, the enzyme required for estrogen synthesis. These drugs are used in the treatment of breast cancer.

ANDROGENS

Testosterone and related androgens are produced in the testis, the adrenal, and, to a small extent, in the ovary. Testosterone is synthesized from progesterone and dehydroepiandrosterone (DHEA). In the plasma, testosterone is partly bound to sex hormone-binding globulin (SHBG), a transport protein. The hormone is converted in several organs (eg, prostate) to **dihydrotestosterone,** which is the active hormone in those tissues. Because of rapid hepatic metabolism, testosterone given by mouth has little effect. It may be given by injection or transdermal patch, or orally active variants may be used (see Table 40–1 and the Drug List).

Many androgens have been synthesized in an effort to increase the anabolic effect (see Effects, below) without increasing androgenic action. **Oxandrolone** and **stanozolol** are examples of drugs that, in laboratory testing, have an increased ratio of anabolic to androgenic action. However, all of the so-called anabolic steroids have full androgenic agonist effects when used in humans.

A. **Mechanism of Action:** Like other steroid hormones, androgens enter cells and bind to cytosolic receptors (Figure 39–2). The hormone-receptor complex enters the nucleus and modulates the expression of certain genes.

B. **Effects:** Testosterone is necessary for normal development of the male fetus and infant and is responsible for the major changes in the male at puberty (growth of penis, larynx, and skeleton; development of facial, pubic, and axillary hair; darkening of skin; enlargement of muscle mass). After puberty, testosterone acts to maintain secondary sex characteristics, fertility and libido. It also acts upon hair cells to cause male-pattern baldness.

   The major effect of androgenic hormones—in addition to development and maintenance of normal male characteristics—is an anabolic action that involves increased muscle size and strength and increased red blood cell production. Excretion of urea nitrogen is reduced, and nitrogen balance becomes more positive. Testosterone also helps maintain normal bone density.

C. **Clinical Use:** The primary clinical use of the androgens is for replacement therapy in hypogonadism (Table 40–1). They have also been used to stimulate red blood cell production in certain anemias and to promote weight gain in patients with wasting syndromes (eg, AIDS patients). The anabolic effects have been exploited illicitly by athletes to increase muscle bulk and strength and perhaps athletic performance.

D. **Toxicity:** Use of androgens by females results in virilization. Paradoxically, excessive doses in men can result in feminization (gynecomastia, testicular shrinkage, infertility) due to feedback inhibition of the pituitary and partly to conversion of the exogenous androgens to estrogens. High doses also cause behavioral effects, including hostility and aggression ("roid rage"). In addition, androgens have caused cholestatic jaundice, elevation of liver enzyme levels, and possibly hepatocellular carcinoma.

ANTIANDROGENS

Reduction of androgen effects is an important mode of therapy for both benign and malignant prostate disease, precocious puberty, hair loss, and hirsutism. Drugs are available that act at several different sites in the androgen pathway (Figure 40–3).

A. Receptor Inhibitors: Flutamide and related drugs are nonsteroidal compounds that act as competitive antagonists at androgen receptors. These drugs are used to decrease the action of endogenous hormones in prostate carcinoma. **Cyproterone** is a steroidal compound with the same action. The drug also has progestational activity that provides negative feedback to the pituitary. It is used for treatment of women with hirsutism. **Spironolactone,** a drug used principally as a potassium-sparing diuretic, also inhibits androgen receptors and is somtimes used in the treatment of hirsutism.

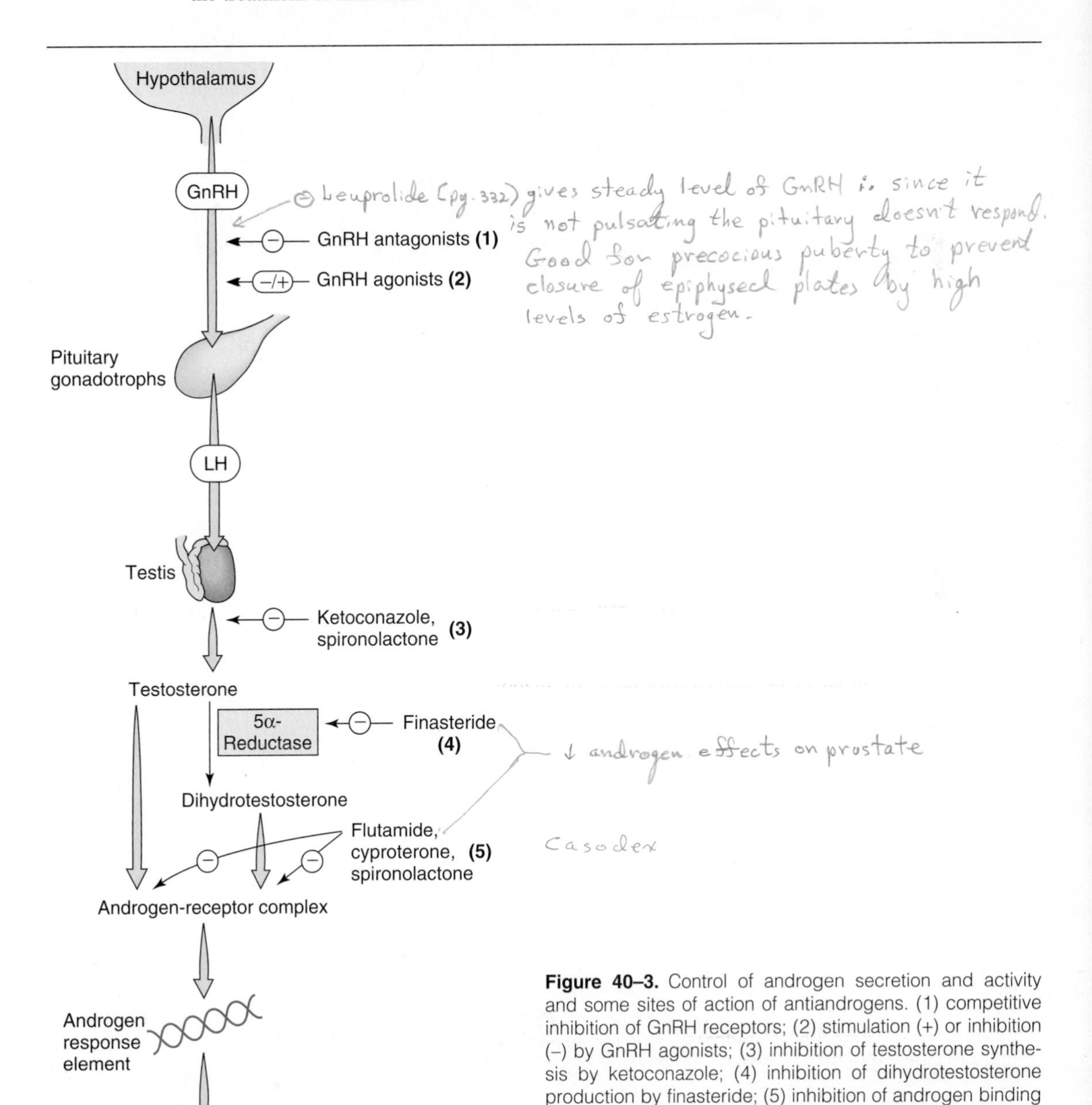

Figure 40–3. Control of androgen secretion and activity and some sites of action of antiandrogens. (1) competitive inhibition of GnRH receptors; (2) stimulation (+) or inhibition (–) by GnRH agonists; (3) inhibition of testosterone synthesis by ketoconazole; (4) inhibition of dihydrotestosterone production by finasteride; (5) inhibition of androgen binding at its receptor by flutamide and other drugs. (Modified and reproduced, with permission, from Katzung BG [editor]: *Basic & Clinical Pharmacology,* 8th ed. McGraw-Hill, 2001.)

B. GnRH Analogs: Reduction of gonadotropins, especially LH, reduces the production of testosterone. This can be effectively accomplished with long-acting depot preparations of **leuprolide** or similar GnRH agonists (Chapter 37). These analogs are used in prostatic carcinoma. During the first week of therapy, an androgen receptor antagonist (eg, flutamide) is added to prevent the tumor flare that can result from the surge in testosterone synthesis caused by the initial agonistic action of the GnRH agonist. Within several weeks, testosterone production falls to normal and then below normal.

C. 5α-Reductase Inhibitors: Testosterone is converted to dihydrotestosterone (DHT) by the enzyme 5α-reductase; some tissues, most notably prostate cells and hair follicles, depend upon DHT rather than testosterone for androgenic stimulation. This enzyme is inhibited by **finasteride,** a drug used to treat benign prostatic hyperplasia and, at a lower dose, to prevent hair loss in men. Because the drug does not interfere with the action of testosterone, it is less likely than other antiandrogens to cause impotence, infertility, and loss of libido.

D. Combined Oral Contraceptives: Combined oral contraceptives exert an antiandrogenic effect when they are used in women with hirsutism that is due to excess production of androgenic steroids. The estrogen in the contraceptive acts in the liver to increase the production of sex hormone binding globulin (SHBG), which in turn acts to reduce the concentration of free androgen in the blood.

E. Inhibitors of Steroid Synthesis: **Ketoconazole,** an antifungal agent, inhibits gonadal and adrenal steroid synthesis. The drug has been used to suppress adrenal steroid synthesis in patients with steroid-responsive metastatic tumors.

DRUG LIST

The following drugs are important members of the groups discussed in this chapter. Prototypes should be learned in detail; features of the major variants should be known well enough to distin-

Subclass	Prototype	Major Variants	Other Significant Agents
Estrogens			
Natural	Estradiol	Conjugated equine estrogens	Estrone, estriol
Synthetic	Ethinyl estradiol	Mestranol	Diethylstilbestrol
SERMs	Tamoxifen, raloxifene		
Partial agonists	Clomiphene		
Aromatase inhibitor	Anastrozole		Letrozole
Progestins			
Natural	Progesterone		
Synthetic	Norgestrel, medroxyprogesterone acetate	Norgestimate	Norethindrone, desogestrel
Partial agonist	Danazol		
Antiprogestin	Mifepristone (RU 486)		
Androgens			
Natural	Testosterone		
Synthetic	Methyltestosterone	Fluoxymesterone	
Anabolic steroid	Oxandrolone		Stanozolol
Antiandrogens			
Receptor antagonist	Flutamide	Cyproterone	Bicalutamide
5α-Reductase inhibitor	Finasteride		
Synthesis inhibitor	Ketoconazole		
Other	GnRH analogs, combined oral contraceptives		

guish the variants from prototypes and from each other; the other significant agents should be recognized as belonging to a specific subclass.

QUESTIONS

DIRECTIONS: Each of the numbered items or incomplete statements in this section is followed by answers or by completions of the statement. Select the ONE lettered answer or completion that is BEST in each case.

1. Which one of the following agents is not used in oral or implantable contraceptives?
(A) Clomiphene
(B) Ethinyl estradiol
(C) Mestranol
(D) Norethindrone
(E) Norgestrel

2. All of the following are recognized effects of combined oral contraceptives EXCEPT
(A) Breakthrough bleeding
(B) Decreased risk of endometrial cancer
(C) Increased risk of ischemic stroke
(D) Increased risk of ovarian cancer
(E) Nausea

3. Which one of the following is not a recognized effect of androgens or anabolic steroids?
(A) Cholestatic jaundice and elevation of AST levels in the blood in adult men
(B) Growth of facial hair in women
(C) Increased milk production in nursing women
(D) Increased muscle bulk
(E) Induction of a growth spurt in pubertal boys

4. A 50-year-old woman with a positive mammogram undergoes lumpectomy and a small carcinoma is removed. Biochemical analysis of the cancer reveals the presence of estrogen and progesterone receptors. After this procedure, she will probably receive
(A) Danazol
(B) Flutamide
(C) Leuprolide
(D) Mifepristone
(E) Tamoxifen

5. A 60-year-old man is found to have a prostate lump and an elevated PSA (prostate-specific antigen) blood test. MRI examination suggests several enlarged lymph nodes in the lower abdomen, and x-ray reveals two radiolucent lesions in the bony pelvis. This patient might benefit from treatment with any of the following EXCEPT
(A) Cyproterone
(B) Flutamide
(C) Ketoconazole
(D) Leuprolide
(E) Mifepristone

6. A young woman complains of severe abdominal pain at the time of menstruation. Careful evaluation indicates the presence of significant endometrial deposits on the pelvic peritoneum. The most appropriate therapy for this patient would be
(A) Flutamide, orally
(B) Medroxyprogesterone acetate by intramuscular injection
(C) Norgestrel as an implant
(D) Oxandrolone by intramuscular injection
(E) Raloxifene orally

7. Diethylstilbestrol should never be used in pregnant women because it is associated with
(A) Development of deep vein thrombosis in the pregnant woman
(B) Feminization of the external genitalia of male offspring
(C) Infertility and development of vaginal cancer in female offspring
(D) Miscarriages
(E) Virilization of the external genitalia of female offspring

8. The unique property of SERMs is that they
   (A) Act as agonists in some tissues and antagonists in other tissues
   (B) Activate a unique plasma membrane-bound receptor
   (C) Have both estrogenic and progestational agonist activity
   (D) Inhibit the aromatase enzyme that is required for estrogen synthesis
   (E) Produce estrogenic effects without binding to estrogen receptors
9. Finasteride has efficacy in the prevention of male-pattern baldness by virtue of its ability to
   (A) Competitively antagonize androgen receptors
   (B) Decrease the release of gonadotropins
   (C) Increase the serum concentration of SHBG
   (D) Inhibit the synthesis of testosterone
   (E) Reduce the production of dihydrotestosterone
10. A 52-year-old postmenopausal patient has evidence of low bone mineral density. She and her physician are considering therapy with raloxifene or a combination of conjugated estrogens and medroxyprogesterone acetate. Which of the following patient characteristics is MOST likely to lead them to select raloxifene?
   (A) Previous hysterectomy
   (B) Recurrent vaginitis
   (C) Rheumatoid arthritis
   (D) Strong family history of breast cancer
   (E) Troublesome hot flushes

ANSWERS

1. Clomiphene, a partial agonist that acts at the pituitary to increase secretion of gonadotropins and thereby to stimulate ovulation, would be of no value as a contraceptive. The answer is **(A).**
2. The oral contraceptives are associated with a decreased risk of both endometrial and ovarian cancer. The answer is **(D).**
3. Androgens, like estrogens, reduce the pituitary release of prolactin and suppress lactation. The answer is **(C).**
4. Tamoxifen has proved useful in adjunctive therapy of breast cancer; the drug decreases the rate of recurrence of cancer. The answer is **(E).**
5. Most antiandrogenic drugs are potentially useful in this androgen-dependent type of tumor. Mifepristone (RU 486) has effects at glucocorticoid and progestin receptors but not at androgen receptors. The answer is **(E).**
6. In endometriosis, suppression of ovarian function and production of gonadal steroids is useful. Intramuscular injection of relatively large doses of medroxyprogesterone acetate provides 3 months of an ovarian suppressive effect due to inhibition of pituitary production of gonadotropins. The answer is **(B).**
7. Diethylstilbestrol (DES) is a nonsteroidal estrogen agonist. Several decades ago, misguided use of the drug in pregnant women appears to have resulted in fetal damage that predisposed female offspring to infertility and a rare form of vaginal cancer. For this reason, the drug should be avoided in pregnant women. Other estrogenic drugs do not appear to have these same effects. While estrogens do increase the risk of deep vein thrombosis, this is not the reason why DES should be avoided. The answer is **(C).**
8. SERMs such as tamoxifen and raloxifene exhibit tissue-specific estrogenic and antiestrogenic effects. The answer is **(A).**
9. Finasteride is an inhibitor of 5α-reductase, the enzyme that converts testosterone to dihydrotestosterone, the principal androgen in androgen-sensitive hair follicles. The answer is **(E).**
10. Conjugated estrogens and raloxifene both improve bone mineral density and protect against osteoporosis. The two advantages of raloxifene over full estrogen receptor agonists is that raloxifene has antagonist effects in breast tissue and lacks an agonistic effect in endometrium. If a patient's uterus was removed by surgery, the difference in the endometrial effect is moot. In patients with a strong family history of breast cancer, raloxifene may be a better choice than a full estrogen agonist for it will not further increase the woman's risk of breast cancer and may even lower her risk. The answer is **(D).**

Skill Keeper Answers: Cytochrome P450 & Oral Contraceptives (see Chapters 4 and 61)

1. Gonadal steroids and their derivatives are metabolized primarily by the cytochrome P450 3A4 (CYP3A4) family of enzymes. Inducers of CYP3A4 include barbiturates, carbamazepine, corticosteroids, griseofulvin, nelfinavir, phenytoin, pioglitazone, rifampin, and rifabutin. The potential reduction in contraceptive efficacy of hormonal contraceptives by carbamazepine and phenytoin are of particular importance because these drugs are known teratogens. St. John's wort, an unregulated herbal product, contains an ingredient that induces CYP3A4 enzymes and can reduce the efficacy of oral contraceptives.
2. To prevent an unwanted pregnancy, it would be advisable to use a combined oral contraceptive pill with a higher dose of estrogen (eg, a formulation containing 50 μg of ethinyl estradiol). Alternatively—or additionally—women may use a barrier form of contraception or switch to an intrauterine device (IUD).

Pancreatic Hormones, Antidiabetic Agents, & Hyperglycemic Drugs — 41

OBJECTIVES

You should be able to:

- Describe the effects of insulin on the liver, on muscle, and on adipose tissue.
- List the types of insulin preparations and their durations of action.
- Describe the major hazards of insulin therapy.
- List the prototypes and describe the mechanisms of action and toxicities of the four major classes of oral antidiabetic agents.
- Give three examples of rational drug combinations for treatment of type 2 diabetes mellitus.
- Describe the clinical uses of glucagon.

CONCEPTS

The islets of Langerhans (the endocrine pancreas) contain at least four different types of endocrine cells, including A (alpha, glucagon-producing), B (beta, insulin-producing), D (delta, somatostatin-producing), and F (PP, pancreatic polypeptide-producing). Of these, the B (insulin-producing) cells are the most numerous.

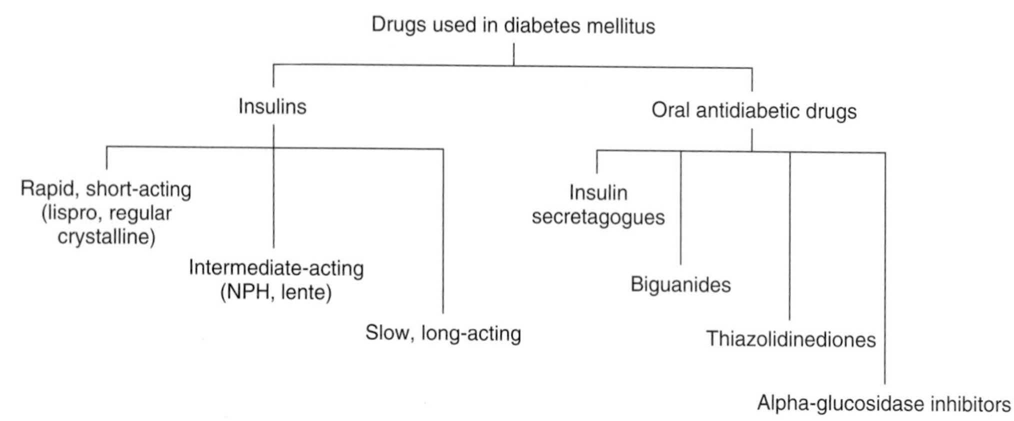

Figure 41–1. Subgroups of hypoglycemic drugs discussed in this chapter.

The most common pancreatic disease requiring pharmacologic therapy is diabetes mellitus, a deficiency of insulin production or effect. Diabetes is treated with several formulations of insulin (all administered parenterally at present) and with four types of oral antidiabetic agents (Figure 41–1).

Glucagon, a hormone that affects the liver, cardiovascular system and gastrointestinal tract, can be used to treat severe hypoglycemia in diabetics.

INSULIN

A. Physiology: Insulin is synthesized as a prohormone, **proinsulin,** an 86-amino-acid single-chain polypeptide. Cleavage of proinsulin and cross-linking result in the two-chain 51-peptide insulin molecule and a 31-amino-acid residual **C-peptide.** Neither proinsulin nor C-peptide appear to have any physiologic actions.

B. Effects: Insulin has extremely important effects in almost every tissue of the body. The insulin receptor, a transmembrane tyrosine kinase, phosphorylates itself and a variety of intracellular proteins when activated by the hormone. The major target organs for insulin action include the following:

1. **Liver:** Insulin increases the storage of glucose as glycogen in the liver. This involves the insertion of additional GLUT 2 glucose transport molecules in cell walls, increased synthesis of the enzymes pyruvate kinase, phosphofructokinase, and glucokinase, and the suppression of several other enzymes. Insulin also decreases protein catabolism.
2. **Muscle:** Insulin stimulates glycogen synthesis and protein synthesis. Glucose transport into muscle cells is facilitated by insertion of additional GLUT 4 transport molecules into cell walls.
3. **Adipose tissue:** Insulin facilitates triglyceride storage by activating plasma lipoprotein lipase, by increasing glucose transport into cells via GLUT 4 transporters, and by reducing intracellular lipolysis.

C. Types of Insulin Available: Human insulin is manufactured by bacterial recombinant DNA technology. Purified porcine insulin is also available in the USA. Because the insulin molecule has a half-life of only a few minutes in the circulation, many preparations for use in diabetes are formulated to release the hormone slowly into the circulation.

The insulin forms available provide four rates of onset and durations of effect: ultra-rapid onset, rapid onset with short-action, intermediate onset and action, and slow onset with long-action (Table 41–1). All insulin preparations contain zinc; the ratio of zinc (and other substances) to insulin influences the rate of release of active hormone from the site of administration, and the duration of action.

1. **Ultra rapid and very short action:** **Insulin lispro** is a recombinant human insulin that contains a transposition of two amino acids, lysine and proline. This transposition alters the physical properties of the peptide so that insulin lispro dissolves more rapidly at its site of

Table 41–1. Insulin: Types and activity.

Pharmacokinetic Type	Species Type	Activity (hours)	
		Peak	Duration
Ultra-rapid-acting			
Insulin lispro	Human, modified	0.25–0.5	3–4
Rapid-acting			
Insulin injection USP (regular, crystalline zinc)	Human, pork	0.5–3	5–7
Intermediate-acting			
NPH insulin (isophane insulin suspension USP)	Human, pork	8–12	18–24
Lente insulin (insulin zinc suspension USP)	Human, pork	8–12	18–24
Long-acting			
Ultralente insulin (insulin zinc suspension extended USP)	Human	8–16	18–28
Ultra-long-acting			
Insulin glargine	Human, modified	No peak	> 24

administration and enters the circulation approximately twice as fast as regular crystalline insulin. It is considered ultra-rapid in onset and is suitable for use immediately before meals. Unlike other insulin preparations, increasing the dose only increases the intensity, not the duration of effect.

2. **Rapid onset and short action: Crystalline zinc (regular) insulin,** a rapid onset preparation, is used intravenously in emergencies, or administered subcutaneously in ordinary maintenance regimens, alone or mixed with intermediate- or long-acting preparations. Before the development of insulin lispro it was the primary rapid onset agent for use in tight control regimens but required administration an hour or more before each meal.
3. **Intermediate onset and action:** These preparations include isophane insulin suspension (NPH insulin) and lente suspension. Both preparations are given by subcutaneous injection; they are not suitable for intravenous use. When mixing intermediate onset insulin with regular insulin, NPH insulin is preferred because lente insulin can retard the onset of action of regular insulin.
4. **Slow onset and long action:** Ultralente insulin is a long-acting insulin. It usually is given in the morning only, or morning and evening to provide maintenance or basal levels for 12–24 hours. This basal insulin level may be supplemented with injections of insulin lispro or regular insulin during the day to meet the requirements of carbohydrate intake. Insulin glargine, a modified form of human insulin, is an ultra-long-acting preparation that provides a peakless basal insulin level that lasts more than 24 hours. Protamine zinc insulin, another long-acting preparation, is no longer available in the USA.

   The time course of effect of these preparations is shown in Figure 41–2.
5. **Insulin delivery systems:** The standard mode of insulin therapy is subcutaneous injection with conventional disposable needles and syringes. Other, more convenient, means of administration are either available or in clinical trials.
   - **a.** Portable pen-sized injectors are used to facilitate subcutaneous injection. Some contain replaceable cartridges whereas others are disposable.
   - **b.** Continuous subcutaneous insulin infusion devices avoid the need for multiple daily injections and provide flexibility in the scheduling of patients' daily activities. Programmable pumps deliver a constant 24-hour basal rate, and manual adjustments in the rate of delivery can be made to accommodate changes in insulin requirements (eg, before meals or exercise).
   - **c.** An inhaled formulation of insulin is in clinical trials. This form may prove effective and convenient for covering mealtime insulin requirements.

D. Hazards of Insulin Use: Diabetic patients who use insulin are subject to two types of complications; hypoglycemia, from excessive insulin effect; and immunologic toxic effects, from the development of antibodies. Hypoglycemia is a very dangerous hazard, because brain damage may result. Prompt administration of glucose (sugar or candy by mouth, glucose by vein) or of glucagon (by intramuscular injection) is essential. Patients with advanced renal disease, the

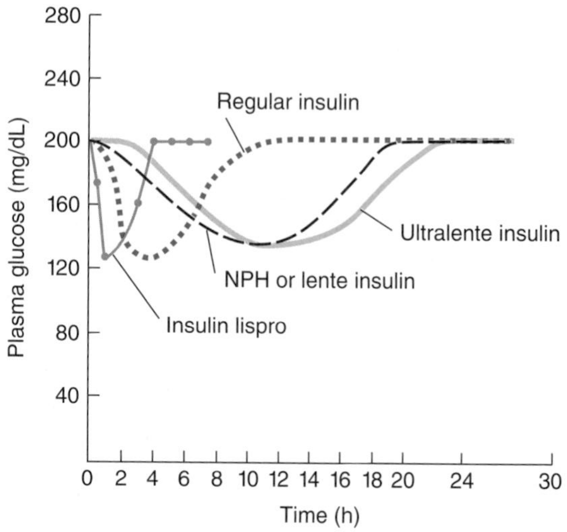

Figure 41–2. Extent and duration of action of various types of insulin (in a fasting diabetic). The durations of action shown are typical of average therapeutic doses; except for insulin lispro, duration increases when dosage is increased. (Reproduced, with permission, from Katzung BG [editor]: *Basic & Clinical Pharmacology,* 8th ed. McGraw-Hill, 2001.)

elderly, and children under 7 years of age are most susceptible to the detrimental effects of hypoglycemia.

The most common and important form of insulin-induced immunologic complication is the formation of insulin antibodies, which results in resistance to the action of the drug or allergic reactions. Human insulins are less antigenic than insulin from animal sources. Lipodystrophy, a change in fatty tissue at the site of injection, was relatively common in the past. Use of more purified, less antigenic forms of insulin has almost eliminated this complication.

ORAL ANTIDIABETIC DRUGS

Four major groups of drugs are used for the oral treatment of diabetes: insulin secretagogues, the biguanides, the thiazolidinediones, and the α-glucosidase inhibitors. Some members of these groups are listed in Table 41–2.

Table 41–2. Representative oral antidiabetic drugs.

Drug	Duration of Action (hours)
Sulfonylureas	
Chlorpropamide	Up to 60
Tolbutamide	6–12
Glimepiride	12–24
Glipizide	10–24
Glyburide	10–24
Meglitinides	
Repaglinide	1–3
Biguanides	
Metformin	10–12
Thiazolidinediones	
Pioglitazone	15–24
Rosiglitazone	> 24
α-Glucosidase inhibitors	
Acarbose	3–4
Miglitol	3–4

A. Insulin Secretagogues:

1. **Mechanism and effects:** The primary action of the insulin secretagogues is to stimulate the release of endogenous insulin. All but one of the insulin secretagogues are sulfonylureas. The sulfonylureas close potassium channels in the pancreatic B cell membrane; channel closure depolarizes the cell and depolarization triggers insulin release. Insulin secretagogues are not effective in patients who lack functional beta cells. These drugs may also reduce glucagon release and increase the number of functional insulin receptors in peripheral tissues. The "second-generation" sulfonylureas **(glyburide, glipizide, glimepiride)** are considerably more potent and used much more commonly than the older agents **(tolbutamide, chlorpropamide, tolazamide, others). Repaglinide** is a new insulin secretagogue from a chemical class known as the meglitinides. It also promotes insulin release by binding to potassium channels in pancreatic B cell membranes. The most notable difference between repaglinide and the sulfonylureas is its rapid onset and short duration of action (Table 41–2). It is taken just before meals for the purpose of controlling postprandial glucose concentrations.
2. **Toxicities:** Adverse effects are relatively uncommon with the sulfonylureas: hypoglycemia due to overdosage, rash (occasionally), and allergy are reported. Chlorpropamide has a long duration of action, and liver or kidney disease may greatly increase the blood levels of the drug. Because of their great potency, hypoglycemia is somewhat more common with glyburide and glipizide. The older sulfonylureas (tolbutamide and chlorpropamide) are extensively bound to serum proteins. Drugs that compete for protein binding may enhance their hypoglycemic effects.

B. Biguanides: The biguanides act by an unknown mechanism to reduce postprandial and fasting glucose levels in patients with type 2 diabetes. Their effects do not depend upon functional islet cells. Proposed mechanisms for their action include reduced hepatic gluconeogenesis, stimulation of glycolysis in peripheral tissues, reduction of glucose absorption from the gastrointestinal tract, and reduction of plasma glucagon levels. Several biguanides are in use overseas. **Metformin** is the primary member of this group in the USA. Unlike the sulfonylureas, the biguanides do not cause hypoglycemia. Their most common toxicity is gastrointestinal distress (nausea, diarrhea), and they can cause lactic acidosis, especially in patients with renal or liver disease, alcoholism, or conditions that predispose to tissue anoxia (eg, chronic cardiopulmonary dysfunction). Metformin also inhibits vitamin B_{12} absorption.

C. Thiazolidinediones:

1. **Mechanism and effects:** Thiazolidinediones increase target tissue sensitivity to insulin. **Troglitazone** was the first thiazolidinedione introduced, but it was removed from the market in several countries because of hepatotoxicity. **Rosiglitazone** and **pioglitazone** appear to carry less risk of serious liver dysfunction. The mechanism of action of the thiazolidinediones is not fully understood but they stimulate the peroxisome proliferator-activated receptor-gamma nuclear receptor (PPAR-γ receptor). This nuclear receptor regulates the transcription of genes encoding proteins involved in carbohydrate and lipid metabolism. The "glitazones" increase glucose uptake in muscle and adipose tissue, inhibit hepatic gluconeogenesis, and have effects on lipid metabolism and the distribution of body fat. Thiazolidinediones reduce both fasting and postprandial hyperglycemia. They are used as monotherapy or in combination with insulin or other oral antidiabetic drugs.
2. **Toxicities:** When these drugs are used alone, hypoglycemia is extremely rare. Thiazolidinediones can cause edema and mild anemia. Pioglitazone and troglitazone appear to induce cytochrome P450 (especially the 3A4 isozyme) and can reduce the serum concentrations of drugs that are metabolized by these enzymes (eg, oral contraceptives, cyclosporine).

D. α-Glucosidase Inhibitors: Acarbose and miglitol are carbohydrate analogs that act within the intestine to inhibit α-glucosidase, an enzyme necessary for the conversion of complex starches, oligosaccharides, and disaccharides to the monosaccharides that can be transported out of the intestinal lumen and into the bloodstream. As a result of slowed absorption, postprandial hyperglycemia is reduced. They have no effect on fasting blood sugar. Both drugs can be used as monotherapy or in combination with other antidiabetic drugs. Their primary adverse effects include flatulence, diarrhea and abdominal pain resulting from increased fermentation of unabsorbed carbohydrate by bacteria in the colon. If a patient who has taken an α-glucosidase inhibitor experiences hypoglycemia, he or she should be treated with oral glucose (dextrose), and not sucrose because the absorption of sucrose will be delayed.

TREATMENT OF DIABETES MELLITUS

Diabetes is diagnosed on the basis of more than one fasting blood sugar determination in excess of 140 mg/dL. Two major forms of the disease have been identified. Type 1 diabetes usually has its onset during childhood and results from an autoimmune reaction that culminates in destruction of the pancreatic B cells. Type 2 diabetes is a progressive disorder characterized by increasing insulin resistance and diminishing insulin secretory capacity. It usually has its onset in adulthood and is frequently associated with obesity. Type 2 diabetes is much more common than type 1 diabetes; it is estimated that type 2 diabetes affects over 20% of all Americans over age 65. The clinical history and course of these two forms differ considerably, but treatment in both cases requires careful attention to diet, to fasting and postprandial blood glucose concentrations, and to serum concentrations of hemoglobin A_{1c}, a glycosylated hemoglobin that serves as a marker of glycemia.

A. Type 1 Diabetes: Therapy of type 1 diabetes involves dietary instruction, parenteral insulin (a mixture of shorter- and longer-acting forms to maintain a stable blood sugar during the day and night), and careful attention by the patient to factors that change insulin requirements: exercise, infections, other forms of stress, and deviations from the regular diet. Recent large clinical studies indicate that tight control of blood sugar—by frequent blood sugar testing and insulin injections—reduces the incidence of vascular complications, including renal and retinal damage. The risk of hypoglycemic reactions is increased in tight control regimens, but not enough to obviate the benefits of better control.

B. Type 2 Diabetes: Since type 2 diabetes is a progressive disease, therapy for an individual patient generally escalates over time. It begins with weight reduction and dietary control. Initial drug therapy usually is monotherapy with a second generation sulfonylurea (glyburide, glipizide or glimepiride), or less commonly, with metformin or a thiazolidinedione. While initial responses to monotherapy usually are good, secondary failure within 5 years is common. Increasingly, oral antidiabetics are being used in combination with each other or with insulin to achieve better glycemic control and minimize toxicity. Since type 2 diabetes involves both insulin resistance and inadequate insulin production, it makes sense to combine an agent that augments insulin's action (metformin, a thiazolidinedione, or an α-glucosidase inhibitor) with one that augments the insulin supplies (insulin secretagogue or insulin). Long-acting drugs (sulfonylureas, metformin, thiazolidinediones, some insulin formulations) help control both fasting and postprandial blood glucose levels whereas short-acting drugs (repaglinide, α-glucosidase inhibitors, regular insulin, and insulin lispro) primarily target postprandial levels. As is the case for type 1 diabetes, recent clinical trials have shown that tight control of blood glucose trials in patients with type 2 diabetes reduces the risk of vascular complications.

Skill Keeper: Diabetes & Hypertension
(see Chapter 11)

Diabetes is linked to hypertension in several important ways. Obesity predisposes patients to hypertension as well as to type 2 diabetes, so many patients suffer from both diseases. Both diseases can damage the kidney and both predispose patients to coronary artery disease. A large clinical trial of patients with type 2 diabetes suggests that poorly controlled hypertension exacerbates the microvascular disease caused by long-standing diabetes. Because of these links, it is important to think about the treatment of hypertension in diabetic patients.

1. Identify the major drug groups used for chronic treatment of essential hypertension.
2. Which of these drug groups have special implications for the treatment of diabetic patients?

The Skill Keeper Answers appear at the end of the chapter.

HYPERGLYCEMIC DRUGS: GLUCAGON

A. Glucagon:

1. **Chemistry, mechanism, and effects:** Glucagon is the product of the A cells of the endocrine pancreas. Like insulin, glucagon is a peptide; but unlike insulin, glucagon acts on G protein-coupled receptors. Activation of glucagon receptors, which are located in heart, smooth muscle, and liver, stimulates adenylyl cyclase and increases intracellular cAMP. This results in increases in the heart rate and the force of contraction, increased hepatic glycogenolysis and gluconeogenesis and relaxation of smooth muscle. The smooth muscle effect is particularly marked in the gut.
2. **Clinical uses:** Glucagon is used to treat severe hypoglycemia in diabetics, but its hyperglycemic action requires intact hepatic glycogen stores. The drug is given intramuscularly or intravenously. Glucagon is also valuable for x-ray studies of the bowel or abdomen when temporary reduction of motility is necessary for optimal visualization. In the management of severe beta-blocker overdose, glucagon may be the most effective method for stimulating the depressed heart, since it increases cardiac cAMP without requiring access to beta receptors.

DRUG LIST

The following drugs are important members of the groups discussed in this chapter. Prototypes should be learned in detail; the other significant agents should be recognized as belonging to a specific subclass.

Subclass	Prototypes	Other Significant Agents
Insulins	Insulin lispro, regular, lente, NPH, ultralente, insulin glargine	
Insulin secretagogues		
Sulfonylureas	Glipizide	Chlorpropamide, tolbutamide, tolazamide, glimepiride, glyburide
Meglitinides	Repaglinide	
Biguanides	Metformin	
Thiazolidinediones	Pioglitazone, rosiglitazone	Troglitazone
α-Glycosidase inhibitors	Acarbose	Miglitol

QUESTIONS

DIRECTIONS: Each of the numbered items or incomplete statements in this section is followed by answers or by completions of the statement. Select the ONE lettered answer or completion that is BEST in each case.

Items 1–2: A 13-year-old boy with type 1 diabetes is brought to the hospital complaining of dizziness. Laboratory findings include severe hyperglycemia, ketoacidosis, and a blood pH of 7.15.

1. In order to achieve rapid control of the severe ketoacidosis in this diabetic boy, the appropriate antidiabetic agent to use is
   (A) Crystalline zinc insulin
   (B) Glyburide
   (C) Isophane (NPH) insulin
   (D) Tolbutamide
   (E) Ultralente insulin
2. The most likely complication of insulin therapy in this patient is
   (A) Dilutional hyponatremia
   (B) Hypoglycemia
   (C) Increased bleeding tendency

(D) Pancreatitis
(E) Severe hypertension

3. A 24-year-old woman with type 1 diabetes wishes to try tight control of her diabetes to improve her long-term prognosis. Which of the following regimens is most appropriate?
(A) Morning injections of mixed lente and ultralente insulins
(B) Evening injections of mixed regular and lente insulins
(C) Morning and evening injections of regular insulin, supplemented by small amounts of lente insulin at mealtimes
(D) Morning injections of ultralente insulin, supplemented by small amounts of insulin lispro at mealtimes
(E) Morning injection of semilente insulin and evening injection of lente insulin

4. Which one of the following drugs does not promote the release of endogenous insulin?
(A) Chlorpropamide
(B) Glipizide
(C) Pioglitazone
(D) Repaglinide
(E) Tolazamide

5. Effects of insulin do not include
(A) Decreased conversion of amino acids into glucose
(B) Decreased gluconeogenesis
(C) Increased glucose transport into cells
(D) Induction of lipoprotein lipase
(E) Stimulation of glycogenolysis

6. A 54-year-old obese patient with type 2 diabetes and a history of alcoholism probably should not receive metformin because it can increase his risk of
(A) A disulfiram-like reaction
(B) Excessive weight gain
(C) Hypoglycemia
(D) Lactic acidosis
(E) Serious hepatotoxicity

7. Which of the following drugs is taken during the first part of a meal for the purpose of delaying the absorption of dietary carbohydrates?
(A) Acarbose
(B) Colestipol
(C) Glipizide
(D) Pioglitazone
(E) Repaglinide

8. The PPAR-γ receptor that is activated by thiazolidinediones increases tissue sensitivity to insulin by
(A) Activating adenylyl cyclase and increasing the intracellular concentration of cAMP
(B) Inactivating a cellular inhibitor of the GLUT 2 glucose transporter
(C) Inhibiting acid glucosidase, a key enzyme in glycogen breakdown pathways
(D) Regulating transcription of genes involved in glucose utilization
(E) Stimulating the activity of a tyrosine kinase that phosphorylates the insulin receptor

9. Which of the following drugs is MOST likely to cause hypoglycemia when used as monotherapy in the treatment of type 2 diabetes?
(A) Acarbose
(B) Glyburide
(C) Metformin
(D) Miglitol
(E) Rosiglitazone

10. Which of the following patients is MOST likely to be treated with intravenous glucagon?
(A) An 18-year-old woman who took an overdose of cocaine and now has a blood pressure of 190/110
(B) A 27-year-old woman with severe diarrhea due to a flare in her inflammatory bowel disease
(C) A 57-year-old female with type 2 diabetes who has not taken her glyburide for the past three days
(D) A 62-year-old man with severe bradycardia and hypotension due to ingestion of an overdose of atenolol
(E) A 74-year-old male with lactic acidosis as a complication of severe infection and shock

DIRECTIONS (Items 11–12): This case history* is followed by discussion questions. Write out brief answers (two to five sentences) and then compare your answers with those given at the end of the Answers section.

An 18-year-old college student was referred to the endocrine clinic at her student health service because a routine urinalysis revealed glycosuria and a random plasma glucose measured subsequently was 250 mg/dL.

The history disclosed that this was the student's first time away from home and that she had had a number of symptoms she attributed to anxiety associated with the move to college. These symptoms included weight loss (5 kg), polydipsia, nocturia, fatigue, and three episodes of vaginal yeast infections in the past 3 months. Before coming to college, she had experienced a series of upper respiratory tract infections. The family history was negative for diabetes, and she was not taking medications.

The physical examination was within normal limits. Her weight was 50 kg, which is in the 20th percentile for her height. The laboratory results were as follows: fasting plasma glucose 280 mg/dL (normal < 115), urine glucose and ketones strongly positive. On the basis of these and other findings, a diagnosis of type 1 diabetes was made.

11. What are the primary therapeutic strategies available in this case?
12. What methods of monitoring and adjusting therapy are available to the patient?

ANSWERS

1. Oral antidiabetic agents are inappropriate in this patient because he has insulin-dependent diabetes. He needs a rapidly acting insulin preparation that can be given intravenously (Table 41–1). The answer is **(A)**.

2. Because of the risk of brain damage, the most important complication of insulin therapy is hypoglycemia. The other choices are not common effects of insulin. The answer is **(B)**.

3. Insulin regimens for close control usually take the form of establishing a basal level of insulin with a small amount of a long-acting preparation (ultralente) and supplementing the insulin levels, when called for by food intake, with short-acting insulin lispro. Less tight control may be achieved with two injections of intermediate-acting insulin per day. Because intake of glucose is mainly during the day, long-acting insulins are usually given in the morning, not at night. The answer is **(D)**.

4. Chlorpropamide, glipizide, and tolazamide are sulfonylureas and repaglinide is a miglitinide. These drugs all promote the release of insulin from pancreatic B cells. In contrast, pioglitazone is a thiazolidinedione that promotes the uptake of glucose by muscle and adipose tissue. The answer is **(C)**.

5. Insulin stimulates the storage of glucose as glycogen. The answer is **(E)**.

6. Biguanides, especially the older drug phenformin, have been associated with lactic acidosis. Thus metformin should be avoided in patients with conditions that increase the risk of lactic acidosis, including alcoholism. The answer is **(D)**.

7. To be absorbed, carbohydrates must be converted into monosaccharides by the action of α-glucosidase enzymes in the gastrointestinal tract. Acarbose inhibits α-glucosidase and, when present during digestion, delays the uptake of carbohydrates. The answer is **(A)**.

8. The PPAR-γ receptor belongs to a family of nuclear receptors. When activated, these receptors translocate to the nucleus where they regulate the transcription of genes encoding proteins involved in the metabolism of carbohydrate and lipids. The answer is **(D)**.

9. The insulin secretagogues, including the sulfonylurea glyburide, can cause hypoglycemia as a result of their ability to increase serum insulin levels. The biguanides, thiazolidinediones and α-glucosidase inhibitors are "euglycemics" that are unlikely to cause hypoglycemia when used alone. The answer is **(B)**.

10. Glucagon acts through cardiac glucagon receptors to stimulate the rate and force of contraction of the heart. Since this bypasses cardiac beta-adrenoceptors, glucagon is useful in the treatment of beta-blocker-induced cardiac depression. The answer is **(D)**.

11. In a young diabetic of low or normal weight with a history of viral infections preceding onset of hyperglycemia, it is likely that the disease is due to loss of functioning pancreatic islet B

* Modified and reproduced, with permission, from Koda-Kimble MA, Rotblatt MD: Diabetes mellitus. In: *Applied Therapeutics*, 3rd ed. Katcher BS, Young LY, Koda-Kimble MA (editors). Applied Therapeutics, 1983.

cells. The diagnosis of insulin deficiency (type 1) diabetes was made in this case. The strategies available in this case are dietary management and insulin. The oral hypoglycemic agents are not useful in type 1 diabetes.

12. Patients must monitor their blood and urine glucose to aid the adjustment of their insulin dosage. The major reason for daily (or even more frequent) adjustment of dosage is that insulin requirement is altered by many factors: diet, exercise, disease, etc. Considerable evidence indicates that close control of blood glucose is associated with a lower incidence of long-term complications of diabetes.

The major adjustments made by most patients are the total number of units of insulin injected and the proportions of rapid-acting and intermediate- or long-acting preparations used.

Skill Keeper Answers: Diabetes & Hypertension (see Chapter 11)

1. The major antihypertensive drug groups are (1) beta-adrenoceptor blockers; (2) $alpha_1$-selective adrenoceptor blockers (eg, prazosin); (3) centrally acting sympathoplegics (eg, clonidine or methyldopa); (4) calcium channel blockers (eg, diltiazem nifedipine, verapamil); (5) angiotensin-converting enzyme (ACE) inhibitors (eg, captopril); (6) angiotensin receptor antagonists (eg, losartan); and (7) thiazide diuretics.
2. ACE inhibitors slow the progression of diabetic nephropathy and help stabilize renal function. Angiotensin receptor antagonists may have similar protective effects in diabetic patients. Beta-adrenoceptor blockers can mask the symptoms of hypoglycemia in diabetic patients. However, many patients with diabetes and cardiovascular disease are successfully treated with these drugs. A large clinical trial showed that control of hypertension decreases diabetes-associated microvascular disease. This trial included many patients being maintained on beta-adrenoceptor blockers. Thiazide diuretics impair the release of insulin and tissue utilization of glucose, so they are not drugs of first choice for patients with diabetes.

42 Drugs That Affect Bone Mineral Homeostasis

OBJECTIVES

You should be able to:

- List the agents useful in the treatment of hypercalcemia.
- Identify the major and minor regulators of bone mineral homeostasis.
- Describe the major effects of parathyroid hormone and vitamin D derivatives on the intestine, the kidney, and bone.

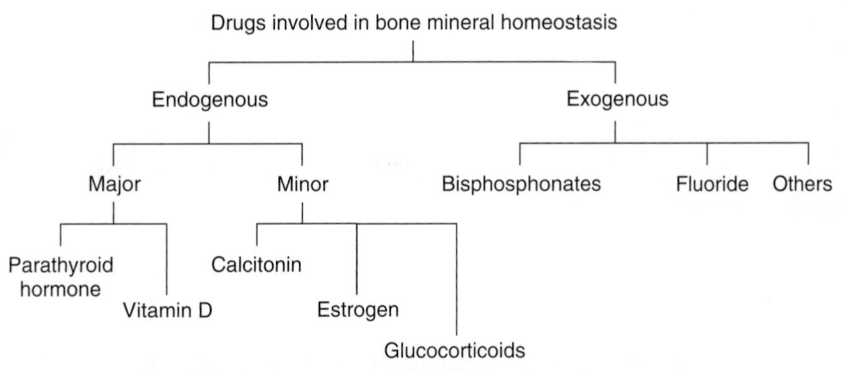

Figure 42–1. Subgroups of drugs discussed in this chapter.

- Describe the therapeutic and toxic effects of vitamin D, calcitonin, and bisphosphonates.
- Recall the effects of adrenal and gonadal steroids on bone structure and the actions of diuretics on serum calcium levels.
- Identify the therapeutic and toxic effects of fluoride ion.

CONCEPTS

Calcium and phosphorus are the two major elements of bone. They are also important in the function of other cells in the body, and bone therefore acts as a storage reservoir. Parathyroid hormone (PTH) and vitamin D are of primary importance in the regulation of bone mineral homeostasis. Calcitonin, glucocorticoids, and estrogens are less important regulators. Exogenous agents used in the treatment of bone mineral disorders (eg, osteoporosis, Paget's disease) include the bisphosphonates, fluoride, and estrogens. (Figure 42–1).

ENDOGENOUS SUBSTANCES

A. Parathyroid Hormone: Parathyroid hormone (PTH), an 84-amino-acid peptide, acts on membrane G protein-coupled receptors to increase cAMP in bone and the renal tubule. At high doses, the hormone increases blood calcium and decreases phosphorus by increasing net bone resorption (Figure 42–2). At low doses (physiologic levels), PTH can increase net bone formation (Table 42–1), and an analog has been used in postmenopausal osteoporosis.

> **Skill Keeper: Diuretics & Calcium**
> **(see Chapter 15)**
>
> The kidney serves as an important regulator of serum calcium concentrations. Several diuretics affect the kidney's handling of filtered calcium.
>
> **1.** Which two classes of diuretics have opposite effects on calcium elimination?
> **2.** What mechanisms are responsible for their effects?
> **3.** What is the clinical importance of these effects?
>
> *The Skill Keeper Answers appear at the end of the chapter.*

B. Vitamin D: Vitamin D, a derivative of 7-dehydrocholesterol, is formed in the skin under the influence of ultraviolet light. Vitamin D is also found in some foods and is commonly used as a food supplement in milk. Active metabolites of vitamin D are formed in the liver (calcifediol)

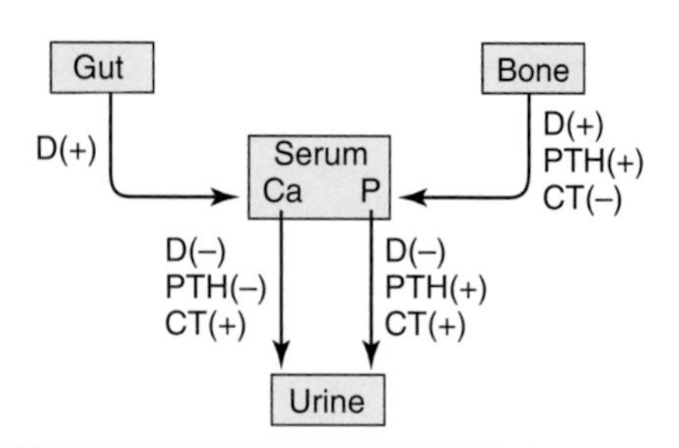

Figure 42–2. Some effects of vitamin D *(D)*, parathyroid hormone *(PTH)*, and calcitonin *(CT)* on calcium and phosphorus metabolism. Vitamin D increases absorption of calcium from both gut and bone, while PTH increases reabsorption from bone. Both vitamin D and parathyroid hormone reduce urinary excretion of calcium. (Reproduced, with permission, from Katzung BG [editor]: *Basic & Clinical Pharmacology,* 8th ed. McGraw-Hill, 2001.)

and the kidney (calcitriol, secalcifediol). They differ in the number of hydroxyl groups on the molecule (Table 42–2). The actions of vitamin D include increased intestinal calcium and phosphorus absorption, decreased renal excretion of these substances, and a net increase in blood levels of both (Figure 42–2; Table 42–1). Bone formation may be increased by secalcifediol (24,25-dihydroxyvitamin D). Vitamin D supplements and synthetic derivatives are used in the treatment of deficiency states, including chronic renal failure, intestinal osteodystrophy, and nutritional rickets. They are also used, in combination with calcium supplementation and hormone replacement therapy, in postmenopausal osteoporosis.

C. Calcitonin: Calcitonin, a peptide hormone secreted by the thyroid gland, decreases bone resorption and serum calcium and phosphate (Figure 42–2). Bone formation is not impaired initially, but ultimately it is reduced. The hormone has been used in conditions in which an acute reduction of serum calcium is needed, eg, Paget's disease and hypercalcemia. While calcitonin is approved for treatment of osteoporosis, it is questionable whether long-term use prevents fractures. Although human calcitonin is available, salmon calcitonin is most often selected for clinical use because of its longer half-life and greater potency. Calcitonin is administered by injection or as a nasal spray.

D. Estrogens: Estrogens and selective estrogen receptor modulators (SERMs; eg, raloxifene) can prevent or delay bone loss in postmenopausal women (Chapter 40). Their action may involve the inhibition of parathyroid hormone-stimulated bone resorption. Because of estrogen's proved efficacy in slowing the progression of osteoporosis, many experts strongly recommend these drugs for general use (unless contraindicated) in postmenopausal women.

E. Glucocorticoids: The glucocorticoids have several effects already referred to (eg, protein catabolism; see Chapter 39) that inhibit bone mineral maintenance. As a result, chronic systemic use of these drugs is a common cause of osteoporosis in adults. However, these hormones are useful in the intermediate-term treatment of hypercalcemia.

Table 42–1. Actions of PTH and vitamin D on intestine, kidney, and bone.*

Organ	PTH	Vitamin D
Intestine	Increased calcium and phosphate absorption (by increased $1,25[OH]_2D$ production)	Increased calcium and phosphate absorption (by $1,25[OH]_2D$)
Kidney	Decreased calcium excretion, increased phosphate excretion	Calcium and phosphate excretion may be decreased by 25(OH)D and $1,25(OH)_2D$
Bone	Calcium and phosphate resorption increased by high doses. Low doses may increase bone formation	Increased calcium and phosphate resorption by $1,25(OH)_2D$. Bone formation may be increased by $24,25(OH)_2D$
Net effect on serum levels	Serum calcium increased, serum phosphate decreased	Serum calcium and phosphate both increased

*Reproduced, with permission, from Katzung BG (editor): *Basic & Clinical Pharmacology,* 8th ed. McGraw-Hill, 2001.

Table 42–2. Vitamin D and its clinically available metabolites and analogs.*

Chemical Name	Generic Name and Abbreviation
Vitamin D_3	Cholecalciferol, D_3
Vitamin D_2	Ergocalciferol, D_2
25-Hydroxyvitamin D_3	Calcifediol, $25(OH)D_3$
1,25-Dihydroxyvitamin D_3	Calcitriol, $1,25(OH)_2D_3$
24,25-Dihydroxyvitamin D_3	Secalcifediol, $24,25(OH)_2D_3$
Dihydrotachysterol	DHT
Calcipotriene	Calcipotriol
1α-Hydroxyvitamin D_2	Doxercalciferol
19-nor-1,25-Dihydroxyvitamin D_2	Paricalcitol

*Reproduced, with permission, from Katzung BG (editor): *Basic & Clinical Pharmacology,* 8th ed. McGraw-Hill, 2001.

EXOGENOUS AGENTS

A. Bisphosphonates: The bisphosphonates (**alendronate, etidronate, pamidronate,** and **risedronate**) are short-chain organic polyphosphate compounds that reduce both the resorption and the formation of bone by an action on the basic hydroxyapatite crystal structure. Chronic bisphosphonate therapy can slow the progress of postmenopausal osteoporosis and reduces fractures. The older drugs (etidronate, pamidronate) cause bone mineralization defects and lose their effectiveness over 12 months. Alendronate and risedronate cause fewer bone problems and are effective for at least 5 years. They are used commonly for treatment of osteoporosis (postmenopausal and glucocorticoid-induced) and for Paget's disease. Alendronate, used in combination with hormone replacement therapy, further increases bone mass in menopausal patients. Oral bioavailability of bisphosphonates is low (< 10%), and food impairs their absorption. Esophageal ulceration may occur. Patients should take the drugs with large quantities of water and avoid situations that permit esophageal reflux.

B. Fluoride: Appropriate concentrations of fluoride ion in drinking water (0.5–1 ppm) or as a dentifrice additive have a well-documented ability to reduce dental caries. Chronic exposure to the ion, especially in high concentrations, may increase new bone synthesis. It is not clear, however, whether this new bone is normal in strength. Clinical trials of fluoride in patients with osteoporosis have not demonstrated a reduction in fractures. Acute toxicity of fluoride (usually caused by ingestion of rat poison) is manifested by gastrointestinal and neurologic symptoms. Chronic toxicity (fluorosis) includes ectopic bone formation and exostoses.

C. Other Drugs with Effects on Calcium and Bone: Plicamycin (mithramycin) is an antibiotic used to reduce serum calcium and bone resorption in Paget's disease and hypercalcemia. Because of the risk of serious toxicity (eg, thrombocytopenia, hemorrhage, hepatic and renal damage), plicamycin is not used commonly and is mainly restricted to short-term treatment of serious hypercalcemia. Several diuretics can affect serum calcium levels (see this chapter's Skill Keeper).

QUESTIONS

DIRECTIONS: Each of the numbered items or incomplete statements in this section is followed by answers or by completions of the statement. Select the ONE lettered answer or completion that is BEST in each case.

1. Which one of the following is LEAST likely to be useful in the therapy of hypercalcemia?
- **(A)** Calcitonin
- **(B)** Glucocorticoids
- **(C)** Plicamycin
- **(D)** Parenteral infusion of phosphate
- **(E)** Thiazide diuretics

2. Characteristics of vitamin D and its metabolites include which one of the following?
   (A) Act to decrease serum levels of calcium
   (B) Activation of their vitamin D receptors increases cellular cAMP
   (C) Calcitriol is the major derivative responsible for increasing intestinal absorption of phosphate.
   (D) Metabolites of vitamin D increase renal excretion of calcium
   (E) Vitamin D deficiency results in Paget's disease
3. Which of the following conditions is an indication for the use of calcitonin?
   (A) Chronic renal failure
   (B) Hypoparathyroidism
   (C) Intestinal osteodystrophy
   (D) Paget's disease
   (E) Rickets

Items 4–6: A 58-year-old postmenopausal woman was sent for dual-energy x-ray absorptiometry to evaluate the bone mineral density of her lumbar spine, femoral neck, and total hip. The test results revealed significantly low bone mineral density in all sites.

4. Chronic use of which of the following medications is MOST likely to have contributed to this woman's osteoporosis?
   (A) Lovastatin
   (B) Metformin
   (C) Prednisone
   (D) Propranolol
   (E) Warfarin
5. Which one of the following agents is least likely to have therapeutic value in the treatment of this woman's osteoporosis?
   (A) Calcium
   (B) Raloxifene
   (C) Risedronate
   (D) Thyroxine
   (E) Vitamin D
6. If this patient began oral therapy with alendronate, she would be advised to drink large quantities of water with the tablets and remain in an upright position for at least 30 minutes and until eating the first meal of the day. These instructions would be given in order to decrease the risk of
   (A) Cholelithiasis
   (B) Diarrhea
   (C) Constipation
   (D) Erosive esophagitis
   (E) Pernicious anemia
7. Clinical uses of vitamin D do not include
   (A) Chronic renal failure
   (B) Hyperparathyroidism
   (C) Intestinal osteodystrophy
   (D) Nutritional rickets
   (E) Osteoporosis
8. Which one of the following drugs, when used chronically, is associated with the development of bone pain and mineralization defects such as osteomalacia?
   (A) Calcitonin
   (B) Dihydrotachysterol
   (C) Ergocalciferol
   (D) Etidronate
   (E) Risedronate

ANSWERS

1. Thiazides increase calcium reabsorption from the urine (see Chapter 15 and the Skill Keeper Answers) and are never used in patients with hypercalcemia. Though it is highly toxic, plicamycin has been used to reduce serum calcium in Paget's disease. The answer is **(E).**

2. Vitamin D increases serum calcium and phosphate, with calcitriol (1,25$[OH]_2$ vitamin D) being the major derivative responsible for promoting their intestinal absorption. Calciferol and calcitriol decrease renal excretion of calcium and phosphate. Parathyroid hormone, not vitamin D, acts via cAMP. The cause of Paget's disease is obscure. The answer is **(C).**
3. Calcitonin is often used in Paget's disease to control hypercalcemia. The answer is **(D).**
4. Long-term therapy with glucocorticoids such as prednisone is associated with a reduction in bone mineral density and an increased risk of fractures. The other drugs are not known to have significant effects upon bone or serum calcium. The answer is **(C).**
5. Bisphosphonates such as risedronate and the selective estrogen receptor modulator raloxifene are approved for treatment of osteoporosis. Patients with osteoporosis also are encouraged to supplement their diets with calcium and vitamin D. Thyroxine does not improve bone mineral density and, in excess, is associated with development of osteoporosis. The answer is **(D).**
6. Chronic use of bisphosphonates such as alendronate has been associated with development of erosive esophagitis, perhaps as a result of direct irritation to the esophageal lining. The risk of this toxicity is reduced by drinking water and by remaining in an upright position after taking the medication. The answer is **(D).**
7. Hyperparathyroidism is associated with hypercalcemia and, if symptoms are significant, is best managed by surgery. Vitamin D (and calcium) supplements are commonly used in postmenopausal patients. Vitamin D may counter the decreased intestinal absorption of calcium that occurs in menopause. The answer is **(B).**
8. Vitamin D supplements are used in diseases of bone and mineral metabolism (eg, intestinal osteodystrophy) that can present with osteomalacia. Older bisphosphonates such as etidronate have only short-term clinical value in osteoporosis or Paget's disease, since their chronic use results in osteomalacia and an increased incidence of bone fractures. The answer is **(D).**

Skill Keeper Answers: Diuretics & Calcium
(see Chapter 15)

1. Loop diuretics (eg, furosemide) and thiazide diuretics exert opposite effects on the renal handling of filtered calcium and have opposite effects on urine calcium concentrations; loop diuretics increase urine concentrations of calcium, whereas the thiazides decrease urine calcium.
2. Loop diuretics inhibit the $Na^+/K^+/2Cl^-$ cotransporter in apical membranes of the thick ascending limb of the loop of Henle (Figure 15–4). Normally, this transporter maintains a lumen-positive potential that serves as the driving force for resorption of Mg^{2+} and Ca^{2+}. When the transporter is inhibited by loop diuretics, the lumen potential is less positive; more Mg^{2+} and Ca^{2+} remain in the tubular fluid, and less Mg^{2+} and Ca^{2+} is returned to the blood. In the distal convoluted tubule, Ca^{2+} is actively resorbed through the concerted action of an apical Ca^{2+} channel and a basolateral Na^+/Ca^{2+} exchanger (Figure 15–5). The system is under control of parathyroid hormone. When the thiazide diuretics inhibit the Na^+/Cl^- transporter in cells that line the distal convoluted tubule, they lower the intracellular concentration of sodium in these cells. This is believed to enhance the Na^+/Ca^{2+} exchange that occurs on the basolateral surface. This, in turn, creates a greater driving force for passage of Ca^{2+} through the calcium channels. The net effect is enhanced resorption of calcium.
3. In patients with hypercalcemia, treatment with a loop diuretic plus saline promotes calcium excretion and helps lower serum calcium. In patients with intact regulatory function, increases in calcium resorption promoted by thiazides have minor impact on serum calcium due to buffering in bone and gut. However, thiazides can unmask hypercalcemia that occurs in diseases that disrupt normal calcium regulation (eg, hyperparathyroidism, sarcoidosis, carcinoma).

Part VIII. Chemotherapeutic Drugs

43 Beta-Lactam Antibiotics & Other Cell Wall Synthesis Inhibitors

OBJECTIVES

You should be able to:

- Describe the mechanism of antibacterial action of beta-lactam antibiotics.
- Describe the mechanisms underlying the resistance of bacteria to beta-lactam antibiotics.
- Identify the important drugs in each subclass of penicillins and describe their antibacterial activity and clinical uses.
- Identify the four subclasses of cephalosporins and describe their antibacterial activities and clinical uses.
- List the major adverse effects of the penicillins and the cephalosporins.
- Identify the important features of aztreonam, imipenem, and meropenem.
- Describe the clinical uses and toxicities of vancomycin, fosfomycin, and bacitracin.

Learn the definitions that follow.

Table 43–1. Definitions.

Term	Definition
Bactericidal	An antimicrobial drug that can eradicate an infection in the absence of host defense mechanisms; kills bacteria
Bacteriostatic	An antimicrobial drug that inhibits microbial growth but requires host defense mechanisms to eradicate the infection; does not kill bacteria
Beta-lactam antibiotics	Drugs with structures containing a beta-lactam ring; includes the penicillins and cephalosporins. This ring must be intact for antimicrobial action
Beta-lactamases	Bacterial enzymes (penicillinases, cephalosporinases) that hydrolyze the beta-lactam ring of certain penicillins and cephalosporins
Minimal inhibitory concentration (MIC)	Lowest concentration of antimicrobial drug capable of inhibiting growth of an organism in a defined growth medium
Penicillin-binding proteins (PBPs)	Bacterial cytoplasmic membrane proteins that act as the initial receptors for penicillins and other beta-lactam antibiotics
Peptidoglycan, murein	Chains of polysaccharides and polypeptides that are cross-linked to form the bacterial cell wall
Selective toxicity	More toxic to the invader than to the host; a property of useful antimicrobial drugs
Transpeptidases	Bacterial enzymes involved in the cross-linking of linear peptidoglycan chains, the final step in cell wall synthesis

CONCEPTS

Penicillins and cephalosporins (Figure 43–1) are the major antibiotics that inhibit bacterial cell wall synthesis. They are called beta-lactams because of the unusual four-member ring that is common to

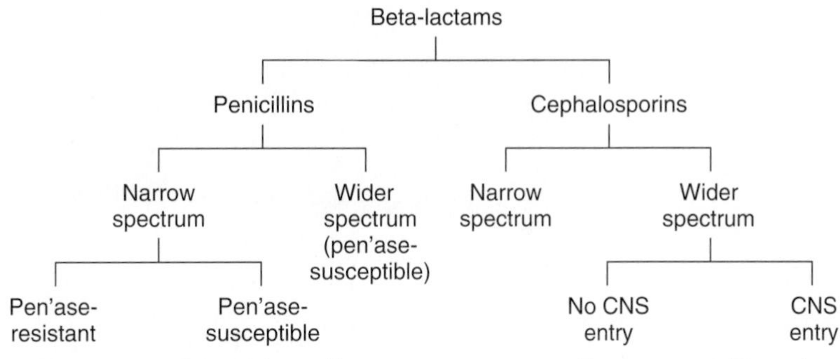

Figure 43–1. Subdivisions of beta-lactam antibiotics (Pen'ase, penicillinase).

all their members. These two large classes of beta-lactams include some of the most effective, widely used, and well-tolerated agents available for the treatment of microbial infections. Vancomycin, fosfomycin, and bacitracin also inhibit cell wall synthesis but for various reasons are not nearly as important as the beta-lactam drugs. The **selective toxicity** of the drugs discussed in this chapter is mainly due to specific actions on the synthesis of a cellular structure that is unique to the microorganism. Over 60 antibiotics that act as cell wall synthesis inhibitors are currently available, with individual spectra of activity that afford a wide range of clinical applications.

The emergence of **microbial resistance** poses a constant challenge to the use of antimicrobial drugs. Mechanisms underlying microbial resistance to cell wall synthesis inhibitors include the production of antibiotic-inactivating enzymes, changes in the structure of target receptors, and decreases in the permeability of microbes' cellular membranes to antibiotics. Strategies designed to combat microbial resistance include the use of adjunctive agents that can protect against antibiotic inactivation, the use of antibiotic combinations, the introduction of new (and often expensive) chemical derivatives of established antibiotics, and efforts to avoid the indiscriminate use or misuse of antibiotics.

PENICILLINS

A. Classification: All penicillins are derivatives of 6-aminopenicillanic acid and contain a beta-lactam ring structure that is essential for antibacterial activity. Penicillin subclasses have additional chemical substituents that confer differences in antimicrobial activity, susceptibility to acid and enzymic hydrolysis, and biodisposition.

B. Pharmacokinetics: Penicillins vary in their resistance to gastric acid and therefore vary in their oral bioavailability. They are polar compounds and are not metabolized extensively. They are usually excreted unchanged in the urine via glomerular filtration and tubular secretion, the latter process being inhibited by probenecid. Ampicillin and nafcillin are excreted partly in the bile. The plasma half-lives of most penicillins vary from one-half to 1 hour. Procaine and benzathine forms of penicillin G are administered intramuscularly and have long plasma half-lives because the active drug is released very slowly into the bloodstream. Most penicillins cross the blood-brain barrier only when the meninges are inflamed.

C. Mechanisms of Action and Resistance: Beta-lactam antibiotics are **bactericidal** drugs. They act to inhibit cell wall synthesis by the following steps (Figure 43–2): (1) binding of the drug to specific receptors **(penicillin-binding proteins; PBPs)** located in the bacterial cytoplasmic membrane; (2) inhibition of **transpeptidase** enzymes that act to cross-link linear peptidoglycan chains which form part of the cell wall; and (3) activation of **autolytic** enzymes that cause lesions in the bacterial cell wall.

Enzymatic hydrolysis of the beta-lactam ring results in loss of antibacterial activity. The formation of **beta-lactamases (penicillinases)** by most staphylococci and many gram-negative organisms is thus a major mechanism of bacterial resistance. Inhibitors of these bacterial enzymes (eg, clavulanic acid, sulbactam, tazobactam) are sometimes used in combination with peni-

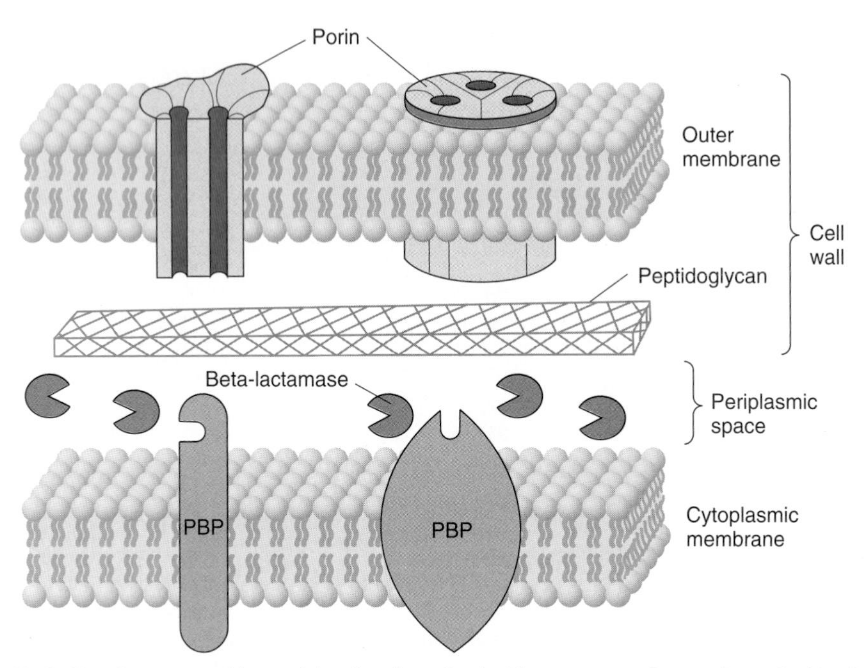

Figure 43–2. Beta-lactams and bacterial cell wall synthesis. The outer membrane shown in this simplified diagram is present only in gram-negative organisms. It is penetrated by proteins (porins) that are permeable to hydrophilic substances such as beta-lactam antibiotics. The peptidoglycan chains (mureins) are cross-linked by transpeptidases located in the cytoplasmic membrane, closely associated with penicillin-binding proteins (PBPs). Beta-lactam antibiotics bind to PBPs and inhibit transpeptidation, the final step in cell wall synthesis. They also activate autolytic enzymes that cause lesions in the cell wall. Beta-lactamases, which inactivate beta-lactam antibiotics, may be present in the periplasmic space or on the outer surface of the cytoplasmic membrane. (Reproduced, with permission, from Katzung BG [editor]: *Basic & Clinical Pharmacology,* 8th ed. McGraw-Hill, 2001.)

cillins to prevent their inactivation. Structural change in target PBPs is another mechanism of resistance and is responsible for methicillin resistance in staphylococci and for resistance to penicillin G in pneumococci. In some gram-negative rods (eg, *Pseudomonas aeruginosa*) changes in the porin structures in the outer membrane may contribute to resistance by impeding access of penicillins to PBPs.

D. Clinical Uses:

1. **Narrow spectrum, penicillinase-susceptible agents:** **Penicillin G** is the prototype of a subclass of penicillins that have a limited spectrum of antibacterial activity and are susceptible to beta-lactamases. Clinical uses include therapy of infections caused by common streptococci, meningococci, gram-positive bacilli, and spirochetes. Many strains of pneumococci are now resistant to penicillins. Most strains of *Staphylococcus aureus* and a significant number of strains of *N gonorrhoeae* are resistant via production of beta-lactamases. While no longer suitable for treatment of gonorrhea, penicillin G remains the drug of choice for syphilis. Activity against enterococci is enhanced by aminoglycoside antibiotics. **Penicillin V** is an oral drug used mainly in oropharyngeal infections.
2. **Very narrow spectrum, penicillinase-resistant drugs:** This subclass of penicillins includes **methicillin** (the prototype), **nafcillin,** and **oxacillin.** Their primary use is in the treatment of known or suspected staphylococcal infections. Methicillin-resistant staphylococci (MRSA) are resistant to other members of this subgroup and may be resistant to multiple antimicrobial drugs.
3. **Wider spectrum, penicillinase-susceptible drugs:**
   a. **Ampicillin and amoxicillin:** These drugs comprise a penicillin subgroup that has a wider spectrum of antibacterial activity than penicillin G but remains susceptible to penicillinases. Their clinical uses include indications similar to penicillin G as well as

infections due to enterococci, *Listeria monocytogenes, Escherichia coli, Proteus mirabilis, Haemophilus influenzae,* and *Moraxella catarrhalis*, though resistant strains occur. When used in combination with inhibitors of penicillinases (clavulanic acid, etc), their antibacterial activity is enhanced. In enterococcal and listerial infections ampicillin is synergistic with aminoglycosides.

b. **Piperacillin and ticarcillin:** These drugs have activity against several gram-negative rods, including pseudomonas, enterobacter, and in some cases klebsiella species. Most drugs in this subgroup have synergistic actions when used with aminoglycosides against such organisms. Piperacillin and ticarcillin are susceptible to penicillinases and are often used in combination with penicillinase inhibitors to enhance their activity.

E. **Toxicity:**

1. **Allergy:** Allergic reactions include urticaria, severe pruritus, fever, joint swelling, hemolytic anemia, nephritis, and anaphylaxis. About 5–10% of persons with a past history of penicillin reaction have an allergic response when given a penicillin again. Methicillin causes nephritis more often than do other penicillins, and nafcillin is associated with neutropenia. Antigenic determinants include degradation products of penicillins such as penicilloic acid. Complete **cross-allergenicity** between different penicillins should be assumed. Ampicillin frequently causes maculopapular skin rash that may not be an allergic reaction.
2. **Gastrointestinal disturbances:** Nausea and diarrhea may occur with oral penicillins, especially with ampicillin. Gastrointestinal upsets may be caused by direct irritation or by overgrowth of gram-positive organisms or yeasts. Ampicillin has been implicated in pseudomembranous colitis.
3. **Cation toxicity:** Toxic effects from Na^+ or K^+ may occur when high doses of penicillin salts are used in patients with cardiovascular or renal disease.

CEPHALOSPORINS

A. **Classification:** The cephalosporins are derivatives of 7-aminocephalosporanic acid and contain the beta-lactam ring structure. Many members of this group are in clinical use. They vary in their antibacterial activity and are designated first-, second-, third-, or fourth-generation drugs according to the order of their introduction into clinical use.

B. **Pharmacokinetics:** Several cephalosporins are available for oral use, but most are administered parenterally. Cephalosporins with side-chains may undergo hepatic metabolism, but the major elimination mechanism for drugs in this class is renal excretion via active tubular secretion. Cefoperazone and ceftriaxone are excreted mainly in the bile. Most first- and second-generation cephalosporins do not enter the cerebrospinal fluid even when the meninges are inflamed.

C. **Mechanisms of Action and Resistance:** Cephalosporins bind to PBPs on bacterial cell membranes to inhibit bacterial cell wall synthesis by mechanisms similar to those of the penicillins. Cephalosporins are bactericidal against susceptible organisms.

Structural differences from penicillins render cephalosporins less susceptible to penicillinases produced by staphylococci, but many bacteria are resistant through the production of other beta-lactamases that can inactivate cephalosporins. Resistance can also result from decreases in membrane permeability to cephalosporins and from changes in PBPs. Methicillin-resistant staphylococci are also resistant to most cephalosporins.

D. **Clinical Uses:**

1. **First-generation drugs:** **Cefazolin** (parenteral) and **cephalexin** (oral) are examples of this subgroup. They are active against gram-positive cocci, including staphylococci and common streptococci. Many strains of *E coli* and *K pneumoniae* are also sensitive. Clinical uses include treatment of infections caused by these organisms and surgical prophylaxis in

selected conditions. These drugs have minimal activity against gram-negative cocci, enterococci, methicillin-resistant staphylococci, and most gram-negative rods.

2. **Second-generation drugs:** Drugs in this subgroup usually have less activity against gram-positive organisms than the first-generation drugs but have an extended gram-negative coverage. Marked differences in activity occur among the drugs in this subgroup. Examples of clinical uses include infections caused by *Bacteroides fragilis* **(cefotetan, cefoxitin)** and by *H influenzae* or *Moraxella catarrhalis* **(cefuroxime, cefaclor).**
3. **Third-generation drugs:** Characteristic features of third-generation drugs (eg, **cefoperazone, cefotaxime**) include increased activity against gram-negative organisms resistant to other beta-lactam drugs and ability to penetrate the blood-brain barrier (except cefoperazone and cefixime). Most are active against enterobacter, providencia, *Serratia marcescens,* and beta-lactamase-producing strains of *H influenzae* and neisseria. Individual drugs also have activity against pseudomonas **(ceftazidime)** and *B fragilis* **(ceftizoxime).** Drugs in this subclass should usually be reserved for treatment of serious infections, eg, bacterial meningitis. **Ceftriaxone** (parenteral) and **cefixime** (oral), currently drugs of choice in gonorrhea, are exceptions. Likewise, in acute otitis media, a single injection of ceftriaxone is as effective as a 10-day course of treatment with amoxicillin or cefaclor.
4. **Fourth-generation drugs: Cefipime** is more resistant to beta-lactamases produced by gram-negative organisms, including enterobacter, haemophilus, and neisseria. Cefipime combines the gram-positive activity of first-generation agents with the wider gram-negative spectrum of third-generation cephalosporins.

E. Toxicity:

1. **Allergy:** Cephalosporins cause a range of allergic reactions from skin rashes to anaphylactic shock. These reactions occur less frequently with cephalosporins than with penicillins. Complete cross-hypersensitivity between different cephalosporins should be assumed. Cross-reactivity between penicillins and cephalosporins is incomplete (5–10%), so penicillin-allergic patients are sometimes treated successfully with a cephalosporin. However, patients with a history of *anaphylaxis* to penicillins should not be treated with a cephalosporin.
2. **Other adverse effects:** Cephalosporins may cause pain at intramuscular injection sites and phlebitis after intravenous administration. They may increase the nephrotoxicity of aminoglycosides when the two are administered together. Drugs containing a methylthiotetrazole group (cefoperazone, cefotetan, moxalactam) cause hypoprothrombinemia and may cause disulfiram-like reactions with ethanol. Moxalactam also decreases platelet function and may cause severe bleeding.

OTHER BETA-LACTAM DRUGS

A. Aztreonam: Aztreonam is a **monobactam** that is resistant to beta-lactamases produced by certain gram-negative rods, including klebsiella, pseudomonas, and serratia. The drug has no activity against gram-positive bacteria or anaerobes. It is an inhibitor of cell wall synthesis, preferentially binding to PBP3, and is synergistic with aminoglycosides.

Aztreonam is administered intravenously and is eliminated via renal tubular secretion. Its half-life is prolonged in renal failure. Adverse effects include gastrointestinal upset with possible superinfection, vertigo and headache, and rare hepatotoxicity. Though skin rash may occur, there is no cross-allergenicity with penicillins.

B. Imipenem and meropenem: These drugs are **carbapenems** (chemically different from penicillins but retaining the beta-lactam ring structure) with low susceptibility to beta-lactamases. The drugs have wide activity against gram-positive cocci (including some penicillin-resistant pneumococci), gram-negative rods, and anaerobes. Imipenem is administered parenterally and is especially useful for infections caused by organisms resistant to other antibiotics. It is currently the drug of choice for infections due to enterobacter.

Imipenem is rapidly inactivated by renal dehydropeptidase I and is administered in fixed combination with cilastatin, an inhibitor of this enzyme. Cilastatin increases the plasma half-life of imipenem and inhibits the formation of a potentially nephrotoxic metabolite.

Adverse effects of imipenem-cilastatin include gastrointestinal distress, skin rash, and, at very high plasma levels, CNS toxicity (confusion, encephalopathy, seizures). There is partial cross-allergenicity with the penicillins. **Meropenem** is similar to imipenem except that it is not metabolized by renal dehydropeptidases and is less likely to cause seizures.

C. **Beta-Lactamase Inhibitors:** **Clavulanic acid, sulbactam,** and **tazobactam** are used in fixed combinations with certain hydrolyzable penicillins. They are most active against plasmid-encoded beta-lactamases such as those produced by gonococci, streptococci, *E coli,* and *H influenzae.* They are not good inhibitors of inducible chromosomal beta-lactamases formed by enterobacter and pseudomonas.

OTHER INHIBITORS OF CELL WALL SYNTHESIS

A. **Vancomycin:** Vancomycin is a bactericidal glycoprotein that binds to the D-Ala-D-Ala terminal of the nascent peptidoglycan pentapeptide side chain and inhibits transglycosylation. This action prevents elongation of the peptidoglycan chain and interferes with cross-linking. Resistance involves a decreased affinity of vancomycin for the binding site due to the replacement of the terminal D-Ala by D-lactate. Vancomycin has a narrow spectrum of activity and is used for serious infections caused by drug-resistant gram-positive organisms, including methicillin-resistant staphylococci (MRSA), penicillin-resistant pneumococci, and *C difficile.*

Vancomycin-resistant enterococci have emerged recently, a potentially serious clinical problem since such organisms usually exhibit multiple drug resistance. Likewise, strains of MRSA have been reported with intermediate resistance to vancomycin, leading to treatment failures. Vancomycin is not absorbed from the gastrointestinal tract and may be given orally for bacterial enterocolitis. When given parenterally, vancomycin penetrates most tissues and is eliminated unchanged in the urine. Dosage modification is mandatory in patients with renal impairment. Toxic effects of vancomycin include chills, fever, phlebitis, ototoxicity, and nephrotoxicity. Rapid intravenous infusion may cause diffuse flushing ("red man syndrome").

B. **Fosfomycin:** Fosfomycin is an antimetabolite inhibitor of cytosolic enolpyruvate transferase. This action prevents the formation of *N*-acetylmuramic acid, an essential precursor molecule for peptidoglycan chain formation. Resistance to fosfomycin occurs via decreased intracellular accumulation of the drug.

Fosfomycin is excreted by the kidney, with urinary levels exceeding the **minimal inhibitory concentrations (MICs)** for many urinary tract pathogens. In a single dose, the drug is less effective than a 7-day course of treatment with fluoroquinolones. With multiple dosing, resistance emerges rapidly and diarrhea is common. Fosfomycin may be synergistic with beta-lactam and quinolone antibiotics in specific infections.

C. **Bacitracin:** Bacitracin is a peptide antibiotic that interferes with a late stage in cell wall synthesis in gram-positive organisms. Because of its marked nephrotoxicity, the drug is limited to topical use.

D. **Cycloserine:** Cycloserine is an antimetabolite that blocks the incorporation of D-Ala into the pentapeptide side chain of the peptidoglycan. Because of its potential neurotoxicity (tremors, seizures, psychosis), cycloserine is only used to treat tuberculosis caused by organisms resistant to first-line antituberculous drugs.

DRUG LIST

The following drugs are important members of the group discussed in this chapter. Prototypes should be learned in detail; features of the major variants should be known well enough to distinguish the variants from prototypes and from each other.

Subclass	Prototype	Major Variants
Penicillins		
Limited spectrum	Penicillin G	Penicillin V
Beta-lactamase-resistant	Methicillin	Nafcillin, oxacillin, cloxacillin
Wider spectrum	Ampicillin, carbenicillin	Amoxicillin, piperacillin, ticarcillin
Cephalosporins		
First-generation	Cefazolin	Cephalexin, cephradine, cephapirin
Second-generation	Cefamandole	Cefaclor, cefotetan, cefoxitin
Third-generation	Cefoperazone	Cefotaxime, ceftazidime, ceftriaxone
Fourth-generation	Cefepime	
Carbapenem	Imipenem	Meropenem
Monobactam	Aztreonam	
Beta-lactamase inhibitors[1]	Clavulanic acid	Sulbactam, tazobactam

[1]Negligible antimicrobial activity when given alone.

QUESTIONS

DIRECTIONS: Each of the numbered items or incomplete statements in this section is followed by answers or by completions of the statement. Select the ONE lettered answer or completion that is BEST in each case.

1. Which one of the following statements about the biodisposition of penicillins and cephalosporins is most accurate?
(A) Oral bioavailability is affected by first-pass hepatic metabolism
(B) Only third-generation cephalosporins cross the blood-brain barrier
(C) Procaine penicillin G is the most commonly used intravenous form of the antibiotic
(D) Renal tubular reabsorption of beta-lactams is inhibited by probenecid
(E) Nafcillin and ceftriaxone are eliminated mainly via biliary secretion

2. The mechanism of antibacterial action of cephalosporins involves
(A) Inhibition of the synthesis of precursors of peptidoglycans
(B) Interference with the synthesis of ergosterol
(C) Inhibition of transpeptidation reactions
(D) Inhibition of beta-lactamases
(E) Binding to cytoplasmic receptor proteins

Items 3–4: A 21-year-old man was seen in a clinic with a complaint of dysuria and urethral discharge of yellow pus. He had a painless clean-based ulcer on the penis and nontender enlargement of the regional lymph nodes. Gram stain of the urethral exudate showed gram-negative diplococci within polymorphonucleocytes. The patient informed the clinic staff that he was unemployed and had not eaten a meal for 2 days.

3. The most appropriate treatment of gonorrhea in this patient is
(A) Amoxicillin orally for 7 days
(B) Ceftriaxone intramuscularly as a single dose
(C) Procaine penicillin G intramuscularly as a single dose plus 1 g of probenecid
(D) Tetracycline orally for 7 days
(E) Vancomycin intramuscularly as a single dose

4. Immunofluorescent microscopic examination of fluid expressed from the penile chancre of this patient revealed treponemes. Since he appears to be infected with *T pallidum,* the best course of action would be to
(A) Treat with spectinomycin
(B) Treat with oral tetracycline
(C) Inject intramuscular benzathine penicillin G
(D) Give a single oral dose of fosfomycin
(E) Give no other antibiotics since drug treatment of gonorrhea provides coverage for incubating syphilis

5. Which one of the following statements about imipenem is most accurate?

(A) The drug has a narrow spectrum of antibacterial action
(B) It is used in fixed combination with sulbactam
(C) Imipenem is highly susceptible to beta-lactamases produced by enterobacter species
(D) In renal dysfunction, dosage reductions are necessary to avoid seizures
(E) Imipenem is active against methicillin-resistant staphylococci

6. An elderly debilitated patient has a fever believed to be due to an infection. He has extensive skin lesions, scrapings of which reveal the presence of large numbers of gram-positive cocci. The most appropriate drug to use for treatment of this patient is
(A) Amoxicillin
(B) Aztreonam
(C) Moxalactam
(D) Nafcillin
(E) Penicillin G

7. A 36-year-old woman recently treated for leukemia is admitted to hospital with malaise, chills, and high fever. Gram stain of blood reveals the presence of gram-negative bacilli. The initial diagnosis is bacteremia, and parenteral antibiotics are indicated. The records of the patient reveal that she had a severe urticarial rash, hypotension, and respiratory difficulty following oral penicillin V about 6 months ago. The most appropriate drug regimen for empiric treatment is
(A) Ampicillin plus sulbactam
(B) Aztreonam
(C) Cefazolin
(D) Imipenem plus cilastatin
(E) Ticarcillin plus clavulanic acid

Items 8–10: A 52-year-old man (weight 70 kg) is brought to the hospital emergency room in a confused and delirious state. He has had an elevated temperature for over 24 hours, during which time he had complained of a severe headache and had suffered from nausea and vomiting. Lumbar puncture reveals an elevated opening pressure, and cerebrospinal fluid findings include elevated protein, decreased glucose, and increased neutrophils. You are informed that the patient has a long history of antibiotic treatment for sinusitis but that currently he is not taking any drugs other than ibuprofen. Gram stain of a smear of cerebrospinal fluid reveals gram-positive diplococci, and a preliminary diagnosis is made of purulent meningitis. The microbiology report informs you that for approximately 15% of *S pneumoniae* isolates in the community, the minimal inhibitory concentration for penicillin G is greater than 2 μg/mL

8. Treatment of this patient should be initiated immediately with
(A) Ampicillin, 2 g intravenously every 6 hours
(B) Cefoperazone, 2 g intravenously every 12 hours
(C) Cefotaxime, 1.5 g intravenously every 6 hours
(D) Nafcillin, 2 g intravenously every 4 hours
(E) Penicillin G, 2 million units intravenously every 4 hours

9. The molecular basis for the resistance of pneumococci to penicillin G is
(A) The production of beta-lactamases
(B) Structural changes in penicillin binding proteins
(C) Decreased intracellular accumulation of penicillin G
(D) Changes in the D-Ala-D-Ala building block of peptidoglycan precursor
(E) Changes in porin structure

10. If this patient had been 82 years old and the Gram stain of the smear of cerebrospinal fluid had revealed gram-positive rods resembling diphtheroids, the antibiotic regimen for empiric treatment would include
(A) Ampicillin
(B) Cefazolin
(C) Moxalactam
(D) Ticarcillin
(E) Vancomycin

11. Which one of the following statements about cefotetan is accurate?
(A) It is active against MRSA strains
(B) It is the drug of choice in community-acquired pneumonia
(C) It is a fourth-generation cephalosporin
(D) It decreases prothrombin time
(E) Its antibacterial spectrum includes *Bacteroides fragilis*

12. A patient needs antibiotic treatment for native valve, culture-positive infective enterococcal endocarditis. His medical history includes a severe anaphylactic reaction to penicillin G during the past year. The best approach would be treatment with
    (A) Amoxicillin/clavulanate
    (B) Aztreonam
    (C) Cefazolin plus gentamicin
    (D) Meropenem
    (E) Vancomycin
13. This drug has activity against many strains of *Pseudomonas aeruginosa.* However, when it is used alone, resistance has emerged during the course of treatment. The drug should not be used in penicillin-allergic patients. Its activity against gram-negative rods is enhanced if it is given in combination with tazobactam.
    (A) Amoxicillin
    (B) Aztreonam
    (C) Imipenem
    (D) Piperacillin
    (E) Vancomycin
14. Which of the following statements about vancomycin is accurate?
    (A) It is bacteriostatic
    (B) It binds to PBPs
    (C) It is not susceptible to penicillinase
    (D) It has the advantage of oral bioavailability
    (E) Staphylococcal enterocolitis occurs commonly with its use
15. Which one of the following statements about ampicillin is false?
    (A) Its activity is enhanced by sulbactam
    (B) It causes maculopapular rashes
    (C) It is the drug of choice for *Listeria monocytogenes* infection
    (D) It eradicates most strains of MRSA
    (E) Pseudomembranous colitis may occur with its use

DIRECTIONS (Items 16–18): This case history* is followed by discussion questions. Write out brief answers (two to five sentences) and then compare your answers with those given at the end of the Answers section.

A 64-year-old man was hospitalized for evaluation and treatment of carcinoma of the tongue. Following a course of chemotherapy, the patient was brought to the operating room for radical neck dissection. He was intubated and given 2 g of cefoxitin intravenously. Ten minutes later, he had developed severe hypotension with a systolic blood pressure of 40–50 mm Hg, wheezing over both lung fields, and urticaria.

The operation was postponed, and the patient was given intravenous epinephrine, dexamethasone, diphenhydramine, and fluids over the next 2 hours. Blood pressure was restored and maintained by intravenous infusion of dopamine. In the intensive care unit, electrocardiography suggested acute cardiac injury; the patient had no history of angina pectoris or heart disease. Subsequent chest x-ray revealed a normal heart size with bilateral pulmonary edema.

16. Why was cefoxitin given at the time of surgery?
17. What type of drug allergy did the patient experience?
18. Why were epinephrine, diphenhydramine, and a corticosteroid administered?

ANSWERS

1. Stability in gastric acid is the main determinant of the oral bioavailability of beta-lactam antibiotics. Cefixime, a third-generation cephalosporin, and cefepime (fourth-generation) both cross the blood-brain barrier. Cefoperazone does not achieve adequate cerebrospinal fluid levels to be useful in bacterial meningitis. Procaine penicillin G is given by intramuscular injec-

---

* Adapted and reproduced, with permission, from Austin SM, Barooah B, Chung SK: Reversible acute cardiac injury during cefoxitin-induced anaphylaxis in a patient with normal coronary arteries. Am J Med 1984;77:729.

tion (not intravenously) and is rarely used now owing to resistance on the part of gonococci and pneumococci. The elimination half-lives of many beta-lactam antibiotics are prolonged by probenecid, which inhibits their proximal tubular secretion. Biliary excretion is the major mode of elimination of nafcillin and ceftriaxone. The answer is **(E).**

2. The cephalosporins bind to PBPs present on the cytoplasmic membrane and act at the transpeptidation stage of cell wall synthesis (the final step) to inhibit peptidoglycan cross-linking. Like penicillins, they also activate autolysins, which break down the bacterial cell wall. Vancomycin is an inhibitor of transglycosylation and, like fosfomycin, interferes with the synthesis of precursor molecules needed for peptidoglycan chain formation. The answer is **(C).**
3. Currently, the treatments of choice for gonorrhea include a single dose of ceftriaxone (intramuscularly) or of cefixime (orally). Note that neither of these third-generation cephalosporins has activity against chlamydia or other organisms responsible for nongonococcal urethritis. Because of the high incidence of beta-lactamase-producing gonococci, the use of penicillin G or amoxicillin is no longer appropriate for gonorrhea. Similarly, many strains of gonococci are resistant to tetracyclines. Other first-line drugs (not listed) for gonorrhea include ciprofloxacin and ofloxacin (see Chapter 46). The answer is **(B).**
4. This patient with gonorrhea also has primary syphilis. The penile chancre, the enlarged non-tender lymph nodes, and the microscopic identification of treponemes in fluid expressed from the lesion are essentials of diagnosis. Serologic tests for syphilis (eg, VDRL) are likely to be positive. While a single dose of ceftriaxone may cure incubating syphilis, it cannot be relied upon for treating primary syphilis. The most appropriate course of action in this patient is to administer a single intramuscular injection of 2.4 million units of benzathine penicillin G. For penicillin-allergic patients oral doxycycline or tetracycline for 15 days is effective in most cases. However, lack of compliance may be a problem with oral therapy. Fosfomycin and spectinomycin have no significant activity against spirochetes. The answer is **(C).**
5. Imipenem has a wide spectrum of activity that includes anaerobes and many beta-lactamase producing gram-negative rods, including enterobacter. The drug is hydrolyzed by renal dehydropeptidases and is given in combination with cilastatin, an inhibitor of this enzyme. The chemical structure of imipenem is related to the beta-lactams, and the drug displays partial cross-allergenicity with the penicillins. Severe CNS toxicity, including seizures, will occur if the dose of imipenem is not reduced in patients with renal impairment. The answer is **(D).**
6. Bacterial lesions of the skin are often caused by staphylococci or streptococci and may lead to systemic infections; they should be treated promptly. Virtually all strains of *S aureus* are penicillinase-producing, so amoxicillin and penicillin G would not be effective. Aztreonam is only active against gram-negative bacilli, and the third-generation cephalosporin (moxalactam) has limited activity against gram-positive organisms. In addition, moxalactam carries the risk of bleeding disorders in elderly debilitated patients. Nafcillin is resistant to penicillinases and has activity against most strains of *S aureus* and common streptococci. The answer is **(D).**
7. Each of the drugs listed has activity against some gram-negative bacilli. All penicillins should be avoided in patients with a history of allergic reactions to any individual penicillin drug. Cephalosporins should also be avoided in patients who have had anaphylaxis or other severe hypersensitivity reactions following use of a penicillin. There is no cross-reactivity between the penicillins and aztreonam. The answer is **(B).**
8. Pneumococcal isolates with a minimal inhibitory concentration for penicillin G of greater than 2 μg/mL are highly resistant. Such strains are not killed by the concentrations of penicillin G or ampicillin that can be achieved in the cerebrospinal fluid. Nafcillin would be of value in a purulent meningitis suspected to be due to staphylococci but has minimal activity against penicillin-resistant pneumococci. Cefotaxime and ceftriaxone (not listed) are the most active cephalosporins against penicillin-resistant pneumococci, and the addition of vancomycin or rifampin is recommended in the case of highly resistant strains. As mentioned above, cefoperazone does not readily cross the blood-brain barrier. The answer is **(C).**
9. Many gram-positive cocci—especially staphylococci—are resistant to penicillin G via the production of penicillinases. Beta-lactamase formation is also the mechanism of resistance of gonococci and many gram-negative rods. Pneumococcal resistance is due to changes in the chemical structures of penicillin-binding proteins located in the bacterial cytoplasmic membrane. A similar mechanism underlies the resistance of staphylococci to methicillin (MRSA strains). Changes in porin structure may play a role in penicillin resistance in gram-negative rods. A structural alteration in the D-Ala-D-Ala component of the pentapeptide side chains of peptidoglycans is the basis for a mechanism of resistance to vancomycin. The answer is **(B).**

10. The presence of diphtheroid-like gram-positive rods in the cerebrospinal fluid smear of an 82-year-old patient is indicative of the presence of *Listeria monocytogenes.* In addition to their role as a potential causative agent in neonatal meningitis, listeria infections are more common in elderly patients and in those who have been treated with immunosuppressive agents. Treatment consists of ampicillin with or without gentamicin. Resistant strains are rare. The answer is **(A).**

11. No currently available cephalosporin agents have activity against MRSA strains, and they are not drugs of choice in community-acquired pneumonia. The second-generation drugs cefotetan and cefoxitin have activity against anaerobes. Cephalosporins containing the methylthiotetrazole ring (cefotetan, cefoperazone, moxalactam) may cause hypoprothrombinemia and disulfiram-like interactions with ethanol. The answer is **(E).**

12. In patients who have had a severe reaction to a penicillin, it is inadvisable to administer a cephalosporin or a carbapenem such as meropenem. Aztreonam has no significant activity against gram-positive cocci, so the logical treatment in this case is vancomycin, often with an aminoglycoside for synergistic activity against enterococci. The answer is **(E).**

13. Several drugs listed have activity against strains of *Pseudomonas aeruginosa,* including aztreonam, imipenem, and piperacillin. When any of these drugs are used as sole agents in pseudomonal infections resistance can emerge rapidly. However, aztreonam is quite safe in patients with established allergy to the penicillins. Piperacillin (not imipenem) has greater activity against beta-lactamase producing gram-negative rods when used with tazobactam. The answer is **(D).**

14. Vancomycin is bactericidal. It acts at an early stage in cell wall synthesis and does not bind to PBPs. It is not absorbed following oral administration and is used by this route in the treatment of colitis caused by *Clostridium difficile* and staphylococci. Vancomycin is not susceptible to beta-lactamases since it is not a beta-lactam. Vancomycin continues to have useful activity against strains of methicillin-resistant staphylococci. The answer is **(C).**

15. Ampicillin disturbs normal microflora and may cause yeast infections and also colitis due to staphylococcal or clostridial species. Maculopapular rashes occur quite frequently during use of ampicillin, especially if the drug is administered to patients with viral infections. Sulbactam (a penicillinase inhibitor) enhances activity, but no penicillin has activity against MRSA strains. The answer is **(D).**

16. Chemoprophylaxis is indicated when the wound infection rate for surgical procedures, under optimal conditions, is 5% or more. This patient had been treated for cancer, possibly with immunosuppressive agents, and may have been at enhanced risk for infection. The cephalosporins are the most frequently used antimicrobial agents for surgical prophylaxis because they have activity against gram-positive cocci and selected gram-negative bacilli that are likely pathogens.

17. The patient experienced a classic type I (immediate) IgE-mediated allergic reaction, which often includes anaphylaxis, urticaria, and angioedema. Antimicrobial drugs—particularly the beta-lactams and sulfonamides—can cause type I reactions. The degree of cross-allergenicity between penicillins and cephalosporins is probably less than 10%. Skin testing with a dilute solution of drug may reveal drug sensitivity but often gives false-negative results.

18. Epinephrine and isoproterenol (via cAMP mechanisms) and theophylline (via cAMP or block of adenosine receptors) inhibit the release of mediators from mast cells and basophils and cause bronchodilation. Diphenhydramine competitively blocks histamine actions at H_1 receptors, actions that would otherwise cause bronchoconstriction and increased capillary permeability. Dexamethasone has multiple cellular effects, including inhibition of IgE-producing clone proliferation, block of T helper cell function, and anti-inflammatory actions. Most of the actions of glucocorticoids result from decreases in the synthesis of cytokines (eg, interleukins, platelet activating factor) or eicosanoids (leukotrienes, prostaglandins).

Chloramphenicol, Tetracyclines, Macrolides, Clindamycin, Streptogramins, & Linezolid

44

OBJECTIVES

You should be able to:

- Describe the mechanisms of action of these inhibitors of bacterial protein synthesis.
- Describe the mechanisms responsible for clinical bacterial resistance to these drugs.
- List the major clinical uses of these drugs.
- Describe the pharmacokinetic features of these agents that are most relevant to their clinical use.
- List the main toxic effects of these drugs

CONCEPTS

The antimicrobial drugs reviewed in this chapter (Figure 44–1) selectively inhibit bacterial protein synthesis. The mechanisms of protein synthesis in microorganisms are not identical to those of mammalian cells. Bacteria have 70S ribosomes, whereas mammalian cells have 80S ribosomes. Differences exist in ribosomal subunits and in the chemical composition and functional specificities of component nucleic acids and proteins. Such differences form the basis for the selective toxicity of these drugs against microorganisms without causing major effects on protein synthesis in mammalian cells.

Chloramphenicol and the tetracyclines were among the first inhibitors of bacterial protein synthesis to be discovered. Because they had a broad spectrum of antibacterial activity and were thought to have low toxicities, they were overused. Many once highly susceptible bacterial species have become resistant, and these drugs are now used for more selected targets. Erythromycin, a macrolide antibiotic, has a narrower spectrum of action but continues to be active against several important pathogens. Azithromycin and clarithromycin are semisynthetic macrolides with some distinctive properties compared with erythromycin. Newer drugs (eg, streptogramins, linezolid) have activity against certain gram-positive bacteria that have developed resistance to older antibiotics.

MECHANISMS OF ACTION

All of the older antibiotics reviewed in this chapter are bacteriostatic inhibitors of protein synthesis acting at the ribosomal level (Figure 44–2). The binding sites for chloramphenicol, macrolides, and

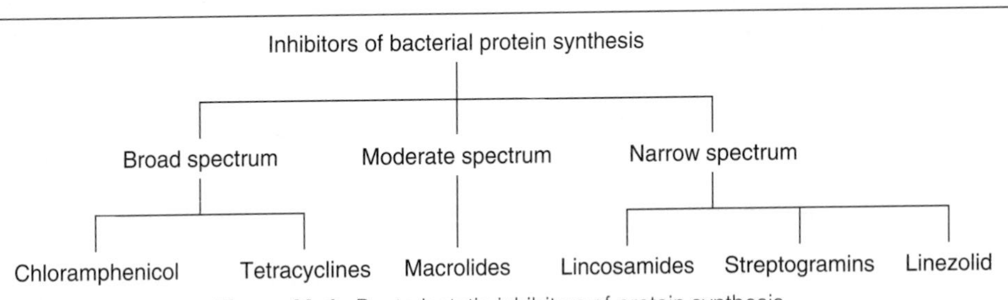

Figure 44–1. Bacteriostatic inhibitors of protein synthesis.

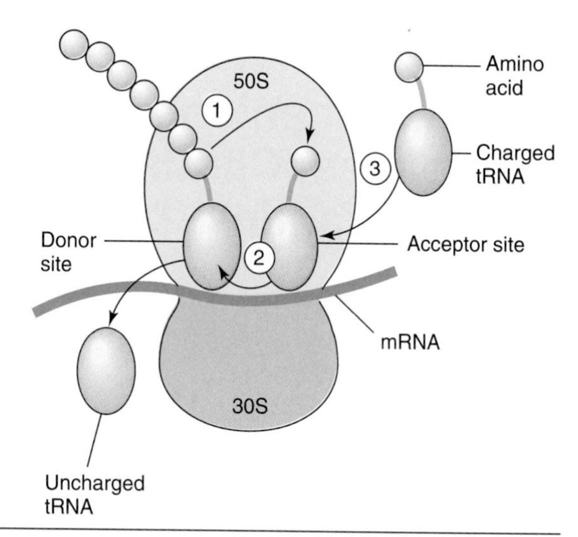

Figure 44–2. Steps in protein synthesis and sites of action of (1) chloramphenicol; (2) macrolides and clindamycin; and (3) tetracyclines. The 70S ribosomal mRNA complex is shown with its 50S and 30S subunits. The peptidyl-tRNA at the donor site donates the growing peptide chain to the aminoacyl-tRNA at the acceptor site in a reaction catalyzed by peptidyl transferase. The tRNA, discharged of its peptide, is released from the donor site to make way for translocation of the newly formed peptidyl-tRNA. The acceptor site is then free to be occupied by the next "charged" aminoacyl-tRNA. See text for additional details. (Reproduced, with permission, from Katzung BG [editor]: *Basic & Clinical Pharmacology,* 8th ed. McGraw-Hill, 2001.)

clindamycin are close to each other on the 50S ribosomal subunit. Chloramphenicol indirectly inhibits transpeptidation (catalyzed by peptidyl transferase) by blocking the binding of the aminoacyl moiety of the charged tRNA molecule to the acceptor site on the ribosome-mRNA complex. Thus, the peptide at the donor site cannot be transferred to its amino acid acceptor. Macrolides and clindamycin block translocation of peptidyl-tRNA from the acceptor site to the donor site. Incoming charged tRNA cannot access the occupied acceptor site, so the next amino acid cannot be added to the nascent peptide chain. Macrolides may also block formation of the initiation complex. Tetracyclines bind to the 30S ribosomal subunit at a site that blocks the binding of amino acid-charged tRNA to the acceptor site of the ribosome-mRNA complex.

Streptogramins are bactericidal for most susceptible organisms. They bind to the 50S ribosomal subunit, constricting the exit channel on the ribosome through which nascent polypeptides are extruded. In addition, transfer RNA (tRNA) synthetase activity is inhibited, leading to a decrease in free tRNA within the cell. Linezolid is mainly bacteriostatic. The drug binds to a unique site on the 50S subunit, inhibiting initiation by blocking formation of the tRNA-ribosome-mRNA ternary complex.

Selective toxicity of these protein synthesis inhibitors against microorganisms may be explained by target differences. Chloramphenicol does not bind to the 80S ribosomal RNA of mammalian cells, though it can inhibit the functions of *mitochondrial* ribosomes, which contain 70S ribosomal RNA. Tetracyclines have little effect on mammalian protein synthesis because an active efflux mechanism prevents their intracellular accumulation.

CHLORAMPHENICOL

A. Classification and Pharmacokinetics: Chloramphenicol has a simple and distinctive structure, and no other antimicrobials have been discovered in this chemical class. It is effective orally as well as parenterally and is distributed throughout all tissues; it readily crosses the placental and blood-brain barriers. The drug undergoes enterohepatic cycling, and a small fraction of the dose is excreted in the urine unchanged. Most of the drug is inactivated by a hepatic glucuronosyltransferase.

B. Antimicrobial Activity: Chloramphenicol has a wide spectrum of antimicrobial activity and is usually bacteriostatic. Some strains of *H influenzae, N meningitidis,* and bacteroides are highly susceptible, and for these organisms chloramphenicol may be bactericidal. It is not active against chlamydia. Resistance to chloramphenicol, which is plasmid-mediated, occurs through the formation of acetyltransferases that inactivate the drug.

C. Clinical Uses: Because of its toxicity, chloramphenicol has very few uses as a systemic drug. It is a backup drug for severe infections caused by salmonella and for the treatment of pneumococcal and meningococcal meningitis in beta-lactam-sensitive persons. Some *H influenzae* strains are resistant to chloramphenicol, and ceftriaxone or another third-generation cephalosporin is usually preferred. Chloramphenicol is sometimes used for rickettsial diseases and for infections caused by anaerobes such as *Bacteroides fragilis.* The drug is commonly used as a topical antimicrobial agent.

D. Toxicity:

1. **Gastrointestinal disturbances:** These may occur from direct irritation and from superinfections, especially candidiasis.
2. **Bone marrow:** Inhibition of red cell maturation leads to a decrease in circulating erythrocytes. This action is dose-dependent and reversible.
3. **Aplastic anemia:** This is a rare idiosyncratic reaction (approximately one case in 25,000–40,000 patients treated). It is usually irreversible and may be fatal.
4. **Gray baby syndrome:** This syndrome occurs in infants and is characterized by cyanosis and cardiovascular collapse. Neonates—especially premature neonates—are deficient in hepatic glucuronosyltransferase, the enzyme required for chloramphenicol elimination. They are therefore very sensitive to doses of this drug that would be tolerated in older infants.
5. **Drug interactions:** Chloramphenicol inhibits the metabolism of several drugs, including phenytoin, coumarins, and tolbutamide.

TETRACYCLINES

A. Classification: Drugs in this class are structural congeners that have a broad range of antimicrobial activity and only minor differences in their activities against specific organisms.

B. Pharmacokinetics: Oral absorption is variable, especially for the older drugs, and may be impaired by foods and multivalent cations (calcium, iron, aluminum). Tetracyclines have a wide tissue distribution and cross the placental barrier. All of the tetracyclines undergo enterohepatic cycling. Doxycycline is excreted mainly in feces; the other drugs are eliminated primarily in the urine. The half-lives of doxycycline and minocycline are longer than those of other tetracyclines.

C. Antibacterial Activity: Tetracyclines are broad-spectrum antibiotics with activity against gram-positive and gram-negative bacteria, rickettsia, chlamydia, mycoplasma, and some protozoa. Susceptible organisms accumulate tetracyclines intracellularly via energy-dependent transport systems in their cell membranes.

Plasmid-mediated resistance to tetracyclines is widespread. Tetracycline-resistant organisms show decreased intracellular accumulation of the drugs. Resistance mechanisms include decreased activity of the uptake systems and the development of mechanisms (efflux pumps) for active extrusion of tetracyclines. Plasmids that include genes involved in the production of efflux pumps for tetracyclines commonly include resistance genes for multiple antibiotics.

D. Clinical Uses:

1. **Primary uses:** Tetracyclines are drugs of first choice in the treatment of infections caused by *Mycoplasma pneumoniae* (in adults), chlamydia, rickettsia, and vibrios.
2. **Secondary uses:** Tetracyclines are alternative drugs in the treatment of syphilis. They are also used in the treatment of respiratory infections caused by susceptible organisms, for prophylaxis against infection in chronic bronchitis, in the treatment of leptospirosis, and in the treatment of acne.
3. **Selective uses:** Specific tetracyclines are used in the treatment of gastrointestinal ulcers caused by *Helicobacter pylori* (tetracycline), in Lyme disease (doxycycline), and in the meningococcal carrier state (minocycline). Doxycycline is also used for the prevention of malaria and in the treatment of amebiasis (Chapter 53). Demeclocycline inhibits the renal actions of ADH and is used in the management of patients with ADH-secreting tumors (Chapter 15).

E. Toxicity:

1. **Gastrointestinal disturbances:** Effects on the gastrointestinal system range from mild nausea and diarrhea to severe, possibly life-threatening colitis. Disturbances in the normal

flora lead to candidiasis (oral and vaginal) and, more rarely, to bacterial superinfections with *S aureus* or *Clostridium difficile.*

2. **Bony structures and teeth:** Fetal exposure to tetracyclines may lead to tooth enamel dysplasia and irregularities in bone growth. While contraindicated in pregnancy, there may be situations where the benefit of tetracyclines may outweigh the risk. Treatment of younger children may cause enamel dysplasia and crown deformation when permanent teeth appear.
3. **Hepatic toxicity:** High doses of tetracyclines, especially in pregnant patients or in patients with preexisting hepatic disease, may impair liver function and lead to hepatic necrosis.
4. **Renal toxicity:** One form of renal tubular acidosis, Fanconi's syndrome, has been attributed to use of outdated tetracyclines. Though not directly nephrotoxic, tetracyclines may exacerbate preexisting renal dysfunction.
5. **Photosensitivity:** Tetracyclines, especially demeclocycline, may cause enhanced skin sensitivity to ultraviolet light.
6. **Vestibular toxicity:** Dose-dependent reversible dizziness and vertigo have been reported with doxycycline and minocycline.

MACROLIDES

A. **Classification and Pharmacokinetics:** The macrolide antibiotics **(erythromycin, azithromycin,** and **clarithromycin)** are large cyclic lactone ring structures with attached sugars. The drugs have good oral bioavailability, but azithromycin absorption is impeded by food. Macrolides distribute to most body tissues, but azithromycin is unique in that the levels achieved in tissues and in phagocytes are considerably higher (tenfold to 100-fold) than those in the plasma. The elimination of erythromycin (via biliary excretion) and clarithromycin (via hepatic metabolism and urinary excretion of intact drug) is fairly rapid (half-life 2–5 hours). Azithromycin is eliminated slowly (half-life 2–4 days), mainly in the urine as unchanged drug.

B. **Antibacterial Activity:** Erythromycin has activity against many species of campylobacter, chlamydia, mycoplasma, legionella, gram-positive cocci, and some gram-negative organisms. The spectrums of activity of azithromycin and clarithromycin are similar but include greater activity against chlamydia, *M avium* complex, and toxoplasma.

Resistance to the macrolides in gram-positive organisms involves production of a methylase that adds a methyl group to the ribosomal binding site. Resistance in enterobacteria is the result of formation of drug-metabolizing esterases. Cross-resistance between the individual macrolides is complete.

C. **Clinical Uses:** Erythromycin is effective in the treatment of infections caused by *Mycoplasma pneumoniae,* corynebacterium, *Chlamydia trachomatis, Legionella pneumophila, Ureaplasma urealyticum,* and *Bordetella pertussis.* The drug is also active against gram-positive cocci, including pneumococci and beta-lactamase-producing staphylococci (but not MRSA strains).

Azithromycin has a similar spectrum of activity but is more active against *H influenzae, M catarrhalis,* and neisseria. Because of its long half-life, a single dose of azithromycin is effective in the treatment of urogenital infections due to *C trachomatis,* and a 4-day course of treatment has been effective in community-acquired pneumonia.

Clarithromycin is approved for prophylaxis against and treatment of *M avium* complex and as a component of drug regimens for ulcers due to *Helicobacter pylori.*

D. **Toxicity:** Adverse effects include gastrointestinal irritation (common), skin rashes, and eosinophilia. A hypersensitivity-based acute cholestatic hepatitis may occur with erythromycin estolate. Hepatitis is rare in children, but there is an increased risk with erythromycin estolate in the pregnant patient. Erythromycin inhibits several forms of hepatic cytochrome P450 and can increase the plasma levels of anticoagulants, carbamazepine, cisapride, digoxin, and theophylline. Cardiac arrhythmias occurred when erythromycin was administered to patients taking astemizole or terfenadine (the two antihistaminic drugs have been discontinued in the USA). Similar drug interactions have also occurred with clarithromycin. The lactone ring structure of azithromycin is slightly different from that of other macrolides, and drug interactions are uncommon since azithromycin does not inhibit hepatic cytochrome P450.

CLINDAMYCIN

A. Classification and Pharmacokinetics: The lincosamides **lincomycin** and **clindamycin** inhibit bacterial protein synthesis via a mechanism similar to that of the macrolides, though they are not chemically related. Mechanisms of resistance include methylation of the binding site on the 50S ribosomal subunit and enzymatic inactivation. Cross-resistance between lincosamides and macrolides is common. Good tissue penetration occurs after oral absorption. The lincosamides are eliminated partly by metabolism and partly by biliary and renal excretion.

B. Clinical Use and Toxicity: The main use of clindamycin is in the treatment of severe infections due to certain anaerobes such as bacteroides. Clindamycin has been used as a backup drug against gram-positive cocci and is currently recommended for prophylaxis of endocarditis in valvular disease patients who are penicillin-allergic. The drug is also active against *Pneumocystis carinii* and *Toxoplasma gondii.* The toxicity of clindamycin includes gastrointestinal irritation, skin rashes, neutropenia, hepatic dysfunction, and possible superinfections such as *C difficile* pseudomembranous colitis.

STREPTOGRAMINS

Quinupristin-dalfopristin, a combination of two streptogramins, is bactericidal (see Mechanism of Action, above) and has a duration of antibacterial activity longer than the half-lives of the two compounds (postantibiotic effects). Antibacterial activity includes penicillin-resistant pneumococci, methicillin-resistant (MRSA) and vancomycin-resistant staphylococci (VRSA), and resistant *Enterococcus faecium.* Administered intravenously, the combination product may cause pain and an arthralgia-myalgia syndrome. Streptogramins are potent inhibitors of CYP3A4 and increase plasma levels of many drugs, including cisapride, cyclosporine, diazepam, nonnucleoside reverse transcriptase inhibitors (NNRTIs), and warfarin.

LINEZOLID

The first of a new class of antibiotics (oxazolidinones), linezolid is active against many drug-resistant gram-positive cocci, including strains resistant to beta-lactams and vancomycin (eg, vancomycin-resistant *Enterococcus faecium*). Linezolid binds to a unique site on the 50S ribosomal subunit, and there is currently no cross-resistance with other protein synthesis inhibitors. Linezolid is available in both oral and parenteral formulations.

DRUG LIST

The following drugs are important members of the groups discussed in this chapter. Prototypes should be learned in detail; features of the major variants should be known well enough to distinguish the variants from the prototypes and from each other; the other significant agents should be recognized as belonging to a specific subclass.

Subclass	Prototype	Major Variants	Other Significant Agents
Chloramphenicol	Chloramphenicol		
Tetracyclines	Tetracycline	Demeclocycline	Doxycycline, minocycline
Macrolides	Erythromycin	Azithromycin	Clarithromycin
Lincosamides	Lincomycin	Clindamycin	
Streptogramins	Quinupristin-dalfopristin		
Oxazoladinones	Linezolid		

QUESTIONS

DIRECTIONS: Each of the numbered items or incomplete statements in this section is followed by answers or by completions of the statement. Select the ONE lettered answer or completion that is BEST in each case.

1. A 2-year-old child is brought to the hospital after ingesting pills that a parent had used for bacterial dysentery when traveling outside the United States. The child has been vomiting for over 24 hours, and has had diarrhea with green stools. He is now lethargic with an ashen color. Other signs and symptoms include hypothermia, hypotension, and abdominal distention. The drug most likely to be the cause of this problem is
(A) Ampicillin
(B) Chloramphenicol
(C) Clindamycin
(D) Doxycycline
(E) Erythromycin

2. The mechanism of antibacterial action of tetracyclines involves
(A) Binding to a component of the 50S ribosomal subunit
(B) Inhibition of translocase activity
(C) Blockade of binding of aminoacyl-tRNA to bacterial ribosomes
(D) Selective inhibition of ribosomal peptidyl transferases
(E) Inhibition of DNA-dependent RNA polymerase

3. A 24-year-old woman has primary syphilis. She has a history of penicillin hypersensitivity, so tetracycline will be used to treat the infection. Which one of the following statements about the proposed drug treatment of this patient is false?
(A) She will have to take the drug for 15 days
(B) She should avoid taking antacids at the same time as she takes the drug
(C) She may experience anorexia and gastrointestinal distress
(D) She should eat plenty of yogurt to prevent vaginal candidiasis
(E) She should call her physician if she develops severe diarrhea

4. Clarithromycin and erythromycin have very similar spectrums of antimicrobial activity. The major advantage of clarithromycin is that it
(A) Eradicates mycoplasmal infections in a single dose
(B) Is active against strains of streptococci that are resistant to erythromycin
(C) Is more active against *Mycobacterium avium* complex
(D) Does not inhibit liver drug-metabolizing enzymes
(E) Acts on methicillin-resistant strains of staphylococci

5. The primary mechanism underlying the resistance of gram-positive organisms to macrolide antibiotics is
(A) Methylation of binding sites on the 50S ribosomal subunit
(B) Formation of esterases that hydrolyze the lactone ring
(C) Increased activity of efflux mechanisms
(D) Formation of drug-inactivating acetyltransferases
(E) Decreased drug permeability of the cytoplasmic membrane

6. A 26-year-old female patient allergic to beta-lactams was treated for gonorrhea at a neighborhood clinic. A single intramuscular injection of spectinomycin was administered, and she was given a prescription for oral doxycycline for 7 days. Two weeks later she returns to the clinic with mucopurulent cervicitis. On questioning she admits that she did not have the prescription filled because she had no money. The best course of action at this point would be to
(A) Give her the money for the prescription
(B) Treat her with a single oral dose of cefixime
(C) Write a prescription for oral erythromycin for 7 days
(D) Treat her with a single oral dose of azithromycin
(E) Delay drug treatment until the infecting organism is identified

7. A 55-year-old patient with a prosthetic heart valve is to undergo a periodontal procedure involving scaling and root planing. Several years ago, the patient had a severe allergic reaction to procaine penicillin G. Regarding prophylaxis against bacterial endocarditis, which one of the following is most appropriate?
(A) No prophylaxis is needed since this patient is in the negligible risk category
(B) Give 600 mg of clindamycin orally 1 hour before the procedure

(C) Give 500 mg of erythromycin orally 1 hour before the procedure and 4 hours after the procedure
(D) Administer intravenous vancomycin prior to the procedure
(E) Give 2 g of amoxicillin orally 1 hour before the procedure

(Items 8–10:) A 24-year-old woman comes to clinic with complaints of dry cough, headache, fever, and malaise which have lasted 3 or 4 days. She appears to have some respiratory difficulty, and chest examination reveals rales but no other obvious signs of pulmonary involvement. However, extensive patchy infiltrates are seen on chest x-ray. Gram stain of expectorated sputum fails to reveal any bacterial pathogens. The patient informs the attending physician that her husband is not sick but that one of her colleagues at work has symptoms similar to those she is experiencing. The patient has no history of serious medical problems. She and her husband have no children and want to start a family when he finishes graduate school. The patient is taking loratadine for allergies, multivitamins, and supplementary iron tablets. She is an avid consumer of coffee and caffeinated beverages. The physician makes an initial diagnosis of community-acquired pneumonia.

8. Regarding the drug management of this patient, which one of the following statements is most accurate?
(A) No antibiotics should be given, since this patient has a viral pneumonia
(B) A single oral dose of clindamycin is indicated
(C) Amoxicillin should be given for 7 days
(D) She should be treated with erythromycin for 14 days
(E) A 7-day course of cefaclor is the best choice in this case

9. If this patient is treated with the macrolide, she should
(A) Temporarily discontinue the antihistamine to prevent cardiotoxicity
(B) Avoid exposure to sunlight
(C) Cut down her consumption of caffeinated beverages
(D) Avoid taking supplementary iron tablets
(E) Have her plasma urea nitrogen or creatinine checked prior to treatment

10. This patient is not an ideal candidate for treatment with tetracycline hydrochloride because
(A) It may cause vaginal candidiasis
(B) Her pulmonary infection may be due to pneumococci
(C) Tetracyclines inhibit hepatic cytochrome P450
(D) Tetracycline has no activity against *M pneumoniae*
(E) The drug causes a high incidence of vestibular dysfunction

11. The appearance of markedly vacuolated, nucleated red cells in the marrow, anemia, and reticulocytopenia are characteristic dose-dependent side effects of
(A) Azithromycin
(B) Chloramphenicol
(C) Clindamycin
(D) Doxycycline
(E) Linezolid

12. In a patient with culture-positive enterococcal endocarditis who has failed to respond to vancomycin because of resistance, the treatment most likely to be effective is
(A) Clarithromycin
(B) Erythromycin
(C) Linezolid
(D) Minocycline
(E) Ticarcillin

13. Which one of the following statements about doxycycline is false?
(A) It is bacteriostatic
(B) It is excreted mainly in the feces
(C) It has a long elimination half-life
(D) It is more active than tetracycline against *Helicobacter pylori*
(E) It is used in Lyme disease

14. Concerning streptogramins, which one of the following statements is false?
(A) They are active versus methicillin-resistant staphylococci
(B) They are excreted mainly in the feces
(C) They induce cytochrome P450
(D) They are associated with postantibiotic effects
(E) They are used in the management of infection with vancomycin-resistant enterococci

15. This inhibitor of bacterial protein synthesis has a narrow spectrum of antibacterial activity. It has been used in the management of abdominal abscess due to *Bacteroides fragilis,* but antibiotic-associated colitis has occurred.
    (A) Chloramphenicol
    (B) Clarithromycin
    (C) Clindamycin
    (D) Minocycline
    (E) Ticarcillin

DIRECTIONS (Items 16–19): This case history* is followed by discussion questions. Write out brief answers (two to five sentences) and then compare your answers with those given at the end of the Answers section.

A 10-year-old girl received erythromycin for a prolonged respiratory tract infection. She continued to have headaches and a stuffy nose; a facial x-ray suggested maxillary sinusitis, which could not be confirmed following sinus puncture. Erythromycin was stopped and she was given amoxicillin (250 mg three times a day) for 10 days.

On the last day of amoxicillin treatment, she developed diarrhea with some abdominal pain but no vomiting. Initially the stools were alternately watery and solid, but later they became mucoid with some blood. After 11 days of these symptoms, she was given loperamide for her diarrhea, and a stool culture was positive for Clostridium difficile.

She was hospitalized, and sigmoidoscopy revealed colitis with pseudomembranes, confirmed histologically. Stool culture was positive for C difficile *and negative for salmonella, shigella, yersinia, and campylobacter. The girl was treated with oral vancomycin, 250 mg four times daily for 7 days and was discharged following rectoscopic examination that proved normal and a negative* C difficile *stool culture.*

16. What was the rationale for the treatment of the upper respiratory tract infections with erythromycin?
17. Why was amoxicillin used to treat the suspected sinusitis?
18. What was the most likely cause of the diarrhea and the overgrowth of *C difficile* in the gastrointestinal tract?
19. Why was oral vancomycin used in this case? What alternative drug treatment should have been employed?

ANSWERS

1. Although the gray baby syndrome was initially described in neonates, a similar syndrome has occurred with overdosage of chloramphenicol in older children and adults, especially those with hepatic dysfunction. The answer is **(B).**
2. Tetracyclines inhibit bacterial protein synthesis by interfering with the binding of aminoacyl-tRNA molecules to bacterial ribosomes. Peptidyl transferase is inhibited by chloramphenicol. The answer is **(C).**
3. The ingestion of foods containing multivalent cations (yogurt contains calcium and magnesium) can interfere with gastrointestinal absorption of tetracyclines and impair their clinical efficacy. The answer is **(D).**
4. Clarithromycin can be administered less frequently than erythromycin, but it is not effective in single doses against susceptible organisms. Organisms resistant to erythromycin, including pneumococci and methicillin-resistant staphylococci, are also resistant to other macrolides. Drug interactions have occurred with clarithromycin through its ability to inhibit cytochrome P450. Clarithromycin is more active than erythromycin against *M avium* complex, *Toxoplasma gondii,* and *H pylori.* The answer is **(C).**
5. Methylase production and methylation of the receptor site accounts for the resistance of gram-positive organisms to macrolide antibiotics. Such enzymes may be inducible by macrolides or constitutive; in the latter case, cross-resistance occurs between macrolides and clindamycin.

* Adapted and reproduced, with permission, from Vesikari T et al: Pseudomembranous colitis with recurring diarrhea and prolonged persistence of *Clostridium difficile* in a 10-year-old girl. Acta Paediatr Scand 1984;73:135.

Esterase formation is a mechanism of macrolide resistance seen in coliforms. Resistance to tetracyclines occurs either from increased activity of efflux mechanisms or changes in cell membrane permeability, leading to decreases in intracellular levels of such drugs. Resistance to chloramphenicol involves plasmid-mediated formation of drug-inactivating acetyltransferases. The answer is **(A).**

6. Cervicitis or urethritis that appears 2–3 weeks after treatment of gonorrhea is often caused by *C trachomatis.* Such infections may have been acquired at the same time as gonorrhea but develop more slowly because of the long incubation period of chlamydial infection. Treatment with oral doxycycline for 7 days would have eradicated *C trachomatis* and most other organisms commonly associated with nongonococcal cervicitis or urethritis. Given the limited compliance of this patient, the best course of action would be the administration (in the clinic) of a single oral dose of azithromycin. In addition, she should encourage her sexual partner to come to the clinic for treatment. The answer is **(D).**

7. This patient is in the high-risk category for bacterial endocarditis and should receive prophylactic antibiotics prior to many dental procedures, including root planing and extractions. The American Heart Association now recommends that clindamycin be used in patients allergic to penicillins. Oral erythromycin is not recommended since it is no more effective than clindamycin and causes more gastrointestinal side effects. Intravenous vancomycin, sometimes with gentamicin, is recommended for prophylaxis in high-risk penicillin-allergic patients undergoing genitourinary and lower gastrointestinal surgical procedures. Complete cross-allergenicity must be assumed between individual penicillins. The answer is **(B).**

8. It is often difficult to establish a definite etiology of pneumonia. The most common pathogens involved in community-acquired pneumonia in an otherwise healthy young adult are *Streptococcus pneumoniae, Mycoplasma pneumoniae,* respiratory viruses, and *Chlamydia pneumoniae.* Empiric antibiotic therapy is initiated in most cases because the physical signs and a Gram stain of sputum do not often indicate a specific etiologic agent. A gradual onset of the condition, with many extrapulmonary symptoms, may be indicative of an atypical pneumonia but does not rule out a bacterial etiology. Erythromycin would provide coverage for both pneumococcal and atypical pathogens (not viral) and should be given for 10–14 days. None of the other antibiotics listed are active against chlamydial or mycoplasmal pathogens. The answer is **(D).**

9. The inhibition of liver cytochrome P450 by erythromycin has led to serious drug interactions. Inhibition of the CYP3A4 isoform of the enzyme has resulted in cardiac arrhythmias with the nonsedating antihistamines astemizole and terfenadine but not with loratadine. However, erythromycin also inhibits the CYP1A2 form of cytochrome P450, which metabolizes methylxanthines. Consequently, cardiac and CNS toxicity may occur with excessive ingestion of caffeine. Unlike the tetracyclines, the oral absorption of erythromycin is not affected by cations and the drug does not cause photosensitivity. Since erythromycin undergoes biliary excretion, there is little reason to assess renal function prior to treatment. The answer is **(C).**

10. Tetracyclines have activity against both chlamydial and mycoplasmal pathogens involved in community-acquired pneumonia. However, their widespread use for minor infections has led to emergence of resistant strains of gram-positive cocci, including *Streptococcus pneumoniae.* Consequently, tetracycline does not provide antibacterial coverage equivalent to that of erythromycin when used empirically in pneumonia. Alterations in normal flora caused by tetracyclines may lead to oral or vaginal candidiasis, but this is not the primary reason why erythromycin is the treatment of choice. The tetracyclines do not inhibit liver drug-metabolizing enzymes. Tetracycline does not cause vestibular dysfunction. The answer is **(B).**

11. Reversible, dose-dependent bone marrow maturation arrest occurs with chloramphenicol. Serum iron concentration increases and blood levels of phenylalanine decrease. These actions are unrelated to the rare occurrence of aplastic anemia. The answer is **(B).**

12. Linezolid is approved for use in vancomycin-resistant enterococcal infections. There are very few alternatives available, and none of the other drugs listed are likely to be effective. The answer is **(C).**

13. The false statement about doxycycline concerns activity against *Helicobacter pylori.* Doxycycline is not more active than tetracycline against this organism and has not been used in any of the proposed regimens that include antimicrobial agents in management of gastrointestinal ulcers thought to be associated with *Helicobacter pylori.* Doxycycline has good bioavailability, effective tissue penetration, and a long half-life. Doxycycline is also more effective against pathogens associated with acute exacerbations of chronic bronchitis (pneumococci, *H influenzae, M catarrhalis*) and has better activity in Lyme disease than other tetracyclines. The answer is **(D).**

14. The combination of quinupristin-dalfopristin is bactericidal against many drug-resistant gram-positive cocci, including MRSA and vancomycin-resistant enterococci (VRE). The drugs are potent *inhibitors* of CYP3A4 and interfere with the metabolism of many other drugs. The answer is **(C).**

15. Of the drugs listed, only chloramphenicol, clindamycin, and ticarcillin (with clavulanic acid) are reliably active against *B fragilis.* Chloramphenicol is a broad-spectrum antibiotic, and ticarcillin inhibits bacterial cell wall synthesis. The answer is **(C).**

16. There is no information in the history of the original upper respiratory tract infection regarding possible or confirmed pathogens or their susceptibility to antimicrobial drugs. Erythromycin has activity against common streptococci, staphylococci (including penicillinase-producing strains), and *Mycoplasma pneumoniae;* this presumably underlies the choice of the drug in this case. Erythromycin may cause gastrointestinal irritation, occasional cholestasis (rare in children), and drug interactions via its inhibition of hepatic cytochrome P450. There is no cross-allergenicity with the penicillin group.

17. The suspected sinusitis had not responded to erythromycin. Since attempts to confirm bacterial infection had failed, amoxicillin therapy was started on empiric grounds. Amoxicillin has activity against many streptococci and some *H influenzae* strains as well as selected gram-negative rods. The drug is not active against penicillinase-producing organisms or *M pneumoniae.* However, these organisms should have been eradicated by the prior treatment with erythromycin.

18. Ampicillin is more likely to cause diarrhea than most other penicillins, partly by direct gastrointestinal irritation and partly by disturbing the normal gut flora. In this case, its close congener, amoxicillin, resulted in diarrhea that persisted more than a week after drug discontinuance, suggesting the possibility of microbial superinfection. This was confirmed by culture of *Clostridium difficile.* This organism causes colitis following therapy with a variety of antibiotics, including clindamycin, the tetracyclines, and beta-lactam agents.

19. When given orally, vancomycin has been effective in the treatment of colitis caused by toxin-producing bacteria, including *C difficile.* However, most infectious disease specialists advocate treatment of pseudomembranous colitis with metronidazole. Oral metronidazole is equally effective, and the cost of treatment is only one-third that of vancomycin. Most importantly, because of the increasing incidence of vancomycin-resistant enterococci and staphylococci, this drug should not be used if an alternative agent is readily available.

45 Aminoglycosides

OBJECTIVES

You should be able to:

- Describe the mechanisms of action of aminoglycoside antibiotics and the mechanisms by which bacterial resistance to this class of drugs occurs.
- List the major clinical applications of aminoglycosides and describe their main toxic effects.
- Describe the pharmacokinetics of this drug class, with special reference to the importance of renal clearance and its relationship to toxicity.

- Understand the concepts of time-dependent and concentration-dependent killing actions of antibiotics and know what is meant by the postantibiotic effect.
- Describe the adverse effects of aminoglycosides

CONCEPTS

A. **Modes of Antibacterial Action:** In the treatment of microbial infections with antibiotics, multiple daily dosage regimens traditionally have been designed to maintain serum concentrations above the minimal inhibitory concentration (MIC) for as long as possible. However, the in vivo effectiveness of some antibiotics, including aminoglycosides, results from a **concentration-dependent** killing action. As the plasma level is increased above the MIC, aminoglycosides kill an increasing proportion of bacteria and do so at a more rapid rate. Other antibiotics, including penicillins and cephalosporins, cause **time-dependent** killing of microorganisms, wherein their in vivo efficacy is directly related to time above MIC and becomes independent of concentration once the MIC has been reached.

Aminoglycosides are also capable of exerting a **postantibiotic effect** such that their killing action continues when their plasma levels have declined below measurable levels. Consequently, aminoglycosides have greater efficacy when administered as a single large dose than when given as multiple smaller doses. The toxicity (in contrast to the antibacterial efficacy) of aminoglycosides depends both on a critical plasma concentration and on the time that such a level is exceeded. The time above such a threshold will be shorter with administration of a single large dose of an aminoglycoside than when multiple smaller doses are given. These concepts form the basis for once-daily aminoglycoside dosing protocols, which can be more effective and less toxic than traditional dosing regimens.

B. **Classification:** The drugs in this class are structurally related amino sugars attached by glycosidic linkages. The main differences among the individual drugs lie in their activities against specific organisms, particularly gram-negative rods.

C. **Pharmacokinetics:** Aminoglycosides are polar compounds and are not absorbed after oral administration. They must be given parenterally for systemic effect and have limited tissue penetration. Glomerular filtration is the major mode of excretion, and plasma levels of these drugs are greatly affected by changes in renal function. Excretion of aminoglycosides is directly proportionate to creatinine clearance, and dosage adjustments must be made in renal insufficiency to avoid toxic accumulation. Monitoring of plasma levels of aminoglycosides can be valuable for safe and effective dosage selection and adjustment. For traditional dosing regimens (two or three times daily), peak serum levels are measured 30–60 minutes after administration and trough levels just before the next dose.

D. **Mechanism of Action:** Aminoglycosides are bactericidal inhibitors of protein synthesis. Their penetration through the bacterial cell envelope is partly dependent on oxygen-dependent active transport, and they have little activity against strict anaerobes. Aminoglycoside transport can be enhanced by cell wall synthesis inhibitors, which may be the basis of antimicrobial synergism. Inside the cell, aminoglycosides bind to the 30S ribosomal subunit and interfere with protein synthesis in at least three ways: (1) they block formation of the initiation complex; (2) they cause misreading of the code on the mRNA template; and (3) they inhibit translocation (Figure 45–1). Aminoglycosides may also disrupt polysomal structure, resulting in nonfunctional monosomes.

E. **Mechanism of Resistance:** The primary mechanism of resistance to aminoglycosides involves the plasmid-mediated formation of inactivating enzymes. These enzymes are **group transferases** that catalyze the acetylation of amine functions and the transfer of phosphoryl or adenylyl groups to the oxygen atoms of hydroxyl groups on the aminoglycoside. Individual aminoglycosides have varying susceptibilities to such enzymes. Currently, **netilmicin** is susceptible to only a few such enzymes, and the drug may be active against more strains of organisms than other aminoglycosides.

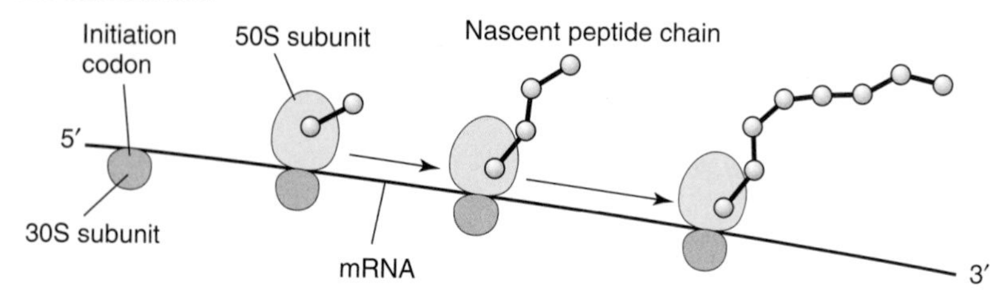

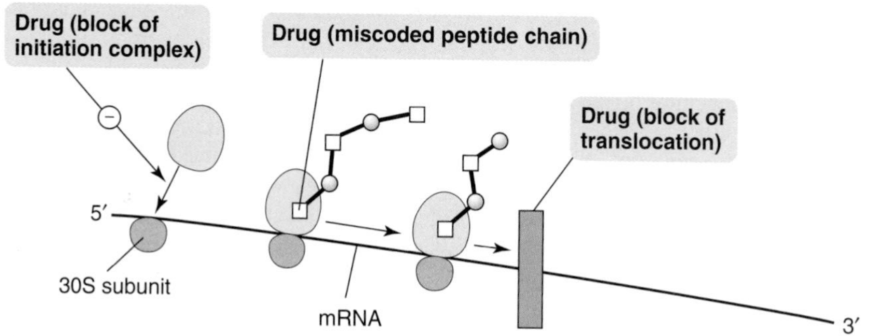

Figure 45–1. Putative mechanisms of action of the aminoglycosides. Normal protein synthesis is shown in the top panel. At least three different aminoglycoside effects have been described, as shown in the bottom panel: block of formation of the initiation complex; miscoding of amino acids in the emerging peptide chain due to misreading of the mRNA; and block of translocation on mRNA. Block of movement of the ribosome may occur after the formation of a single initiation complex, resulting in an mRNA chain with only a single ribosome on it, a so-called monosome.

F. Clinical Uses:

1. **Primary uses:** Three aminoglycosides (gentamicin, tobramycin, amikacin) are important drugs for the treatment of serious infections caused by aerobic gram-negative bacteria, including *E coli* and enterobacter, klebsiella, proteus, pseudomonas, and serratia species (Table 45–1). Drug choice depends on susceptibility patterns. Antibacterial synergy may occur when aminoglycosides are used in combination with beta-lactam antibiotics. Examples include their combined use in the treatment of serious pseudomonal and enterococcal infections.
2. **Other indications:**
   a. **Streptomycin:** Streptomycin is used in the treatment of tuberculosis, plague, and tularemia. Because of the risk of ototoxicity, streptomycin should not be used when other drugs will serve.
   b. **Neomycin:** Owing to its toxic potential, neomycin is only used topically or locally, eg, in the gastrointestinal tract.
   c. **Netilmicin:** Usually reserved for treatment of serious infections caused by organisms resistant to the other aminoglycosides.

Table 45–1. Clinical applications of the aminoglycosides.

Drug	Application
Gentamicin, amikacin, tobramycin, netilmicin	Serious infections with aerobic gram-negative bacteria, including *E coli,* and enterobacter, klebsiella, proteus, pseudomonas, and serratia
Streptomycin	Tuberculosis; rarely plague, brucellosis, tularemia, and infective endocarditis
Neomycin, kanamycin	Bowel sterilization, skin infections
Spectinomycin	Gonorrhea

d. **Spectinomycin:** Spectinomycin is an aminocyclitol related to the aminoglycosides. It is a backup drug, administered intramuscularly as a single dose for the treatment of gonorrhea.

G. **Toxicity:**

1. **Ototoxicity:** Auditory or vestibular damage (or both) may occur with any aminoglycoside and may be irreversible. Auditory impairment is more likely with amikacin and kanamycin; vestibular dysfunction is more likely with gentamicin and tobramycin. Ototoxicity risk is proportionate to the plasma levels and thus is especially high if dosage is not appropriately modified in a patient with renal dysfunction. Ototoxicity may be increased by the use of loop diuretics. Since ototoxicity has been reported following fetal exposure, the aminoglycosides are contraindicated in pregnancy unless their potential benefits are judged to outweigh risk.
2. **Nephrotoxicity:** Renal toxicity usually takes the form of acute tubular necrosis. This adverse effect, which is often reversible, is more common in elderly patients and in those concurrently receiving amphotericin B, cephalosporins, or vancomycin. Gentamicin and tobramycin are the most nephrotoxic.
3. **Neuromuscular blockade:** Though rare, a curare-like block may occur at high doses of aminoglycosides and may result in respiratory paralysis. It is usually reversible by treatment with calcium and neostigmine, but ventilatory support may be required.
4. **Skin reactions:** Allergic skin reactions may occur in patients, and contact dermatitis may occur in personnel handling the drug. Neomycin is the agent most likely to cause this adverse effect.

Skill Keeper: Nephrotoxicity

One of the characteristics of aminoglycoside antibiotics is their nephrotoxic potential. What other drugs can you identify that are known to have adverse effects on renal function? *The Skill Keeper Answer appears at the end of the chapter.*

DRUG LIST

The following drugs are important members of the group discussed in this chapter. Prototypes should be learned in detail; features of the major variants should be known well enough to distinguish the variants from the prototypes and from each other; the other significant agents should be recognized as belonging to a specific subclass.

Subclass	Prototype	Major Variants	Other Significant Agents
Aminoglycosides Systemic	Gentamicin	Tobramycin	Amikacin, netilmicin, streptomycin
Local	Neomycin		Gentamicin, kanamycin
Aminocyclitols	Spectinomycin		

QUESTIONS

DIRECTIONS: Each of the numbered items or incomplete statements in this section is followed by answers or by completions of the statement. Select the ONE lettered answer or completion that is BEST in each case.

1. Which one of the following statements about the mechanism of action of aminoglycosides is false?
   (A) They induce misreading of the code on the mRNA template
   (B) They promote polysome instability

(C) They inhibit peptidyl transferase
(D) They block the formation of the initiation complex
(E) They are bactericidal inhibitors of protein synthesis

2. A 70-kg patient with creatinine clearance of greater than 90 mL/min has a gram-negative infection. Amikacin is administered intramuscularly at a dose of 5 mg/kg every 8 hours, and the patient begins to respond. After 2 days, creatinine clearance declines to 30 mL/min. Assuming that no information is available about amikacin plasma levels, what would be the most reasonable approach to management of the patient at this point?
   (A) Decrease the daily dose to a total of 100 mg
   (B) Decrease the dosage to 120 mg every 8 hours
   (C) Maintain the patient on the present dosage and test auditory function
   (D) Administer 5 mg/kg every 12 hours
   (E) Discontinue amikacin and switch to gentamicin
3. Which one of the following statements about the clinical uses of the aminoglycosides is false?
   (A) Owing to their polar nature, aminoglycosides are not absorbed following oral administration
   (B) Aminoglycosides are often used in combination with cephalosporins in the empiric treatment of life-threatening bacterial infections
   (C) Netilmycin is more likely to be effective than streptomycin in the treatment of a hospital-acquired infection caused by *Serratia marcescens*
   (D) The spectrum of antimicrobial activity of aminoglycosides includes *Bacteroides fragilis*
   (E) Gentamicin is used with ampicillin for synergistic effects in the treatment of enterococcal endocarditis
4. Which one of the following statements about bacterial resistance to aminoglycosides is most accurate?
   (A) Resistance is due to the production of peptidyl transferases
   (B) Bacteria resistant to aminoglycosides have characteristic alterations in the pathway of folic acid synthesis
   (C) Emergence of resistance during the course of drug treatment is common
   (D) Clinical resistance mainly occurs through plasmid-mediated formation of group transferase enzymes
   (E) Staphylococci resistant to methicillin (MRSA) are usually sensitive to aminoglycosides
5. Which one of the following antibiotics is likely to be the MOST effective agent in the treatment of an infection due to enterococci if used in conjunction with penicillin G?
   (A) Amikacin
   (B) Gentamicin
   (C) Netilmicin
   (D) Streptomycin
   (E) Tobramycin
6. Regarding the antibacterial action of gentamicin, which one of the following statements is most accurate?
   (A) Efficacy is directly proportionate to the time that the plasma level of the drug is greater than the minimal inhibitory concentration
   (B) The antibacterial action of gentamicin is not concentration-dependent
   (C) Gentamicin continues to exert antibacterial effects even after plasma levels decrease below detectable levels
   (D) Antibacterial activity is often reduced by the presence of an inhibitor of cell wall synthesis
   (E) The antibacterial action of gentamicin is time-dependent
7. An adult patient (weight 70 kg) has bacteremia suspected to be due to a gram-negative rod. Tobramycin is to be administered using a once-daily dosing regimen, and the loading dose must be calculated to achieve a peak plasma level of 20 mg/L. Assume that the patient has normal renal function. Pharmacokinetic parameters of tobramycin in this patient are: V_d = 20 L; $t_{1/2}$ = 3 hours; and CL = 80 mL/min. What loading dose should be given?
   (A) 100 mg
   (B) 200 mg
   (C) 300 mg
   (D) 400 mg
   (E) 800 mg

8. Which one of the following drugs is most likely to be effective against multidrug-resistant strains of *M tuberculosis,* including those resistant to streptomycin?
 (A) Amikacin
 (B) Clarithromycin
 (C) Gentamicin
 (D) Meropenem
 (E) Spectinomycin

9. A 57-year-old man is seen in a hospital emergency room complaining of pain in and behind the right ear. Physical examination shows edema of the external otic canal with purulent exudate and weakness of the muscles on the right side of the face. There are no obvious signs of systemic infection. The patient informs the physician that he is a diabetic, taking glipizide daily but no insulin. He is also taking a "baby" aspirin daily but no other drugs. Gram stain of the exudate from the ear shows many polymorphonucleocytes and gram-negative rods. Samples of the exudate are sent to the microbiology laboratory for culture and drug susceptibilty testing. A preliminary diagnosis is made of external otitis. At this point, which of the following is most appropriate?
 (A) Analgesics should be prescribed for pain, but antibiotics should be withheld pending the results of cultures
 (B) The patient should be sent home with a prescription for oral cefaclor
 (C) The patient should be hospitalized and treatment started with gentamicin plus ticarcillin
 (D) The patient should be hospitalized and treatment started with intravenous imipenem-cilastatin
 (E) The patient should be hospitalized and treatment started with spectinomycin

10. Regarding the toxicity of gentamicin, which one of the following statements is most accurate?
 (A) Ototoxicity is reduced if loop diuretics are used to facilitate gentamicin excretion
 (B) Systemic neomycin is usually safer than gentamicin
 (C) Gentamicin is more likely to cause ototoxic effects than renal damage
 (D) With traditional dosage regimens, the earliest sign of nephrotoxicity is a reduced creatinine clearance
 (E) Ototoxicity due to gentamicin is usually irreversible and manifests itself as vestibular dysfunction

11. Which one of the following statements about neomycin is accurate?
 (A) Adjunctive use in treatment of tuberculosis
 (B) Drug of choice in Rocky Mountain spotted fever
 (C) Least nephrotoxic aminoglycoside
 (D) Metabolized by hepatic enzymes
 (E) Used in hepatic coma

12. Streptomycin has no useful activity in the treatment of
 (A) Bubonic plague
 (B) Brucellosis
 (C) Lyme disease
 (D) Tuberculosis
 (E) Tularemia

13. This drug has a spectrum of activity and pharmacokinetic properties almost identical to those of gentamicin. However, the drug in question shows poor activity in combination with penicillin against enterococci.
 (A) Amikacin
 (B) Erythromycin
 (C) Netilmycin
 (D) Spectinomycin
 (E) Tobramycin

14. Your 23-year-old female patient is pregnant and has gonorrhea. The past medical history includes anaphylaxis following exposure to amoxicillin. Worried about compliance, you would like to treat this patient with a single dose, so you choose
 (A) Cefixime
 (B) Ceftriaxone
 (C) Ciprofloxacin
 (D) Spectinomycin
 (E) Tetracycline

15. In the empiric treatment of severe bacterial infections of unidentified etiology, this drug, often used in combination with an aminoglycoside, provides coverage against many staphylococci
    (A) Amoxicillin
    (B) Clavulanic acid
    (C) Erythromycin
    (D) Nafcillin
    (E) Tetracycline
16. Which one of the following statements about "once daily" dosing with aminoglycosides is false?
    (A) It is convenient for outpatient therapy
    (B) Adjustment of dosage is less important in renal insufficiency
    (C) Less nursing time is required
    (D) It is often less toxic than conventional (multiple) dosing regimens
    (E) Under-dosing is less of a problem

DIRECTIONS (Items 17–20): This case history is followed by discussion questions. Write out brief answers (two to five sentences) and then compare your answers with those given at the end of the Answers section.

A 28-year-old male intravenous drug abuser comes to the emergency room complaining of fever, chills, and palpitations that have lasted for over 6 hours. He states that he last used IV heroin 24 hours prior to seeking medical attention. Physical examination reveals a disheveled male with multiple tattoos who is hyperthermic and sweating profusely. The pulse is 120/min and blood pressure is 100/50 mm Hg. Lungs and pharynx are clear. A right-sided 2/6 diastolic rumble is detected on cardiovascular examination; fingernail examination reveals no splinter hemorrhages (no emboli). Pertinent laboratory values are WBC 18,000/μL, creatinine 1.1 mg/dL. Blood samples are sent to the microbiology laboratory for culture. A preliminary diagnosis is made of bacterial endocarditis, right-sided as anticipated in an intravenous drug abuser. The patient is hospitalized and treated empirically with antibiotics. The most likely infecting organism in this patient is Staphylococcus aureus, *but antibiotic coverage is advisable for streptococci, enterococci, and possibly gram-negative bacteria such as* Pseudomonas aeruginosa.

17. What antibiotic regimen is appropriate for the presumptive treatment of bacterial endocarditis in this patient?
18. If this patient is allergic to beta-lactam antibiotics, what alternative antibiotic regimen is suitable?
19. How will you monitor therapy?
20. What newer antibiotics may be useful if this infection was due to a staphylococcal strain resistant to conventional antibiotics?

ANSWERS

1. Aminoglycosides are bactericidal inhibitors of protein synthesis binding to specific components of the 30S ribosomal subunit. Their actions include block of the formation of the initiation complex, miscoding, and polysomal break-up. Peptidyl transferase is inhibited by chloramphenicol, not aminoglycosides. The answer is **(C)**.
2. Monitoring plasma drug levels is important when aminoglycosides are used. In this case the patient seems to be improving, so a decrease of the amikacin dose in proportion to decreased creatinine clearance is most appropriate. Since creatinine clearance is only one-third of the starting value, a dose reduction should be made to one-third of that given initially. The answer is **(B)**.
3. The intracellular accumulation of aminoglycoside by bacteria is oxygen-dependent. Anaerobic bacteria are inherently resistant. The answer is **(D)**.
4. Clinical resistance to aminoglycosides results from the formation of drug-metabolizing transferases. The emergence of resistance during drug treatment is rare. Aminoglycosides are not active against staphylococci resistant to methicillin. The answer is **(D)**.
5. When used in combination with penicillin G, streptomycin continues to be a useful agent for treating enterococcal infections. About 15% of enterococcal isolates that are resistant to gen-

tamicin and the other systemic aminoglycosides remain susceptible to streptomycin. The answer is **(D)**.

6. The antibacterial action of aminoglycosides is concentration-dependent rather than time-dependent. The activity of the drug continues to increase as its plasma level rises above the minimal inhibitory concentration (MIC). When the plasma level of gentamicin falls below the MIC, the drug continues to exert antibacterial effects for several hours, exerting a postantibiotic effect. Inhibitors of bacterial cell wall synthesis often exert synergistic effects with aminoglycosides, possibly by increasing the intracellular accumulation of the aminoglycoside. The answer is **(C)**.
7. The loading dose of any drug is calculated by multiplying the desired plasma concentration (mg/L) by the volume of distribution (L). The answer is **(D)**.
8. Strains of multidrug-resistant *M tuberculosis* resistant to streptomycin are usually susceptible to amikacin. None of the other drugs listed (including gentamicin) have significant antitubercular activity. In the treatment of tuberculosis, amikacin and streptomycin are backup drugs and if used are always used in combination regimens with other antitubercular agents. The answer is **(A)**.
9. The diabetic patient with external otitis is at special risk because of the danger of spread to the middle ear and possibly the meninges, so hospitalization is advisable. Based on the Gram stain, the likely pathogens include *E coli* and *Pseudomonas aeruginosa,* and coverage must be provided for these and possibly other gram-negative rods. The combination of an aminoglycoside plus a wider-spectrum penicillin is most suitable in this case and is synergistic against many pseudomonas strains. Imipenem-cilastatin is also possible, but resistant strains of *Pseudomonas aeruginosa* have emerged during treatment. Cefaclor is used for otitis media in ambulatory patients but lacks antipseudomonal activity. The answer is **(C)**.
10. The incidence of nephrotoxic effects with gentamicin is two to three times greater than the incidence of ototoxicity. With traditional dosage regimens, the first indication of potential nephrotoxicity is an increase in trough serum levels of aminoglycosides, which is followed by an increase in blood creatinine. While ototoxicity due to gentamicin usually involves irreversible effects on vestibular function, hearing loss can also occur. Ototoxicity is enhanced by loop diuretics. The answer is **(E)**.
11. When used parenterally, neomycin causes renal damage and ototoxicity. It is used topically and for local actions, including gastrointestinal tract infections and sterilization prior to bowel surgery. In hepatic coma, neomycin is used (with decreased protein intake) to suppress coliform bacteria, thus reducing ammonia intoxication. The answer is **(E)**.
12. Streptomycin is the drug of choice for treatment of plague and tularemia and has important adjunctive value in tuberculosis. Gentamicin (plus tetracycline) is usually preferred in brucellosis, but streptomycin is a backup drug. Aminoglycosides have minimal activity in Lyme disease, which is usually treated with either doxycycline or amoxicillin. The answer is **(C)**.
13. Tobramycin is almost identical to gentamicin in both its pharmacodynamic and pharmacokinetic properties. However, it is much less active than either gentamicin or streptomycin when used in combination with a penicillin in the treatment of enterococcal endocarditis. The answer is **(E)**.
14. Spectinomycin (2 g intramuscularly) is the appropriate choice in this case. Avoid cephalosporins in patients with a history of severe hypersensitivity to penicillins, and avoid fluoroquinolones (see Chapter 46) in pregnancy. Tetracyclines have been used in the past for gonorrhea but not as single doses, and they too should be avoided in pregnancy. The answer is **(D)**.
15. In most cases involving the empiric use of aminoglycosides, coverage for possible staphylococcal infection would involve combined use with nafcillin or a cephalosporin (not listed). Amoxicillin is susceptible to penicillinases produced by most staphylococci, and though clavulanic acid is an inhibitor of these enzymes it would not be used independently of a penicillin. Many staphylococcal strains are resistant to tetracyclines. The answer is **(D)**.
16. In "once-daily dosing" with aminoglycosides, the selection of an appropriate dose is particularly critical in patients with renal insufficiency. The aminoglycosides are eliminated by the kidney in proportion to creatinine clearance. Knowledge of the degree of insufficiency, based on plasma creatinine (or BUN), is essential for estimation of the appropriate single daily dose of an aminoglycoside. The answer is **(B)**.
17. Staphylococci are the most common cause of endocarditis in IV drug abusers. A triple-antibiotic regimen of ampicillin, nafcillin, and gentamicin is appropriate if there is no hypersensitiv-

ity to penicillins. Nafcillin provides coverage for staphylococci (but not MRSA strains); ampicillin plus gentamicin are synergistic against enterococci and possibly *S viridans;* gentamicin provides coverage for gram-negative aerobic bacteria.

18. Vancomycin plus gentamicin is an alternative regimen in cases of penicillin allergy, or if MRSA strains are suspected or identified.

19. Treatment of this patient will involve the monitoring of his fever and leukocytosis, the results of blood culture, his renal function, and his auditory and vestibular function.

20. Quinupristin-dalfopristin and linezolid are newer drugs with activity against gram-positive cocci resistant to vancomycin and conventional antibiotics.

Skill Keeper Answer: Nephrotoxicity

Drugs with nephrotoxic potential include ACE inhibitors, acetazolamide, aminoglycosides, aspirin, amphotericin B, cyclosporine, furosemide, gold salts, lithium, methicillin, methoxyflurane, NSAIDs, pentamidine, sulfonamides, tetracyclines (degraded), thiazides, and triamterene.

46 Sulfonamides, Trimethoprim, & Fluoroquinolones

OBJECTIVES

You should be able to:

- Describe the mechanisms of antibacterial action of sulfonamides and trimethoprim on bacterial folic acid synthesis and the mechanisms involved in bacterial resistance to the antifolate drugs.
- List the major clinical uses of sulfonamides and trimethoprim, singly and in combination, and describe their pharmacokinetic properties and toxic effects.
- Describe the mechanisms of action of the fluoroquinolone antibiotics and the mechanisms involved in bacterial resistance to these agents.
- List the major clinical uses of fluoroquinolones and describe their pharmacokinetic properties and toxic effects.

Learn the definitions that follow.

Table 46–1. Definitions.

Term	Definition
Antimetabolite	A drug that through chemical similarity is able to interfere with the role of an endogenous compound in cellular metabolism. The term includes antibacterial agents that inhibit bacterial folic acid metabolism
Sequential blockade	The combined action of two drugs that inhibit sequential steps in a pathway of bacterial metabolism

CONCEPTS

Sulfonamides and trimethoprim are examples of drugs that act as **antimetabolites.** Having chemical structures close to those of naturally occurring compounds, they are able to interfere with folic acid synthesis, which is critical to many microorganisms. Sulfonamides (structural congeners of para-aminobenzoic acid) inhibit dihydropteroic acid synthase, an early step in folic acid synthesis. Trimethoprim (an analog of dihydrofolic acid) inhibits the enzyme dihydrofolate reductase, which converts dihydrofolic acid to an active form, tetrahydrofolic acid. The combination of a sulfonamide and trimethoprim causes a sequential blockade of folic acid synthesis, resulting in a bactericidal and synergistic action.

The development of fluoroquinolones in the mid 1980s represented an important advance, since these drugs have a broad spectrum of antimicrobial activity that includes strains of many common pathogens resistant to older antibiotics. Fluoroquinolones have good oral bioavailability and cause few side effects—characteristics that have contributed to their widespread use during the past decade. Unfortunately, the emergence of resistant strains of formerly susceptible organisms (eg, staphylococci and streptococci) is starting to reduce the clinical value of those fluoroquinolones that have been in use for a decade or more.

ANTIFOLATE DRUGS

A. Classification and Pharmacokinetics:

1. **Sulfonamides:** The sulfonamides are weakly acidic compounds that have a common chemical nucleus resembling *p*-aminobenzoic acid (PABA). Members of this group differ mainly in their pharmacokinetic properties and clinical uses. Pharmacokinetic features include modest tissue penetration, hepatic metabolism, and excretion of both intact drug and acetylated metabolites in the urine. Solubility may be decreased in acidic urine, resulting in precipitation of the drug or its metabolites. Because of the solubility limitation, a combination of three separate sulfonamides **(triple sulfa)** has been used to reduce the likelihood that any one drug will precipitate. The sulfonamides may be classified as short-acting (eg, sulfisoxazole), intermediate-acting (eg, sulfamethoxazole), and long-acting (eg, sulfadoxine). Sulfonamides bind to plasma proteins at sites shared by bilirubin and by other drugs.
2. **Trimethoprim:** This drug is structurally similar to folic acid. It is a weak base and is trapped in acidic environments, reaching high concentrations in prostatic and vaginal fluids. (The trapping of a congener, pyrimethamine, is illustrated in Figure 1–1). A large fraction of trimethoprim is excreted unchanged in the urine. The half-life of this drug is similar to that of sulfamethoxazole (10–12 hours).

B. Mechanisms of Action:

1. **Sulfonamides:** The sulfonamides are bacteriostatic inhibitors of folic acid synthesis. As antimetabolites of PABA, they are competitive inhibitors of dihydropteroate synthase (Figure 46–1). They can also act as substrates for this enzyme, resulting in the synthesis of nonfunctional forms of folic acid. The selective toxicity of sulfonamides results from the inability of mammalian cells to synthesize folic acid; they must use preformed folic acid that is present in the diet.

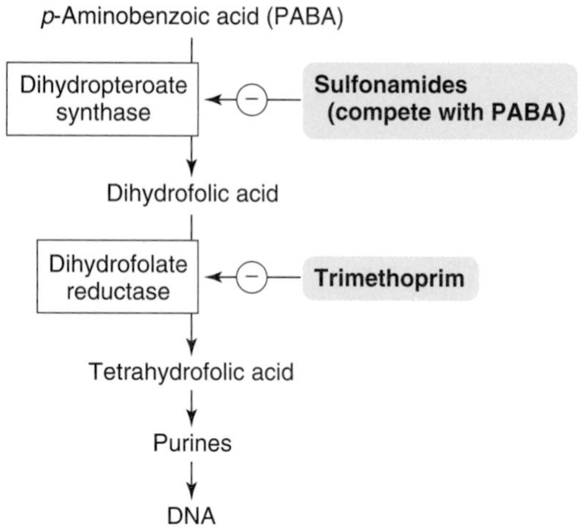

p-Aminobenzoic acid (PABA)
Dihydropteroate synthase ← (−) — **Sulfonamides (compete with PABA)**
Dihydrofolic acid
Dihydrofolate reductase ← (−) — **Trimethoprim**
Tetrahydrofolic acid
Purines
DNA

Figure 46–1. Inhibitory effects of sulfonamides and trimethoprim on folic acid synthesis. Inhibition of two successive steps in the formation of tetrahydrofolic acid constitutes sequential blockade and results in antibacterial synergy. (Modified and reproduced, with permission, from Katzung BG [editor]: *Basic & Clinical Pharmacology,* 8th ed. McGraw-Hill, 2001.)

2. **Trimethoprim:** Trimethoprim is a selective inhibitor of bacterial dihydrofolate reductase that prevents formation of the active tetrahydro form of folic acid (Figure 46–1). Bacterial dihydrofolate reductase is four to five orders of magnitude more sensitive to inhibition by trimethoprim than the mammalian enzyme.
3. **Trimethoprim plus sulfamethoxazole:** When the two drugs are used in combination, antimicrobial synergy results from the **sequential blockade** of folate synthesis (Figure 46–1). The drug combination is bactericidal against susceptible organisms.

C. **Resistance:** Bacterial resistance to sulfonamides is common and may be plasmid-mediated. It can result from decreased intracellular accumulation of the drugs, increased production of PABA by bacteria, or a decrease in the sensitivity of dihydropteroate synthase to the sulfonamides. Clinical resistance to trimethoprim most commonly results from the production of dihydrofolate reductase that has a reduced affinity for the drug.

D. **Clinical Use:**

1. **Sulfonamides:** The sulfonamides are active against gram-positive and gram-negative organisms, chlamydia, and nocardia. Specific members of the sulfonamide group are used by the following routes for the conditions indicated:
   a. **Simple urinary tract infections:** Oral (eg, triple sulfa, sulfisoxazole).
   b. **Ocular infections:** Topical (eg, sulfacetamide).
   c. **Burn infections:** Topical (eg, mafenide, silver sulfadiazine).
   d. **Ulcerative colitis, rheumatoid arthritis:** Oral (eg, sulfasalazine).
2. **Trimethoprim and sulfamethoxazole (TMP-SMZ):** This important drug combination is currently accepted treatment for complicated urinary tract infections and for respiratory, ear, and sinus infections due to *H influenzae* and *Moraxella catarrhalis.* In the immunocompromised patient, TMP-SMZ is used for infections due to *Aeromonas hydrophila* and is the drug of choice for prevention and treatment of pneumocystis pneumonia. TMP-SMZ is a possible backup drug for typhoid fever and shigellosis and has been used in the treatment of infections caused by methicillin-resistant staphylococci and *Listeria monocytogenes.*

E. **Toxicity of Sulfonamides:**

1. **Hypersensitivity:** Allergic reactions, including skin rashes and fever, occur commonly. Cross-allergenicity between the individual sulfonamides should be assumed and may also occur with chemically related drugs (eg, oral hypoglycemics, thiazides). Exfoliative dermatitis, polyarteritis nodosa, and Stevens-Johnson syndrome have occurred rarely.
2. **Gastrointestinal:** Nausea, vomiting, and diarrhea occur commonly. Mild hepatic dysfunction can occur, but hepatitis is uncommon.
3. **Hematotoxicity:** Though such effects are rare, sulfonamides can cause granulocytopenia, thrombocytopenia, and aplastic anemia. Acute hemolysis may occur in persons with glucose-6-phosphate dehydrogenase deficiency.

4. **Nephrotoxicity:** Sulfonamides may precipitate in the urine at acidic pH, causing crystalluria and hematuria.
5. **Drug interactions:** Competition with warfarin and methotrexate for plasma protein binding transiently increases the plasma levels of these drugs. Sulfonamides can displace bilirubin from plasma proteins, with the risk of kernicterus in the neonate if used in the third trimester of pregnancy.

F. **Toxicity of Trimethoprim:** Trimethoprim may cause the predictable adverse effects of an antifolate drug, including megaloblastic anemia, leukopenia, and granulocytopenia. These effects are usually ameliorated by supplementary folinic acid. The combination of trimethoprim-sulfamethoxazole may cause any of the adverse effects associated with the sulfonamides. AIDS patients given TMP-SMZ have a high incidence of adverse effects, including fever, rashes, leukopenia, and diarrhea.

FLUOROQUINOLONES

A. **Classification and Pharmacokinetics:** The original fluoroquinolone is **norfloxacin;** others in the group include **ciprofloxacin, ofloxacin, levofloxacin, lomefloxacin,** and **sparfloxacin.** All of the drugs have good oral bioavailability (antacids may interfere) and penetrate most body tissues. However, norfloxacin does not achieve adequate plasma levels for use in most systemic infections. Elimination of most fluoroquinolones is through the kidneys via active tubular secretion (which can be blocked by probenecid). Dosage reductions are usually needed in renal dysfunction. Moxifloxacin, sparfloxacin, and trovafloxacin are eliminated partly by hepatic metabolism and also by biliary excretion. Half-lives of fluoroquinolones are usually in the range of 3–8 hours, but the drugs eliminated by nonrenal routes have half-lives in the 10- to 20-hour range.

B. **Mechanism of Action:** The fluoroquinolones interfere with bacterial DNA synthesis by inhibiting topoisomerase II (DNA gyrase) and topoisomerase IV. They block the relaxation of supercoiled DNA that is catalyzed by DNA gyrase—a step required for normal transcription and duplication. Inhibition of topoisomerase IV by fluoroquinolones interferes with the separation of replicated chromosomal DNA during cell division. Fluoroquinolones are usually bactericidal against susceptible organisms.

C. **Resistance:** Fluoroquinolone resistance occurs during treatment with a frequency of about one in 10^8 organisms, especially in staphylococci, pseudomonas, and serratia. Mechanisms of resistance include decreased intracellular accumulation of the drug and changes in the sensitivity of target enzymes via point mutations in the fluoroquinolone binding regions. In coliforms, changes in DNA gyrase sensitivity are most important, while in gram-positive cocci resistance is mainly due to changes in the sensitivity of topoisomerase IV.

D. **Clinical Use:** Fluoroquinolones are effective in the treatment of infections of the urogenital and gastrointestinal tracts caused by gram-negative organisms, including gonococci, *E coli, Klebsiella pneumoniae, Campylobacter jejuni,* enterobacter, *Pseudomonas aeruginosa,* salmonella, and shigella. They have been used widely for respiratory tract, skin, and soft tissue infections, but their effectiveness is now variable because of the emergence of resistance. Ciprofloxacin and ofloxacin are alternatives to third-generation cephalosporins in gonorrhea, administered in single oral doses. Ofloxacin will eradicate accompanying organisms such as chlamydia, but a 7-day course of treatment is required. Levofloxacin has good activity against organisms associated with community-acquired pneumonia, including atypicals such as *Mycoplasma pneumoniae.* Sparfloxacin has increased activity against gram-positive organisms, including penicillin-resistant pneumococci. Moxifloxacin and trovafloxacin have the widest spectrum of activity, which includes both gram-positive and gram-negative organisms and anaerobic bacteria. Fluoroquinolones have also been used in the meningococcal carrier state, in the treatment of tuberculosis, and in prophylactic management of neutropenic patients.

E. **Toxicity:** Gastrointestinal distress is the most common side effect. The fluoroquinolones may cause skin rashes, headache, dizziness, insomnia, abnormal liver function tests, phototoxicity, and tendonitis. Superinfections due to *C albicans* and streptococci have occurred. The fluoroquinolones are not recommended for use in children or in pregnancy because they have caused cartilage problems in developing animals. Fluoroquinolones may increase the plasma levels of theophylline and other methylxanthines, enhancing their toxicity. Sparfloxacin prolongs the QT interval, with possible risk of cardiac arrhythmias, and the drug is associated with a high incidence of photosensitivity. Trovafloxacin has hepatotoxic potential.

Skill Keeper: Prolongation of the QT Interval (see Chapter 14)

Grepafloxacin was withdrawn from clinical use in the USA because of serious cardiotoxicity. Sparfloxacin, currently available, is contraindicated in patients taking drugs that prolong the QT interval. What other drugs can you recall that have this characteristic effect to increase the duration of the ventricular action potential? *The Skill Keeper Answer appears at the end of the chapter.*

DRUG LIST

The following drugs are important members of the group discussed in this chapter. Prototypes should be learned in detail; features of the major variants should be known well enough to distinguish the variants from the prototypes and from each other; the other significant agents should be recognized as belonging to a specific subclass.

Subclass	Prototype	Major Variants	Other Significant Agents
Sulfonamides			
Oral agents	Sulfisoxazole	Triple sulfa, sulfamethoxazole	Sulfadiazine
Local agents, drugs for special applications	Sulfacetamide, sulfasalazine, mafenide		
Combination	Trimethoprim-sulfamethoxazole		Pyrimethamine-sulfadoxine
Folate reductase inhibitors	Trimethoprim		Pyrimethamine
Fluoroquinolones	Ciprofloxacin	Levofloxacin, ofloxacin	Moxifloxacin, sparfloxacin, trovafloxacin

QUESTIONS

DIRECTIONS: Each of the numbered items or incomplete statements in this section is followed by answers or by completions of the statement. Select the ONE lettered answer or completion that is BEST in each case.

1. Which one of the following statements about sulfonamides is false?
(A) Sulfonamides inhibit bacterial dihydrofolate reductase
(B) Dysfunction of the basal ganglia may occur in the newborn if sulfonamides are administered late in pregnancy
(C) Cross-allergenicity may occur between sulfonamides and thiazides
(D) Sulfonamide crystalluria is most likely to occur at low urinary pH
(E) Sulfonamides are antimetabolites of PABA

2. The combination of trimethoprim and sulfamethoxazole is effective against which one of the following opportunistic infections in the AIDS patient?
(A) Disseminated herpes simplex
(B) Cryptococcal meningitis
(C) Toxoplasmosis

(D) Oral candidiasis
(E) Tuberculosis

3. A 24-year-old woman has returned from a vacation abroad suffering from traveler's diarrhea and her problem has not responded to antidiarrheal drugs. A pathogenic gram-negative bacillus is suspected. Which one of the following drugs is most likely to be effective in the treatment of this patient?
   (A) Ampicillin
   (B) Levofloxacin
   (C) Sulfacetamide
   (D) Trimethoprim
   (E) Vancomycin
4. Which one of the following statements about the clinical use of sulfonamides is false?
   (A) Resistant bacterial strains may have decreased intracellular accumulation of sulfonamides
   (B) Sulfonamides have activity against *C trachomatis* and can be used topically for the treatment of chlamydial infections of the eye
   (C) Sulfonamides are effective in Rocky Mountain spotted fever in patients allergic to tetracyclines
   (D) A sulfonamide is unlikely to be effective as the sole antibacterial agent in the treatment of chronic prostatitis
   (E) Some strains of bacteria become resistant because of increased production of PABA
5. A 31-year-old man has gonorrhea. He has no drug allergies, but he recalls that a few years ago while in Africa he had acute hemolysis following use of an antimalarial drug. The physician is concerned that the patient has an accompanying urethritis due to *C trachomatis,* though no cultures or enzyme tests have been performed. Which of the following drugs is most likely to be effective against gonococci and to eradicate *C trachomatis* in this patient?
   (A) Cefixime
   (B) Ciprofloxacin
   (C) Ofloxacin
   (D) Spectinomycin
   (E) Sulfamethoxazole
6. Which of the following statements about the fluoroquinolones is false?
   (A) Antacids may decrease the oral bioavailability of fluoroquinolones
   (B) Pneumococcal resistance to fluoroquinolones may involve changes in topoisomerase IV
   (C) Modification of fluoroquinolone dosage is required in patients if creatinine clearance is less than 50 mL/min
   (D) A fluoroquinolone is the drug of choice for treatment of an uncomplicated urinary tract infection in a 10-year-old girl
   (E) Fluoroquinolones inhibit relaxation of positively supercoiled DNA
7. A 55-year-old man complains of periodic bouts of diarrhea with lower abdominal cramping and intermittent rectal bleeding. Seen in the clinic he appears well-nourished, with blood pressure in the normal range. Examination reveals moderate abdominal pain and tenderness. His current medications are limited to ibuprofen for "tennis elbow" and loperamide for his diarrhea. He has no other significant medical history. Sigmoidoscopy reveals mucosal edema, friability, and some pus. Laboratory findings include mild anemia and decreased serum albumin. Microbiologic examination via stool cultures and mucosal biopsies do not reveal any evidence for bacterial, amebic, or cytomegalovirus involvement. A preliminary diagnosis is made of mild to moderate ulcerative colitis. The most appropriate drug to use in this patient is
   (A) Ciprofloxacin
   (B) Ganciclovir
   (C) Metronidazole
   (D) Sulfasalazine
   (E) Trimethoprim-sulfamethoxazole
8. The mechanism by which sulfasalazine exerts its primary action in ulcerative colitis is inhibition of
   (A) Folic acid synthesis
   (B) The formation of leukotrienes and prostaglandins

(C) Phospholipase C
(D) Proton pump activity
(E) The formation of interleukins

9. Which one of the following statements about the combination of trimethoprim plus sulfamethoxazole is false?
   (A) This combination is effective in the treatment of pneumonia due to *Pneumocystis carinii*
   (B) The drugs produce a sequential blockade of folic acid synthesis
   (C) Fever and pancytopenia occur frequently when these drugs are used in AIDS patients
   (D) The combination is appropriate for the treatment of streptococcal pharyngitis
   (E) The combination is effective in the management of acute exacerbations of chronic bronchitis
10. Which one of the following adverse effects is most likely to occur with sulfonamides?
   (A) Neurologic effects, including headache, dizziness, and lethargy
   (B) Hematuria
   (C) Fanconi's aminoaciduria syndrome
   (D) Kernicterus in the newborn
   (E) Skin reactions
11. This drug is the preferred agent for treatment of nocardiosis and, in combination with pyrimethamine, is prophylactic against *Pneumocystis carinii* infections in AIDS patients.
   (A) Ampicillin
   (B) Clindamycin
   (C) Norfloxacin
   (D) Sulfadiazine
   (E) Trimethoprim
12. Which one of the following statements about sulfisoxazole is false?
   (A) It is active against organisms associated with middle ear infections
   (B) Clinical antagonism occurs if it is used with inhibitors of dihydrofolate reductase
   (C) It is often used for "first-time" urinary tract infections
   (D) It is the most water-soluble of the sulfonamide group of drugs
   (E) It has a potential for hypersensitivity reactions
13. Supplementary folinic acid may prevent anemia in folate-deficient persons who use this drug; it is a weak base, and achieves tissue levels similar to those in plasma
   (A) Ciprofloxacin
   (B) Norfloxacin
   (C) Sulfacetamide
   (D) Trimethoprim
   (E) Trovafloxacin
14. It is now recommended that trovafloxacin be reserved for treatment of life-threatening infections because
   (A) Bacterial resistance to the drug is very common
   (B) Complete liver failure has occurred
   (C) It is very expensive
   (D) Its use is associated with torsade de pointes
   (E) Nephrotoxicity is dose-limiting
15. The overall incidence of phototoxicity due to this drug is approximately 8%. Reactions have been reported following indirect exposure to sunlight through window glass.
   (A) Norfloxacin
   (B) Sparfloxacin
   (C) Sulfadiazine
   (D) Trimethoprim
   (E) Trimethoprim-sulfamethoxazole

DIRECTIONS (Items 16–18): This case history is followed by discussion questions. Write out brief answers (two to five sentences) and then compare your answers with those given at the end of the Answers section.

A 26-year-old woman, otherwise healthy, complains of burning on urination. She has had a slight fever for the past 24 hours, with "backache." On physical examination, her temperature is elevated but her blood pressure and pulse are within normal limits. Abdominal examination is normal, but she has back and right-sided flank tenderness. Pelvic examination reveals no cervical motion tenderness. Laboratory data include an elevated white count, leukocytes in the urine, and the Gram stain of uncentrifuged urine reveals gram-negative rods. Blood is sent to the microbiology laboratory for culture. A presumptive diagnosis is made of pyelonephritis due to Escherichia coli *or a related gram-negative bacteria.*

16. If the symptoms are not severe and the patient can tolerate oral medications, she could be treated as an outpatient. What antibiotics would be most appropriate in this case?

17. What antibiotics would be appropriate for parenteral treatment if this patient is ill enough to be hospitalized and cannot tolerate oral drugs?

18. What antibiotics should be avoided if this patient is pregnant?

ANSWERS

1. Make sure you know the specific enzymes in bacterial folic acid synthesis that are inhibited by sulfonamides and trimethoprim: Sulfonamides inhibit dihydropteroate synthase; dihydrofolate reductase is inhibited by trimethoprim. The answer is **(A).**

2. Trimethoprim-sulfamethoxazole is not effective in the treatment of infections due to viruses, fungi, or mycobacteria. However, the drug combination is active against certain protozoans, including toxoplasma, and can be used for both prevention and treatment of toxoplasmosis in the AIDS patient. The answer is **(C).**

3. The fluoroquinolones are very effective in diarrhea caused by bacterial pathogens, including *E coli,* shigella and salmonella. None of the other drugs listed would be appropriate. Many coliforms are now resistant to ampicillin. Sulfacetamide is a topical agent used for bacterial conjunctivitis. While trimethoprim is available as a single drug, resistance may emerge during treatment unless it is used for urinary tract infections, where high concentrations are achieved. Vancomycin has no activity against gram-negative bacilli. The answer is **(B).**

4. Sulfonamides have minimal therapeutic actions in rickettsial infections. Chloramphenicol may be used for Rocky Mountain spotted fever in patients with established allergy or other contraindication to tetracyclines. The answer is **(C).**

5. While cefixime in a single oral dose is effective in gonorrhea, it has no activity against organisms causing nongonococcal urethritis. Both ciprofloxacin and spectinomycin are active against gonococci, but neither drug will eradicate a urogenital chlamydial infection. However, another fluoroquinolone, ofloxacin, is effective in both gonorrhea and chlamydial urethritis. In practice, this patient would best be treated by single oral doses of cefixime and azithromycin (not listed). Sulfamethoxazole would not be useful and may cause an acute hemolytic episode in this patient. The answer is **(C).**

6. The fluoroquinolones should not be used to treat uncomplicated first-time urinary tract infections. In this child, the infection is almost certainly due to a strain of *E coli* that is sensitive to many other drugs, including beta-lactam antibiotics. In addition, because of possible effects on cartilage, fluoroquinolones are not recommended for use in patients under the age of 18 years. The answer is **(D).**

7. Oral antimicrobial agents sometimes have beneficial effects in inflammatory bowel disease. However, in the absence of any evidence pointing toward a definite microbial cause for the colitis in this patient, a drug that decreases inflammation is indicated. Sulfasalazine has significant anti-inflammatory action, and its oral use results in symptomatic improvement in 50–75% of patients. The drug is also used for its anti-inflammatory effects in rheumatoid arthritis. The answer is **(D).**

8. Sulfasalazine is degraded by intestinal flora to sulfapyridine and 5-aminosalicylate (mesalamine). Release of high concentrations of salicylate in the colon exerts anti-inflammatory action, the major benefit of the use of sulfasalazine in ulcerative colitis (and presumably rheumatoid arthritis). Mesalamine is an inhibitor of cyclooxygenases and lipoxygenases, decreasing the formation of inflammatory eicosanoids. The answer is **(B).**

9. The combination of trimethoprim and sulfamethoxazole is often effective in respiratory infections due to susceptible *S pneumoniae* and *H influenzae.* However, in streptococcal pharyngitis the organisms are not eradicated. The answer is **(D).**

10. The most common adverse effect of sulfonamides is a skin rash due to hypersensitivity. CNS effects and hematuria occur less frequently. Sulfonamides are usually avoided in the third trimester of pregnancy or in neonates, so kernicterus is rare. Fanconi's syndrome, characterized by low back pain, aminoaciduria, polydipsia, and polyuria, is associated with the use of outdated tetracyclines. The answer is **(E).**

11. Sulfadiazine is the preferred drug in nocardiosis. In combination with pyrimethamine (an effective dihydrofolate reductase inhibitor in protozoa), sulfadiazine is effective in toxoplasmosis and is prophylactic against pneumocystis pneumonia in the AIDS patient. However, trimethoprim-sulfamethoxazole is more commonly used for the latter purpose. The answer is **(D).**

12. Sulfisoxazole is very soluble in urine and is commonly used for the treatment of acute uncomplicated urinary tract infections. The drug is also active against some common causative agents of otitis media, including *H influenzae* and pneumococci. For the treatment of otitis media, sulfisoxazole is usually given in a fixed-ratio combination with erythromycin. The answer is **(B).**

13. Trimethoprim is the only weak base listed (fluoroquinolones and sulfonamides are acidic compounds), and its high lipid solubility at blood pH allows penetration of the drug into prostatic and vaginal fluid to reach levels similar to those in plasma. Leukopenia and thrombocytopenia may occur in folate deficiency when the drug is used alone or in combination with sulfamethoxazole. Fluoroquinolones do not exacerbate symptoms of folic acid deficiency. The answer is **(D).**

14. In a small number of patients the use of trovafloxacin has been associated with severe liver injury which has culminated in death or the need for liver transplant. The risk of hepatotoxicity increases with more than 2 weeks of treatment. The answer is **(B).**

15. Each of the drugs listed has the potential to cause phototoxicity. However, sparfloxacin is distinctive in terms of the frequency of such reactions. Sunscreens may not be protective, and patients are at risk for up to 5 days after the last dose. The answer is **(B).**

16. In an acute uncomplicated pyelonephritis, a 7-day course of oral fluoroquinolones (eg, ciprofloxacin) is a primary choice. Backup drugs, which may require a 14-day course of treatment, include amoxicillin-clavulanate, an oral cephalosporin (eg, cephalexin), or TMP-SMZ.

17. Primary antibiotics used in hospitalized patients with acute pyelonephritis include intravenous fluoroquinolone, or ampicillin plus gentamicin, or a third-generation cephalosporin. Treatment is usually for 14 days.

18. Fluoroquinolones are not approved for use during pregnancy. Gentamicin should only be used if it is judged that the benefit outweighs the risk. TMP-SMZ should be used guardedly in the third trimester of pregnancy. Beta-lactam antibiotics are safe in pregnancy.

Skill Keeper Answer: Prolongation of the QT Interval (see Chapter 14)

The most important drugs that prolong the QT interval are antiarrhythmics. These include drugs from class IA and class III, including amiodarone, bretylium, disopyramide, procainamide, quinidine and sotalol. You may recall that though group IA drugs are classified as Na^+ channel blockers, they also block K^+ channels and prolong the duration of the ventricular action potential.

Antimycobacterial Drugs 47

OBJECTIVES

You should be able to:

- Describe the special problems associated with chemotherapy of mycobacterial infections.
- Describe the pharmacodynamic and pharmacokinetic properties of the first-line drugs used in tuberculosis (isoniazid, ethambutol, pyrazinamide, rifampin, and streptomycin).
- Identify the second-line drugs used in tuberculosis and list their limitations.
- Identify the drugs used in leprosy and in atypical mycobacterial diseases and describe their major toxic effects.

CONCEPTS

The chemotherapy of infections caused by *Mycobacterium tuberculosis, M leprae,* and *M avium-intracellulare* is complicated by numerous factors, including (1) limited information about the mechanisms of antimycobacterial drug actions; (2) the development of resistance; (3) the intracellular location of mycobacteria; and (4) the chronic nature of mycobacterial disease, which requires protracted drug treatment and is associated with drug toxicities. Chemotherapy of mycobacterial infections almost always involves the use of **drug combinations** to delay the emergence of resistance and to enhance antimycobacterial efficacy. The major drugs used in tuberculosis are **isoniazid (INH), rifampin, ethambutol, pyrazinamide,** and **streptomycin.** Actions of these agents on *M tuberculosis* are bactericidal or bacteriostatic depending on drug concentration and strain susceptibility. Suppression of *M avium-intracellulare* in the immunocompromised patient also requires multidrug treatment. The primary drug for leprosy is **dapsone,** commonly given with **rifampin** or **clofazimine** (or both). The subgroups of drugs used in these conditions are shown in Figure 47–1.

DRUGS FOR TUBERCULOSIS

A. Isoniazid:

1. Mechanisms: Isoniazid (INH) is a structural congener of pyridoxine. Its mechanism of action involves inhibition of enzymes required for the synthesis of mycolic acids and mycobacterial cell walls. Resistance can emerge rapidly if the drug is used alone. High-level resistance is associated with deletion in the *katG* gene that codes for a catalase involved in the bioactivation of INH. Low-level resistance occurs via deletions in the *inhA* gene that codes for the target acyl carrier protein.

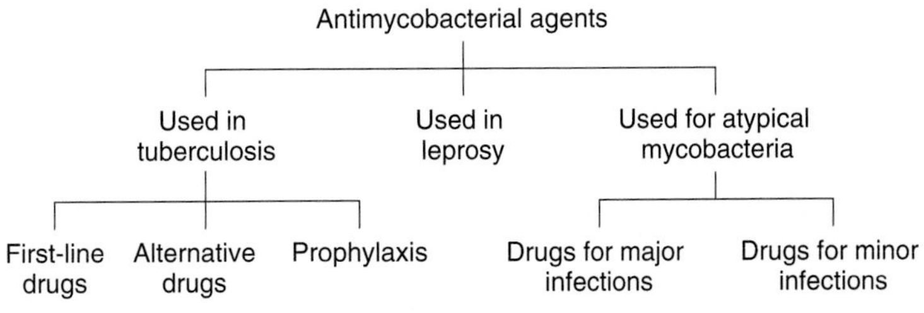

Figure 47–1. Subgroups of drugs discussed in this chapter.

2. **Pharmacokinetics:** INH is well absorbed orally and penetrates cells to act on intracellular mycobacteria. The liver metabolism of INH is by acetylation and is under genetic control. Patients may be fast or slow inactivators of the drug. The proportion of fast acetylators is higher among people of Asian origin (including Native Americans) than those of European or African origin. Fast acetylators require higher dosage than slow acetylators for equivalent therapeutic effects.
3. **Clinical use:** INH is the single most important drug used in tuberculosis and is a component of most drug combination regimens. In the prophylactic management of skin test converters and for close contacts of patients with active disease, INH is given as the sole drug.
4. **Toxicity and interactions:** Neurotoxic effects are common and include peripheral neuritis, restlessness, muscle twitching, and insomnia. These effects can be alleviated (without blocking the antibacterial effect) by administration of pyridoxine. INH is hepatotoxic and may cause abnormal liver function tests, jaundice, and hepatitis. Fortunately, hepatotoxicity is rare in children. INH may inhibit the hepatic metabolism of drugs, eg, phenytoin. Hemolysis has occurred in patients with glucose-6-phosphate dehydrogenase deficiency. A lupus-like syndrome has been reported.

Skill Keeper: Genotypic Variations in Drug Metabolism (see Chapter 4)

Genotypic variants occur with regard to the metabolism of isoniazid. What other drugs exhibit such variation, and what enzymes are involved in their metabolism? What are the clinical consequences of genetic polymorphisms in drug metabolism? *The Skill Keeper Answer appears at the end of the chapter.*

B. Rifampin:

1. **Mechanisms:** Rifampin—a derivative of rifamycin—is bactericidal against *M tuberculosis.* The drug inhibits DNA-dependent RNA polymerase (encoded by the *rpo* gene) in *M tuberculosis* and many other microorganisms. Resistance via changes in drug sensitivity of the polymerase emerges rapidly if the drug is used alone.
2. **Pharmacokinetics:** When given orally, rifampin is well absorbed and is distributed to most body tissues, including the CNS. The drug undergoes enterohepatic cycling and is partially metabolized in the liver. Both free drug and metabolites (which are orange-colored) are eliminated mainly in the feces.
3. **Clinical uses:** In tuberculosis, rifampin is always used in combination with other drugs. In leprosy, rifampin given monthly delays the emergence of resistance to dapsone. Rifampin can be used as the sole drug in prophylaxis against tuberculosis in INH-intolerant patients or close contacts of patients with INH-resistant strains of the organism. Other uses of rifampin include the meningococcal and staphylococcal carrier states.
4. **Toxicity and interactions:** Rifampin commonly causes light chain proteinuria and may impair antibody responses. Occasional side effects include skin rashes, thrombocytopenia, nephritis, and liver dysfunction. If given less often than twice weekly, rifampin may cause a flu-like syndrome and anemia. Rifampin strongly induces liver drug-metabolizing enzymes and enhances the elimination rate of many drugs including anticonvulsants, contraceptive steroids, cyclosporine, ketoconazole, methadone, and warfarin.

C. Ethambutol:

1. **Mechanisms:** Ethambutol inhibits arabinosyl transferases (encoded by the *embCAB* operon) involved in the synthesis of arabinogalactan, a component of mycobacterial cell walls. Resistance occurs rapidly via mutations in the *emb* gene if the drug is used alone.
2. **Pharmacokinetics:** The drug is well absorbed orally and distributed to most tissues, including the CNS. A large fraction is eliminated unchanged in the urine. Dose reduction is necessary in renal failure.
3. **Clinical use:** The only use of ethambutol is in tuberculosis, and it is always given in combination with other drugs.
4. **Toxicity:** The most common adverse effects are dose-dependent visual disturbances, in-

cluding decreased visual acuity, red-green color blindness, optic neuritis, and possible retinal damage (from prolonged use at high doses). Most of these effects regress when the drug is stopped. Other neurotoxic effects include headache, confusion, and peripheral neuritis.

D. Pyrazinamide:

1. **Mechanisms:** The mechanism of action of pyrazinamide is not known; however, its bacteriostatic action appears to require metabolic conversion via pyrazinamidases (encoded by the *pncA* gene) present in *M tuberculosis.* Resistant mycobacteria lack these enzymes, and resistance develops rapidly if the drug is used alone. There is minimal cross-resistance with other antimycobacterial drugs.
2. **Pharmacokinetics:** Pyrazinamide is well absorbed orally and penetrates most body tissues, including the CNS. The drug is partly metabolized to pyrazinoic acid, and both parent molecule and metabolite are excreted in the urine. The plasma half-life of pyrazinamide is increased in hepatic or renal failure.
3. **Clinical use:** The combined use of pyrazinamide with other antituberculous drugs is an important factor in the success of "short-course" treatment regimens.
4. **Toxicity:** Approximately 40% of patients develop nongouty polyarthralgia. Hyperuricemia occurs commonly but is usually asymptomatic. Other adverse effects include myalgia, gastrointestinal irritation, maculopapular rash, hepatic dysfunction, porphyria, and photosensitivity reactions.

E. Streptomycin: This aminoglycoside is now used more frequently than hitherto because of the growing prevalence of drug-resistant strains of *M tuberculosis.* Streptomycin is used principally in drug combinations for the treatment of life-threatening tuberculous disease, including meningitis, miliary dissemination, and severe organ tuberculosis. The pharmacodynamic and pharmacokinetic properties of streptomycin are similar to those of other aminoglycosides (see Chapter 45).

F. Alternative Drugs: The second-line antimycobacterial drugs are used in cases that are resistant to first-line agents; they are considered second-line drugs because they are no more effective, and their toxicities are often more serious than those of the major drugs.

1. **Amikacin** is indicated for treatment of tuberculosis suspected to be caused by streptomycin-resistant or multidrug-resistant mycobacterial strains. To avoid emergence of resistance, amikacin should always be used in combination drug regimens.
2. **Ciprofloxacin** and **ofloxacin** are often active against strains of *M tuberculosis* resistant to first-line agents. The fluoroquinolones should always be used in combination regimens with two or more other active agents.
3. **Ethionamide** is a congener of INH, but cross-resistance does not occur. The major disadvantage of ethionamide is severe gastrointestinal irritation and adverse neurologic effects at doses needed to achieve effective plasma levels.
4. ***p*-Aminosalicylic acid (PAS)** is now rarely used because primary resistance is common. In addition, its toxicity includes gastrointestinal irritation, peptic ulceration, hypersensitivity reactions, and effects on kidney, liver, and thyroid function.
5. Other drugs of limited use because of their toxicity include **capreomycin** (ototoxicity, renal dysfunction) and **cycloserine** (peripheral neuropathy, CNS dysfunction).

DRUGS FOR LEPROSY

A. Sulfones: Dapsone (diaminodiphenylsulfone) remains the most active drug against *M leprae.* The mechanism of action of sulfones may involve inhibition of folic acid synthesis. Resistance can develop, especially if low doses are given. Dapsone can be given orally, penetrates tissues well, undergoes enterohepatic cycling, and is eliminated in the urine, partly as acetylated metabolites. Common adverse effects include gastrointestinal irritation, fever, skin rashes, and methemoglobinemia. Hemolysis may occur, especially in patients with glucose-6-phosphate dehydrogenase deficiency.

Acedapsone is a repository form of dapsone that provides inhibitory plasma concentrations for several months. In addition to its use in leprosy, dapsone is an alternative drug for the treatment of *Pneumocystis carinii* pneumonia in AIDS patients.

B. Other Agents: Alternative drugs for leprosy include rifampin (see above) and **clofazimine.** Clofazimine is given in cases of dapsone resistance or intolerance. The drug causes gastrointestinal irritation and marked skin discoloration.

DRUGS FOR ATYPICAL MYCOBACTERIAL INFECTIONS

Infections due to atypical mycobacteria (eg, *M marinum, M avium-intracellulare, M ulcerans*), though sometimes asymptomatic, may be treated with the described antimycobacterial drugs (eg, ethambutol, rifampin) or with other antibiotics (eg, erythromycin, amikacin).

M avium complex (MAC) is a cause of disseminated infections in AIDS patients. Currently, clarithromycin or azithromycin is recommended for prophylaxis in patients with CD4 counts less than 50/μL. Treatment of MAC infections requires a combination of drugs, one favored regimen consisting of azithromycin or clarithromycin with ethambutol and rifabutin, a congener of rifampin.

DRUG LIST

The following drugs are important members of the group discussed in this chapter. Prototypes should be learned in detail; other significant agents should be recognized as belonging to a specific subclass.

Subclass	Prototype	Other Significant Agents
Drugs for tuberculosis		
Pyridines	Isoniazid	Ethionamide, pyrazinamide
Rifamycins	Rifampin	Rifabutin
Diamines	Ethambutol	
Aminoglycosides	Streptomycin	Amikacin
Others		Ciprofloxacin, ofloxacin, aminosalicylic acid, capreomycin, cycloserine, viomycin
Drugs for leprosy		
Sulfones	Dapsone	Acedapsone
Phenazines	Clofazimine	
Thiosemicarbazones	Amithiozone	
Drugs for *M avium* complex		A combination of azithromycin or clarithromycin with ethambutol, with or without rifabutin, is favored.

QUESTIONS

DIRECTIONS: Each of the numbered items or incomplete statements in this section is followed by answers or by completions of the statement. Select the ONE lettered answer or completion that is BEST in each case.

1. The primary reason for the use of drug combinations in the treatment of tuberculosis is to
(A) Ensure patient compliance with the drug regimen
(B) Reduce the incidence of adverse effects
(C) Enhance activity against metabolically inactive mycobacteria
(D) Delay or prevent the emergence of resistance
(E) Provide prophylaxis against other bacterial infections

Items 2–5: A 21-year-old woman from Thailand has been staying with family members in California for the past 3 months and is looking after her sister's preschool children during the day. Since she has difficulty with the English language, her sister escorts her to the emergency room of a local hospital. She tells the staff that the patient has been feeling very tired for the past month, has a poor appetite, and has lost weight. Two weeks ago she had symptoms of the "flu," with fever and night sweats. The patient has been feeling better lately except for a cough that produces a greenish sputum, sometimes specked with blood. With the exception of rales in the left upper lobe, the physical examination of the patient is unremarkable and she does not seem to be acutely ill. Laboratory values show a white count of 12,000/μL and a hematocrit of 33%. Chest x-ray reveals an infiltrate in the left upper lobe with a possible cavity. A Gram-stained smear of the sputum shows mixed flora with no dominance. An acid-fast stain reveals many thin rods of pinkish hue. A preliminary diagnosis is made of pulmonary tuberculosis. Sputum is sent to the laboratory for culture.

2. At this point, the most appropriate course of action is to
- **(A)** Send the patient home to await the culture results
- **(B)** Prescribe isoniazid for prophylaxis and send the patient home to await culture results
- **(C)** Start outpatient treatment with isoniazid and rifampin
- **(D)** Hospitalize the patient and start treatment with four antimycobacterial drugs
- **(E)** Hospitalize the patient and start treatment with isoniazid, rifampin, and ethambutol

3. When treatment is started, which one of the following drug regimens should be initiated in this patient?
- **(A)** Amikacin, isoniazid, pyrazinamide, streptomycin
- **(B)** Ciprofloxacin, cycloserine, isoniazid, PAS
- **(C)** Ethambutol, isoniazid, rifabutin, streptomycin
- **(D)** Ethambutol, pyrazinamide, rifampin, streptomycin
- **(E)** Isoniazid, rifampin, pyrazinamide, ethambutol

4. Which of the following statements concerning the possible use of isoniazid (INH) in this patient is false?
- **(A)** She may experience flushing, palpitations, sweating, and dyspnea after ingestion of tyramine-containing foods
- **(B)** Persons from Southeast Asia require lower maintenance doses of INH than most other persons in the USA
- **(C)** She should take pyridoxine daily
- **(D)** Symptoms of peripheral neuritis may occur during treatment
- **(E)** Her risk of developing hepatitis due to INH is less than 0.5%

5. On her release from hospital, the patient is advised not to rely solely on oral contraceptives to avoid pregnancy since they may be less effective while she is being maintained on antimycobacterial drugs. The agent most likely to interfere with the action of oral contraceptives is
- **(A)** Ethambutol
- **(B)** Isoniazid
- **(C)** Pyrazinamide
- **(D)** Rifampin
- **(E)** Streptomycin

6. The mechanism of high-level INH resistance of *M tuberculosis* is
- **(A)** Formation of drug-inactivating *N*-acetyltransferase
- **(B)** Reduced expression of the *katG* gene
- **(C)** Decreased intracellular accumulation of INH
- **(D)** Mutation in the *inhA* gene
- **(E)** Change in the pathway of mycolic acid synthesis

7. Which one of the following statements concerning drugs used in leprosy is false?
- **(A)** The mechanism of action of dapsone probably involves inhibition of folic acid synthesis
- **(B)** Single intramuscular injections of acedapsone maintain inhibitory levels of dapsone in tissues for up to 3 months
- **(C)** Monthly doses of rifampin delay the emergence of resistance to dapsone
- **(D)** Clofazimine should not be given to patients who are intolerant of dapsone or who fail to improve during treatment with dapsone
- **(E)** Clofazimine may cause changes in skin color

8. A patient with AIDS and a CD4 cell count of 100/μL has persistent fever and weight loss associated with invasive pulmonary disease that is due to *M avium* complex. Optimal management of this patient is to
- **(A)** Treat with rifabutin, since it prevents the development of MAC bacteremia
- **(B)** Select an antibiotic regimen based on drug susceptibility of the cultured organism
- **(C)** Start treatment with INH and pyrazinamide
- **(D)** Treat the patient with clarithromycin, ethambutol, and rifabutin
- **(E)** Treat with trimethoprim-sulfamethoxazole

9. A patient with pulmonary tuberculosis due to an INH-susceptible strain of *M tuberculosis* has been treated with INH, rifampin, and pyrazinamide for a total of 2 months. If the pyrazinamide is stopped at this time, treatment should be continued with INH and rifampin for a further minimum time period of

(A) 2 months
(B) 4 months
(C) 6 months
(D) 12 months
(E) 18 months

10. A 10-year-old boy has uncomplicated pulmonary tuberculosis. After initial hospitalization, he is now being treated at home with isoniazid, rifampin, and ethambutol. Which one of the following statements about this case is false?

(A) Caregivers should not worry about orange-colored tears if he cries
(B) Periodic tests of liver function should be considered
(C) Pyridoxine should be administered
(D) His mother (who takes care of him) should receive INH prophylaxis, but this is inadvisable for his younger siblings
(E) The boy may develop symptoms similar to those of influenza

11. This drug has been used prophylactically in contacts of children with infection due to *Haemophilus influenzae* type B. It is also prophylactic in meningococcal and staphylococcal carrier states. While the drug eliminates a majority of meningococci from carriers, highly resistant strains may be selected out during treatment.

(A) Ciprofloxacin
(B) Clofazimine
(C) Dapsone
(D) Rifampin
(E) Streptomycin

12. Which one of the following statements about ethambutol is false?

(A) Action against mycobacteria involves inhibition of arabinosyl transferases
(B) Decreases in visual acuity are dose-dependent
(C) Ocular toxicity is prevented by thiamine
(D) The drug is relatively contraindicated in very young children
(E) Resistance involves mutations in the *emb* gene

13. Once-weekly administration of this antibiotic has prophylactic activity against bacteremia due to *M avium* complex in AIDS patients.

(A) Azithromycin
(B) Clarithromycin
(C) Isoniazid
(D) Kanamycin
(E) Rifabutin

14. Which one of the following statements about pyrazinamide is false?

(A) It is bioactivated by enzymes encoded by the *pncA* gene
(B) One should discontinue treatment immediately if hyperuricemia occurs
(C) There is minimal cross-resistance with INH
(D) Polyarthralgia is a common adverse effect
(E) The drug is relatively contraindicated in patients with porphyric disease

15. Which one of the following drugs is most likely to cause loss of equilibrium and auditory damage?

(A) Amikacin
(B) Ethambutol
(C) Isoniazid
(D) Para-aminosalicylic acid
(E) Rifabutin

DIRECTIONS (Items 16–18): This case history is followed by discussion questions. Write out brief answers (two to five sentences) and then compare your answers with those given at the end of the Answers section.

A 32-year-old male who works as a nurse in an AIDS clinic comes to an internist with complaints of weakness, fever, chills, and night sweats. During the past 2 months, he has lost weight and has developed a cough productive of whitish-yellow sputum. He mentions contact with a patient 3 months ago who had tuberculosis and is worried that he has become infected. His history includes BCG vac-

cination as a child. The man is HIV antibody-negative and is not engaged in risky sexual behavior. Physical examination reveals mild cervical adenopathy and rales at the right lung base with dullness to percussion. Chest x-ray reveals a right lower lobe infiltrate. Sputum is positive for acid-fast bacilli and is sent to the laboratory for culture. A diagnosis is made of primary pulmonary tuberculosis.

16. What is the most appropriate drug regimen if resistance to INH is known to exceed 4%?
17. What factors influence the risk of multidrug-resistant tuberculosis?
18. What is the most appropriate drug regimen if there is known resistance to both INH and rifampin?

ANSWERS

1. While it is sometimes possible to achieve synergistic effects against mycobacteria with drug combinations, the primary reason for their use is to delay the emergence of resistance. The answer is **(D).**

2. Despite the fact that this patient does not appear to be acutely ill, she should be treated with four drugs that have activity against *M tuberculosis.* This is because organisms infecting patients from Southeast Asia are commonly INH-resistant and coverage must be provided with three other antituberculosis drugs in addition to isoniazid. This patient should be hospitalized for several reasons, including potential difficulties with compliance regarding the drug regimen and the fact that young children are in the home where she is living. The answer is **(D).**

3. Sputum cultures will not be available for several weeks, and no information is available regarding drug susceptibility of the organism at this stage. For optimum coverage, the initial regimen should include INH, rifampin, pyrazinamide, and ethambutol. INH-resistant organisms are usually sensitive to both rifampin and pyrazinamide. Streptomycin is usually reserved for use in severe forms of tuberculosis or for infections known to be resistant to first-line drugs. Likewise, amikacin and ciprofloxacin are possible agents for treatment of multidrug-resistant strains of *M tuberculosis.* Cycloserine, PAS, and rifabutin are alternative second-line drugs that may be used in cases of failed response to more conventional agents. The answer is **(E).**

4. Peripheral neuropathy caused by INH is due to pyridoxine deficiency. It is more common in the diabetic, malnourished, or AIDS patient and can be prevented by a daily dose of 25–50 mg of pyridoxine. INH can inhibit monoamine oxidase type A and has caused tyramine reactions. Hepatotoxicity is age-dependent, with an incidence of 0.3% in patients aged 21–35 years and greater than 2% in patients over the age of 50 years. Patients from Pacific Rim countries do not require lower doses of INH. Fast acetylators, including Native Americans, may require higher doses of the drug than others. The answer is **(B).**

5. Rifampin induces the formation of several microsomal drug-metabolizing enzymes, including cytochrome P450 isoforms. This action increases the rate of elimination of a number of drugs, including anticoagulants, ketoconazole, methadone, and steroids present in oral contraceptives. The pharmacologic activity of these drugs can be reduced in patients taking rifampin. The answer is **(D).**

6. Mutations in the *katG* gene result in the underproduction of mycobacterial catalase, an enzyme that bioactivates INH, facilitating its interaction with its target, keto-acyl carrier protein synthetase. The result is high-level resistance to isoniazid but without cross-resistance to pyrazinamide. Mutations in the *inhA* gene result in low-level resistance, with cross-resistance to pyrazinamide. The answer is **(B).**

7. Clofazimine is not related chemically to dapsone, and there is little cross-resistance. The drug is used in sulfone-resistant leprosy and for patients who are unable to tolerate dapsone. The answer is **(D).**

8. Combinations of antibiotics are essential for suppression of disease caused by *M avium* complex in the AIDS patient, and treatment should be started before culture results are available. While rifabutin is prophylactic against MAC bacteremia, when it is used as sole therapy in active disease, resistant strains of the organism emerge rapidly.

MAC is much less susceptible than *M tuberculosis* to conventional antimycobacterial drugs. Both isoniazid and pyrazinamide have minimal activity against MAC. Currently, the optimum regimen consists of clarithromycin (or azithromycin) with ethambutol and rifabutin. The answer is **(D).**

9. The duration of antimycobacterial drug therapy depends on the severity and location of the infection, the drug susceptibility characteristics of the infecting organism, and the effectiveness of the individual drugs used in the combination regimens. In pulmonary tuberculosis, treatment with INH, rifampin, and pyrazinamide should be continued for a total of 6 months, with pyrazinamide included for the first 2 months only. If pyrazinamide is not used during the first 2 months, INH and rifampin must be given for a total of 9 months. The answer is **(B).**

10. Hepatic dysfunction due to INH is rare in patients under 20 years of age. However, periodic tests of liver function may be advisable in younger patients who are also receiving rifampin, especially if higher doses of these drugs are used. Prophylaxis with INH is advisable for all household members and very close contacts of patients with active tuberculosis, especially children. A flu-like syndrome has occurred following intermittent high-dose administration of rifampin. The answer is **(D).**

11. Resistance emerges rapidly when rifampin is used as a single agent in the treatment of bacterial infections. It is an effective prophylactic and is used as a back-up drug to INH to prevent tuberculosis. However, when rifampin is used to treat the meningococcal carrier state, up to 10% of treated carriers may harbor rifampin-resistant organisms. The answer is **(D).**

12. Ocular toxicity due to ethambutol is dose-dependent and is usually reversible when the drug is discontinued. Thiamine is not protective. Periodic testing of visual acuity is advisable during treatment. Ethambutol is relatively contraindicated in children too young for assessment of their visual acuity and red-green color discrimination. The answer is **(C).**

13. Owing to its long elimination half-life (3–4 days), weekly administration of azithromycin has proved to be equivalent to daily administration of clarithromycin when used for prophylaxis against *M avium* complex in AIDS patients. The answer is **(A).**

14. The most common adverse effect of pyrazinamide is polyarthralgia. The drug uniformly causes hyperuricemia, but this is not a reason to halt therapy even though the drug may provoke acute gouty arthritis in susceptible individuals. The answer is **(B).**

15. Ototoxicity is characteristic of the aminoglycoside antibiotics. Many multidrug-resistant strains of mycobacteria remain susceptible to amikacin, and there is no cross-resistance with streptomycin. While disturbances of equilibrium may occur with overdosage, PAS does not cause hearing loss. The answer is **(A).**

16. For known resistance to isoniazid (or if the patient cannot tolerate the drug), the currently recommended regimen involves directly observed therapy (DOT) with rifampin plus ethambutol plus pyrazinamide for 18 months (< 12 months after a negative sputum culture is reported).

17. Multidrug-resistant tuberculosis (MDR-TB) is defined as resistance to two or more drugs. Risk factors include living in an area of over 4% INH resistance; recent immigration from Asia or Latin America; and a history of treatment of tuberculosis without rifampin.

18. In the case of resistance to both INH and rifampin, initial regimens still include both drugs plus ethambutol, pyrazinamide, streptomycin (or other aminoglycoside), and a fluoroquinolone. Continuation therapy should include at least three drugs shown to be active in vitro against the infecting strain. The appropriate duration of therapy has not been established.

Skill Keeper Answer: Genotypic Variations in Drug Metabolism (see Chapter 4)

Enzyme	Drugs	Clinical Consequences
Aldehyde dehydrogenase	Ethanol	Facial flushing, cardiovascular symptoms in Asians with low enzyme activity
N-Acetyltransferase	Izoniazid	Increased dose requirement in fast acetylators; increased peripheral neuropathy in slow acetylators
N-Acetyltransferase	Hydralazine, procainamide	Increased risk of lupus-like syndrome in slow acetylators; possible increased cardiotoxicity with procainamide in fast acetylators
Pseudocholinesterase	Succinylcholine	Deficiencies may lead to prolonged apnea

Though not described in the text, genetic polymorphisms occur in isoforms of cytochrome P450. Variants in the CYP2D6 isoform have been implicated in excessive responses to codeine and nortriptyline, and variants in CYP2C9 may be responsible for unusual sensitivity to the anticoagulant effects of warfarin.

Antifungal Agents

48

OBJECTIVES

You should be able to:

- Describe the mechanisms of action of the major drugs used for fungal infections.
- Describe the clinical uses and pharmacokinetics of amphotericin B, flucytosine, fluconazole, itraconazole, ketoconazole, griseofulvin, and terbinafine.
- Identify the toxic effects of the major antifungal drugs.
- Identify the main topical antifungal agents.

CONCEPTS

Fungal infections are difficult to treat, particularly in the immunocompromised or neutropenic patient. Most fungi are resistant to conventional antimicrobial agents, and only a few drugs are available for the treatment of systemic fungal diseases. Amphotericin B and the azoles (fluconazole, itraconazole, and ketoconazole) are useful in systemic infections and are selectively toxic to fungi because they interact with ergosterol or inhibit its synthesis. Ergosterol is a sterol that is unique to the fungal cell membrane; the predominant sterol of human cells is cholesterol.

DRUGS FOR SYSTEMIC FUNGAL INFECTIONS (Figure 48–1)

A. **Amphotericin B:**
   1. **Classification and pharmacokinetics:** Amphotericin B is a polyene antibiotic related to nystatin. Amphotericin is poorly absorbed from the gastrointestinal tract and is usually administered intravenously as a colloidal suspension, or in some cases in a lipid formulation. The drug is widely distributed to all tissues except the CNS. Elimination is mainly via slow hepatic metabolism; the half-life is approximately 2 weeks. A small fraction of the drug is excreted in the urine, dosage modification is necessary only in extreme renal dysfunction. Amphotericin B is not dialyzable.
   2. **Mechanism of action:** The fungicidal action of amphotericin B is due to its effects on the permeability and transport properties of fungal membranes. Polyenes are molecules with both hydrophilic and lipophilic characteristics, ie, they are amphipathic. They bind to **ergosterol,** a sterol specific to fungal cell membranes, and cause the formation of artificial pores (Figure 48–2). Resistance can occur via a decreased level of—or a structural change in—membrane ergosterol.
   3. **Clinical uses:** Amphotericin B is the most important of the drugs available for the treatment of systemic mycoses and is often used for initial induction regimens prior to follow-up treatment with an azole. It has the widest antifungal spectrum of any agent and remains the drug of choice for most systemic infections caused by aspergillus, *Candida albicans,* cryptococcus,

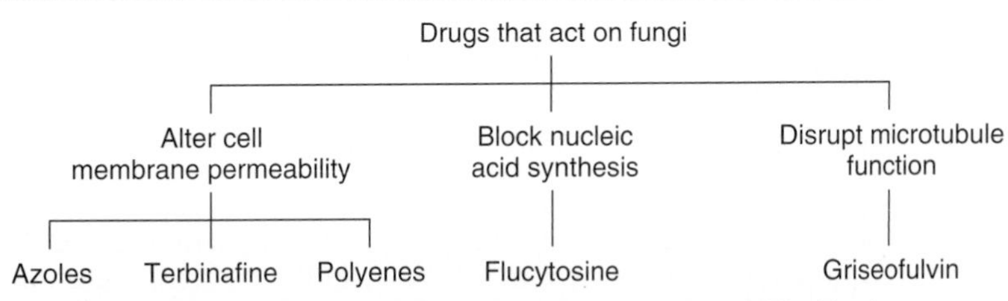

Figure 48–1. Subgroups of the antifungal drugs discussed in this chapter.

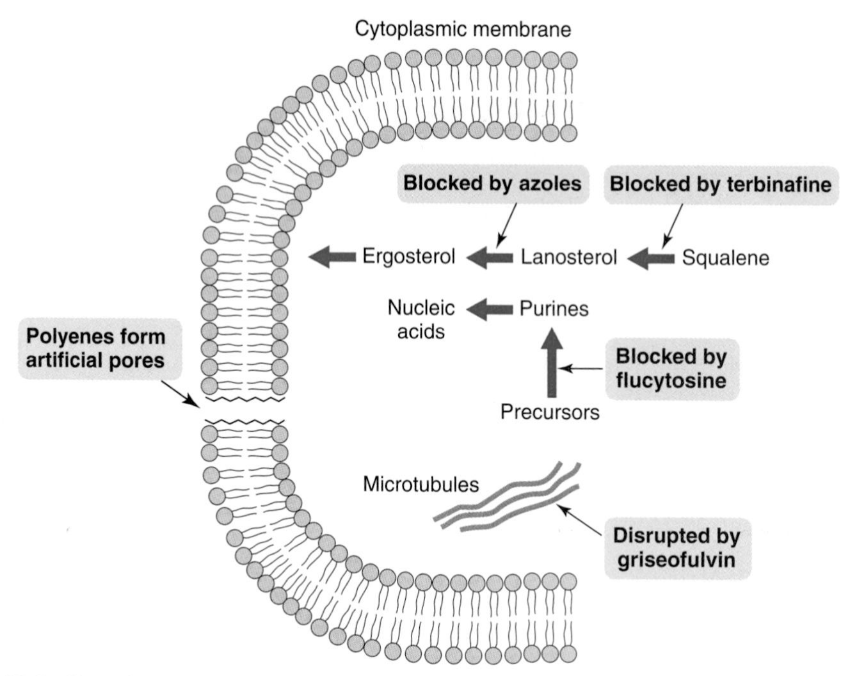

Figure 48–2. Sites of action of some antifungal drugs. The cell cytoplasmic membrane shown is that of a typical fungus. Because ergosterol is not a component of mammalian membranes, significant selective toxicity is achieved with the azole drugs.

histoplasma, and mucor. Amphotericin B is usually given by slow intravenous infusion, but in fungal meningitis intrathecal administration, though dangerous, has been employed.

4. **Toxicity:**
   a. **Infusion-related:** Adverse effects related to intravenous infusion commonly include fever, chills, muscle spasms, vomiting, and a shock-like fall in blood pressure. These effects may be attenuated by a slow infusion rate and by premedication with antihistamines, antipyretics, meperidine, or glucocorticoids.
   b. **Dose-limiting:** Amphotericin B decreases the glomerular filtration rate and causes renal tubular acidosis with magnesium and potassium wasting. Anemia may result from decreases in the renal formation of erythropoietin. While concomitant saline infusion may reduce renal damage, the nephrotoxic effects of the drug are dose-limiting. Dose reduction (with lowered toxicity) is possible in some infections when amphotericin B is used with flucytosine. Liposomal formulations of amphotericin B have reduced nephrotoxic effects, possibly due to decreased binding of the drug to renal cells.
   c. **Neurotoxicity:** Intrathecal administration of the drug may cause seizures and neurologic damage.

B. Flucytosine (5-Fluorocytosine, 5-FC):

1. **Classification and pharmacokinetics:** 5-FC is a pyrimidine antimetabolite related to the anticancer drug 5-fluorouracil. It is effective orally and is distributed to most body tissues, including the CNS. The drug is eliminated intact in the urine, and the dose must be reduced in patients with renal impairment.
2. **Mechanism of action:** Flucytosine is accumulated in fungal cells by the action of a membrane permease and converted by cytosine deaminase to 5-FU, an inhibitor of thymidylate synthase (Figure 48–2). Selective toxicity occurs because mammalian cells have low levels of permease and deaminase. Resistance can occur rapidly and involves decreased activity of the fungal permeases or deaminases. When 5-FC is given with amphotericin B, emergence of resistance is decreased and synergistic antifungal effects may occur.
3. **Clinical uses:** The antifungal spectrum of 5-FC is narrow; its clinical use is limited to the treatment, in combination with amphotericin B, of infections due to *Cryptococcus neoformans* and possibly systemic candidal infections.

4. **Toxicity:** Prolonged high plasma levels of flucytosine cause reversible bone marrow depression, alopecia, and liver dysfunction.

C. **Azole Antifungal Agents:**

1. **Classification and pharmacokinetics:** The azoles used for systemic mycoses include **ketoconazole, fluconazole, itraconazole,** and **voriconazole.** Oral bioavailability is variable (normal gastric acidity is required). Fluconazole and voriconazole are more reliably absorbed via the oral route than the other azoles. The drugs are distributed to most body tissues, but with the exception of fluconazole, drug levels achieved in the CNS are low. Liver metabolism is responsible for the elimination of ketoconazole, itraconazole, and voriconazole. Fluconazole is eliminated by the kidneys, largely in unchanged form.
2. **Mechanism of action:** The azoles interfere with fungal cell membrane permeability by inhibiting the synthesis of ergosterol. These drugs act at the step of 14α-demethylation of lanosterol, which is catalyzed by a cytochrome P450 isozyme. With increasing use of azole antifungals, especially for long-term prophylaxis in immunocompromised and neutropenic patients, resistance is occurring, possibly via changes in the sensitivity of the target enzymes.
3. **Clinical uses:**
   a. **Ketoconazole:** Ketoconazole has a narrow antifungal spectrum and is considered to be a backup drug for systemic infections caused by certain blastomyces, coccidioides, and histoplasma. Ketoconazole has been used commonly for chronic mucocutaneous candidiasis and when given orally is also effective against dermatophytes.
   b. **Fluconazole:** Fluconazole is a drug of choice in esophageal and oropharyngeal candidiasis and for most infections due to coccidioides. A single oral dose usually eradicates vaginal candidiasis. Fluconazole is now the drug of choice for initial and secondary prophylaxis against cryptococcal meningitis and is an alternative drug of choice (with amphotericin B) in treatment of active disease due to *Cryptococcus neoformans.* The drug is also equivalent to amphotericin B in candidemia.
   c. **Itraconazole:** This azole is currently the drug of choice for systemic infections due to blastomyces and sporothrix and for subcutaneous chromoblastomycosis. Itraconazole is an alternative agent in the treatment of infections caused by aspergillus, coccidioides, cryptococcus, and histoplasma. In esophageal candidiasis the drug is active against some strains resistant to fluconazole. Itraconazole is also active in dermatophytoses.
   d. **Voriconazole:** Voriconazole is a new azole with an even wider spectrum of fungal activity than itraconazole. Its clinical usefulness and toxic potential remain to be established.
4. **Toxicity:** Adverse effects of the azoles include vomiting, diarrhea, rash, and sometimes hepatotoxicity (especially in patients with preexisting liver dysfunction). Ketoconazole inhibits hepatic cytochrome P450 isozymes and may increase the plasma levels of other drugs, including anticoagulants, cyclosporine, oral hypoglycemics, and phenytoin. The same inhibition of drug metabolism is responsible for life-threatening cardiotoxicity when cisapride is used concomitantly with ketoconazole. Inhibition of cytochrome P450 isoforms by ketoconazole interferes with the synthesis of adrenal and gonadal steroids and may lead to gynecomastia, menstrual irregularities, and infertility. The newer azoles appear to be more selective inhibitors of fungal cytochrome P450. While they are less likely than ketoconazole to cause endocrine dysfunction, their inhibitory effects on liver drug-metabolizing enzymes have resulted in drug interactions.

Skill Keeper: Inhibitors of Cytochromes P450
(see Chapters 4 and 61)

Ketoconazole has the unenviable reputation of association with multiple drug interactions due to its inhibition of cytochromes P450 involved in drug metabolism.

1. How many drugs can you identify that have their metabolism via such enzymes inhibited by ketoconazole?
2. How many other drugs that inhibit hepatic cytochromes P450 can you recall?

The Skill Keeper Answers appear at the end of the chapter.

SYSTEMIC DRUGS FOR SUPERFICIAL FUNGAL INFECTIONS

A. Griseofulvin:

1. **Pharmacokinetics:** Oral absorption of griseofulvin depends on the physical state of the drug—ultramicrosize formulations, which have finer crystals or particles, are more effectively absorbed—and is aided by high-fat foods. The drug is distributed to the stratum corneum, where it binds to keratin. Biliary excretion is responsible for its elimination.
2. **Mechanism of action:** Griseofulvin interferes with microtubule function in dermatophytes (Figure 48–2) and may also inhibit the synthesis and polymerization of nucleic acids. Sensitive dermatophytes take up the drug by an energy-dependent mechanism, and resistance can occur via decrease in this transport.
3. **Clinical uses and toxicity:** The drug is indicated for severe dermatophytoses of the skin, hair, and nails. Adverse effects include headaches, mental confusion, gastrointestinal irritation, photosensitivity, and changes in liver function. A drug interaction may enhance coumarin metabolism, resulting in decreased anticoagulant effect.

B. Terbinafine:

1. **Mechanism of action:** Terbinafine inhibits a fungal enzyme, squalene epoxidase. It causes accumulation of toxic levels of squalene, which can interfere with ergosterol synthesis. Terbinafine is fungicidal.
2. **Clinical uses and toxicity:** Like griseofulvin, terbinafine accumulates in keratin, but it is much more effective than griseofulvin in onychomycosis. Adverse effects include gastrointestinal upsets, rash, headache, and taste disturbances. Terbinafine does not inhibit cytochrome P450.

C. Azoles:

1. **Pulse dosing:** All three of the azoles used for systemic antifungal infections have activity against dermatophytes. Pulse or intermittent dosing with itraconazole is as effective in onychomycoses as continuous dosing because the drug persists in the nails for several months. Typically, treatment for 1 week is followed by 3 weeks without drug. Advantages of pulse dosing include a lower incidence of side effects and major cost savings. Similar dosing regimens may be applicable to fluconazole and terbinafine.

TOPICAL DRUGS FOR SUPERFICIAL FUNGAL INFECTIONS

A number of antifungal drugs are used topically for superficial infections caused by *C albicans* and dermatophytes. **Nystatin** is a polyene antibiotic (related to amphotericin) that disrupts fungal membranes by binding to ergosterol. Nystatin is commonly used topically to suppress local candida infections and has been used orally to eradicate gastrointestinal fungi in patients with impaired defense mechanisms. Other topical antifungal agents include the azole compounds **miconazole** and **clotrimazole** and the nonazoles **haloprogin, tolnaftate,** and **undecylenic acid.**

DRUG LIST

The following drugs are important members of the group discussed in this chapter. Prototypes should be learned in detail; the other significant agents should be recognized as belonging to a specific subclass.

Subclass	Prototype	Other Significant Agents
Drugs for systemic mycoses		
Polyenes	Amphotericin B	
Azoles	Ketoconazole	Fluconazole, itraconazole, voriconazole
Pyrimidine	Flucytosine	
Systemic drugs for superficial infections	Griseofulvin	Terbinafine, ketoconazole, fluconazole, itraconazole
Drugs for topical or local use	Nystatin	Miconazole, clotrimazole, tolnaftate

QUESTIONS

DIRECTIONS: Each of the numbered items or incomplete statements in this section is followed by answers or by completions of the statement. Select the ONE lettered answer or completion that is BEST in each case.

1. Chemical interactions between this drug and cell membrane components can result in the formation of pores lined by hydrophilic groups present in the drug molecule.
- **(A)** Dactinomycin
- **(B)** Griseofulvin
- **(C)** Fluconazole
- **(D)** Nystatin
- **(E)** Terbinafine

2. Which one of the following statements about fluconazole is most accurate?
- **(A)** It is highly effective in treatment of aspergillosis
- **(B)** It does not penetrate the blood-brain barrier
- **(C)** Its oral bioavailability is less than that of ketoconazole
- **(D)** It inhibits demethylation of lanosterol
- **(E)** It is a potent inhibitor of hepatic drug-metabolizing enzymes

Items 3–6: A 20-year-old woman with leukemia was undergoing chemotherapy with intravenous antineoplastic drugs. During treatment she developed a systemic infection due to an opportunistic pathogen. There was no erythema or edema at the catheter insertion site. A white vaginal discharge was observed. After appropriate specimens were obtained for culture, empiric antibiotic therapy was started with gentamicin, nafcillin, and ticarcillin intravenously. This regimen was maintained for 72 hours, during which time the patient's condition did not improve significantly. Her throat was sore, and white plaques had appeared in her pharynx. On day 4, none of the cultures had shown any bacterial growth, but both the blood and urine cultures grew out *Candida albicans.*

3. At this point, the best course of action is to
- **(A)** Continue current antibiotics and start flucytosine
- **(B)** Stop current antibiotics and start ketoconazole
- **(C)** Continue current antibiotics and start amphotericin B
- **(D)** Continue current antibiotics and start griseofulvin
- **(E)** Stop current antibiotics and start amphotericin B

4. If given amphotericin B, the patient should be premedicated with
- **(A)** Diphenhydramine
- **(B)** Ibuprofen
- **(C)** Prednisone
- **(D)** Any or all of the above
- **(E)** None of the above

5. The dose-limiting toxicity of amphotericin B is
- **(A)** Myelosuppression
- **(B)** Infusion-related adverse effects
- **(C)** Renal tubular acidosis
- **(D)** Hypotension
- **(E)** Hepatitis

6. The opportunistic candidal infection in this patient could have been prevented by administration of
- **(A)** Fluconazole
- **(B)** Itraconazole
- **(C)** Ketoconazole
- **(D)** Nystatin
- **(E)** None of the above

Items 7–8: An African-American man living on the East Coast was transferred by his employer to California for 6 months. On his return he complains of having influenza-like symptoms with fever and a cough. He also has red, tender nodules on his shins. His physician suspects that these symptoms are due to coccidioidomycosis, contracted during his stay in California.

7. This patient should be treated immediately with
- **(A)** None of the following drugs
- **(B)** Amphotericin B
- **(C)** Griseofulvin

(D) Itraconazole
(E) Ketoconazole

8. Which of the following is the drug of choice if this patient is suffering from persistent lung lesions or disseminated disease due to *Coccidioides immitis*?
(A) Amphotericin B
(B) Fluconazole
(C) Ketoconazole
(D) Itraconazole
(E) Terbinafine

9. Which one of the following drugs is LEAST likely to be effective in the treatment of esophageal candidiasis if it is used by the oral route?
(A) Amphotericin B
(B) Clotrimazole
(C) Fluconazole
(D) Griseofulvin
(E) Ketoconazole

10. Which one of the following statements about flucytosine is accurate?
(A) It is bioactivated by fungal cytosine deaminase
(B) It does not cross the blood-brain barrier
(C) It inhibits cytochrome P450
(D) It is useful in esophageal candidiasis
(E) It has a wide spectrum of antifungal activity

11. Cardiac arrhythmias have occurred when this drug was used by patients taking the gastrointestinal promotility agent cisapride.
(A) Amphotericin B
(B) Clotrimazole
(C) Griseofulvin
(D) Ketoconazole
(E) Voriconazole

12. Which one of the following statements about terbinafine is false?
(A) Its activity is restricted to dermatophytes
(B) It is effective in onychomycosis
(C) It inhibits squalene epoxidase
(D) It is only used topically
(E) Rifampin may increase its clearance

13. Which one of the following drugs is most appropriate for oral use in vaginal candidiasis?
(A) Clotrimazole
(B) Griseofulvin
(C) Fluconazole
(D) Flucytosine
(E) Nystatin

14. Regarding the recently introduced lipid formulations of amphotericin B, which one of the following statements is accurate?
(A) Affinity of amphotericin B for these lipids is greater than affinity for ergosterol
(B) They are less expensive to use than conventional amphotericin B
(C) They are more effective in fungal infections because they increase tissue uptake of amphotericin B
(D) They may decrease nephrotoxicity of amphotericin B
(E) They have wider spectrums of antifungal activity than conventional formulations of amphotericin B

DIRECTIONS (Items 15–17): This case history is followed by discussion questions. Write out brief answers (two to five sentences) and then compare your answers with those given at the end of the Answers section.

Induction chemotherapy for acute myelocytic leukemia was initiated in a hospitalized 29-year-old male patient. Seven days later he developed a fever with cough and abdominal pain. An indwelling central catheter had been in place for a week, but there was no fluctuance or tenderness at the catheter site. The patient had painful mucosal ulcerations, significant alopecia, and his white cell count was 200/μL. The lungs and chest were clear, and the abdomen was soft and nontender. Blood and urine cultures were sent to the laboratory for culture, and parenteral antimicrobial treatment was initiated (day 7). One day later, the patient temporarily defervesced, but the fevers returned on the following day (day 9). Chest x-ray was negative, the white count was 350/μL, and both blood and urine cultures were negative for pathogens. Nonetheless, the attending physician added another antibiotic to the regimen to cover for drug-resistant staphylococci. On day 11, fever was unabated despite therapy with multiple antibacterial drugs. At this point, candidiasis was suspected and appropriate treatment was started. During the following week, the fever subsided and the patient's neutropenia was alleviated by treatment with erythropoietin and sargramostim.

15. Since the portal of entry of a pathogen could not be positively identified, the patient was treated empirically (day 7) to cover for microorganisms known to cause systemic infections in a hospitalized patient with neutropenia. Such pathogens include Enterobacteriaceae, *Pseudomonas aeruginosa,* and staphylococci. What antibiotic regimen would be appropriate to cover for such microorganisms?

16. What drugs would be used to cover for opportunistic infections due to drug-resistant staphylococci in the hospitalized neutropenic patient?

17. What antifungal agents are used for treatment of candidiasis in the neutropenic patient?

ANSWERS

1. The polyene antifungal drugs are amphipathic molecules that can interact with ergosterol in fungal cell membranes to form artificial pores. In these structures, the lipophilic groups on the drug molecule are arranged on the outside of the pore and the hydrophilic regions are located on the inside. The fungicidal action of amphotericin B and nystatin derives from this interaction, which results in leakage of intracellular constituents. The answer is **(D).**

2. The only azoles with activity against aspergillus are itraconazole and voriconazole. Fluconazole is the best-absorbed member of the azole group by the oral route and the only one that readily penetrates into cerebrospinal fluid. Fluconazole has minimal effects on hepatic cytochrome P450. The answer is **(D).**

3. The antibiotic regimen should be stopped on the grounds that the condition of the patient did not improve after 3 days of such treatment, the cultures were negative for bacteria, the clinical picture suggested that the patient had a candidal infection, and the blood culture results confirmed a fungal infection. The answer is **(E).**

4. Infusion-related adverse effects of amphotericin B include chills and fevers (the "shake and bake" syndrome), muscle spasms, nausea, headache, and hypotension. Antipyretics, antihistamines, and glucocorticoids have all been shown to be helpful. The administration of a 1 mg test dose of amphotericin B is sometimes useful in predicting the severity of infusion-related toxicity. The answer is **(D).**

5. Renal toxicity is dose-limiting with amphotericin B. Azotemia is commonplace and sometimes is severe enough to warrant dialysis. Decreases in glomerular filtration rate may be reversible, but irreversible damage can occur, presenting as renal tubular acidosis with hypokalemia and hypomagnesemia. The answer is **(C).**

6. In the case of opportunistic candidal infections in the immunocompromised patient, no prophylactic drugs have been shown to be effective. Prophylaxis against other fungi may be effective in some instances, including suppression of cryptococcal meningitis in AIDS patients with fluconazole. However, prophylactic use of azoles may be contributory to the development of fungal resistance. The answer is **(E).**

7. A travel history can be important in the diagnosis of fungal disease. If this patient has a fungal infection of the lungs, it is probably due to *C immitis,* which is endemic in dry regions of the western United States. Pulmonary symptoms of coccidioidomycosis are usually self-limiting, and drug therapy is not commonly required. The presence of tender red nodules on extensor surfaces is a good prognostic sign. Erythema nodosum is a delayed hypersensitivity response to fungal antigens. No organisms are present in the lesions, and it is not a sign of disseminated disease. The answer is **(A).**

8. In progressive or disseminated forms of coccidioidomycosis, systemic antifungal drug treatment is needed. Until recently, amphotericin B was the recommended therapy, but fluconazole is now considered to be the drug of choice. Note that the risk of dissemination is much greater in blacks (10% incidence) and in pregnant women during the third trimester. The answer is **(B).**

9. Griseofulvin has no activity against *Candida albicans* and is not effective in the treatment of systemic or superficial infections caused by such organisms. "Swish and swallow" formulations of clotrimazole and nystatin have been used commonly, and a similar formulation of amphotericin B is now available for use in resistant candidiasis. Most of the azoles are effective in esophageal candidiasis. The answer is **(D).**

10. Flucytosine is converted via fungal cytosine deaminase to the antimetabolite fluorouracil, which causes inhibition of thymidylate synthase. Flucytosine enters the cerebrospinal fluid and has been used in combination with amphotericin B in cryptococcal meningitis. The drug has a narrow spectrum of antifungal activity and is not effective in esophageal candidiasis. The answer is **(A).**

11. Cardiotoxicity occurred when ketoconazole was used by patients taking astemizole or terfenadine, a drug interaction that led to the withdrawal of the two nonsedating antihistamines in the United States. The same type of drug interaction has been reported between ketoconazole and cisapride as a result of the ability of ketoconazole to inhibit hepatic drug-metabolizing enzymes. The answer is **(D).**

12. Terbinafine has a unique action to inhibit squalene epoxidase, causing the intracellular accumulation of squalene to toxic levels. An antidermatophytic agent, terbinafine is used orally and is highly effective in onychomycosis. Its clearance from the body via hepatic metabolism is markedly increased by rifampin. The answer is **(D).**

13. Clotrimazole and nystatin may be used topically (not orally) for vaginal candidiasis. The activity of griseofulvin is limited to dermatophytes. Fluconazole in a single oral dose is usually effective in vaginal candidiasis. The answer is **(C).**

14. Damage to renal tubular cells during treatment with amphotericin B is dose-limiting. Liposomal formulations of amphotericin B result in decreased accumulation of the drug in tissues, including the kidney. As a result, nephrotoxicity is decreased. With some lipid formulations, infusion-related toxicity may also be reduced. Lipid formulations do not have a wider antifungal spectrum; their daily cost ranges from 10 to 40 times more than conventional formulations of amphotericin B. The answer is **(D).**

15. Nosocomial infections occur commonly in the hospitalized neutropenic patient and are a leading cause of death. At the earliest sign of infection, empiric therapy is often instituted with antibiotics that provide coverage against potential bacterial pathogens. Such drugs include imipenem-cilastatin (or meropenem), cefipime (a fourth-generation cephalosporin), or an extended-spectrum penicillin (eg, ticarcillin) in combination with an aminoglycoside. If infection due to staphylococci is suspected, nafcillin or vancomycin is included in the antibiotic regimen. None of the above drugs have activity against fungi!

16. *Staphylococcus epidermidis* and *S aureus* are common pathogens associated with infection originating from intravenous lines. Most strains of these organisms responsible for hospital-acquired infections are resistant to methicillin. Vancomycin remains the drug of choice for both MRSA and MRSE. Quinupristin-dalfopristin is usually effective in the case of staphylococci resistant to vancomycin.

17. No bacterial or fungal pathogen was identified. Resolution of the infection following treatment with an antifungal agent suggests that the bloodstream was infected with *Candida albicans,* a relatively common pathogen in the neutropenic patient. Intravenous fluconazole (for 7 days) is usually the treatment of choice, switching to oral therapy until neutropenia resolves or signs and symptoms of candidiasis disappear. Amphotericin B with or without flucytosine is currently an alternative regimen for management of candidiasis in neutropenic patients.

Skill Keeper Answers: Inhibitors of Cytochromes P450 (see Chapters 4 and 61)

1. A sampling of commonly used drugs with cytochrome P450-mediated metabolism inhibited by ketoconazole or other azoles includes chlordiazepoxide, cisapride, cyclosporine, didanosine, fluoxetine, loratadine, lovastatin, methadone, nifedipine, phenytoin, quinidine, theophylline, verapamil, warfarin, and zolpidem.
2. Other drugs that inhibit hepatic cytochromes P450 include chloramphenicol, cimetidine, clarithromycin, disulfiram, erythromycin, ethanol, grapefruit juice (contains furanocoumarins), ethinyl estradiol, fluconazole, isoniazid, itraconazole, MAO inhibitors, phenylbutazone, and secobarbital.

Antiviral Chemotherapy & Prophylaxis 49

OBJECTIVES

You should be able to:

- Identify the main steps in viral replication.
- Describe the mechanisms of action and of resistance of the major antiherpes drugs.
- Describe the pharmacokinetic properties, the clinical uses, and the toxic effects of the antiherpes drugs.
- Describe the mechanisms of action and of resistance of the major antiretroviral drugs.
- Describe the pharmacokinetic properties, the clinical uses, and the toxic effects of the antiretroviral drugs.
- Identify the significant antiviral properties of amantadine, neuraminidase inhibitors, interferons, and ribavirin.

CONCEPTS

Most clinically useful antiviral agents exert their actions on viral replication, either at the stage of nucleic acid synthesis or the stage of late protein synthesis and processing (Figure 49–1). Most of the drugs active against herpes viruses and against the human immunodeficiency virus (HIV) are antimetabolites, structurally similar to naturally occurring compounds. In order to interfere with viral nucleic acid synthesis or the late synthesis of viral proteins, antimetabolites must first undergo conversion to active forms, usually triphosphate derivatives. For example, drugs such as **zidovudine**

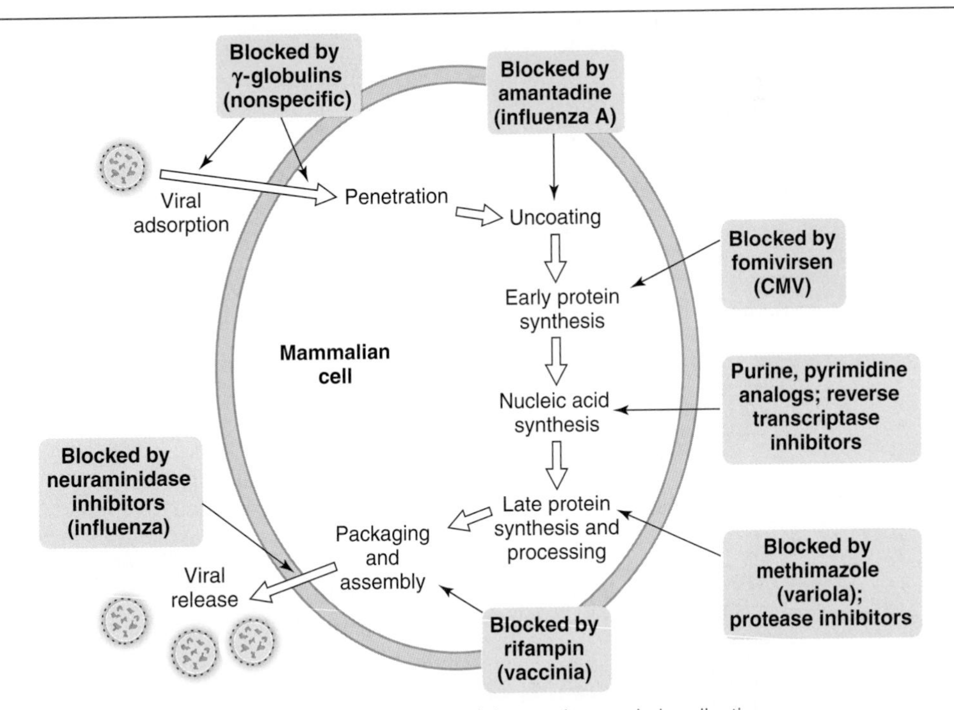

Figure 49–1. The major sites of drug action on viral replication.

(AZT) undergo phosphorylation by host cell kinases to form nucleotide analogs that may inhibit viral DNA polymerases (Figure 49–2). Selective toxicity results because viral DNA polymerases are more sensitive to inhibition by these antimetabolites than are mammalian polymerases. **Acyclovir** is more selectively toxic than the drugs that require phosphorylation only by host cell enzymes. This increased selectivity is partly a result of initial phosphorylation of acyclovir by a *viral* thymidine kinase that is absent in uninfected cells (Figure 49–2, top).

One of the most important recent trends in viral chemotherapy has been combination therapy. The strategy is similar to that of cancer chemotherapy, where treatment with combinations of drugs can result in greater effectiveness and prevent or delay the emergence of resistance. The limited success of monotherapy in treatment of HIV disease has been the major stimulus to combination antiviral chemotherapy. The current approach to treatment of infection with HIV is the initiation of treatment with three drugs—if possible, before symptoms appear. Such combinations usually include two nucleoside reverse transcriptase inhibitors (NRTIs) plus an inhibitor of HIV protease (PI). In some combination regimens, a nonnucleoside reverse transcriptase inhibitor (NNRTI) has been used in place of a protease inhibitor. Highly active antiretroviral therapy (HAART) involving drug combinations can slow or reverse the increases in viral RNA load that normally accompany progression of disease. In many AIDS patients, HAART slows or reverses the decline in CD4 cells and decreases the incidence of opportunistic infections.

ANTIHERPES DRUGS

A. Acyclovir (Acycloguanosine):

1. **Mechanisms:** Acyclovir is a guanosine analog active against herpes simplex virus (HSV) and varicella-zoster (VZV) virus. The drug is activated to form acyclovir triphosphate, a competitive substrate for DNA polymerase, leading to chain termination following its incorporation into viral DNA (Figure 49–2). Resistance of herpes simplex virus can involve changes in viral DNA polymerase. However, many resistant strains of HSV (TK^- strains) lack thymidine kinase, the enzyme involved in the initial *viral-specific* phosphorylation of acyclovir. Such strains are cross-resistant to famciclovir, ganciclovir, and valacyclovir.
2. **Pharmacokinetics:** Acyclovir can be administered by the topical, oral, and intravenous routes. Renal excretion is the major route of elimination of acyclovir and dosage should be reduced in patients with renal impairment.
3. **Clinical uses and toxicity:** Oral acyclovir is used for treatment of mucocutaneous and genital herpes lesions and for prophylaxis in AIDS and in other immunocompromised patients (eg, those undergoing organ transplantation). The oral drug is well tolerated but may cause gastrointestinal distress and headache. Intravenous administration is used for severe herpes disease (including encephalitis) and for neonatal HSV infection. Toxic effects with parenteral administration include delirium, tremor, seizures, hypotension, and nephrotoxicity. Acyclovir has no significant toxicity on the bone marrow.

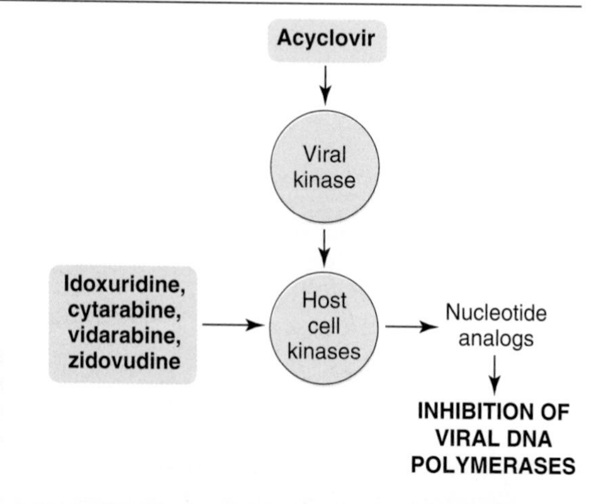

Figure 49–2. Antiviral actions of purine and pyrimidine analogs. Acyclovir (top) is metabolized first by viral kinase to an intermediate. This intermediate and the drugs shown on the left are then metabolized by host cell kinases to nucleotide analogs that inhibit viral replication.

4. **Acyclovir congeners:** Several new antiviral agents have characteristics similar to acyclovir. **Famciclovir** is a prodrug converted to penciclovir by first-pass metabolism in the liver. Used orally in genital herpes and for herpes zoster, famciclovir is well tolerated and is similar to acyclovir in its pharmacokinetic properties. **Penciclovir** also undergoes activation by viral thymidine kinase, and the triphosphate form inhibits DNA polymerase but does not cause chain termination. **Valacyclovir** is converted to acyclovir by hepatic metabolism after oral administration and reaches plasma levels three to five times greater than those achieved by acyclovir. Valacyclovir has a longer duration of action than acyclovir but is otherwise identical. None of the acyclovir congeners have activity against TK^- strains of HSV.

B. Foscarnet:

1. **Mechanisms:** Foscarnet is a phosphonoformate derivative that does not require phosphorylation for antiviral activity. Though it is not an antimetabolite, foscarnet inhibits viral RNA polymerase, DNA polymerase, and HIV reverse transcriptase. A known mechanism of resistance involves point mutations in the DNA polymerase gene.
2. **Pharmacokinetics:** Foscarnet is given intravenously and penetrates well into tissues, including the CNS. Up to one-third of a dose may be deposited in bone. The drug undergoes renal elimination in direct proportion to creatinine clearance.
3. **Clinical uses and toxicity:** The drug is used for prophylaxis and treatment of cytomegalovirus (CMV) infections (including CMV retinitis) and has activity against ganciclovir-resistant strains of this virus (Table 49–1). Foscarnet inhibits herpes DNA polymerase in acyclovir-resistant strains that are thymidine kinase-deficient and may suppress such resistant herpetic infections in patients with AIDS. Adverse effects include nephrotoxicity (30% incidence) with disturbances in electrolyte balance (especially hypocalcemia), genitourinary ulceration, and CNS effects (headache, hallucinations, seizures).

C. Ganciclovir:

1. **Mechanisms:** Ganciclovir, a guanine derivative, is triphosphorylated to form a nucleotide that inhibits DNA polymerases of CMV and HSV but does not cause chain termination. The first phosphorylation step is catalyzed by virus-specific enzymes in both CMV-infected and HSV-infected cells. CMV resistance mechanisms include changes in DNA polymerase and mutations in the gene that codes for the activating viral phosphotransferase. Thymidine kinase-deficient HSV strains are resistant to ganciclovir.
2. **Pharmacokinetics:** Ganciclovir is usually given intravenously and penetrates well into tissues, including the eye and the CNS. The drug undergoes renal elimination in direct proportion to creatinine clearance. Although oral bioavailability is less than 10%, an oral formulation is available for maintenance therapy.
3. **Clinical uses and toxicity:** Ganciclovir is used for the prophylaxis and treatment of CMV retinitis and other CMV infections in immunocompromised patients. Systemic toxic effects include leukopenia, thrombocytopenia, mucositis, hepatic dysfunction, and seizures. The drug may cause severe neutropenia when used with zidovudine or other myelosuppressive agents.

Table 49–1. Major clinical uses of antiviral drugs.

Virus	Drugs or Regimen of Choice	Alternative Drugs or Regimens
CMV	Ganciclovir	Foscarnet, cidofovir
HBV, HCV	Interferon alfa-2b	Lamivudine (adjunctive)
HSV	Acyclovir	Foscarnet, ganciclovir, cidofovir, vidarabine
HIV	Two NRTIs[1] plus a protease inhibitor	Two NRTIs plus an NNRTI[2]
Influenza A	Amantadine	Rimantadine
Influenza A and B	Oseltamivir	Zanamivir
RSV	Ribavirin	
VZV	Acyclovir	Foscarnet

[1]Nucleoside reverse transcriptase inhibitor.
[2]Nonnucleoside reverse transcriptase inhibitor.

D. Cidofovir:

1. **Mechanisms and pharmacokinetics:** Cidofovir is activated exclusively by host cell kinases and inhibits DNA polymerases of HSV, CMV, adenovirus, and papillomavirus. Resistance is due to mutations in the DNA polymerase gene. The drug has been used by intravenous and topical administration and by intravitreal injection. Cidofovir undergoes renal elimination in proportion to creatinine clearance.
2. **Clinical uses and toxicity:** Cidofovir is effective in CMV retinitis. It may also be valuable in mucocutaneous HSV infections, including those resistant to acyclovir, and in genital warts. Nephrotoxicity is the major dose-limiting toxicity.

E. Other Antiherpes Drugs:

1. **Vidarabine:** Vidarabine is an adenine analog and has activity against HSV, VZV, and CMV. Its use for systemic infections is limited by rapid metabolic inactivation and by marked toxic potential. However, it has been used intravenously for severe HSV infections, including those resistant to acyclovir, and it also prevents the dissemination of varicella-zoster virus in immunocompromised patients. Vidarabine is used topically for herpes keratitis, but it has no effect on genital lesions. Toxic effects with systemic use include gastrointestinal irritation, paresthesias, tremor, convulsions, and hepatic dysfunction. Vidarabine is teratogenic in animals.
2. **Sorivudine:** Sorivudine is a pyrimidine analog with activity against HSV-1, VZV, and EBV. This investigational drug is approximately 1000 times more potent than acyclovir against HSV strains. However, thymidine kinase-deficient strains of HSV are resistant to sorivudine.
3. **Idoxuridine and trifluridine:** These pyrimidine analogs are used topically in herpes keratitis. They are too toxic for systemic use.
4. **Fomivirsen:** Fomivirsen is an antisense oligonucleotide that binds to mRNA of CMV, inhibiting early protein synthesis. The drug is injected intravitreally for treatment of CMV retinitis.

ANTI-HIV AGENTS: NUCLEOSIDE REVERSE TRANSCRIPTASE INHIBITORS (NRTIs)

A. Zidovudine (ZDV):

1. **Mechanisms:** Formerly called azidothymidine (AZT), zidovudine is a nucleoside requiring phosphorylation by host cell kinases to form a nucleotide analog that both inhibits reverse transcriptase of HIV-1 and HIV-2 and causes chain termination in viral DNA. Resistance—common in patients with advanced HIV infection—is due to mutations at several sites on the *pol* gene which encodes for several proteins, including reverse transcriptase.
2. **Pharmacokinetics:** Zidovudine is active orally (with 60% bioavailability) and is distributed to most tissues, including the CNS. Elimination of the drug involves both hepatic metabolism to glucuronides and renal excretion. Dosage reduction is necessary in uremic patients and those with cirrhosis. The half-life of zidovudine is 1–3 hours.
3. **Clinical use:** Zidovudine continues to be the most frequently used reverse transcriptase inhibitor in combination drug regimens (HAART). It is of value also in prophylaxis against HIV infection through accidental needlesticks and in prophylaxis against vertical transmission from mother to neonate.
4. **Toxicity:** The primary toxicity is bone marrow suppression leading to anemia and neutropenia, which may require transfusions. Bone marrow toxicity is additive with other myelosuppressants. Gastrointestinal distress, thrombocytopenia, headaches, myalgia, acute cholestatic hepatitis, agitation, and insomnia may also occur.
5. **Drug interactions:** Drugs that undergo hepatic glucuronidation, including acetaminophen, benzodiazepines, cimetidine, and sulfonamides, may increase plasma levels of zidovudine. Metabolism of zidovudine may also be inhibited by azole antifungals and by protease inhibitors. Rifampin increases the clearance of zidovudine.

B. Didanosine (ddI):

1. **Mechanisms:** Didanosine is an analog of deoxyadenosine that is activated by host cell kinases to a triphosphate form which inhibits reverse transcriptase and causes chain termination. Resistant strains are associated with point mutations of the *pol* gene, and there is com-

plete cross-resistance with zalcitabine (ddC) but only partial cross-resistance with zidovudine.

2. **Pharmacokinetics and clinical use:** Oral bioavailability of ddI is reduced by food and by chelating agents. The drug is eliminated by glomerular filtration and active tubular secretion, and the dose must be reduced in patients with renal dysfunction. Didanosine is used in HAART combination drug regimens.
3. **Toxicity:** Pancreatitis is dose-limiting and occurs more frequently in alcoholic patients and those with hypertriglyceridemia. Other adverse effects include peripheral neuropathy, diarrhea, hepatic dysfunction, hyperuricemia, and CNS effects.

C. Zalcitabine (ddC):

1. **Mechanisms:** Zalcitabine is a pyrimidine nucleoside with mechanisms of action and resistance similar to those of other NRTIs. Depending on specific sites of mutation on the *pol* gene, resistance may emerge to ddC alone or cross-resistance between other RT inhibitors may occur.
2. **Pharmacokinetics and clinical use:** Zalcitabine has high oral bioavailability. Dosage adjustment is needed in patients with renal insufficiency. Zalcitabine is always used in combination with other anti-HIV drugs.
3. **Toxicity:** Dose-dependent peripheral neuropathy is the major adverse effect of ddC. Pancreatitis, esophageal ulceration, stomatitis, and arthralgias may also occur.

D. Lamivudine (3TC):

1. **Mechanisms:** Like other NRTIs, lamivudine requires activation by host cell kinases and the drug is active against HIV-1, including strains resistant to zidovudine. Lamivudine is also effective in hepatitis B, and HBV nucleic acid is undetectable after treatment for 12 weeks.
2. **Pharmacokinetics and clinical uses:** Lamivudine is used orally in HAART regimens for HIV and adjunctively with interferon alpha in HBV infection. Dosage adjustment is needed in patients with renal insufficiency.
3. **Toxicity:** Adverse effects of lamivudine are usually mild and include gastrointestinal distress, headache, insomnia, and fatigue.

E. Stavudine (d4T):

1. **Mechanisms:** Stavudine is a thymidine analog. Depending on specific sites of mutation on the reverse transcriptase gene, resistance may emerge to stavudine alone, or cross-resistance between other NRTIs may occur.
2. **Pharmacokinetics and clinical uses:** Stavudine is used in HAART regimens. The drug has good oral bioavailability and penetrates most tissues, including the CNS. Dosage adjustment is needed in renal insufficiency.
3. **Toxicity:** Peripheral neuropathy is dose-limiting.

F. Abacavir:

1. **Mechanisms:** Abacavir is a guanosine analog with mechanisms similar to those of other NRTIs.
2. **Pharmacokinetics and clinical uses:** There is good oral bioavailability, with metabolism via alcohol dehydrogenase and glucuronosyltransferase. Abacavir has been used in combinations with zidovudine and lamivudine.
3. **Toxicity:** Severe hypersensitivity reactions involving multiple organ systems may occur, occasionally with lethal outcome.

ANTI-HIV AGENTS: NONNUCLEOSIDE REVERSE TRANSCRIPTASE INHIBITORS (NNRTIs)

A. Mechanisms: NNRTIs bind to a site on reverse transcriptase different from the binding site of NRTIs. Nonnucleoside drugs do not require phosphorylation to be active and do not compete with nucleoside triphosphates. There is no cross-resistance with NRTIs. Resistance due to mutations in the *pol* gene occur very rapidly if these agents are used as monotherapy.

B. Nevirapine: Nevirapine is currently used in alternative combination regimens and is effective in preventing HIV vertical transmission when given as single doses to mothers at the onset of labor and to the neonate. Hypersensitivity reactions with nevirapine include Stevens-Johnson syndrome and a life-threatening toxic epidermal necrolysis. Nevirapine is metabolized by CYP3A4, and its blood levels are increased by cimetidine and macrolide antibiotics and decreased by enzyme inducers such as rifampin.

C. Delavirdine: Drug interactions are a major problem with delavirdine, which is metabolized by both CYP3A4 and CYP2D6. Its blood levels are decreased by antacids, ddI, phenytoin, rifampin, and nelfinavir. Conversely, the blood levels of delavirdine are increased by azole antifungals and macrolide antibiotics. Delavirdine increases plasma levels of several benzodiazepines, nifedipine, protease inhibitors, quinidine, and warfarin. Delavirdine causes skin rash in up to 20% of patients, and the drug should be avoided in pregnancy since it is teratogenic in animals.

D. Efavirenz: This NNRTI has been shown to be effective in HIV treatment when used in combination with two NRTIs. Efavirenz is metabolized by hepatic cytochromes P450 and is frequently involved in drug interactions. Toxicity of efavirenz includes CNS dysfunction, skin rash, and elevations of plasma cholesterol. The drug should be avoided in pregnancy since fetal abnormalities have been reported in animals.

ANTI-HIV AGENTS: PROTEASE INHIBITORS

A. Indinavir:

1. **Mechanisms:** Indinavir inhibits HIV-1 protease, an enzyme that cleaves viral precursor proteins and is critical to the production of mature infectious virions. The protease is encoded by the *pol* gene, and resistance to indinavir is mediated by multiple point mutations. Up to 70% of indinavir-resistant strains are cross-resistant with ritonavir.
2. **Pharmacokinetics and clinical use:** Oral bioavailability is good except in the presence of food. Clearance is mainly via the liver, with about 10% renal excretion. Like the other protease inhibitors, indinavir is used in drug combinations, most often with two NRTIs.
3. **Toxicity:** Nausea, diarrhea, thrombocytopenia, hyperbilirubinemia, and nephrolithiasis occur. To reduce renal damage, it is important to maintain good hydration. Indinavir is a substrate for and an inhibitor of the cytochrome P450 isoform CYP3A4 and is implicated in drug interactions. Serum levels of indinavir are increased by azole antifungals and decreased by rifamycins. Indinavir increases the serum levels of antihistamines, benzodiazepines, and rifampin.

B. Ritonavir:

1. **Mechanisms:** Mechanisms of action and resistance are quite similar to those of indinavir.
2. **Pharmacokinetics:** Oral bioavailability is good, and the drug should be taken with meals. Clearance is mainly via the liver, and dosage reduction is necessary in patients with hepatic impairment.
3. **Toxicity:** The most common adverse effects of the drug are gastrointestinal irritation and a bitter taste. Paresthesias and elevations of hepatic aminotransferases and triglycerides in the plasma also occur. Drugs that increase the activity of the cytochrome P450 isoform CYP3A4 (anticonvulsants, rifamycins) reduce serum levels of ritonavir, and drugs that inhibit this enzyme (azole antifungals, cimetidine, erythromycin) elevate serum levels of the antiviral drug. Ritonavir inhibits the metabolism of a wide range of drugs, including erythromycin, dronabinol, ketoconazole, prednisone, rifampin, and saquinavir.

C. Other Protease Inhibitors:

1. **Saquinavir:** Mechanisms of action and resistance of saquinavir are similar to those of the other protease inhibitors. The drug is usually taken with food to decrease gastrointestinal distress and to improve its oral bioavailability (10–15%). Saquinavir may cause headache and neutropenia. The drug is involved in many interactions. Saquinavir plasma levels are increased by azole antifungals, clarithromycin, grapefruit juice, indinavir, and ritonavir. Drugs that induce CYP3A4 decrease plasma levels of saquinavir.

2. **Nelfinavir:** This protease inhibitor is both an inducer and an inhibitor of hepatic cytochromes P450, so drug interactions are common. Its major adverse effect is a dose-limiting diarrhea.
3. **Amprenavir:** Amprenavir is a newer protease inhibitor that appears to be effective when used in combination with two NRTIs. It is an inhibitor of hepatic cytochromes P450. Skin rash occurs, in some cases leading to the Stevens-Johnson syndrome.

D. **Effects on Carbohydrate and Lipid Metabolism:** The use of protease inhibitors in HAART drug combinations has led to the development of disorders in carbohydrate and lipid metabolism. It has been suggested that this is due to the inhibition of lipid-regulating proteins which have active sites with structural homology to that of HIV protease. The syndrome includes hyperglycemia and insulin resistance or hyperlipidemia, with altered body fat distribution. Buffalo hump, gynecomastia, and truncal obesity may occur with facial and peripheral lipodystrophy. The syndrome has been observed with protease inhibitors used in HAART regimens, with an incidence of 30–50% and a median onset time of approximately 1 year's duration of treatment.

MISCELLANEOUS ANTIVIRAL AGENTS

A. **Amantadine and Rimantadine:**
1. **Mechanisms:** Amantadine and rimantadine inhibit the first steps in replication of the influenza A and rubella viruses (Figure 49–1). These steps involve viral adsorption to the host cell membrane, penetration into the cell via endocytosis, and viral particle uncapping. The inhibitory action of these drugs may be due to their alkaline reaction, which raises the endosomal pH. At low concentrations, amantadine also binds to a specific protein in the surface coat of the influenza virus to prevent fusion. Drug-resistant influenza A virus mutants can emerge and infect contacts of patients in treatment.
2. **Clinical uses and toxicity:** These drugs are prophylactic against influenza A virus infection with 80% efficacy. They can reduce the duration of symptoms if given within 48 hours after contact. Toxic effects include gastrointestinal irritation, dizziness, ataxia, and slurred speech. Rimantadine's activity is no greater than that of amantadine, but it has a longer half-life and requires no dosage adjustment in renal failure.

B. **Oseltamivir and Zanamivir:**
1. **Mechanisms:** These drugs are inhibitors of neuraminidase produced by influenza A and B. This viral enzyme cleaves sialic acid residues from viral proteins and surface proteins of infected cells, preventing clumping of newly released virions and sticking to cells that are already infected. By preventing these actions, neuraminidase inhibitors impede viral spread. Decreased susceptibility to the drugs is associated with mutations in viral neuraminidase.
2. **Clinical use and toxicity:** Oseltamivir is a prodrug used orally, activated in the gut and the liver. Zanamivir is administered intranasally. The drugs decrease the time to alleviation of influenza symptoms by a day or so and are more effective if used within 24 hours after onset of symptoms.

C. **Interferons:**
1. **Mechanisms:** Interferons are glycoproteins produced in human leukocytes (IFN-α), fibroblasts (IFN-β), and immune cells (IFN-γ). They exert multiple actions that affect viral RNA and DNA synthesis. Interferons induce the formation of enzymes, including a protein kinase that phosphorylates a factor which blocks peptide chain initiation, a phosphodiesterase that degrades terminal nucleotides of tRNA, and enzymes that activate RNase.
2. **Clinical use and toxicity:** Interferon alpha is approved for use in chronic hepatitis A and B infections, Kaposi's sarcoma, papillomatosis, and topically for genital warts. Another possible use of interferons is to prevent herpes zoster virus dissemination in cancer patients. Toxic effects include dose-limiting neutropenia, gastrointestinal irritation, fatigue, myalgia, mental confusion, and a reversible cardiomyopathy.

D. **Ribavirin:**
1. **Mechanisms:** Although the precise antiviral mechanism of ribavirin is not known, the

drug inhibits guanosine triphosphate formation, prevents capping of viral mRNA, and can block RNA-dependent RNA polymerases.

2. **Clinical use and toxicity:** Ribavirin is used in aerosol form for respiratory syncytial virus infections. Early intravenous administration decreases mortality in Lassa fever and other viral hemorrhagic fevers. Ribavirin has recently been shown to have efficacy in treatment of hepatitis C viral infections. Aerosol ribavirin may cause conjunctival or bronchial irritation. Systemic use results in dose-dependent myelosuppression. Ribavirin is a known human teratogen, absolutely contraindicated in pregnancy.

E. **Topical Antiviral Drugs:** Several antiviral agents with marked systemic toxicity (bone marrow, hepatic, renal) are used mainly as topical drugs for herpes simplex eye infections, including keratitis. These drugs include three antimetabolites: **idoxuridine, cytarabine,** and **trifluorothymidine.**

DRUG LIST

The following drugs are important members of the group discussed in this chapter. Prototypes should be learned in detail; features of the other significant agents should be known well enough to distinguish them from the prototypes and from each other.

Subclass	Prototype	Other Significant Agents
Antiherpes drugs		
Topical	Idoxuridine	Trifluridine
Systemic (HSV, VZV)	Acyclovir	Famciclovir, valacyclovir
Systemic (CMV)	Ganciclovir	Foscarnet, cidofovir
Anti-HIV drugs		
Nucleoside reverse transcriptase inhibitors	Zidovudine	Didanosine, lamivudine, stavudine, zalcitabine
Nonnucleoside reverse transcriptase inhibitors	Nevirapine	Delavirdine, efavirenz
Protease inhibitors	Indinavir	Amprenavir, nelfinavir, ritonavir, saquinavir
Anti-influenza drugs		
Inhibitors of viral uncoating	Amantadine	Rimantadine
Neuraminidase inhibitors	Zanamivir	Oseltamivir
Miscellaneous antiviral drugs	Interferons, ribavirin	

QUESTIONS

DIRECTIONS: Each of the numbered items or incomplete statements in this section is followed by answers or by completions of the statement. Select the ONE lettered answer or completion that is BEST in each case.

1. Which one of the following statements about the mechanisms of action of antiviral drugs is LEAST accurate?
   (A) The initial step in activation of famciclovir in HSV-infected cells is its phosphorylation by viral thymidine kinase
   (B) The reverse transcriptase of HIV is 30–50 times more sensitive to inhibition by indinavir than host cell DNA polymerases
   (C) Ganciclovir inhibits viral DNA polymerase but does not cause chain termination
   (D) Increased activity of host cell phosphodiesterases that degrade tRNA is one of the antiviral actions of interferons
   (E) Foscarnet has no requirement for activation by phosphorylation

Items 2–3: A 30-year-old male patient who is HIV-positive has a CD4 count of 500/μL and a viral RNA load of 5000/mL. His treatment involves a three-drug antiviral regimen consisting of zidovudine, didanosine, and ritonavir. Because of weight loss, he is taking dronabinol. Nystatin had been used for oral candidiasis, but for the past week the patient has been taking ketoconazole. He now complains of anorexia, nausea and vomiting, and abdominal pain. His abdomen is tender in the epigastric area. Laboratory results reveal an amylase activity of 220 units/L, and a preliminary diagnosis is made of acute pancreatitis.

2. If this patient has acute pancreatitis, the drug most likely to be responsible is
(A) Didanosine
(B) Dronabinol
(C) Ketoconazole
(D) Saquinavir
(E) Zidovudine

3. In the further treatment of this patient, the drug causing the pancreatitis should be withdrawn and replaced by
(A) Cidofovir
(B) Foscarnet
(C) Indinavir
(D) Ribavirin
(E) Zalcitabine

4. Which one of the following statements about antiviral agents is LEAST accurate?
(A) Interferons may prevent dissemination of herpes zoster in cancer patients and reduce CMV shedding after renal transplantation
(B) The oral absorption of acyclovir is slow and incomplete, but this process is not affected by foods
(C) Dosage modification of amantadine is required in renal insufficiency
(D) Peripheral neuropathy is the major dose-limiting toxic effect of ganciclovir
(E) Topical use of vidarabine requires caution during pregnancy because systemic absorption occurs, and the drug is potentially mutagenic and teratogenic

5. In an accidental needlestick, an unknown quantity of blood from an AIDS patient is injected into a nurse. The most recent laboratory report on the AIDS patient shows a CD4 count of 20/μL and a viral RNA load of greater than 10^7 copies/mL. The most appropriate course of action regarding treatment of the nurse is to
(A) Monitor the nurse's blood to see if HIV transmission has occurred
(B) Treat him with full doses of zidovudine for 2 weeks
(C) Treat him with full doses of zidovudine for 4 weeks
(D) Add acyclovir to the 4-week zidovudine regimen
(E) Administer zidovudine with lamivudine for 4 weeks

Items 6–7: A patient with AIDS has a CD4 count of 45/μL. He is being maintained on a three-drug regimen of indinavir, zalcitabine, and zidovudine. For prophylaxis against opportunistic infections, he is also receiving cidofovir, fluconazole, rifabutin, and trimethoprim-sulfamethoxazole.

6. The drug most likely to suppress herpetic infections in this patient and provide prophylaxis against CMV retinitis is
(A) Cidofovir
(B) Fluconazole
(C) Indinavir
(D) Rifabutin
(E) Zalcitabine

7. The plasma levels of indinavir in this patient will be considerably lower than those achieved if indinavir is given as the sole drug. The reason for this is that
(A) Cidofovir increases the renal clearance of other drugs
(B) Indinavir has to be taken with meals
(C) Rifabutin increases liver drug-metabolizing enzymes
(D) Sulfamethoxazole displaces indinavir from plasma proteins
(E) Zidovudine slows gastric emptying

8. Which of the following drugs is most likely to cause additive anemia and neutropenia if administered to an AIDS patient taking zidovudine?
(A) Acyclovir
(B) Amantadine
(C) Ganciclovir

(D) Pentamidine
(E) Stavudine

Items 9–10: A 27-year-old nursing mother is diagnosed as suffering from genital herpes. She has a prior history of this viral infection. Previously she responded to a drug used topically. Apart from her current problem, she is in good health.

9. Which of the following drugs is most likely to be prescribed at this time?
(A) Acyclovir
(B) Amantadine
(C) Foscarnet
(D) Ritonavir
(E) Trifluridine

10. Which one of the following statements about the drug management of genital herpes in this patient is LEAST accurate?
(A) Topical administration of the antiviral drug will provide minimal clinical benefit
(B) Oral use of the antiviral drug will reduce pain and shorten the duration of disease manifestations
(C) It is probably advisable to terminate use of the antiviral drug if she becomes pregnant
(D) Prompt intravenous treatment with the antiviral drug will prevent recurrent disease
(E) She should not breast-feed the infant while taking the antiviral drug

11. The antiviral actions of this drug include inhibition of both RNA and DNA synthesis. The drug is used for the treatment of severe respiratory syncytial virus infections in neonates.
(A) Amantadine
(B) Amprenavir
(C) Foscarnet
(D) Ribavirin
(E) Ritonavir

12. Regarding interferon alpha, which one of the following statements is LEAST accurate?
(A) At the start of treatment, most patients experience flu-like symptoms
(B) Indications include treatment of genital warts
(C) It is used in the management of hepatitis C
(D) Lamivudine interferes with its activity against hepatitis B
(E) Toxicity includes bone marrow suppression

13. Over 90% of this drug is excreted in the urine in intact form. Because its urinary solubility is low, patients should be well hydrated to prevent nephrotoxicity.
(A) Acyclovir
(B) Amantadine
(C) Indinavir
(D) Zanamivir
(E) Zidovudine

14. Used in the prophylaxis and treatment of infection due to influenza viruses, this drug facilitates clumping of mature virions and their adhesion to infected cells.
(A) Amantadine
(B) Efavirenz
(C) Oseltamivir
(D) Rimantadine
(E) Saquinavir

15. Which one of the following statements about stavudine is accurate?
(A) Bone marrow suppression is dose-limiting
(B) It causes marked neurotoxicity
(C) It inhibits HIV protease
(D) It is a nonnucleoside reverse transcriptase inhibitor
(E) Resistance occurs via mutations in the gene that codes for thymidine kinase

DIRECTIONS (Items 16–20): This case history is followed by discussion questions. Write out brief answers (two to five sentences) and then compare your answers with those given at the end of the Answers section.

A 28-year-old male patient with HIV infection who was being treated as an outpatient with zidovudine and didanosine came to an AIDS clinic with complaints of abdominal pain, nausea, and *vomiting. At his last visit, the CD4 count was > 500/μL and the viral load was < 500 vRNA copies/mL. Current laboratory data included amylase 240 units/L, creatinine 1 mg/dL, CD4 < 400/μL, and viral load > 5000 vRNA copies/mL. At this point the drug regimen was changed to zidovudine plus lamivudine.*

The patient's gastrointestinal symptoms diminished, but several months later the patient complained of feeling weak and presented with symptoms of thrush. At this time his CD4 count was 300/μL, viral load was 11,000 copies/mL, and a tuberculin skin test was positive. The attending physician prescribed clotrimazole troches, isoniazid plus pyridoxine, and indinavir to supplement the combination of zidovudine and lamivudine.

During the next few months, the viral load declined to 6000 vRNA copies/mL and then stabilized, but the CD4 count dropped to 150/μL, at which point two more agents were added to his drug regimen to prevent opportunistic infections. Unfortunately, the patient developed a gastric ulcer and had to be treated with bismuth subsalicylate, metronidazole, and tetracycline for Helicobacter pylori.

Ultimately the viral load of the patient began to increase, and when the CD4 count of the patient decreased to 40/μL three more drugs were prescribed. By this time, 11 drugs were being administered to slow disease progression and to manage or prevent opportunistic infections.

16. Why was didanosine discontinued and replaced by lamivudine when the patient complained of abdominal pain? What drug class do these anti-HIV agents represent?

17. What other antiretroviral drug classes are available for treatment of HIV infection? Is the initial treatment afforded this patient an example of highly active antiretroviral therapy (HAART)?

18. What type of drug is indinavir? What are its anticipated adverse effects?

19. Which prophylactic drugs were most likely to have been administered when the CD4 count dropped below 200/μL, and what infections might they prevent?

20. Which other drugs were likely to have been administered when the CD4 count dropped below 50/μL, and why might they be needed?

ANSWERS

1. Indinavir is an inhibitor of HIV protease and has no significant effect on reverse transcriptase. Note that initial monophosphorylation by viral thymidine kinase is not only a characteristic of the activation of acyclovir but also of its congeners famciclovir and valacyclovir. The answer is **(B)**.

2. Gastrointestinal problems occur with most antiviral drugs used in the HIV-positive patient, and acute pancreatitis has been reported for several reverse transcriptase inhibitors. However, didanosine is the drug most likely to be responsible, since its most characteristic adverse effect is a dose-limiting acute pancreatitis. Other risk factors that are relative contraindications to didanosine are advanced AIDS, hypertriglyceridemia, and alcoholism. The answer is **(A)**.

3. Cidofovir, foscarnet, and ribavirin have minimal activity against retroviruses and would not be useful components of a three-drug anti-HIV regimen. Use of a second protease inhibitor (indinavir) has not yet been shown to be as effective as regimens that include two reverse transcriptase inhibitors and will greatly increase the possibility of drug interactions. Standard HAART protocols include one NRTI from group A (zidovudine, stavudine) and one from group B (didanosine, lamivudine, zalcitabine). Since didanosine must be discontinued, zalcitabine would be the best choice for replacement in this case. The answer is **(E)**.

4. The adverse effects of ganciclovir are similar to those caused by radiation therapy. The major dose-limiting adverse effects—myelosuppression, gastrointestinal distress, and mucositis—occur commonly. The toxic effects of ganciclovir are enhanced by concomitant administration of other drugs that suppress bone marrow. The answer is **(D)**.

5. The viral RNA titer in the blood from the AIDS patient in this case is very high, and this needlestick must be considered as a high risk situation. While full doses of zidovudine for 4 weeks has been shown to have prophylactic value, in high-risk situations combination regimens are favored. Optimal prophylaxis in this case might best be provided by the combination of zidovudine with lamivudine (basic regimen), and some experts in the field would advise the further addition of a protease inhibitor (expanded regimen). The answer is **(E)**.

6. Foscarnet and ganciclovir have been the most commonly used drugs for prevention and treatment of CMV infections in the immunocompromised patient. Foscarnet has activity also against thymidine kinase-deficient strains of HSV. Cidofovir is very effective in CMV retinitis and has good activity against many strains of HSV, including those resistant to acyclovir. The answer is **(A).**

7. Drug interactions can be severe in the immunocompromised patient, since many of the drugs administered can influence the pharmacokinetic properties of other drugs. Rifabutin, like rifampin, acts as an inducer of several isoforms of hepatic cytochrome P450. This action can result in an increased clearance of other drugs, including indinavir, with negative effects on their effectiveness. Cidofovir is more likely to decrease the renal clearance of other drugs, since nephrotoxicity is dose-limiting. The answer is **(C).**
8. Like zidovudine, ganciclovir is myelosuppressant, and over 40% of patients who are treated with the drug as a single agent develop granulocytopenia or thrombocytopenia. When the two drugs are coadministered, there is a much higher incidence of anemia and neutropenia. Colony-stimulating factors may be needed if the two drugs must be given together. None of the other drugs listed have significant hematotoxicity. The answer is **(C).**
9. Three of the drugs listed (acyclovir, foscarnet, trifluridine) are active against strains of herpes simplex virus. Foscarnet is not used in genital infections (HSV-2) because clinical efficacy has not been established and the drug causes many toxic effects. Trifluridine is used topically, but only for herpes keratoconjunctivitis (HSV-1). The answer is **(A).**
10. First episodes of genital HSV usually respond to the topical use of acyclovir, but oral or parenteral administration is necessary to treat recurrent disease. Acyclovir treatment by any mode of administration does not eradicate latent herpes and will not prevent recurrence of the disease. Note that the drug is secreted in breast milk and—while there are no reports of human teratogenicity—acyclovir is a potential mutagen. The answer is **(D).**
11. The antiviral actions of ribavirin include inhibition of RNA polymerases, inhibition of DNA and RNA synthesis, and interference with viral coating. Ribavirin is used by aerosol inhalation for respiratory syncytial virus infections in premature infants and children with cardiopulmonary disease. The answer is **(D).**
12. Headache, fever, chills, and muscle aches are common side effects of treatment with interferons. Indications include hepatitis B and C, Kaposi's sarcoma, and human papilloma virus. Lamivudine has adjunctive value when used with interferon alpha in the treatment of hepatitis B. Interferons may also cause neurotoxicity, cardiovascular dysfunction, and bone marrow depression. The answer is **(D).**
13. Acyclovir is eliminated in the urine by glomerular filtration and by active tubular secretion, which is inhibited by probenecid. Nephrotoxic effects, including hematuria and crystalluria, are enhanced in patients who are dehydrated or who have preexisting renal dysfunction. Adequate hydration is equally important in the case of indinavir, since it causes nephrolithiasis. However, more than 80% of a dose of indinavir is eliminated via hepatic metabolism. The answer is **(A).**
14. Oseltamivir and zanamivir (not listed) are inhibitors of neuraminidase produced by influenza A and B. They prevent the trimming of sialic acid residues from viral proteins, facilitating their clumping and adhesion to host cells that are already infected. The answer is **(C).**
15. Stavudine (d4T) is a nucleoside reverse transcriptase inhibitor. While it has only minor hematotoxic potential, the drug is markedly neurotoxic, causing dose-limiting peripheral neuropathy. Resistance occurs via mutations in the *pol* gene, which encodes for several proteins including reverse transcriptase. The answer is **(B).**
16. In the initial management of this patient, two nucleoside reverse transcriptase inhibitors (NRTIs) were administered. Hematologic suppression is a major adverse effect of zidovudine, while peripheral neuropathy and pancreatitis are important toxicities of didanosine. The gastrointestinal symptoms, together with the elevated amylase levels, were the reasons for discontinuance of didanosine and the substitution of another nucleoside reverse transcriptase inhibitor (lamivudine) in the drug regimen. See answer to question 3, above.
17. In addition to NRTIs, the two other important classes of antiretroviral drugs available are the protease inhibitors and the nonnucleoside reverse transcriptase inhibitors (NNRTIs). Most authorities recommend initiation of antiretroviral therapy in treatment-naive patients with viral RNA loads above 10,000 copies/mL even if the CD4 cell count is normal. Preferred highly active antiretroviral therapy (HAART) combines one drug from the class of protease inhibitors with two NRTIs. Alternatively, one NNRTI may be combined with two NRTIs.
18. The availability of quantitative measures of viral RNA permits direct measurement and monitoring of antiviral drug effects. Since the viral load was increasing despite the administration of two NRTIs, a protease inhibitor (indinavir) was added to the anti-HIV drug regimen. The

adverse effects of indinavir include kidney stones (which may be diminished by full hydration), hyperbilirubinemia, and drug interactions due to inhibition of hepatic cytochrome P450.

19. When the CD4 count of this patient fell below 200/μL, prophylaxis against pneumocystis pneumonia was instituted. The currently recommended therapy is double-strength trimethoprim-sulfamethoxazole or dapsone. Alternative prophylactic regimens include aerosolic pentamidine, dapsone plus pyrimethamine, and atovaquone. Primary prophylaxis against toxoplasmosis is normally recommended with CD4 cell counts below 100/μL in AIDS patients who are IgG antibody-positive. Trimethoprim-sulfamethoxazole plus dapsone is also prophylactic against toxoplasmosis. With the continued decline in CD4 cells, exacerbation of candidal infection may occur despite use of clotrimazole troches, necessitating treatment with fluconazole or itraconazole.

20. When the CD4 count of an HIV patient falls below 50/μL, there are several possible drug scenarios. Prophylaxis is recommended against *M avium-intracellulare* with azithromycin or clarithromycin. In the event of infection, the recommended treatment regimen is clarithromycin plus ethambutol plus rifabutin. Ganciclovir (or foscarnet) may be given prophylactically if the patient is seropositive for CMV or for treatment if he develops retinitis. Note that in many AIDS patients, HAART is effective in suppressing CMV viremia without specific CMV therapy. Finally, the disease progression in this particular patient raises the possibility of the need for drug treatment of tubercular disease or of infections caused by other opportunistic pathogens.

Miscellaneous Antimicrobial Agents & Urinary Antiseptics 50

OBJECTIVES

You should be able to:

- Describe the antibacterial actions, clinical uses and toxicities of metronidazole, mupirocin, and polymyxins.
- Identify nitrofurantoin, methenamine, and nalidixic acid as urinary antiseptics and describe their toxic effects.
- List the compounds used as antiseptics and disinfectants and describe their advantages and disadvantages.

Learn the definitions that follow.

Table 50–1. Definitions.

Term	Definition
Antiseptic	An agent used to inhibit bacterial growth in vitro and in vivo
Disinfectant	An agent used to kill microorganisms in an inanimate environment
Sterilization	Procedures that kill microorganisms on instruments and dressings; methods include autoclaving, dry heat, and exposure to ethylene oxide
Chlorine demand	The amount of chlorine bound to organic matter in water and thus unavailable for antimicrobial activity

MISCELLANEOUS ANTIMICROBIAL AGENTS

A. Metronidazole:

1. **Mechanisms:** Metronidazole is an imidazole derivative with activity against protozoa and bacteria. The drug undergoes a reductive bioactivation of its nitro group by ferredoxin (present in anaerobic parasites) to form reactive cytotoxic products that interfere with nucleic acid synthesis.
2. **Pharmacokinetics:** Metronidazole is effective orally and is distributed widely to tissues, achieving CSF levels similar to those in the blood. The drug can also be given intravenously and is available in topical formulations. Elimination of metronidazole requires hepatic metabolism and dosage reduction may be needed in patients with liver dysfunction.
3. **Clinical use:** As an antibacterial agent, metronidazole has greatest activity against bacteroides and clostridia. It is the drug of choice for treatment of pseudomembranous colitis due to *C difficile* and is effective in anaerobic or mixed intra-abdominal infections and in brain abscess. Metronidazole is also used for infections involving *Gardnerella vaginalis* and in regimens for the eradication of *Helicobacter pylori* in gastric ulcers. As an antiprotozoal drug, metronidazole is the drug of choice in trichomoniasis and in the treatment of intestinal amebiasis and amebic hepatic abscess.
4. **Toxicity:** Adverse effects include gastrointestinal irritation, headache, and dark coloration of urine. More serious toxicity includes leukopenia, dizziness, and ataxia. Drug interactions with metronidazole include a disulfiram-like reaction with ethanol and potentiation of coumarin anticoagulant effects. Although it is not contraindicated in pregnancy, the drug should be used with caution.

B. Mupirocin:

1. **Mechanisms:** Mupirocin is a fermentation product of *Pseudomonas fluorescens* and is unrelated to any other antimicrobial drug. It acts on gram-positive cocci and inhibits protein synthesis by specifically binding to isoleucyl-tRNA synthetase.
2. **Pharmacokinetics and clinical use:** Mupirocin is used topically and is not absorbed. This drug is indicated for impetigo caused by staphylococci (including methicillin-resistant strains), beta-hemolytic streptococci, and *Streptococcus pyogenes*. It is also used intranasally to eliminate staphylococcal carriage by patients and medical personnel.
3. **Toxicity:** Local itching and burning sensations are common. Mupirocin may also cause rash, erythema, and contact dermatitis.

C. Polymyxins:

1. **Mechanisms:** The polymyxins are polypeptides that are bactericidal against gram-negative bacteria. These drugs interact with a specific lipopolysaccharide component of the outer cell membrane that is also a binding site for calcium. Membrane lipid structure is distorted, with an increase in permeability to polar molecules, resulting in marked changes in cell metabolism.
2. **Clinical use:** Because of toxicity, the clinical applications of the polymyxins are limited to topical therapy of resistant gram-negative infections, including those caused by enterobacter and pseudomonas. These drugs are occasionally administered into infected cavities, eg, the joints and the pleural and peritoneal cavities.
3. **Toxicity:** If absorbed into the systemic circulation, adverse effects include neurotoxicity (paresthesias, dizziness, ataxia) and acute renal tubular necrosis (hematuria, proteinuria, nitrogen retention).

URINARY ANTISEPTICS

Urinary antiseptics are oral drugs that are rapidly excreted into the urine and act there to suppress bacteriuria. The drugs lack systemic antibacterial effects but may be toxic. Urinary antiseptics are often administered with acidifying agents, because low pH is an independent inhibitor of bacterial growth in urine.

A. Nitrofurantoin: This drug is active against many urinary tract pathogens (but not proteus or pseudomonas), and resistance emerges slowly. Single daily doses of the drug can prevent recurrent urinary tract infections. The drug is active orally and is excreted in the urine via filtration and secretion; toxic levels may occur in the blood of patients with renal dysfunction. Adverse effects of nitrofurantoin include gastrointestinal irritation, skin rashes, phototoxicity, neuropathies, and hemolysis in patients with glucose-6-phosphate dehydrogenase deficiency.

B. Nalidixic Acid: This quinolone drug acts against many gram-negative organisms (but not proteus or pseudomonas) by mechanisms that may involve acidification or inhibition of DNA gyrase. Resistance emerges rapidly. The drug is active orally and is excreted in the urine partly unchanged and partly as the inactive glucuronide. Toxic effects include gastrointestinal irritation, glycosuria, skin rashes, phototoxicity, visual disturbances, and CNS stimulation.

C. Methenamine: Methenamine mandelate and methenamine hippurate combine urine acidification with the release of the antibacterial compound formaldehyde at pH levels below 5.5. These drugs are not usually active against proteus because those organisms alkalinize the urine. Insoluble complexes form between formaldehyde and sulfonamides, and the drugs should not be used together.

DISINFECTANTS & ANTISEPTICS

Although the terms are often used interchangeably, a **disinfectant** is a compound that is used to kill microorganisms in an inanimate environment, whereas an **antiseptic** is one that is used to inhibit bacterial growth both in vitro and in contact with the surfaces of living tissues. Disinfectants and antiseptics do not have selective toxicity, and their clinical use is therefore limited. Most antiseptics delay wound healing.

A. Alcohols, Aldehydes, and Acids: **Ethanol** (70%) and **isopropanol** (70–90%) are effective skin antiseptics because they denature microbial proteins. **Formaldehyde,** which also denatures proteins, is too irritating for topical use but is a disinfectant for instruments. **Acetic acid** (1%) is used in surgical dressings and has activity against gram-negative bacteria, including pseudomonas, when used as a urinary irrigant and in the external ear. **Salicylic acid** and **undecylenic acid** are useful in the treatment of dermatophyte infections.

B. Halogens: **Iodine tincture** is an effective antiseptic for intact skin and, although it can cause dermatitis, is commonly used in preparing the skin before taking blood samples. Iodine complexed with povidone **(povidone-iodine)** is widely used, particularly as a preoperative skin antiseptic, but solutions can become contaminated with aerobic gram-negative bacteria.

Hypochlorous acid, formed when **chlorine** dissolves in water, is antimicrobial. This is the basis for the use of chlorine and **halazone** in water purification. Organic matter binds chlorine, thus preventing antimicrobial actions. In a given water sample, this process is referred to as the **"chlorine demand,"** since the chlorine-binding capacity of the organic material must be exceeded before bacterial killing is accomplished. Many preparations of chlorine for water purification do not eradicate all bacteria or entamoeba cysts.

Sodium hypochlorite is the active component in household bleach, a 1:10 dilution of which is recommended by the Centers for Disease Control and Prevention for the disinfection of blood spills that may contain HIV or hepatitis B virus (HBV).

C. Oxidizing Agents: **Hydrogen peroxide** exerts a short-lived antimicrobial action through the release of molecular oxygen. The agent is used as a mouthwash, for cleansing wounds, and for disinfection of contact lenses. **Potassium permanganate** is an effective bactericidal agent but has the disadvantage of causing persistent brown stains on skin and clothing.

D. Heavy Metals: **Mercury** and **silver** precipitate proteins and inactivate sulfhydryl groups of enzymes but are used rarely because of toxicity. Organic mercurials such as **nitromersol** and **thimerosal** frequently cause hypersensitivity reactions but continue to be used as preservatives for vaccines, antitoxins, and immune sera. **Merbromin** is a weak antiseptic and stains tissues a bright red color. In the past **silver nitrate** was commonly used for prevention of neonatal gonococcal ophthalmia, but it has been largely replaced by topical antibiotics. **Silver sulfadiazine** (a sulfonamide) is used to decrease bacterial colonization in burns.

E. Chlorinated Phenols: Owing to its toxicity **phenol** itself is used only as a disinfectant of inanimate objects. Mixtures of phenolic derivatives are used in antiseptics but can cause skin irritation. **Hexachlorophene** has been widely used in surgical scrub routines and in deodorant soaps, where it forms antibacterial deposits on the skin, decreasing the population of resident bacteria. Repeated use on the skin in infants can lead to absorption of the drug, resulting in CNS white matter degeneration. Antiseptic soaps may also contain other chlorinated phenols such as **triclocarban** and **chlorhexidine.** Chlorhexidine is mainly active against gram-positive cocci and is commonly used in hospital scrub routines to cleanse skin sites. All antiseptic soaps may cause allergies or photosensitization.

Lindane (gamma benzene hexachloride) is used to treat infestations with mites or lice and also as an agricultural insecticide. The agent can be absorbed through the skin; if excessive amounts are applied, toxic effects, including blood dyscrasias and convulsions, may occur.

F. Cationic Surfactants: **Benzalkonium chloride** and **cetylpyridinium chloride** are used as disinfectants of surgical instruments and surfaces such as floors and benchtops. Since they are effective against most bacteria and fungi and are not irritating, they are also used as antiseptics. However, when used on the skin, the antimicrobial action of these agents is antagonized by soaps and multivalent cations. The CDC has recommended that benzalkonium chloride and similar quaternary compounds *not* be used as antiseptics because outbreaks of infection have resulted from growth of gram-negative bacteria (eg, pseudomonas) in such antiseptic solutions.

DRUG LIST

The following drugs are important members of the group discussed in this chapter. Prototypes should be learned in detail; features of the major variants should be known well enough to distinguish the variants from prototypes and from each other.

Subclass	Prototype	Major Variants
Miscellaneous antimicrobials		
Nitroimidazole	Metronidazole	
Pseudomonic acid	Mupirocin	
Basic peptides	Polymyxin B	Polymyxin E
Urinary tract antiseptics		
Quinolones	Nalidixic acid	Cinoxacin
Methenamine salts	Methenamine mandelate	Methenamine hippurate
Nitrofurans	Nitrofurantoin	
Disinfectants and antiseptics		
Alcohols, aldehydes, and acids	Ethanol, formaldehyde, acetic acid	Isopropanol, glutaraldehyde, salicylic acid
Halogens	Iodine, chlorine	Povidone-iodine, halazone, sodium hypochlorite (household bleach)
Heavy metals	Silver nitrate, mercury bichloride	Silver sulfadiazine, nitromersol, thimerosal
Chlorinated phenols	Hexachlorophene	Triclocarban, chlorhexidine
Cationic surfactants	Benzalkonium chloride	Cetylpyridinium chloride

QUESTIONS

DIRECTIONS: Each of the numbered items or incomplete statements in this section is followed by answers or by completions of the statement. Select the ONE lettered answer or completion that is BEST in each case.

1. Infections due to gram-negative bacilli have occurred when this agent has been used as a skin antiseptic.

(A) Acetic acid

(B) Benzalkonium chloride
(C) Hexachlorophene
(D) Merbromin
(E) Thimerosal

Items 2–3: A young woman is brought to a hospital emergency room with intense abdominal pain of 2 days' duration. The pain has spread to the right lower quadrant and is accompanied by nausea, vomiting and fever. In the emergency room her blood pressure is 85/45, pulse 120/min, and temperature 40 °C. Her abdomen has a board-like rigidity with diffuse pain to palpation. Laboratory values include: WBC 20,000/μL and creatinine 1.5 mg/dL. Following abdominal x-rays, a preliminary diagnosis is made of abdominal sepsis, possibly due to bowel perforation. After appropriate samples are sent to the laboratory for culture, the patient is hospitalized and antimicrobial therapy is started with intravenous ampicillin and gentamicin.

2. Regarding the treatment of this patient which one of the following statements is most accurate?
(A) Cultures are pointless, since this is probably a mixed infection
(B) A Gram stain of the blood would provide positive identification of the specific organism involved in this infection
(C) A drug active against anaerobes should be included in the antibiotic regimen
(D) Empiric antimicrobial therapy of abdominal sepsis should always include a third-generation cephalosporin
(E) The combination of ampicillin and gentamicin provides good coverage for all likely pathogens

3. If the antibiotic regimen in this patient is modified to include metronidazole
(A) The patient should be monitored for candidiasis
(B) Gentamicin should be excluded from the regimen
(C) Metronidazole should not be used intravenously
(D) Ampicillin should be excluded from the regimen
(E) Coverage will be extended to methicillin-resistant staphylococci

4. Which one of the following compounds is used topically to treat scabies and pediculosis?
(A) Lindane
(B) Mupirocin
(C) Nitrofurazone
(D) Polymyxin B
(E) Silver sulfadiazine

5. Methenamine salts are used as urinary antiseptics. The reason why they lack systemic antibacterial action is that they are
(A) Not absorbed into the systemic circulation following oral ingestion
(B) Rapidly metabolized by liver drug-metabolizing enzymes
(C) Converted to formaldehyde only at low urinary pH
(D) Substrates for active tubular secretion
(E) Over 98% bound to plasma proteins

6. Which one of the following statements about the actions of antimicrobial agents is LEAST accurate?
(A) Polymyxins act as cationic detergents to disrupt bacterial cell membranes
(B) Resistance to nitrofurantoin emerges rapidly, and there is cross-resistance with sulfonamides
(C) Salicylic acid has useful antidermatophyte activity when applied topically
(D) Neonatal gonococcal ophthalmia can be prevented by silver nitrate
(E) Isoleucyl tRNA synthetase is inhibited by mupirocin

7. Which one of the following antiseptics *promotes* wound healing?
(A) Cetylpyridium chloride
(B) Chlorhexidine
(C) Hexachlorophene
(D) Iodine
(E) None of the above

8. A 22-year-old man with gonorrhea is to be treated with cefixime and will need another drug to provide coverage for possible urethritis due to *C trachomatis.* Which one of the following drugs is LEAST likely to be effective in nongonococcal urethritis?
(A) Azithromycin
(B) Ciprofloxacin

(C) Erythromycin
(D) Nitrofurantoin
(E) Tetracycline

9. A patient with AIDS has an extremely high viral RNA titer. While blood is being drawn from this patient, the syringe is accidentally dropped, contaminating the floor, which is made of porous material. The best way to deal with this is to
(A) Completely replace the contaminated part of the floor
(B) Clean the floor with soap and water
(C) Seal the room and decontaminate with ethylene oxide
(D) Clean the floor with a 10% solution of household bleach
(E) Neutralize the spill with a solution of potassium permanganate

DIRECTIONS (Items 10–16): The matching questions in this section consist of a list of lettered options followed by several numbered items. For each numbered item, select the ONE lettered option that is most closely associated with it. Each lettered option may be selected once, more than once, or not at all.

(A) Benzalkonium chloride
(B) Chlorhexidine
(C) Formaldehyde
(D) Halazone
(E) Hexachlorophene
(F) Methenamine
(G) Metronidazole
(H) Nalidixic acid
(I) Nitrofurantoin
(J) Polymyxin B
(K) Salicylic acid

10. This compound is used in tablet form to purify drinking water. If a large quantity of organic material is present, cysts of *Entamoeba histolytica* may not be eradicated.

11. This agent has activity against gram-negative bacteria in urinary tract infections, but resistance may develop during the course of treatment. There is cross-resistance with cinoxacin. The drug has no useful systemic antibacterial effects.

12. Daily use of this substituted phenol results in a bacteriostatic deposit on the skin. The compound may be absorbed and has caused neurotoxic effects in neonates when used as an antistaphylococcal agent.

13. Neuropathies are more likely to occur with this agent when it is used in patients with renal dysfunction. The drug may cause acute hemolysis in patients with G6PD deficiency.

14. This agent is commonly incorporated into soaps used for skin antisepsis and surgical scrub procedures. The compound has minimal activity against pseudomonas and serratia.

15. A urinary antiseptic, this agent is not effective in the treatment of urinary tract infections caused by proteus. Mutual antagonism may occur if this drug is used concomitantly with sulfonamides.

16. Consumption of ethanol together with this drug will cause nausea, vomiting, abdominal cramps, flushing and headache in some patients.

DIRECTIONS (Items 17–20): This case history* is followed by discussion questions. Write out brief answers (two to five sentences) and then compare your answers with those given at the end of the Answers section.

After returning from a trip to Mexico, a 41-year-old woman residing in New York had a week-long bout of diarrhea that resolved spontaneously. She did not feel well for the next 4 months, and abdominal discomfort then became severe, and fever (without bowel symptoms) occurred. There was no history of jaundice, gallstones, or hepatitis, but acute cholecystitis was suspected; the patient was admitted to the hospital for what proved to be a normal oral cholecystogram.

Following the x-ray studies, diarrhea occurred again. She was referred to another institution and

* Modified and reproduced, with permission, from Strum WB: Persistent pain, fever after a trip to Mexico. Hosp Pract (Off Ed) 1984 Oct;19:86.

was initially treated with metronidazole, ampicillin, and gentamicin for presumed amebic liver abscesses or acute cholecystitis with liver abscesses. Subsequently, a serologic test for amebic infection was positive, and liver and spleen scans confirmed the presence of abscesses. Based on these findings, gentamicin and ampicillin were discontinued.

The patient's symptoms improved with a 10-day course of oral metronidazole and tetracycline. She became afebrile, and serologic tests for amebic infection reverted to negative. Oral iodoquinol was given for 3 weeks, and follow-up examinations showed resolution of the abscess cavities and no recurrence of symptoms.

17. What are the most likely causes of diarrhea in a tourist following a trip to a Central American country? Should such cases of traveler's diarrhea be routinely treated with antibiotics?

18. What antimicrobial activity is anticipated for ampicillin and gentamicin as used in this case?

19. Why was metronidazole treatment continued after discontinuance of the above antibiotics? What does tetracycline add to the therapeutic regimen?

20. What was the rationale for the 3 weeks of oral treatment with iodoquinol?

ANSWERS

1. Pseudomonas and other gram-negative bacteria have caused infections following the use of cationic surfactants, partly because they form a film on the skin under which microorganisms can survive. In addition, some gram-negative bacilli are able to grow in solutions containing benzalkonium salts. Bacterial growth may also occur in solutions of povidone-iodine. The answer is **(B).**

2. Abdominal sepsis is commonly a mixed infection with the most likely pathogens being *Bacteroides fragilis*, Enterobacteriaceae, and *Enterococcus faecalis.* An antibiotic regimen that includes only ampicillin and gentamicin will not control *B fragilis.* Empiric treatment in this case should include a drug active against this pathogen—eg, metronidazole, cefoxitin, cefotetan, clindamycin, or imipenem. The answer is **(C).**

3. Fungal superinfections, especially from *Candida albicans,* occur quite frequently during treatment with metronidazole. In most cases of abdominal sepsis metronidazole would be given by slow intravenous infusion. Both ampicillin and gentamicin should be maintained until the infection is controlled, at which time surgery is indicated. Metronidazole has no activity against aerobes. The combination of ampicillin, gentamicin, and metronidazole does not provide coverage for methicillin-resistant staphylococci. The answer is **(A).**

4. Of the agents listed, only lindane is an effective scabicide and pediculicide. There is some concern about the systemic absorption of topically applied lindane, which may cause neurotoxicity. Accidental ingestion in children has caused seizures. The answer is **(A).**

5. Below pH 5.5, methenamine releases formaldehyde, which is antibacterial. This pH is achieved in the urine but nowhere else in the body. Ascorbic acid is sometimes given with methenamine salts to ensure a low urinary pH. The answer is **(C).**

6. Clinical drug resistance emerges very slowly when nitrofurantoin is used as a urinary antiseptic. There is no cross-resistance between the drug and other drugs used in the treatment of bacterial infections of the urinary tract. The answer is **(B).**

7. No antiseptic in current use is able to promote wound healing, and most agents do the opposite. In general, cleansing of abrasions and superficial wounds with soap and water is just as effective as and less damaging than the application of topical antiseptics. The answer is **(E).**

8. Urinary tract infections due to *C trachomatis* are likely to respond to all of the drugs listed except nitrofurantoin. However, nitrofurantoin is effective against many bacterial urinary tract pathogens with the exception of *Pseudomonas aeruginosa* and strains of proteus. The answer is **(D).**

9. Household bleach contains sodium hypochlorite. A 1:10 dilution of bleach is effective for disinfection of a direct blood spill on a porous surface. In addition to inactivating HIV, sodium hypochlorite solutions have disinfectant activity against other viruses including hepatitis B virus. The answer is **(D).**

10. The addition of 4–8 mg of halazone per liter will sterilize most water samples in about 30 minutes but will not kill cysts of *Entamoeba histolytica*. The answer is **(D).**

11. Nalidixic acid, a quinolone, is structurally related to cinoxacin. Both drugs are used in the treatment of urinary tract infections, and cross-resistance may occur. Quinolone derivatives may lower seizure threshold in susceptible individuals. The answer is **(H).**

12. Repeated bathing of newborns with hexachlorophene to prevent staphylococcal colonization may permit systemic absorption, which leads to neurotoxic effects (eg, spongiform degeneration of white matter). The answer is **(E).**
13. Acute hemolytic reactions in G6PD deficiency occur with drugs that are oxidizing agents, including antimalarials, nalidixic acid, sulfonamides, and the nitrofurans. Severe polyneuropathies, with both motor and sensory nerve degeneration, may occur with nitrofurantoin. These reactions are more likely to occur in patients with renal dysfunction. The answer is **(I).**
14. Chlorhexidine is a biguanide that disrupts bacterial cytoplasmic membranes, especially of gram-positive organisms. The agent is less effective against pseudomonas and serratia. Hospital uses include hand-washing, wound cleansing, and preparation of skin sites for operative procedures. The answer is **(B).**
15. The activity of methenamine as a urinary antiseptic is mainly due to the release of formaldehyde at acidic pH. Sulfonamides may form insoluble complexes with formaldehyde, resulting in mutual antagonism. Proteus organisms alkalinize the urine, preventing the release of formaldehyde. The answer is **(F).**
16. Metronidazole inhibits aldehyde dehydrogenase and may cause a disulfiram-like reaction in patients who consume alcoholic beverages while taking the drug. The answer is **(G).**
17. The most common causes of traveler's diarrhea are infections due to coliform bacteria and viruses. Most such infections are self-limiting, and fluid and electrolyte replacement is usually adequate treatment. Antibiotics (eg, doxycycline, trimethoprim-sulfamethoxazole) are useful prophylactic agents against such organisms but are ineffective in gastrointestinal infections due to viruses and only minimally effective against intestinal protozoans.
18. Ampicillin and gentamicin were included in the drug regimen on the basis of a possible bacterial involvement in acute cholecystitis, a component of the initial clinical diagnosis. Neither drug is active against amebic infection. Ampicillin would provide coverage for streptococci (including enterococci) and selected gram-negative enteric organisms, and gentamicin is active against aerobic gram-negative rods. Neither drug has good activity against gram-negative anaerobes, and anaerobic bacteria are a major cause of bacterial liver abscess.
19. The confirmed diagnosis of amebic disease justified therapy with metronidazole, which is effective in most cases of extraluminal amebiasis. Oral tetracycline is an inhibitor of bacteria that are associated with *Entamoeba histolytica* in the gut.
20. Iodoquinol (and diloxanide furoate) are not effective in severe intestinal amebiasis or in amebic hepatic abscess. These drugs are used in asymptomatic intestinal amebiasis, to treat concurrent intestinal infection, and to totally eradicate the protozoan to prevent disease recurrence (see Chapter 53).

Clinical Use of Antimicrobials

51

OBJECTIVES

You should be able to:

- List the steps that should be taken prior to the initiation of empiric antimicrobial therapy.
- Describe the importance of susceptibility testing and analyses of serum drug levels or bactericidal titers in antimicrobial chemotherapy.
- Identify the antimicrobial drugs that require major modifications of dosage when renal or hepatic function change, or when dialysis is used.
- List the reasons for use of antimicrobial drugs in combination and the probable mechanisms involved in drug synergy.
- Describe the principles underlying valid antimicrobial chemoprophylaxis and give examples of commonly used surgical and nonsurgical prophylaxis.

Learn the definitions that follow.

Table 51–1. Definitions.

Term	Definition
Antimicrobial prophylaxis	The use of antimicrobial drugs to decrease the risk of infection
Combination antimicrobial drug therapy	The use of two or more drugs together to increase efficacy more than can be accomplished with the use of a single agent
Empiric (presumptive) antimicrobial therapy	Initiation of drug treatment prior to identification of a specific pathogen
Minimum inhibitory concentration (MIC)	An estimate of the drug sensitivity of pathogens for comparison with anticipated levels in blood or tissues
Postantibiotic effect	Antibacterial effect that persists after drug concentration falls below the minimum inhibitory concentration
Susceptibility testing	Laboratory methods to determine the sensitivity of the isolated pathogen to antimicrobial drugs

CONCEPTS

A. **Guidelines for Antimicrobial Therapy:** Empiric antimicrobial therapy is antimicrobial therapy that is begun before a specific pathogen has been identified and is based on the presumption of an infection that requires immediate drug treatment. Prior to initiation of such therapy, accepted practice involves making a clinical diagnosis of microbial infection, obtaining specimens for laboratory analyses, making a microbiologic diagnosis, deciding whether treatment should precede the results of laboratory tests, and, finally, selecting the optimal drug or drugs. A variety of publications provide annually updated lists of antimicrobial drugs of choice for specific pathogens. Such lists can provide a useful guide to empiric therapy based on presumptive microbiologic diagnosis. Table 51–2 sets forth the current drugs of choice and alternative agents for various common pathogens.

B. **Principles of Antimicrobial Therapy:** Antimicrobial therapy in established infections is guided by the following principles:

1. **Susceptibility testing:** The results of susceptibility testing establish the drug sensitivity of the organism. These results usually predict the **minimum inhibitory concentrations**

Table 51–2. Examples of empiric antimicrobial therapy based on microbiologic etiology.

Pathogen	Drugs of First Choice	Alternative Drugs
Gram-positive cocci		
Pneumococcus	Penicillin G, ampicillin, if susceptible, otherwise vancomycin ± rifampin	Cephalosporin, fluoroquinolone, macrolide
Streptococcus (common)	Penicillin G, ampicillin	Cephalosporin, macrolide
Staphylococcus (penicillinase-producing)	Penicillinase-resistant penicillin	Cephalosporin, vancomycin, macrolide
Staphylococcus (methicillin-resistant)	Vancomycin	TMP-SMZ. VRSA[1]: linezolid or streptogramin
Enterococcus faecalis	Penicillin G plus gentamicin	Vancomycin plus gentamicin
Gram-negative cocci		
Gonococcus	Ceftriaxone, cefixime	Ciprofloxacin, ofloxacin, spectinomycin
Meningococcus	Penicillin G, ampicillin	Cefotaxime, cefuroxime, chloramphenicol
Gram-negative rods		
E coli, proteus, klebsiella	Cephalosporin, fluoroquinolone, TMP-SMZ	Aminoglycoside, extended-spectrum penicillin
Shigella and salmonella	Fluoroquinolone	TMP-SMZ, ampicillin, third-generation cephalosporin
Enterobacter, citrobacter, serratia	Imipenem, TMP-SMZ, fluoroquinolone	Extended-spectrum penicillin, aminoglycoside
Haemophilus	Cefuroxime or third-generation cephalosporin	TMP-SMZ, ampicillin, chloramphenicol
Pseudomonas aeruginosa	Aminoglycoside plus extended-spectrum penicillin	Ceftazidime, aztreonam, imipenem
Bacteroides fragilis	Metronidazole, clindamycin	Imipenem, cefotetan or cefoxitin, chloramphenicol, ampicillin-sulbactam
Miscellaneous		
Mycoplasma pneumoniae	Macrolide or fluoroquinolone	Doxycycline
Treponema pallidum	Penicillin G	Erythromycin, tetracycline

[1]Vancomycin-resistant Staphylococcus aureus

(MICs) of a drug for comparison with anticipated blood or tissue levels. The two most common methods of susceptibility testing are disk diffusion (Kirby-Bauer) and broth dilution. For some bacteria (eg, gonococci, enterococci, *H influenzae*), a direct test for beta-lactamase can be substituted, since susceptibility patterns are identical for all strains except for the production of beta-lactamase.

2. **Drug concentration in blood:** The measurement of drug concentration in the blood may be appropriate when using agents with a low therapeutic index (eg, aminoglycosides, vancomycin) and when investigating poor clinical response to a drug treatment regimen.
3. **Serum bactericidal titers:** In certain infections in which host defenses may contribute minimally to cure, the estimation of serum bactericidal titers can confirm the appropriateness of choice of drug and dosage. Serial dilutions of serum are incubated with standardized quantities of the pathogen isolated from the patient; killing at a dilution of 1:8 is generally considered satisfactory.
4. **Route of administration:** Parenteral therapy is preferred in most cases of serious microbial infections. Chloramphenicol, the fluoroquinolones, and trimethoprim-sulfamethoxazole (TMP-SMZ) may be effective orally.
5. **Monitoring of therapeutic response:** Therapeutic responses to drug therapy should be monitored clinically and microbiologically to detect the development of resistance or superinfections. The duration of drug therapy required depends on the pathogen (eg, longer courses of therapy are required for infections due to fungi or mycobacteria), the site of infection (eg, endocarditis and osteomyelitis require longer duration of treatment), and the immunocompetence of the patient.
6. **Clinical failure of antimicrobial therapy:** Inadequate clinical or microbiologic response to antimicrobial therapy can result from laboratory testing errors, problems with the drug

(eg, incorrect choice, poor tissue penetration, inadequate dose), the patient (poor host defenses, undrained abscesses), or the pathogen (resistance, superinfection).

C. Factors Influencing Antimicrobial Drug Use:

1. **Bactericidal versus bacteriostatic actions:** Antibiotics classified as bacteriostatic include clindamycin, macrolides, sulfonamides, and tetracyclines. For bacteriostatic drugs, the concentrations that inhibit growth are much lower than those which kill bacteria. Antibiotics classified as bactericidal include the aminoglycosides, beta-lactams, fluoroquinolones, metronidazole, most antimycobacterial agents, and vancomycin. For such drugs there is little difference between the concentrations that inhibit growth and those that kill bacteria. Bactericidal drugs are preferred for the treatment of infections in patients with impaired defense mechanisms, especially immunocompromised patients.

   Some bactericidal agents (aminoglycosides, fluoroquinolones) cause **concentration-dependent** killing. Maximizing peak blood levels of such drugs increases the rate and the extent of their bactericidal effects. This is one of the factors responsible for the clinical effectiveness of high-dose, once-daily administration of aminoglycosides. Other bactericidal agents (beta-lactams, vancomycin) cause **time-dependent** killing. Their killing action is independent of drug concentration and continues only while blood levels are maintained above the minimal bactericidal concentration (MBC).

   Inhibition of bacterial growth that continues after antibiotic blood concentrations have fallen to low levels is called the **postantibiotic effect (PAE).** The mechanisms of PAE are unclear but may reflect the lag time required by bacteria to synthesize new enzymes and cellular components, the possible persistence of antibiotic at the target site, or an enhanced susceptibility of bacteria to phagocytic and other defense mechanisms. PAE may be another factor contributory to the clinical effectiveness of high-dose, once-daily administration of aminoglycosides.
2. **Drug elimination mechanisms:** Changes in hepatic and renal function—and the use of dialysis—can influence the pharmacokinetics of antimicrobials and may necessitate dosage modifications. The major mechanisms of elimination of commonly used antimicrobial drugs are shown in Table 51–3. In anuria (creatinine clearance < 5 mL/min), the elimination half-life of drugs that are eliminated by the kidney is markedly increased, usually necessitating major reductions in drug dosage. Erythromycin, clindamycin, chloramphenicol, rifampin, and ketoconazole are notable exceptions, requiring no change in dosage in renal failure. In patients with biliary dysfunction or cirrhosis, reductions in dosage may be required for drugs that undergo hepatic elimination. Dialysis, especially hemodialysis, may markedly decrease the plasma levels of many antimicrobials; supplementary doses of such drugs may be required to reestablish effective plasma levels following these procedures. Drugs that are *not* removed from the blood by hemodialysis include amphotericin B, cefonicid, cefoperazone, ceftriaxone, erythromycin, nafcillin, tetracyclines, and vancomycin.
3. **Pregnancy and the neonate:** Antimicrobial therapy during pregnancy and the neonatal period requires special consideration. Tetracyclines cause tooth enamel dysplasia and inhibition of bone growth. Sulfonamides, by displacing bilirubin from serum albumin, may cause kernicterus in the neonate. Chloramphenicol may cause the gray baby syndrome. Other drugs that should be used with extreme caution during pregnancy include most antiviral and antifungal agents. The fluoroquinolones are not recommended for use in pregnancy or in children because of possible effects on growing cartilage.

Table 51–3. Elimination of commonly used antimicrobial agents.

Mode of Elimination	Drugs or Drug Groups
Renal	Acyclovir, aminoglycosides, amphotericin B, most cephalosporins, fluconazole, imipenem, most penicillins, most quinolones, sulfonamides, tetracyclines (except doxycycline), TMP-SMZ, vancomycin
Hepatic	Amphotericin B, ampicillin, cefoperazone, chloramphenicol, clindamycin, erythromycin, isoniazid, ketoconazole, nafcillin, rifampin
Hemodialysis	Acyclovir (and most antiviral agents), aminoglycosides, cephalosporins (not cefonicid, cefoperazone, ceftriaxone), penicillins (not nafcillin), sulfonamides

4. **Drug interactions:** Interactions sometimes occur between antimicrobials and other drugs (see also Chapter 61). Interactions include enhanced nephrotoxicity or ototoxicity when aminoglycosides are given with loop diuretics, vancomycin, or cisplatin. Several drug interactions with sulfonamides are based on competition for plasma protein binding; these include excessive hypoglycemia with sulfonylureas and increased hypoprothrombinemia with warfarin. Disulfiram-like reactions to ethanol occur with metronidazole, with TMP-SMZ, and with several cephalosporins (see Chapter 43). Erythromycin inhibits the hepatic metabolism of a number of drugs, including clozapine, lidocaine, loratadine, phenytoin, quinidine, sildenafil, theophylline, and warfarin. The azole antifungals (eg, ketoconazole) inhibit the metabolism of caffeine, carbamazepine, cyclosporine, HMG-CoA reductase inhibitors, methadone, oral contraceptives, phenytoin, sildenafil, verapamil, and zidovudine. Rifampin, an inducer of hepatic drug-metabolizing enzymes, decreases the effects of digoxin, ketoconazole, oral contraceptives, propranolol, quinidine, and warfarin.

D. **Antimicrobial Drug Combinations:** Therapy with multiple antimicrobials may be indicated in the following clinical situations.

1. **Emergency situations:** In severe infections (eg, sepsis, meningitis), combinations of antimicrobial drugs are used empirically to suppress all of the most likely pathogens.
2. **To delay resistance:** The combined use of drugs is valid in situations where the rapid emergence of resistance impairs the chances for cure. For this reason, combined drug therapy is especially important in the treatment of tuberculosis.
3. **Mixed infections:** Multiple organisms may be involved in some infections. For example, peritoneal infections may be caused by several pathogens (eg, anaerobes and coliforms); a combination of drugs may be required to achieve coverage. Skin infections are often due to mixed bacterial, fungal, or viral pathogens.
4. **To achieve synergistic effects:** The use of a drug combination against a specific pathogen may result in an effect greater than that achieved with a single drug. Examples include the use of penicillins with gentamicin in enterococcal endocarditis, the use of an extended-spectrum penicillin plus an aminoglycoside in *Pseudomonas aeruginosa* infections, and the combined use of amphotericin B and flucytosine in cryptococcal meningitis.

   In terms of bactericidal actions, the outcome of the combined use of two antimicrobials may be indifference, synergism, potentiation, or antagonism (see Chapter 61). Such actions are more readily demonstrated in vitro than at the clinical level. Some mechanisms that may account for synergism follow.

   a. **Sequential blockade:** The combined use of drugs may cause inhibition of two or more steps in a metabolic pathway. For example, trimethoprim and sulfamethoxazole (TMP-SMZ) block different steps in the formation of tetrahydrofolic acid.
   b. **Blockade of drug-inactivating enzymes:** Clavulanic acid, sulbactam, and tazobactam inhibit penicillinases and are often combined with penicillinase-sensitive beta-lactam drugs.
   c. **Enhanced drug uptake:** Increased permeability to aminoglycosides after exposure of certain bacteria to cell wall-inhibiting antimicrobials (eg, beta-lactams) is thought to underlie some synergistic effects.

E. **Antimicrobial Chemoprophylaxis:** The general principles of antimicrobial chemoprophylaxis can be summarized as follows: (1) Prophylaxis should always be directed toward a **specific pathogen;** (2) **no resistance** should develop during the period of drug use; (3) prophylactic drug use should be of **limited duration;** (4) conventional **therapeutic doses** should be employed; and (5) prophylaxis should be employed only in situations of documented **drug efficacy.**

Examples of common clinical situations in which nonsurgical antimicrobial prophylaxis is effective are given in Table 51–4. Nonsurgical prophylaxis, mentioned in earlier chapters, includes the prevention of CMV and HIV infections, influenza, meningococcal infections, and tuberculosis. Though somewhat less effective, antimicrobial prophylaxis is also commonly used for animal or human bite wounds and chronic bronchitis. Severely leukopenic patients are often given prophylactic antibiotics.

Prophylaxis against postsurgical infections should be limited to procedures that are associated with infection in more than 5% of untreated cases under optimal conditions. Prophylaxis should embody the principles listed above, with drug selection based on the most likely infect-

Table 51–4. Examples of nonsurgical antimicrobial prophylaxis with established efficacy.

Disease Prevented	Subjects for Prophylaxis	Drugs	Comments
Endocarditis	Dental or oral procedures in high-risk patients[1]	Amoxicillin (PO) or ampicillin (IV)	In penicillin hypersensitivity: clindamycin (PO), or vancomycin (IV)
Genital herpes	Recurrent infections (more than four episodes per year)	Acyclovir	Excellent efficacy
Gonorrhea	Contacts of index case	Cefixime or ceftriaxone	Ciprofloxacin and ofloxacin are alternatives
	Newborn	Silver nitrate	
Otitis media	Recurrent infection	Amoxicillin	Good efficacy
Rheumatic fever	History of rheumatic fever or rheumatic heart disease	Benzathine penicillin G	Excellent efficacy
Urinary tract infections	Recurrent infection	TMP-SMZ	Alternatively, treat each episode

[1]Risk factors include prosthetic heart valves, congenital cardiac malformations, prior endocarditis, rheumatic valvular dysfunction, and mitral valve prolapse with valvular regurgitation.

ing organism and treatment initiated just prior to surgery and continued throughout the procedure. A first-generation cephalosporin (eg, cefazolin) is often selected. Cefoxitin or cefotetan may be used for surgical patients at risk for infection due to anaerobic bacteria. Situations in which surgical prophylaxis is of benefit (or commonly used) include gastrointestinal procedures, vaginal hysterectomy, cesarean section, joint replacement, open fracture surgery, and dental procedures in patients with valvular disease or prostheses.

QUESTIONS

DIRECTIONS: Each of the numbered items or incomplete statements in this section is followed by answers or by completions of the statement. Select the ONE lettered answer or completion that is BEST in each case.

Items 1–3: A hospitalized AIDS patient is receiving antiretroviral drugs but no antimicrobial prophylaxis. He develops sepsis with fever, suspected to be caused by a gram-negative bacillus. Treatment will include antibiotics, and the drugs under consideration include aminoglycosides, cephalosporins, fluoroquinolones, and imipenem.

1. Antimicrobial treatment of this severely immune-depressed patient should *not* be initiated before
- **(A)** The pathogen has been identified by the microbiology laboratory
- **(B)** Specimens have been taken for laboratory tests and examinations
- **(C)** The results of a Gram stain are available
- **(D)** Antipyretic drugs have been given to reduce body temperature
- **(E)** The results of antibacterial drug susceptibility tests are available

2. If gentamicin is used systemically in the treatment of this patient, monitoring of serum drug level may be advised because
- **(A)** If administered orally, the drug is unstable in gastric acid
- **(B)** The drug's antibacterial action will be antagonized by cephalosporins
- **(C)** Gentamicin is hematotoxic
- **(D)** The drug will not readily penetrate into the cerebrospinal fluid
- **(E)** Gentamicin has a narrow therapeutic window

3. A combination of drugs might be given to this patient to provide coverage against multiple organisms or to obtain a synergistic action. Examples of antimicrobial drug synergism established at the clinical level do *not* include
- **(A)** Amphotericin B and flucytosine in cryptococcal meningitis

(B) Carbenicillin and gentamicin in pseudomonal infections
(C) Penicillin and tetracycline in bacterial meningitis
(D) Penicillin and vancomycin in enterococcal infections
(E) Trimethoprim and sulfamethoxazole in coliform infections

Items 4–5: A 27-year-old pregnant patient with a past history of pyelonephritis has developed a severe upper respiratory tract infection that appears to be due to a bacterial pathogen. The woman is hospitalized and an antibacterial agent is to be selected for treatment.

4. Assuming that the physician is concerned about the effects of renal impairment on drug dosage in this patient, which one of the following drugs is LEAST likely to require dosage reduction, even if creatinine clearance is less than 10 mL/min?
(A) Ampicillin
(B) Cefazolin
(C) Clindamycin
(D) Tetracycline
(E) Trimethoprim-sulfamethoxazole

5. Which one of the following antibacterial agents appears to be quite safe for the treatment of infections in the pregnant patient?
(A) Azithromycin
(B) Clarithromycin
(C) Erythromycin
(D) Sulfadiazine
(E) Tetracycline

6. A common drug interaction that occurs with the use of antimicrobial drugs, particularly drugs that have a wide antibacterial spectrum of activity, is
(A) Disulfiram-like reactions when ethanol is ingested
(B) Increased ototoxicity if administered to a patient on furosemide
(C) Enhancement of the anticoagulant effects of warfarin
(D) Increased adverse effects if acetaminophen is administered as an antipyretic
(E) Hypertension with ingestion of red wine and cheese

7. There is no evidence that antimicrobial prophylaxis is of established benefit in
(A) Contacts of the index case in mycoplasmal pneumonia
(B) "Traveler's diarrhea"
(C) Contacts of the index case in gonorrhea
(D) Recurrent urinary tract infection
(E) Tuberculin convertors

8. Which one of the following is not an established mechanism of antimicrobial drug synergy?
(A) Drugs A and B block successive steps in a bacterial metabolic pathway
(B) Drug A promotes the accumulation of drug B within the bacterium
(C) Drug A induces enzymes that convert drug B to a more polar form
(D) Drug A inhibits an enzyme that inactivates drug B

Items 9–10: A 48-year-old patient is scheduled for a vaginal hysterectomy. An antimicrobial drug will be used for prophylaxis against postoperative infection. It is proposed that cefazolin, a first-generation cephalosporin, be given intravenously at the normal therapeutic dose immediately prior to surgery and continued until the patient is released from the hospital.

9. Which one of the following statements about the proposed drug management of this patient is LEAST accurate?
(A) Without prophylaxis, the infection rate following this procedure exceeds 5% under optimal conditions
(B) This drug will not be effective against bacteroides
(C) Probable pathogens do not become rapidly resistant to this drug
(D) Nosocomial (hospital-acquired) infection will be prevented by treatment throughout the period of hospitalization
(E) Prophylaxis has documented efficacy in this type of surgical procedure

10. If the above patient had been scheduled for elective colonic surgery, optimal prophylaxis against infection would be achieved by mechanical bowel preparation and the use of
(A) Intravenous cefotetan
(B) Oral ampicillin
(C) Oral neomycin and erythromycin

(D) Intravenous third-generation cephalosporin
(E) Oral fluoroquinolone

11. Which one of the following antimicrobial drugs is LEAST likely to affect the hepatic metabolism of other drugs?
(A) Ampicillin
(B) Chloramphenicol
(C) Erythromycin
(D) Ketoconazole
(E) Rifampin

12. Which one of the following antimicrobial drugs does not require supplementation of dosage following hemodialysis?
(A) Ampicillin
(B) Cefazolin
(C) Ganciclovir
(D) Tobramycin
(E) Vancomycin

13. The persistent suppression of bacterial growth that may occur following limited exposure to some antimicrobial drugs is called
(A) Time-dependent killing
(B) The postantibiotic effect
(C) Clinical synergy
(D) Concentration-dependent killing
(E) Sequential blockade

14. If ampicillin and piperacillin are used in combination in the treatment of infections due to *Pseudomonas aeruginosa* antagonism may occur. The most likely explanation is that
(A) The two drugs form an insoluble complex
(B) Piperacillin blocks the attachment of ampicillin to penicillin-binding proteins
(C) Ampicillin induces beta-lactamase production
(D) Autolytic enzymes are inhibited by piperacillin
(E) Ampicillin is bacteriostatic

DIRECTIONS (Items 15–20): This case history* is followed by discussion questions. Write out brief answers (two to five sentences) and then compare your answers with those given at the end of the Answers section.

A 42-month-old child was brought to a hospital emergency room with fever and signs suggestive of bacterial meningitis. Two months earlier, she had been treated for otitis media with cefaclor and had developed an urticarial rash. There was no record of vaccination against Haemophilus influenzae *type b. On hospitalization, the child was treated with ampicillin and chloramphenicol for 72 hours and then placed on chloramphenicol alone on the basis of the results of microbiology laboratory tests.*

After 10 days of antibiotic treatment, the patient was afebrile and cerebrospinal fluid was sterile, with normal protein and glucose levels. Drug treatment was discontinued, but after 2 days she developed vomiting and fever to 40.5 °C. Cerebrospinal fluid culture was sterile, but counterimmunoelectrophoresis (CIE) was positive for H influenzae *type b polyribosylribitol phosphate antigen.*

The patient was treated for 10 days with ceftriaxone and remained afebrile after the second day. At completion of therapy, cerebrospinal fluid was sterile, CIE was negative, and the white cell count and protein levels were returning toward the normal range.

15. Why was antibiotic treatment started before microbiologic laboratory examinations were completed?

16. What is the recommended antibiotic regimen for initial management of suspected bacterial meningitis in a child of this age?

17. Why was ampicillin therapy stopped after 3 days?

18. What is the most likely cause of the apparent relapse after discontinuance of chloramphenicol?

19. What was the basis for the use of ceftriaxone?

20. What prophylaxis (if any) should be given to the close contacts of this child?

---

* Adapted from: Ampicillin and chloramphenicol resistance in systemic *Haemophilus influenzae* disease. MMWR Morb Mortal Wkly Rep 1984;33:35.

ANSWERS

1. To delay therapy until laboratory results are available is inappropriate in serious bacterial infections, but specimens for possible microbial identification must be obtained before drugs are administered. The answer is **(B)**.
2. Monitoring plasma aminoglycoside levels is important because these drugs have a low therapeutic index; toxicity occurs when plasma levels are only three to four times higher than their minimal inhibitory concentrations. Decreases in renal function may elevate the plasma levels of aminoglycosides to toxic levels within a few hours. The answer is **(E)**.
3. Combinations of antimicrobial drugs are not always synergistic. In the treatment of bacterial meningitis, two drugs may *not* be better than one. For example, the combination of penicillin and a tetracycline cures fewer patients with pneumococcal meningitis than the same dose of penicillin used alone. The answer is **(C)**.
4. Antimicrobial drugs that are eliminated via hepatic metabolism or biliary excretion include erythromycin, cefoperazone, clindamycin, doxycycline, isoniazid, ketoconazole, and nafcillin. The answer is **(C)**.
5. Several groups of antimicrobial drugs are relatively safe in pregnancy, including penicillins and cephalosporins. While the macrolide azithromycin appears to be safe, the use of the estolate form of erythromycin is associated with an increased incidence of cholestasis in the pregnant patient. Studies in animals have shown that clarithromycin is potentially embryotoxic. The answer is **(A)**.
6. Disturbance of the gut microbial flora often leads to decreased availability of vitamin K, with enhancement of the anticoagulant effects of coumarins. The answer is **(C)**. (Can you name the drugs in the other drug interactions listed?)
7. Tetracycline has been administered to subjects exposed to mycoplasmal pneumonia, but the effectiveness of such treatment has not been documented. The answer is **(A)**.
8. Increased activity of enzymes that make drugs more polar is likely to inactivate an antimicrobial drug and will not lead to increased antibacterial activity. Specific examples of mechanisms that *do* result in synergy include **(A)** the combination of trimethoprim and sulfamethoxazole; **(B)** the combination of a penicillin and an aminoglycoside; and **(D)** the combination of clavulanic acid and amoxicillin. The answer is **(C)**.
9. With few exceptions, the prophylactic use of antibiotics in surgery should not extend beyond the duration of the procedure. Following routine surgical procedures, the risk of superinfection (from disturbances in microbial flora) *increases* in a hospitalized patient if prophylaxis is prolonged; there is also more likelihood of drug toxicity. The answer is **(D)**.
10. Second-generation cephalosporins, including cefoxitin and cefotetan, are more active than cefazolin against bowel anaerobes such as *B fragilis* and are sometimes used for prophylaxis in "dirty" surgical procedures. However, for elective bowel surgery, most authorities favor the oral use of neomycin together with a poorly absorbed formulation of erythromycin. In cases of bowel perforation, the use of a second- or third-generation cephalosporin is more appropriate. The answer is **(C)**.
11. Chloramphenicol, ketoconazole, and erythromycin can inhibit the hepatic metabolism of various drugs. Rifampin is an inducer of liver microsomal drug-metabolizing enzymes. The answer is **(A)**.
12. Vancomycin is not removed from the blood during hemodialysis, and no change in dosage is required. The answer is **(E)**.
13. Many antibiotics continue to exert effects on the growth of bacteria when blood levels are lower than those which are normally thought of as the minimal inhibitory concentration. This is called the postantibiotic effect (PAE). The PAE may contribute to the clinical effectiveness of antibiotics, especially in the case of bactericidal agents such as aminoglycosides, which exert concentration-dependent killing. For example, once-daily dosing with an aminoglycoside is as effective as conventional dosage regimens and is less likely to cause toxicity. The answer is **(B)**.
14. Gram-negative rods such as enterobacter and *Pseudomonas aeruginosa* have inducible beta-lactamases. Several beta-lactam antibiotics, including ampicillin, cefoxitin, and imipenem, are potent inducers of beta-lactamase production. When such inducers are used in combination with a hydrolyzable penicillin (eg, piperacillin), antagonism may result. The answer is **(C)**.
15. The principal justification for empiric, antimicrobial therapy is that the infection is best treated early to avoid serious morbidity or death. Suspected bacterial meningitis is a classic example

of the need to initiate therapy immediately—after relevant samples have been taken for culture and sensitivity determination—on the basis of the clinical diagnosis and the initial microbiologic diagnosis. The latter should include the history, physical signs, and Gram stain.

16. The most likely pathogens involved in bacterial meningitis in children above the age of 3 months are *S pneumoniae* and meningococci. Meningitis due to *H influenzae* type b has become less common since the introduction of protein-conjugated vaccines. However, coverage may be necessary if there is no record of vaccination. Most infectious disease specialists would *start* treatment of suspected bacterial meningitis in children with a third-generation cephalosporin such as ceftriaxone or cefotaxime (plus dexamethasone). Chloramphenicol is now considered to be a backup drug in suspected bacterial meningitis and possibly useful in cases of hypersensitivity to cephalosporins. Ampicillin would provide coverage for *Listeria monocytogenes,* but this organism would be a rare pathogen in an immunocompetent child of this age.

17. The microbiology laboratory confirmed *H influenzae* type b and demonstrated that the isolate was beta-lactamase-positive. Ampicillin is inactivated by penicillinases unless used in combination with an inhibitor of such enzymes. Beta-lactamase-producing isolates of *H influenzae* type b are not resistant to chloramphenicol or to third-generation cephalosporins.

18. Although the cerebrospinal fluid was apparently sterile, the counterimmunoelectrophoresis analysis suggests a relapse caused by *H influenzae* type b owing to inadequate treatment with chloramphenicol or development of resistance.

19. The third-generation cephalosporins cefotaxime and ceftriaxone are effective in the empiric treatment of bacterial meningitis caused by most strains of meningococci, pneumococci, and *H influenzae.* However, the prevalence of drug-resistant *S pneumoniae* can influence empiric therapy and may necessitate the addition of vancomycin. Note that some isolates of *H influenzae* are now resistant to both ampicillin and chloramphenicol.

20. Rifampin is recommended for household or day care contacts of the index case with meningitis due to *H influenzae* type b, and the drug would also be prophylactic for close contacts of meningococcal meningitis.

Basic Principles of Antiparasitic Chemotherapy 52

OBJECTIVES

You should be able to:

- Describe the mechanisms of drugs whose targets are enzymes unique to parasites, ie, not found in host cells.
- Describe the mechanisms of drugs whose targets are enzymes indispensable to parasites but not to their hosts.
- Describe the mechanisms of drugs whose targets are biochemical functions common to host and parasite cells.

Learn the definitions that follow.

Table 52–1. Definitions.

Term	Definition
Glycosome	A membrane-bound intracellular organelle in trypanosomes that contains glycolytic enzymes
Hydrogenosome	A membrane-bound intracellular organelle in certain anaerobic protozoans that contains hydrogenase
Salvage enzymes	Nucleoside phosphotransferases involved in the salvage of purines and pyrimidines in protozoans
Sequential blockade	Actions of two or more drugs that interfere with sequential steps in a metabolic pathway
Suicide substrate	A chemical that forms a stable complex with an enzyme leading to its irreversible inhibition; suicide compounds are chemically related to natural enzyme substrates

CONCEPTS

Rational approaches to antiparasite chemotherapy utilize the principle of **selective toxicity,** which exploits biochemical and physiologic differences between parasite and host cells. Many antiparasitic agents target enzymes that are unique to—or indispensable to—parasites; other drugs affect cellular functions common to both host and parasite cells (Table 52–2).

A. Mechanisms Involving Enzymes Unique to Parasites: These enzymes are not found in the host's cells.

1. **Dihydropteroate synthase:** Sporozoans (eg, plasmodium, toxoplasma, and eimeria species) lack the ability to utilize exogenous folate and therefore possess enzymes for its synthesis; these enzymes can be inhibited by drugs. **Sulfonamides,** which are antimetabolites of PABA, inhibit dihydropteroate synthase. **Sequential blockade** can be achieved with a sulfonamide and an inhibitor of dihydrofolate reductase (eg, pyrimethamine); such drug combinations are effective in malaria and toxoplasmosis.

Table 52–2. Identified targets and mechanisms of action of some antiparasitic drugs.

Mechanism	Parasites	Examples of Drugs
Act on enzymes specific to parasites		
Dihydropteroate synthase	Sporozoa	Sulfonamides, sulfones
Pyruvate-ferredoxin oxidoreductase	Anaerobic protozoa	Nitroimidazoles
Nucleoside phosphotransferase	Flagellated protozoa	Allopurinol riboside
Trypanothione reductase	Kinetoplastida	Nifurtimox, melarsoprol
Act on enzymes indispensable to parasites		
Purine phosphoribosyl transferase	Protozoa	Allopurinol
Ornithine decarboxylase	Protozoa	α-Difluoromethylornithine
Glycolytic enzymes	Kinetoplastida	Glycerol plus salicylhydroxamic acid and suramin
Act on functions common to both host and parasites[1]		
Dihydrofolate reductase	Eimeria, plasmodia, toxoplasma	Pyrimethamine
Thiamine transporter	Coccidia	Amprolium
Mitochondrial electron transporter	Coccidia	4-Hydroxyquinolines
Microtubules	Helminths	Benzimidazoles
Neurotransmission, muscle contraction	Helminths and ectoparasites	Levamisole, piperazines, avermectins, milbemycins

[1]Differences in the structures of regulatory macromolecules among parasites and host cells and differences in drug access may account for the selective toxicities of drugs in this subgroup.

2. **Pyruvate-ferredoxin oxidoreductase:** Certain anaerobic protozoans (trichomonas, entamoeba) lack mitochondria and possess a pyruvate-ferredoxin oxidoreductase of low redox potential that generates acetyl-CoA via electron transport. In trichomonal flagellates, this enzyme is coupled to a hydrogenase located in hydrogenosomes. Under anaerobic conditions, electron transport results in formation of hydrogen. The system also transfers electrons from pyruvate to the nitro groups of nitroimidazoles (eg, **metronidazole**), forming cytotoxic products that inhibit growth by binding to the parasite's proteins and DNA.
3. **Nucleoside phosphotransferases:** Protozoan parasites depend critically on purine salvage pathways because these organisms are unable to synthesize purine nucleotides de novo. In leishmania, purine nucleoside phosphotransferase (a salvage enzyme that transfers phosphate groups to the 5′ position of purine nucleosides) also phosphorylates purine nucleoside analogs such as **allopurinol riboside, formycin B,** and **thiopurinol riboside.** The triphosphate derivatives of these drugs may be incorporated into nucleic acids or may inhibit enzymes in purine metabolism. Toxicity is low because mammalian cells lack this salvage enzyme.
4. **Trypanothione reductase:** In the protozoans known as kinetoplastidans, glutathione exists largely in the form of trypanothione, a unique conjugate with spermidine. Trypanothione, via the action of a specific trypanothione reductase, plays a central role in maintaining the reduced state of intracellular thiols and is essential for the survival of such parasites. **Nifurtimox** and certain trivalent arsenicals used as antitrypanosomal agents inhibit trypanothione reductase.

B. Mechanisms Involving Enzymes Indispensable to Parasites: These enzymes are present in the host as well as the parasite, but they are essential only to the parasite.

1. **Purine phosphoribosyl transferases:** Hypoxanthine-guanine phosphoribosyltransferase (HGPRTase) is a key enzyme in purine synthesis in many parasites, including leishmania, schistosoma, and trypanosoma species. **Allopurinol** is a good substrate for this enzyme in certain parasites (but not for the mammalian enzyme); the drug is metabolized to the ribotide, which is incorporated after phosphorylation into RNA forms that interfere with normal growth. Purine salvage in giardia depends critically on adenine phosphoribosyltransferase and guanine phosphoribosyltransferase. Unlike mammalian forms of these enzymes, the parasitic enzymes do not utilize hypoxanthine, xanthine, or adenine as substrates and are thus amenable to inhibition by a designed inhibitor.
2. **Ornithine decarboxylase:** This enzyme controls the formation of the polyamine, putrescine, and appears to be more critical for the growth of certain parasites than for the growth of mammalian cells. **Alpha-difluoromethylornithine (DFMO)** is a suicide substrate of ornithine decarboxylase and has antiparasitic activity against trypanosoma, plasmodium, and giardia species. In *T brucei,* DFMO transforms the organism into a nondividing form that can be eliminated by the host immune system.
3. **Glycolytic enzymes:** The bloodstream form of the African trypanosome *T brucei* is entirely dependent on glycolysis for generation of ATP. The enzymes involved are arranged in close proximity to each other in glycosomes. Glycerol-3-phosphate oxidase is a key enzyme that can be inhibited by **salicylhydroxamic acid,** bringing the parasite into an anaerobic state. The addition of glycerol inhibits the reversed glycerol kinase reaction, stops glycolysis, and results in the death of the parasite. Biogenesis of glycosomes may also be a target for antiparasitic drugs. **Suramin,** a very large polar molecule, binds to glycolytic enzymes and may prevent the incorporation of the enzymes into the glycosome.

C. Mechanisms Involving Biochemical Functions Common to Host and Parasite: Several processes that occur in both parasites and hosts are nevertheless more susceptible to inhibition in the parasite.

1. **Dihydrofolate reductase:** Dihydrofolate reductase (DHFR) is a classic target in antimicrobial and cancer chemotherapy. The enzyme is also a useful therapeutic target in plasmodium, toxoplasma, and eimeria species. **Pyrimethamine** inhibits DHFR in all three species of parasites. However, in the case of *P falciparum,* point mutations in the gene that codes for DHFR have rendered the enzyme less susceptible to pyrimethamine.
2. **Thiamin transporter:** Carbohydrate metabolism is the primary energy source in coccidia. Inhibition of the cellular transport of thiamin by the structurally similar agent **amprolium** leads to a deficiency of this cofactor in coccidia.

3. **Mitochondrial electron transporter: 4-Hydroxyquinoline** drugs with anticoccidial effects interact with components of the respiratory chain that are specific to eimeria species and inhibit electron transport in the mitochondria of these organisms. Mitochondrial respiration in other parasites and in mammals is not inhibited by these drugs.
4. **Microtubules:** The microtubules of the cytoskeleton and mitotic spindle consist of tubulin polymers. These tubulins are heterogeneous among species. Structural features of alpha-tubulins in helminths may account for the selective toxicity of benzimidazole drugs (eg, **mebendazole**). These agents bind to microtubules in helminths to block transport processes.
5. **Neurotransmission and muscle contraction:** The antiparasitic effect of nicotinic agonist drugs (eg, **levamisole, pyrantel pamoate**) in nematodes is caused by stimulation of neuromuscular transmission, which leads to muscle contraction. **Piperazine** acts as a GABA receptor agonist in nematodes, causing flaccid paralysis; facilitation of the actions of GABA appears to underlie the actions of **milbemycins** and **avermectins.** These natural products do not cross the blood-brain barrier in mammalian hosts and are relatively nontoxic. **Praziquantel,** an antischistosomal and antitapeworm agent, stimulates Ca^{2+} entry into muscles of these parasites and causes unphysiologic contraction.

QUESTIONS

DIRECTIONS: Each of the numbered items or incomplete statements in this section is followed by answers or by completions of the statement. Select the ONE lettered answer or completion that is BEST in each case.

1. Certain anaerobic protozoan parasites lack mitochondria and generate energy-rich compounds, such as acetyl-CoA, by means of enzymes present in organelles called hydrogenosomes. An important enzyme involved in this process is
   (A) Cytochrome P450
   (B) Glycerol-3-phosphate oxidase
   (C) Hypoxanthine-guanine phosphoribosyltransferase
   (D) Pyruvate-ferredoxin oxidoreductase
   (E) Thymidylate synthase
2. Which of the following compounds is a good substrate for hypoxanthine-guanine phosphoribosyltransferase in trypanosomes (but not mammals) and is eventually converted into metabolites that are incorporated into RNA?
   (A) Allopurinol
   (B) Alpha-difluoromethylornithine
   (C) Glycerol
   (D) Mebendazole
   (E) Salicylhydroxamic acid
3. One chemotherapeutic strategy used to eradicate the bloodstream form of African trypanosomes is based on the absolute dependence of the organism on
   (A) Cytochrome-dependent electron transfer
   (B) Dihydropteroate synthesis
   (C) Glycolysis
   (D) Lactate dehydrogenase
   (E) Mitochondrial respiration
4. Which of the following drugs enhances GABA actions on the neuromuscular junctions of nematodes and arthropods?
   (A) Glutamic acid
   (B) Ivermectin
   (C) Picrotoxin
   (D) Pyrantel pamoate
   (E) Pyrimethamine
5. Which of the following drugs is an antimetabolite that inhibits a trypanosomal enzyme involved in putrescine synthesis?
   (A) Alpha-difluoromethylornithine
   (B) Alpha-fluorodeoxyuridine

(C) Metronidazole
(D) Polymyxin
(E) Thiopurinol riboside

6. All of the following statements about the mechanisms of action of antiparasitic drugs are accurate EXCEPT
(A) 4-Hydroxyquinolines inhibit phospholipase C
(B) Mebendazole binds to tubulins to alter the transport functions of microtubules
(C) Metronidazole is activated in the parasite to a cytotoxic product
(D) Salicylhydroxamic acid is an inhibitor of glycerol-3-phosphate oxidase
(E) Sulfonamides inhibit 7,8-dihydropteroate synthase

7. Which one of the following enzymes is not unique to parasites?
(A) Dihydropteridine pyrophosphokinase
(B) Hypoxanthine-guanine phosphoribosyltransferase
(C) Lanosterol demethylase
(D) Purine nucleoside phosphotransferase
(E) Trypanothione reductase

8. Which one of the following statements about specific antiparasitic drugs is LEAST accurate?
(A) Amprolium is an inhibitor of thiamin transport in eimeria species
(B) Allopurinol riboside is a potent inhibitor of mitochondrial electron transfer
(C) Sulfadoxine is an inhibitor of dihydropteroate synthase in the malaria parasite
(D) Suramin binds to glycolytic enzymes and prevents their incorporation into glycosomes
(E) The mechanism of action of diloxanide furoate in amebiasis is unknown

ANSWERS

1. In *T vaginalis,* conversion of pyruvate to acetyl-CoA takes place via the actions of pyruvate-ferredoxin oxidoreductase. The answer is **(D).**

2. Allopurinol is a good substrate for HGPRTase in trypanosomes but not mammals. Recall that allopurinol is also an inhibitor of xanthine oxidase and is used in gout and cancer chemotherapy. The answer is **(A).**

3. Glycolytic enzyme inhibitors (such as salicylhydroxamic acid) that inhibit glycerol-3-phosphate oxidase may be selectively toxic to African trypanosomes. The answer is **(C).**

4. Several antiparasitic drugs enhance GABA neurotransmission in nematodes and arthropods and cause muscle paralysis. These drugs include piperazine, milbemycins, and avermectins (eg, ivermectin). The answer is **(B).**

5. DFMO is a suicide inhibitor of ornithine decarboxylase. Although it also inhibits mammalian ornithine decarboxylase, DMFO is less toxic to the host because of more rapid turnover and replacement of the irreversibly inhibited enzyme in the host than in parasites. The answer is **(A).**

6. The anticoccidial 4-aminoquinolines inhibit mitochondrial respiration in eimeria species, probably through interaction with a component between NADH oxidase and cytochrome b in the electron transport chain. The answer is **(A).**

7. HGPRTase, an enzyme involved in purine salvage, is present in both parasites and mammals. Note that in leishmania and *T cruzi,* ergosterol is an essential component of their plasma membranes. In such species the antifungal azoles inhibit a cytochrome P450 isoform that converts lanosterol to ergosterol via demethylation. The answer is **(B).**

8. Leishmania species possess the unique salvage enzyme, purine nucleoside phosphotransferase. This enzyme phosphorylates allopurinol riboside to form the corresponding nucleotide, which interferes with purine and nucleic acid metabolism. The answer is **(B).**

53 Antiprotozoal Drugs

OBJECTIVES

You should be able to:

- List the major groups of antiprotozoal drugs.
- Describe the pharmacodynamic and pharmacokinetic properties of the major antimalarial drugs (chloroquine, mefloquine, quinine, primaquine, and the antifolate agents).
- Describe the pharmacodynamic and pharmacokinetic properties of the major amebicides (diloxanide, emetine, iodoquinol, and metronidazole). List other clinical applications of metronidazole.
- Identify the drugs useful for prophylaxis and treatment of pneumocystosis and toxoplasmosis and know their toxic effects.
- Identify the major drugs used for trypanosomiasis and leishmaniasis and know their toxic effects.

CONCEPTS

DRUGS FOR MALARIA

Malaria parasites have a complex life cycle that permits drug action at several points. Plasmodium species that infect humans *(P falciparum, P malariae, P ovale, P vivax)* are spread by the female *Anopheles* mosquito and, after inoculation into the human host, undergo a primary developmental stage in the liver (primary tissue phase). They then enter the blood and parasitize erythrocytes (erythrocytic phase). *P falciparum* and *P malariae* have only one cycle of liver cell invasion; thereafter, multiplication is confined to erythrocytes. The other species have a dormant hepatic stage (in which they become **hypnozoites**) that is responsible for recurrent infections and relapses after apparent recovery of the host from the initial infection.

Primary **tissue schizonticides** (eg, primaquine) kill schizonts in the liver soon after infection, whereas **blood schizonticides** (eg, chloroquine, quinine) kill these parasitic forms only in the erythrocyte. Antimalarial drugs may exert multiple actions. Primaquine is **gametocidal,** since it kills gametes in the blood; the drug also destroys the secondary exoerythrocytic (liver) schizonts that cause the relapsing fevers of malaria. **Sporonticides** (proguanil, pyrimethamine) prevent sporogony and multiplication in the mosquito (Table 53–1).

A. Chloroquine:

1. Classification and pharmacokinetics: Chloroquine is a 4-aminoquinoline derivative. The drug is rapidly absorbed when given orally, is widely distributed to tissues, and has an

Table 53–1. Drugs used in malaria.

Drug	Use in Acute Attacks?	Use for Eradication of Liver Stages?	Use for Prophylaxis?
Chloroquine	Yes	No	Yes, except in regions where *P falciparum* is resistant
Quinine, mefloquine	Yes, in resistant *P falciparum*	No	Yes, mefloquine is used in regions with chloroquine-resistant *P falciparum*
Primaquine	No	Yes *(P vivax, P ovale)*	Yes, but only if exposed to *P vivax* or *P ovale*
Antifols	Yes, but only in resistant *P falciparum*	No	Not usually advised

extremely large volume of distribution. Antacids may decrease oral absorption of the drug. Chloroquine is excreted largely unchanged in the urine.

2. **Mechanism of action:** Chloroquine prevents polymerization of the hemoglobin breakdown product heme into hemozoin. Intracellular accumulation of heme is toxic to the parasite. Chloroquine is a weak base and may buffer intracellular pH, thereby inhibiting cellular invasion by parasitic organisms. The selective toxicity of the drug is due to an energy-dependent carrier mechanism in parasitized cells. Chloroquine-resistant parasites are able to expel the drug via a membrane P-glycoprotein pump.
3. **Clinical use:** Chloroquine is the drug of choice for acute attacks of nonfalciparum and sensitive falciparum malaria and as a chemosuppressant, except in regions where *P falciparum* is resistant. The drug is solely a blood schizonticide and will not eradicate secondary tissue schizonts. Chloroquine has been used in amebic liver disease in combination with metronidazole and in autoimmune disorders including rheumatoid arthritis.
4. **Toxicity:** At low doses, chloroquine causes gastrointestinal irritation, skin rash, and headaches. High doses may cause severe skin lesions, peripheral neuropathies, myocardial depression, retinal damage, auditory impairment, and toxic psychosis. Chloroquine may also precipitate porphyria attacks.

B. Quinine:

1. **Classification and pharmacokinetics:** Quinine is the principal alkaloid derived from the bark of the cinchona tree. Quinine is rapidly absorbed orally and is metabolized before renal excretion. Intravenous administration of quinine is possible in severe infections.
2. **Mechanism of action:** Quinine complexes with double-stranded DNA to prevent strand separation, resulting in block of DNA replication and transcription to RNA. Quinine is a blood schizonticide and has no effect on liver stages of the malaria parasite.
3. **Clinical use:** The main use of quinine is in *P falciparum* infections resistant to chloroquine. Quinine is sometimes used with doxycycline to shorten the duration of therapy and limit toxicity. Quinidine, the dextrorotatory stereoisomer of quinine, is used intravenously in the USA for treatment of severe falciparum malaria. To delay emergence of resistance, the drugs should not be used routinely for prophylaxis.
4. **Toxicity:** Quinine commonly causes **cinchonism,** whose symptoms include gastrointestinal distress, headache, vertigo, blurred vision, and tinnitus. Severe overdose results in disturbances in cardiac conduction that resemble quinidine toxicity. Hematotoxic effects occur, including hemolysis in glucose-6-phosphate dehydrogenase-deficient patients. **Blackwater fever** (intravascular hemolysis) is a rare and sometimes fatal complication in quinine-sensitized persons. Quinine is an FDA Pregnancy Risk category X drug, contraindicated in pregnancy.

C. Mefloquine:

1. **Classification and pharmacokinetics:** Mefloquine is a synthetic 4-quinoline derivative chemically related to quinine. Because of local irritation, mefloquine can only be given orally, though it is subject to variable absorption. Its mechanism of action is not known.
2. **Clinical use:** Recommended by the CDC for prophylaxis in all malarious areas except those with no chloroquine resistance.
3. **Toxicity:** Mefloquine is less toxic than quinine; its adverse effects include gastrointestinal distress, skin rash, headache, and dizziness. At high doses, mefloquine may cause neurologic symptoms and seizures.

D. Primaquine:

1. **Classification and pharmacokinetics:** Primaquine is a synthetic 8-aminoquinoline. Absorption is complete after oral administration and is followed by extensive metabolism.
2. **Mechanism of action:** Primaquine forms quinoline-quinone metabolites, which are electron-transferring redox compounds that act as cellular oxidants. The drug is a tissue schizonticide and also limits malaria transmission by acting as a gametocide.
3. **Clinical use:** Primaquine is used to eradicate liver stages of *P vivax* and *P ovale* and should be used in conjunction with a blood schizonticide. Though not active alone in acute attacks of vivax and ovale malaria, a 14-day course of primaquine is standard following initial treatment with chloroquine.
4. **Toxicity:** Primaquine is usually well tolerated but may cause gastrointestinal distress,

pruritus, headaches, and methemoglobinemia. More serious toxicity involves hemolysis in glucose-6-phosphate dehydrogenase-deficient patients.

E. **Antifolate Drugs:**
1. **Classification and pharmacokinetics:** The antifolate group includes pyrimethamine, proguanil, sulfadoxine, and dapsone. All of these drugs are absorbed orally and are excreted in the urine, partly in unchanged form. Proguanil has a shorter half-life (12–16 hours) than other drugs in this subclass (half-life > 100 hours).
2. **Mechanisms of action:** Sulfonamides act as antimetabolites of PABA and block folic acid synthesis in certain protozoans by inhibiting dihydropteroate synthase. Proguanil (chloroguanide) is bioactivated to cycloguanil. Pyrimethamine and cycloguanil are selective inhibitors of protozoan dihydrofolate reductases. The combination of pyrimethamine with sulfadoxine has synergistic antimalarial effects through the **sequential blockade** of two steps in folic acid synthesis.
3. **Clinical use:** The antifols are blood schizonticides that act mainly against *P falciparum.* Pyrimethamine with sulfadoxine in fixed combination (Fansidar) is used in the treatment of chloroquine-resistant forms of this species, although the onset of activity is slow. Many strains of *P falciparum* are now resistant to antifols, and the drugs are not commonly used for prophylaxis because of their toxicities.
4. **Toxicity:** The toxic effects of sulfonamides include skin rashes, gastrointestinal distress, hemolysis, kidney damage, and drug interactions caused by competition for plasma protein binding sites. Pyrimethamine may cause folic acid deficiency when used in high doses.

DRUGS FOR AMEBIASIS

Tissue amebicides **(chloroquine, emetines, metronidazole)** act on organisms in the bowel wall and the liver; luminal amebicides **(diloxanide furoate, iodoquinol, paromomycin)** act only in the lumen of the bowel. The choice of a drug depends on the form of amebiasis. For asymptomatic disease, diloxanide furoate is the first choice. For mild to severe intestinal infection, metronidazole is used with diloxanide furoate or iodoquinol. The latter regimen, plus chloroquine, is recommended in amebic liver abscess (Table 53–2). The mechanisms of amebicidal action of most drugs in this subclass are unknown.

A. **Diloxanide Furoate:** This drug is commonly used as the sole agent for the treatment of asymptomatic amebiasis, and is also useful in mild intestinal disease when used with other drugs. Diloxanide furoate is converted in the gut to the diloxanide freebase form, which is the active amebicide. Toxic effects are mild and are usually restricted to gastrointestinal symptoms.

B. **Emetines:** Emetine and dehydroemetine inhibit protein synthesis by blocking ribosomal movement along messenger RNA. These alkaloids are used as backup drugs for treatment of severe intestinal or hepatic amebiasis in hospitalized patients. Emetines are given parenterally. The drugs may cause severe toxicity, including gastrointestinal distress, muscle weakness, and cardiovascular dysfunction (arrhythmias and congestive heart failure).

C. **Iodoquinol:** Iodoquinol, a halogenated hydroxyquinoline, is an orally active luminal amebicide used as an alternative drug for mild-to-severe intestinal infections. Adverse gastrointestinal

Table 53–2. Drugs used in the treatment of amebiasis.*

Disease Form	Drug of Choice	Alternative Drug
Asymptomatic intestinal	Diloxanide furoate	Iodoquinol, paromomycin
Mild to severe intestinal	Metronidazole plus diloxanide or iodoquinol	Diloxanide (plus doxycycline), chloroquine, paromomycin
Hepatic abscess	Metronidazole plus diloxanide, followed by chloroquine	Emetines, followed by chloroquine plus diloxanide

*Adapted, with permission, from Katzung BG (editor): *Basic & Clinical Pharmacology,* 8th ed. McGraw-Hill, 2001.

effects are common but usually mild. Systemic absorption after high doses may lead to thyroid enlargement and neurotoxic effects, including peripheral neuropathy and visual dysfunction.

D. Metronidazole:

1. **Pharmacokinetics:** Metronidazole is effective orally and distributed widely to tissues. Elimination of the drug requires hepatic metabolism.
2. **Mechanism of action:** Metronidazole undergoes a reductive bioactivation of its nitro group by ferredoxin (present in anaerobic parasites) to form reactive cytotoxic products.
3. **Clinical use:** Metronidazole is the drug of choice in severe intestinal wall disease and in hepatic abscess and other extraintestinal amebic disease. Metronidazole is commonly used with a luminal amebicide. Other important clinical uses of metronidazole include treatment of trichomoniasis, giardiasis, and infections caused by *Gardnerella vaginalis* and anaerobic bacteria *(B fragilis, C difficile).*
4. **Toxicity:** Adverse effects of metronidazole include gastrointestinal irritation, headache, and dark coloration of urine. More serious toxicity includes leukopenia, dizziness, and ataxia. Drug interactions with metronidazole include a disulfiram-like reaction with ethanol and potentiation of coumarin anticoagulant effects. Safety of metronidazole in pregnancy and in nursing mothers has not been established.

E. Paromomycin: This drug is an aminoglycoside antibiotic used as a second-line luminal amebicide. It may also have some efficacy against cryptosporidiosis in the AIDS patient. Adverse gastrointestinal effects are common, and systemic absorption may lead to headaches, dizziness, rashes, and arthralgia. Tetracyclines (eg, doxycycline) are sometimes used with a luminal amebicide in mild intestinal disease.

DRUGS FOR PNEUMOCYSTOSIS & TOXOPLASMOSIS

A. Pentamidine:

1. **Mechanism of action:** Pentamidine's mechanism of action is unknown but may involve inhibition of glycolysis or interference with nucleic acid metabolism of protozoans and fungi. Preferential accumulation of the drug by susceptible parasites may account for its selective toxicity.
2. **Clinical use:** Aerosol pentamidine (once monthly) can be used in primary and secondary prophylaxis, though oral TMP-SMZ is usually preferred. Daily intravenous or intramuscular administration of the drug for 21 days is needed in the treatment of active pneumocystosis in the HIV-infected patient. Pentamidine is also used in trypanosomiasis (see below).
3. **Toxicity:** Severe adverse effects follow parenteral use including respiratory stimulation followed by depression, hypotension due to peripheral vasodilation, hypoglycemia, anemia, neutropenia, hepatitis, and pancreatitis. Systemic toxicity is minimal when pentamidine is used by inhalation.

B. Trimethoprim-Sulfamethoxazole (TMP-SMZ):

1. **Clinical use:** TMP-SMZ is the first choice in prophylaxis and treatment of pneumocystis pneumonia (PCP). Prophylaxis in AIDS patients is recommended when the CD4 count drops below 200 cells/μL. Oral treatment with the double-strength formulation three times weekly is usually effective. The same regimen of TMP-SMZ is prophylactic against toxoplasmosis and infections due to *Isospora belli.* For treatment of active PCP, daily oral or intravenous administration of TMP-SMZ is required.
2. **Toxicity:** Adverse effects due to TMP-SMZ occur in up to 50% of AIDS patients. Toxicity includes gastrointestinal distress, rash, fever, neutropenia, and thrombocytopenia. These effects may be serious enough to warrant discontinuance of TMP-SMZ and substitution of alternative drugs. (See Chapter 46 for additional information on TMP-SMZ.)

C. Antifols: Pyrimethamine and Sulfonamides:

1. **Clinical use:** The combination of pyrimethamine with sulfadiazine has synergistic activity against *Toxoplasma gondii* through the **sequential blockade** of two steps in folic acid synthesis. Pyrimethamine plus sulfadiazine is a regimen of choice for prophylaxis against toxoplasmosis and is an alternative to TMP-SMZ or pentamidine in prophylaxis against

pneumocystis pneumonia in the AIDS patient. For treatment of active toxoplasmosis, the drug combination is given daily for 3–4 weeks, with folinic acid to offset hematologic toxicity. For patients allergic to sulfonamides, clindamycin can be used in combination with pyrimethamine. For toxoplasma encephalitis in AIDS, high-dose treatment with pyrimethamine plus sulfadiazine (or clindamycin) must be maintained for at least 6 weeks.

2. **Toxicity:** High doses of pyrimethamine plus sulfadiazine are associated with gastric irritation, glossitis, neurologic symptoms (headache, insomnia, tremors, seizures), and hematotoxicity (megaloblastic anemia, thrombocytopenia). Antibiotic-associated colitis may occur during treatment with clindamycin.

D. Atovaquone:

1. **Mechanism and pharmacokinetics:** Atovaquone inhibits mitochondrial electron transport and probably folate metabolism. Used orally, it is poorly absorbed and should be given with food to maximize bioavailability. Most of the drug is eliminated in the feces in unchanged form.
2. **Clinical use and toxicity:** Atovaquone is approved for use in mild to moderate pneumocystis pneumonia. It is less effective than TMP-SMZ or pentamidine, but is better tolerated. Adverse effects include rash, cough, nausea, vomiting, diarrhea, fever, and abnormal liver function tests.

E. Miscellaneous Agents: Other alternative drug regimens for the treatment of pneumocystis pneumonia include trimethoprim plus dapsone, primaquine plus clindamycin, and trimetrexate plus leucovorin.

DRUGS FOR TRYPANOSOMIASIS

A. Pentamidine: Pentamidine is commonly used in the hemolymphatic stages of disease caused by *Trypanosoma gambiense* and *T rhodesiense.* Because it does not cross the blood-brain barrier, pentamidine is not used in later stages of trypanosomiasis. Other clinical uses include pneumocystosis and treatment of the kala azar form of leishmaniasis (Table 53–3).

B. Melarsoprol: This drug is an organic arsenical that inhibits enzyme sulfhydryl groups. Because it enters the CNS, melarsoprol is the drug of choice in African sleeping sickness. Melarsoprol is given parenterally because it causes gastrointestinal irritation; it may also cause a reactive encephalopathy that can be fatal.

C. Nifurtimox: This drug is a nitrofurazone derivative that inhibits the parasite-unique enzyme trypanothione reductase. Nifurtimox is the drug of choice in American trypanosomiasis and has also been effective in mucocutaneous leishmaniasis. The drug causes severe toxicity, including allergies, gastrointestinal irritation, and CNS effects.

Table 53–3. Drugs used in the treatment of other protozoal infections.

Drug	Primary Indications
Melarsoprol	Drug of choice in African sleeping sickness (late, CNS stage of trypanosomiasis); also used in mucocutaneous forms of the disease
Nifurtimox	Trypanosomiasis due to *T cruzi*
Pentamidine	Hemolymphatic stage of trypanosomiasis; also used in *Pneumocystis carinii* pneumonia
Pyrimethamine plus sulfadiazine	Drug combination of choice in toxoplasmosis
Sodium stibogluconate	Drug of choice for leishmaniasis (all species)
Suramin	Drug of choice for hemolymphatic stage of trypanosomiasis *(T brucei gambiense, T rhodesiense)*
Trimethoprim-sulfamethoxazole	Drug combination of choice in *Pneumocystis carinii* infections

D. Suramin: This polyanionic compound is a drug of choice for the early hemolymphatic stages of African trypanosomiasis (before CNS involvement). It is also an alternative to ivermectin in the treatment of onchocerciasis (see Chapter 54). Suramin is used parenterally and causes skin rashes, gastrointestinal distress, and neurologic complications.

DRUGS FOR LEISHMANIASIS

Leishmania, parasitic protozoa transmitted by flesh-eating flies, cause various diseases ranging from cutaneous or mucocutaneous lesions to splenic and hepatic enlargement with fever. **Sodium stibogluconate** (pentavalent antimony), the primary drug in all forms of the disease, appears to kill the parasite by inhibition of glycolysis or effects on nucleic acid metabolism. Alternative agents include pentamidine (for visceral leishmaniasis), metronidazole (for cutaneous lesions), and amphotericin B (for mucocutaneous leishmaniasis).

DRUG LIST

See Tables 53–1, 53–2, and 53–3.

QUESTIONS

DIRECTIONS: Each of the numbered items or incomplete statements in this section is followed by answers or by completions of the statement. Select the ONE lettered answer or completion that is BEST in each case.

1. Which one of the following statements about antimalarial drugs is LEAST accurate?
- **(A)** A combination of primaquine and clindamycin is an alternative drug regimen for *Pneumocystis carinii* pneumonia
- **(B)** Chloroquine is a blood schizonticide but does not affect secondary tissue schizonts
- **(C)** Mefloquine destroys secondary exoerythrocytic schizonts
- **(D)** Primaquine acts primarily on exoerythrocytic stages of the malarial life cycle
- **(E)** Proguanil is converted to a reactive metabolite that is sporonticidal

2. Which of the following antimalarial drugs causes a dose-dependent toxic state that includes flushed and sweaty skin, dizziness, nausea, diarrhea, tinnitus, blurred vision, and impaired hearing?
- **(A)** Amodiaquine
- **(B)** Primaquine
- **(C)** Pyrimethamine
- **(D)** Quinine
- **(E)** Sulfadoxine

3. Plasmodial resistance to chloroquine is due to
- **(A)** Change in receptor structure
- **(B)** Decreased carrier-mediated drug transport
- **(C)** Increase in the activity of DNA repair mechanisms
- **(D)** Induction of inactivating enzymes
- **(E)** Inhibition of dihydrofolate reductase

Items 4–6: A photographer traveled in a jungle region where chloroquine-resistant *P falciparum* is endemic. She took a drug for prophylaxis but nevertheless developed a severe attack of *P vivax* malaria.

4. The drug she took for prophylaxis was probably
- **(A)** Chloroquine
- **(B)** Mefloquine
- **(C)** Primaquine
- **(D)** Proguanil
- **(E)** Pyrimethamine

5. Which of the following drugs should be used for oral treatment of the photographer's acute attack of *P vivax* malaria?

(A) Chloroquine
(B) Mefloquine
(C) Primaquine
(D) Pyrimethamine-sulfadoxine
(E) Quinine

6. Which of the following drugs should be given later in order to eradicate schizonts and latent hypnozoites in the patient's liver?
(A) Chloroquine
(B) Mefloquine
(C) Primaquine
(D) Proguanil
(E) Quinine

7. Which one of the following statements about amebicides is LEAST accurate?
(A) Diloxanide furoate is a luminal amebicide
(B) Emetine is contraindicated in pregnancy and in patients with cardiac disease
(C) Metronidazole has little activity in the gut lumen
(D) Paromomycin is effective in extraintestinal amebiasis
(E) Systemic use of iodoquinol may cause thyroid enlargement and peripheral neuropathy

Items 8–9: A male patient presents with lower abdominal discomfort, flatulence, and occasional diarrhea. A diagnosis is made of intestinal amebiasis and *E histolytica* is identified in his diarrheal stools. An oral drug is prescribed and reduces his intestinal symptoms. Later he presents with severe dysentery, right upper quadrant pain, weight loss, fever, and an enlarged liver. Amebic liver abscess is diagnosed and the patient is hospitalized. He has a past history of drug treatment for a tachyarrhythmia but is not taking antiarrhythmic drugs at present.

8. The preferred treatment that he *should* have received for the initial symptoms (which were indicative of mild-to-moderate intestinal infection) is
(A) Diloxanide furoate
(B) Emetine
(C) Metronidazole
(D) Metronidazole plus diloxanide furoate
(E) Tetracycline

9. The drug regimen most likely to be effective in treating the hepatic abscess in this patient and in eradicating intestinal infection is
(A) Chloroquine alone
(B) Diloxanide furoate plus iodoquinol
(C) Emetine plus diloxanide furoate plus chloroquine
(D) Metronidazole plus chloroquine plus iodoquinol
(E) Paromomycin plus mefloquine

10. Which one of the following statements about antiprotozoal drugs is LEAST accurate?
(A) Blackwater fever occurs in patients sensitized to chloroquine
(B) Intravenous injection of pentamidine produces a sharp fall in blood pressure that is only partially blocked by atropine
(C) Metronidazole is the drug of choice for trichomoniasis
(D) Nifurtimox is selectively toxic to some protozoans because it inhibits trypanothione reductase
(E) Pyrimethamine is synergistic with sulfadoxine against malarial parasites (sequential blockade)

11. This drug is the antimalarial agent most commonly associated with causing an acute hemolytic reaction in patients with glucose-6-phosphate dehydrogenase deficiency.
(A) Chloroquine
(B) Clindamycin
(C) Mefloquine
(D) Primaquine
(E) Quinine

12. Following a back-packing trip in the mountains, a 24-year-old man develops diarrhea. He acknowledges drinking stream water without purification and you suspect he is showing symptoms of giardiasis. Since you know that laboratory detection of cysts or trophozoites in the feces can be difficult, you decide to treat the patient empirically with

(A) Chloroquine
(B) Emetine
(C) Metronidazole
(D) Pentamidine
(E) TMP-SMZ

13. This drug can clear trypanosomes from the blood and lymph nodes and is active in the late CNS stages of African sleeping sickness.
(A) Emetine
(B) Melarsoprol
(C) Nifurtimox
(D) Pentamidine
(E) Suramin

14. Metronidazole is LEAST likely to be effective in the treatment of
(A) Amebiasis
(B) Giardiasis
(C) Pneumocystosis
(D) Pseudomembranous colitis
(E) Trichomoniasis

15. Which one of the following drugs is recommended as a single agent for oral treatment of uncomplicated malaria due to chloroquine-resistant *P falciparum* strains?
(A) Doxycycline
(B) Iodoquinol
(C) Primaquine
(D) Proguanil
(E) Quinine

ANSWERS

1. Mefloquine has many properties similar to those of quinine. Both drugs are effective blood schizonticides, and both have minimal effects on the secondary exoerythrocytic (liver) schizonts that cause the relapsing fevers of malaria. The answer is **(C)**.

2. These dose-related symptoms are characteristic adverse effects of cinchona alkaloids (quinine, quinidine) and are termed cinchonism. The answer is **(D)**.

3. Resistance occurs through decreases in the activity of a carrier-mediated transport system. The answer is **(B)**.

4. Mefloquine is the preferred drug for prophylaxis in regions of the world where chloroquine-resistant *P falciparum* is endemic. One dose of mefloquine weekly starting before travel and continuing until 4 weeks after leaving the region is the preferred regimen. Doxycycline is an alternative drug for this indication. Another alternative for prophylaxis is chloroquine plus proguanil. The answer is **(B)**.

5. Chloroquine is the drug of choice for the oral treatment of an acute attack of malaria due to *P vivax* but will not eradicate exoerythrocytic forms of the parasite. Quinine or quinidine is used for the parenteral treatment of acute attacks. The answer is **(A)**.

6. Primaquine is the only antimalarial drug that reliably acts on tissue schizonts in liver cells. Starting about day 4 following an acute attack, primaquine should be given daily for 2 weeks. The answer is **(C)**.

7. Paromomycin is an aminoglycoside antibiotic used as a back-up drug in the treatment of amebiasis. The drug acts only on organisms in the lumen of the bowel because the aminoglycosides are not absorbed when given orally. The answer is **(D)**.

8. Metronidazole plus a luminal amebicide is the treatment of choice in mild to moderate amebic colitis. Diloxanide furoate is commonly used as the sole agent in asymptomatic intestinal infection. The answer is **(D)**.

9. Metronidazole given for 10 days is effective as monotherapy in many cases of hepatic abscess and has the dual advantage of being both amebicidal and active against anaerobic bacteria. However, treatment failures can occur and follow-up therapy with chloroquine is highly recommended. Luminal amebicides should also be given to eradicate intestinal infection. Treatment with emetine is contraindicated in patients with a history of cardiac disease. The answer is **(D)**.

10. Massive intravascular hemolysis (blackwater fever) is now a rare complication of the treatment of malaria with quinine. Blackwater fever does not occur in the few patients who may be sensitive to chloroquine. The answer is **(A).**
11. Primaquine is the prototypical drug that induces hemolysis in persons deficient in glucose-6-phosphate dehydrogenase. It may also occur, less frequently, during treatment with chloroquine or quinine. The answer is **(D).**
12. Giardiasis is a common intestinal protozoan infection caused by *Giardia lamblia.* A large number of infections result from fecal contamination of food or water. Metronidazole is the drug of choice in the USA. The answer is **(C).**
13. In the advanced stages of African sleeping sickness melarsoprol is the drug of choice because, unlike pentamidine or suramin, it effectively enters the CNS. Nifurtimox is the most commonly used drug for Chagas' disease. The answer is **(B).**
14. Metronidazole is the drug of first choice for all of the conditions listed except pneumocystosis. The answer is **(C).**
15. Quinine sulfate is the standard drug for oral treatment of acute attacks of malaria due to chloroquine-resistant *P falciparum.* It should be used in combination with one or more other antimalarial drugs such as doxycycline, clindamycin, or pyrimethamine plus sulfadiazine. The answer is **(E).**

Anthelmintic Drugs 54

OBJECTIVES

You should be able to:

- Identify the drugs of choice for treatment of common infections caused by nematodes, trematodes, and cestodes.
- Describe the mechanisms of action (if known), the important pharmacokinetic features, and the major toxic effects of these drugs.
- Describe the main features of important back-up anthelmintics.

CONCEPTS

Anthelmintic drugs have diverse chemical structures, mechanisms of action, and properties. Most were discovered by empiric screening methods; many act against specific parasites, and few are devoid of significant toxicity to host cells. In addition to the direct toxicity of the drugs, reactions to dead and dying parasites may cause serious toxicity in patients. In the text that follows, the drugs are divided into three groups on the basis of the type of helminth primarily affected (nematodes, trematodes, and cestodes). The drugs of choice and alternative agents for selected important helminthic infections are listed in Table 54–1.

DRUGS THAT ACT AGAINST NEMATODES

The medically important intestinal nematodes responsive to drug therapy include *Enterobius vermicularis* (pinworm), *Trichuris trichiuria* (whipworm), *Ascaris lumbricoides* (roundworm), ancyclostoma and necator species (hookworms), and *Strongyloides stercoralis* (threadworm). Over one billion persons worldwide are estimated to be infected by intestinal nematodes. Pinworm infections

Table 54–1. Major helminthic infections and the drugs used to treat them.

Infecting Organism	Drugs of Choice	Alternative Drugs
Nematodes		
Ascaris lumbricoides (roundworm)	Pyrantel pamoate, mebendazole	Albendazole, levamisole, piperazine
Necator americanus, Ancylostoma duodenale (hookworm)	Pyrantel pamoate, mebendazole	Albendazole, levamisole
Trichuris trichiura (whipworm)	Mebendazole	Albendazole, pyrantel pamoate
Strongyloides stercoralis (threadworm)	Ivermectin	Thiabendazole, albendazole
Enterobius vermicularis (pinworm)	Mebendazole, pyrantel pamoate	Albendazole
Larva migrans	Thiabendazole	Albendazole, diethylcarbamazine
Wuchereria bancrofti, Brugia malayi	Diethylcarbamazine	Ivermectin
Onchocerca volvulus	Ivermectin	Suramin, diethylecarbamazine
Trematodes (flukes)		
Schistosoma haematobium	Praziquantel	Metrifonate
Schistosoma mansoni	Praziquantel	Oxamniquine
Schistosoma japonicum	Praziquantel	None
Paragonimus westermani	Praziquantel	Bithionol
Fasciola hepatica	Bithionol	Praziquantel, emetine, dehydroemetine
Cestodes (tapeworms)		
Taenia saginata	Niclosamide, praziquantel	Mebendazole
Taenia solium	Niclosamide, praziquantel	
Diphyllobothrium latum	Niclosamide, praziquantel	
Cysticercosis	Albendazole	Praziquantel
Echinococcus granulosus (hydatid disease)	Albendazole	Mebendazole

are common throughout the United States, while the hookworm and threadworm are endemic in the southern United States.

Tissue nematodes responsive to drug therapy include ancyclostoma species, which cause cutaneous larva migrans, seen primarily in the southern USA. Species of dracunculus, onchocerca, toxocara, and *Wuchereria bancrofti* (the cause of filariasis) are all responsive to drug treatment. The number of persons worldwide estimated to be infected by tissue nematodes exceeds 0.5 billion.

A. **Albendazole:**
   1. **Mechanisms:** The mechanism of action of albendazole is unclear. The drug blocks glucose uptake in both larval and adult parasites, which leads to decreased formation of ATP and subsequent parasite immobilization. The actions of albendazole may also include inhibition of microtubule assembly, as has been described for mebendazole and thiabendazole.
   2. **Clinical use:** Albendazole has a wide anthelmintic spectrum. It is an alternative drug for larva migrans, for ascariasis, and for infections caused by roundworms, whipworms, hookworms, pinworms, and threadworms. Albendazole is also active against the pork tapeworm in the larval stage.
   3. **Toxicity:** Albendazole has few toxic effects during short courses of therapy. Reversible leukopenia, alopecia, and changes in liver enzymes may occur with prolonged use. Long-term animal toxicity studies report bone marrow suppression and fetal toxicity.

B. **Diethylcarbamazine:**
   1. **Mechanisms:** Diethylcarbamazine immobilizes microfilariae by an unknown mechanism, increasing their susceptibility to host defense mechanisms.
   2. **Clinical use:** Diethylcarbamazine is the drug of choice for filariasis and an alternative

drug, when used in combination with suramin, for onchocerciasis. Microfilariae are killed more readily than adult worms. The drug is rapidly absorbed from the gut and is excreted in the urine.

3. **Toxicity:** Adverse effects include headache, malaise, weakness, and anorexia. Reactions to proteins released by dying filariae include fever, rashes, ocular damage, joint and muscle pain, and lymphangitis. In onchocerciasis, the **Mazzotti reaction** includes most of these symptoms as well as hypotension, pyrexia, respiratory distress, and prostration.

C. Ivermectin:

1. **Mechanisms:** Ivermectin intensifies GABA-mediated neurotransmission in nematodes and causes immobilization of parasites, facilitating their removal by the reticuloendothelial system. Selective toxicity results because in humans GABA is a neurotransmitter only in the CNS, and ivermectin does not cross the blood-brain barrier.
2. **Clinical use:** Ivermectin is the drug of choice for onchocerciasis, acts more slowly than diethylcarbamazine, and causes fewer systemic and ocular reactions. Ivermectin is also the drug of first choice for strongyloidiasis and an alternative agent in filariasis.
3. **Toxicity:** Single-dose oral treatment in onchocerciasis results in Mazzotti reactions that include fever, headache, dizziness, rashes, pruritus, tachycardia, hypotension, and pain in joints, muscles, and lymph glands. These symptoms are usually of short duration, and most can be controlled with antihistamines and nonsteroidal anti-inflammatory drugs.

D. Mebendazole:

1. **Mechanism:** Mebendazole acts by selectively inhibiting microtubule synthesis and glucose uptake in nematodes.
2. **Clinical use:** Mebendazole is a drug of choice for pinworm and whipworm infections. It is one of two drugs of choice (with pyrantel pamoate) for roundworm and for combined infections with ascarids and hookworm. Mebendazole can also be used as a backup drug in certain cestode and trematode infections. Less than 10% of the drug is absorbed systemically after oral use, and this portion is metabolized rapidly.
3. **Toxicity:** Mebendazole toxicity is limited to gastrointestinal irritation. However, the drug is contraindicated in pregnancy because of possible embryotoxicity.

E. Piperazine:

1. **Mechanism:** Piperazine paralyzes ascaris by acting as an agonist at GABA receptors. The paralyzed roundworms are expelled live by normal peristalsis.
2. **Clinical use:** Piperazine is an alternative drug for ascariasis.
3. **Toxicity:** Mild gastrointestinal irritation is the most common side effect. Piperazine should not be used in patients with seizure disorders.

F. Pyrantel Pamoate:

1. **Mechanism:** Pyrantel pamoate and its congener, **oxantel pamoate,** stimulate nicotinic receptors present at neuromuscular junctions of nematodes. Contraction of muscles occurs, followed by a depolarization-induced paralysis.
2. **Clinical use:** Pyrantel pamoate is one of two drugs of choice (with mebendazole) for infections due to hookworm, pinworm, and roundworm. The drug is poorly absorbed when given orally.
3. **Toxicity:** Adverse effects are minor but include gastrointestinal distress, headache, and weakness.

G. Thiabendazole:

1. **Mechanism:** Thiabendazole is a structural congener of mebendazole and has a similar action on microtubules.
2. **Clinical use:** Thiabendazole is a drug of choice for visceral forms of larva migrans and is an effective drug for treatment of strongyloidiasis, cutaneous larva migrans, and threadworm infections. Thiabendazole is rapidly absorbed from the gut and is metabolized by liver enzymes. The drug has anti-inflammatory and immunorestorative actions in the host.
3. **Toxicity:** Thiabendazole's toxic effects include gastrointestinal irritation, headache, dizziness, drowsiness, leukopenia, hematuria, and allergic reactions, including intrahepatic

cholestasis. Reactions caused by dying parasites include fever, chills, lymphadenopathy, and skin rash.

Skill Keeper: Antimicrobial Chemotherapy in Pregnancy

Mebendazole is widely used for the treatment of nematode infections but is contraindicated in the pregnant patient because of possible embryotoxicity. Think back over the drugs used for the treatment of bacterial, fungal, protozoal, and viral infections.

1. Which drugs can you recall where the risk in pregnancy is greater than the benefit?
2. Which drugs can you recall that are nominally contraindicated in pregnancy but might be used if the benefit was judged to outweigh the risk?

The Skill Keeper Answers appear at the end of the chapter.

DRUGS THAT ACT AGAINST TREMATODES

The medically important trematodes include schistosoma species (blood flukes, estimated to affect over 150 million persons, worldwide), *Clonorchis sinensis* (liver fluke, endemic in Southeast Asia), and *Paragonimus westermani* (lung fluke, endemic to both Asia and the Indian subcontinent). With few exceptions, fluke infections respond well to praziquantel.

A. Praziquantel:

1. **Mechanism:** Praziquantel increases membrane permeability to calcium, causing marked contraction initially and then paralysis of trematode muscles; this is followed by vacuolization and parasite death.
2. **Clinical use:** Praziquantel has a wide anthelmintic spectrum that includes activity in both trematode and cestode infections. It is the drug of choice in schistosomiasis (all species), clonorchiasis, and paragonimiasis and for infections caused by small and large intestinal flukes. The drug is active against immature and adult schistosomal forms. Praziquantel is also one of two drugs of choice (with niclosamide) for infections due to cestodes (all common tapeworms) and in the treatment of cysticercosis.
3. **Pharmacokinetics:** Absorption from the gut is rapid, and the drug is metabolized by the liver to inactive products.
4. **Toxicity:** Common adverse effects include headache, dizziness, malaise, and, less frequently, gastrointestinal irritation, skin rash, and fever. Praziquantel is contraindicated in ocular cysticercosis.

B. Bithionol:

1. **Clinical use:** Bithionol is the drug of choice for treatment of fascioliasis (sheep liver fluke) and an alternative agent in paragonimiasis. The mechanism of action of the drug is unknown. Bithionol is orally effective and is eliminated in the urine.
2. **Toxicity:** Common adverse effects include nausea and vomiting, diarrhea and abdominal cramps, dizziness, headache, and phototoxicity. Less frequently, pyrexia, tinnitus, proteinuria, and leukopenia may occur.

C. Metrifonate: Metrifonate is an organophosphate prodrug that is converted in the body to the cholinesterase inhibitor dichlorvos. The active metabolite acts solely against *Schistosoma haematobium* (the cause of bilharziasis). Toxic effects occur from excess cholinergic stimulation.

D. Oxamniquine: Oxamniquine is effective solely in *Schistosoma mansoni* infections, acting on male immature forms and adult schistosomal forms. Dizziness is a common adverse effect; headache, gastrointestinal irritation, and pruritus may also occur. Reactions to dying parasites include eosinophilia, urticaria, and pulmonary infiltrates. It is not advisable to use the drug in pregnancy or in patients with a past history of seizure disorders.

DRUGS THAT ACT AGAINST CESTODES (TAPEWORMS)

The four medically important cestodes are *Taenia saginata* (beef tapeworm), *Taenia solium* (pork tapeworm, which can cause cysticerci in the brain and the eyes), *Diphyllobothrium latum* (fish tapeworm), and *Echinococcus granulosus* (dog tapeworm, which can cause hydatid cysts in the liver, lungs, and brain). The primary drugs for treatment of cestode infections are praziquantel (see above) and niclosamide.

A. Niclosamide:

1. **Mechanism:** Niclosamide may act by uncoupling oxidative phosphorylation or by activating ATPases.
2. **Clinical use:** Niclosamide is one of two drugs of choice (with praziquantel) for infections caused by beef, pork, and fish tapeworm infections. However, it is not effective in cysticercosis (for which albendazole or praziquantel is used) or hydatid disease caused by *Echinococcus granulosus* (for which albendazole is used). Scoleces and cestode segments are killed, but ova are not. Niclosamide is effective in the treatment of infections due to small and large intestinal flukes.
3. **Toxicity:** Toxic effects are usually mild but include gastrointestinal distress, headache, rash, and fever. Some of these effects may result from systemic absorption of antigens from disintegrating parasites.

DRUG LIST

See Table 54–1.

QUESTIONS

DIRECTIONS: Each of the numbered items or incomplete statements in this section is followed by answers or by completions of the statement. Select the ONE lettered answer or completion that is BEST in each case.

1. All of the following drugs are active against nematodes. Which one causes muscle paralysis by activating receptors for the inhibitory transmitter GABA?
   (A) Albendazole
   (B) Diethylcarbamazine
   (C) Mebendazole
   (D) Piperazine
   (E) Pyrantel pamoate
2. A patient with a tapeworm infection is to be treated with niclosamide. Which one of the following statements concerning the use of the drug is LEAST accurate?
   (A) The drug is not effective against the dog tapeworm.
   (B) Niclosamide is active against taenia species and *Diphyllobothrium latum*
   (C) The patient probably became infected by eating raw or undercooked meat or fish
   (D) Niclosamide is only effective against intestinal worms
   (E) The drug will kill ova of the parasite
3. A missionary from Chicago is sent to work in a geographic region of a Central American country where *Onchocerca volvulus* is endemic. Infections due to this tissue nematode (onchocerciasis) are a major cause of "river blindness," since microfilariae migrate through subcutaneous tissues and concentrate in the eyes. Which one of the following drugs can be used prophylactically to prevent onchocerciasis?
   (A) Bithionol
   (B) Ivermectin
   (C) Niclosamide
   (D) Oxamniquine
   (E) Suramin
4. A nonindigenous individual who develops onchocerciasis in an endemic region would normally be treated with ivermectin and is likely to experience the Mazzotti reaction. Which one of the following statements concerning this reaction is LEAST accurate?

(A) The Mazzotti reaction is more intense in expatriate adults than indigenous adults
(B) Symptoms usually include headache, weakness, rash, muscle aches, hypotension, and peripheral edema
(C) The reaction is due to drug toxicity
(D) NSAIDs and steroids relieve symptoms of the reaction
(E) The reaction is due to killing of microfilariae

5. Which one of the following statements about pyrantel pamoate is LEAST accurate?
(A) It is highly effective in pinworm infections
(B) Its action at the neuromuscular junction is similar to that of succinylcholine
(C) Toxicity mainly concerns the gastrointestinal tract because little of an oral dose is absorbed
(D) The drug is equivalent in efficacy to niclosamide in the treatment of tapeworm infections
(E) The drug kills adult worms in the colon but not the eggs

6. A student studying medicine at a Caribbean university develops fever, chills, and diarrhea due to *S mansoni,* and oxamniquine is prescribed. Which one of the following statements about the proposed therapy is accurate?
(A) It is not effective in late stages of the disease
(B) If the patient has a history of seizure disorders, hospitalization is recommended during treatment
(C) The drug is effective in other forms of schistosomiasis
(D) Oxamniquine is safe to use in pregnancy
(E) The drug blocks GABA receptors in trematodes

7. A 22-year-old Korean male has recently moved to Minnesota. He has symptoms of clonorchiasis (anorexia, upper abdominal pain, eosinophilia), presumably contracted in his homeland where the Oriental liver fluke is endemic. He also has symptoms of diphyllobothriasis (abdominal discomfort, diarrhea, megaloblastic anemia), probably due to consumption of raw fish from lakes near the Canadian border. Which one of the following drugs is most likely to be effective in the treatment of both clonorchiasis and diphyllobothriasis in this patient?
(A) Albendazole
(B) Ivermectin
(C) Levamisole
(D) Niclosamide
(E) Praziquantel

8. Which one of the following infections due to helminths is LEAST likely to respond to treatment with praziquantel?
(A) Hydatid disease
(B) Opisthorchiasis
(C) Paragonimiasis
(D) Pork tapeworm infection
(E) Schistosomiasis

Items 9–10: A sheepherder who lives most of the year in the mountains of eastern Nevada is hospitalized with liver cysts (hydatid disease) attributed to infection with *Echinococcus granulosus,* the dog tapeworm. He refuses to undergo surgery for removal of the cysts.

9. Which one of the following drugs is most likely to be of some help in this situation?
(A) Albendazole
(B) Ivermectin
(C) Niclosamide
(D) Oxamniquine
(E) Suramin

10. Since the patient will have to undergo drug treatment for many months, he should be monitored for toxicity to the
(A) Gonads
(B) Kidney
(C) Liver
(D) Peripheral nerves
(E) Retina

11. Which one of the following adverse effects occurs with the use of mebendazole during intestinal nematode therapy?

(A) Cholestatic jaundice
(B) Corneal opacities
(C) Mazzotti reactions
(D) Peripheral neuropathy
(E) None of the above

12. A malnourished 12-year-old child who lives in a rural area of the southern United States presents with weakness, fever, cough, abdominal pain, and eosinophilia. His mother tells you that she has seen long, thin worms in the child's stools, sometimes with blood. A presumptive diagnosis of ascariasis is confirmed by the presence of the ova of *A lumbricoides* in the stools. However, microscopy also reveals that the stools contain the eggs of *Necator americanus*. The drug most likely to be effective in the treatment of this child is
(A) Diethylcarbamazine
(B) Ivermectin
(C) Mebendazole
(D) Niclosamide
(E) Praziquantel

DIRECTIONS (Items 13–17): This case history* is followed by discussion questions. Write out brief answers (two to five sentences) and then compare your answers with those given at the end of the Answers section.

A 20-year-old woman in good health planned to visit Kenya in a travel and study program. She was immunized against tetanus, typhoid, cholera, and yellow fever, received immune globulin intramuscular (IGIM), and in Kenya took chloroquine and Fansidar (pyrimethamine-sulfadoxine) for malaria prophylaxis. After 10 weeks, she was one of 15 students (of 18 in the original group) to become ill, with fever, abdominal pain, and nonbloody diarrhea. Five days later, she developed severe back pain and then rapidly lost ability to walk. Stool examination showed ova of Schistosoma mansoni, *and she was diagnosed as having schistosomiasis with transverse myelitis.*

She was treated with oxamniquine and transported to the USA, where evaluation showed flaccid paralysis and decreased sensation of touch and of temperature over the skin of the legs. Cerebrospinal fluid examination showed pleocytosis and protein elevation. Serologic tests for mycoplasma and viral pathogens were negative. A myelogram showed no masses amenable to surgical removal.

The patient was treated with praziquantel and large doses of dexamethasone. Motor function and sensation improved with treatment, and within a month she was ambulating with assistance in a rehabilitation center.

13. Why was this patient taking both chloroquine and pyrimethamine-sulfadoxine for malaria prophylaxis?
14. Why was oxamniquine used for the initial treatment of schistosomiasis in this case? What are its anticipated adverse effects?
15. How does praziquantel differ from other drugs used in schistosomiasis? What is known about its mechanism of action?
16. What are the anticipated adverse effects of praziquantel?
17. Why was dexamethasone administered?

ANSWERS

1. Piperazine and ivermectin (not listed in the question) both cause muscle paralysis in nematodes by acting through GABA receptors. Pyrantel pamoate relaxes muscles by blocking nicotinic receptors. Diethylcarbamazine also causes muscle relaxation, but the mechanism is un-

* Adapted from: Acute schistosomiasis with transverse myelitis in American students returning from Kenya. MMWR Morb Mortal Wkly Rep 1984;33:445.

known. The benzimidazoles (albendazole, mebendazole) bind to alpha-tubulins in helminths to block transport processes. The answer is **(D).**

2. Niclosamide is often used to treat tapeworm infections since it is usually effective in a single dose. It is minimally absorbed from the gastrointestinal tract and causes few side effects. The drug kills scoleces and cestode segments, but ova are not affected. The answer is **(E).**
3. Ivermectin prevents onchocerciasis and is the drug of choice in the individual and mass treatment of the disease. The only other drugs effective against *Onchocerca volvulus* are suramin and diethylcarbamazine (not listed in the question). The World Health Organization no longer recommends diethylcarbamazine for onchocerciasis, since it is less effective and more toxic than ivermectin. Suramin is toxic to the kidney, liver, and nervous system and would not be used prophylactically in this case. The answer is **(B).**
4. The Mazzotti reaction is due to the killing action of ivermectin on microfilariae and its intensity correlates with skin microfilaria load. It occurs more frequently and with greater severity in nonindigenous persons than in the indigenous inhabitants of endemic areas. The reaction will occur with any drug capable of killing microfilariae, and it is not a drug toxicity. The answer is **(C).**
5. Pyrantel pamoate is equivalent to mebendazole in the treatment of pinworm infections, but it is not effective in the treatment of infections caused by cestodes. The answer is **(D).**
6. Oxamniquine may cause seizures, especially in persons with a past history of convulsive disorders. Such persons should be hospitalized or treated with praziquantel. Oxamniquine is effective in all stages of disease caused by *S mansoni,* including advanced hepatosplenomegaly. It has been used extensively for mass treatment. The drug is not effective in other schistosomal diseases, and it is contraindicated in pregnancy. The answer is **(B).**
7. Praziquantel is the drug of first choice for infections caused by the Oriental liver fluke and by the fish tapeworm. Both types of infection are transmitted mainly via the consumption of raw fish. Niclosamide is one of two drugs of choice for fish tapeworm infections (with praziquantel), but it is not active against *Clonorchis sinensis.* Albendazole is not effective in fish tapeworm infections but is useful in the pork tapeworm larval stage (cysticercosis). The answer is **(E).**
8. Praziquantel has a wide spectrum of activity that includes many cestodes and trematodes. However, in hydatid disease the drug has marginal efficacy because it does not affect the inner germinal membrane of *Echinococcus granulosus* present in hydatid cysts. The answer is **(A).**
9. The optimal treatment of hydatid cysts is their surgical removal. Albendazole has been used—at high doses for 3 months or longer—for liver hydatid cysts. However, the cure rate, judged by shrinkage or disappearance of cysts, is less than 40%. The answer is **(A).**
10. Elevations of aminotransferase occur most frequently (15–20% incidence) during long-term therapy with mebendazole. Jaundice has been reported in a few patients. With the exception of liver function, none of the other organ systems listed require periodic monitoring. The answer is **(C).**
11. Doses of mebendazole required for intestinal nematode therapy are almost free of adverse effects even in the malnourished or debilitated patient. Gastrointestinal distress may occur in children with ascariasis who are heavily parasitized, together with a slight headache or dizziness. The answer is **(E).**
12. Mebendazole and pyrantel pamoate (not listed in this question) are drugs of choice for the treatment of combined infections due to hookworm and roundworm. If this patient is also infected with *Trichuris trichiura* (whipworm), mebendazole would be more effective than pyrantel pamoate. The answer is **(C).**
13. Chloroquine-resistant *P falciparum* is endemic in many regions of Africa, including Kenya, and the prophylactic use of chloroquine as a sole agent will not prevent infection. While pyrimethamine-sulfadoxine has been used prophylactically, it is not the drug of choice. Weekly doses of mefloquine one week before entering an endemic area, during the sojourn, and for 4 weeks after leaving, is the preferred method.
14. Oxamniquine is active against mature and immature forms of *Schistosoma mansoni* (but not other schistosomes), though resistance can occur. The initial use of the drug was presumably based on identification of the parasite ova in stools, this drug's ease of administration (it is orally effective), and—perhaps—its availability. Adverse effects of oxamniquine include dizziness, headache, drowsiness, gastrointestinal irritation, and pruritus. Effects probably due

to dying parasites include eosinophilia, pulmonary infiltrates, and urticaria. At high doses, oxamniquine may cause hallucinations and seizures.

15. Praziquantel is the drug of choice for infections caused by all species of schistosomes. The agent increases the permeability of the parasite cell membrane to calcium, causing initial contraction and then paralysis of its musculature. The tegmen becomes vacuolized and disintegrates, causing parasite death.
16. The most common toxic effects of praziquantel are malaise, headache, dizziness, gastrointestinal irritation, urticaria, and fever. Some of these effects may be caused by dying parasites.
17. Corticosteroids are used to suppress host immune responses and inflammation, including reactions to eggs deposited in the venules in and around the spinal cord.

Skill Keeper Answers: Antimicrobial Chemotherapy in Pregnancy

1. A drug is designated (by the FDA) as Pregnancy Risk Category **X** if the risk of its use in pregnancy is judged to be greater than any possible benefit. Such drugs have been established to cause fetal abnormalities or miscarriage in humans. This category includes the antiviral agent ribavirin and the antimalarial drug quinine. Ethionamide and thalidomide, which have been used in mycobacterial infections, are also category **X** drugs.
2. For drugs in FDA Pregnancy Risk Category **D** there is evidence of human risk, but their potential benefit may outweigh such risk. In other words, they are not *absolutely* contraindicated in pregnancy. The most important drugs in this category are the aminoglycosides (eg, gentamicin) and the tetracyclines. Though they are not category **D** drugs, fluoroquinolones are not approved by the FDA for use in pregnancy, and many other drugs should be used with caution—or avoided if alternatives are available.

55 Cancer Chemotherapy

OBJECTIVES

You should be able to:

- Describe the relevance of cell cycle kinetics to the modes of action and clinical uses of anticancer drugs.
- Identify the major subclasses of anticancer drugs, describe the mechanisms of action of the main drugs in each subclass, and describe the mechanisms by which tumor cells develop drug resistance.
- Identify the drugs used in regimens for treatment of the more common neoplastic diseases and describe their pharmacokinetics and their toxic effects.
- Understand the rationale underlying the strategies of combination drug chemotherapy and rescue therapies.

Learn the definitions that follow.

Table 55–1. Definitions.

Term	Definition
Cell cycle-specific (CCS) drug	An anticancer agent that acts selectively on tumor stem cells when they are traversing the cell cycle and not when they are in the G_0, or resting, phase
Cell cycle-nonspecific (CCNS) drug	An anticancer agent that acts on tumor stem cells when they are traversing the cell cycle and when they are in the resting phase
Log-kill hypothesis	A concept used in cancer chemotherapy to mean that anticancer drugs kill a fixed proportion of a tumor cell population, not a fixed number of tumor cells. For example, a 1-log-kill will decrease a tumor cell population by one order of magnitude, ie, 90% of the cells will be eradicated
Growth fraction	The proportion of cells in a tumor population that are actively dividing
Rescue therapy	The administration of endogenous metabolites to counteract the effects of anticancer drugs on normal (nonneoplastic) cells

CONCEPTS

The treatment of cancer requires a variety of different types of drugs acting on several different targets (Figure 55–1).

CANCER CELL CYCLE KINETICS

A. Cell Cycle Kinetics: Cancer cell population kinetics and the cancer cell cycle are important determinants of the actions and clinical uses of anticancer drugs. Some anticancer drugs act specifically on tumor cells undergoing cycling (cell cycle-specific [CCS] drugs), and others (cell cycle-nonspecific [CCNS] drugs) kill tumor cells in both cycling and resting phases of the cell cycle. CCS drugs are usually most active in a specific phase of the cell cycle (Figure 55–2). CCS drugs are particularly effective when a large proportion of the tumor cells are proliferating (ie, when the growth fraction is high).

B. The Log-Kill Hypothesis: Cytotoxic drugs act with first-order kinetics, a given dose killing a constant *proportion* of a cell population rather than a constant *number* of cells. The log-kill hypothesis proposes that the magnitude of tumor cell kill by anticancer drugs is a logarithmic function. For example, a 3-log-kill dose of an effective drug will reduce a cancer cell population of 10^{12} cells to 10^9 (a total kill of $10^{12} - 10^9$, or 999×10^9 cells); the same dose would reduce a starting population of 10^6 cells to 10^3 cells (a kill of 999×10^3 cells). In both cases, the dose reduces the numbers of cells by three orders of magnitude, or "3 logs."

C. Resistance to Anticancer Drugs: Drug resistance is a major problem in cancer chemotherapy. Mechanisms of resistance include the following.

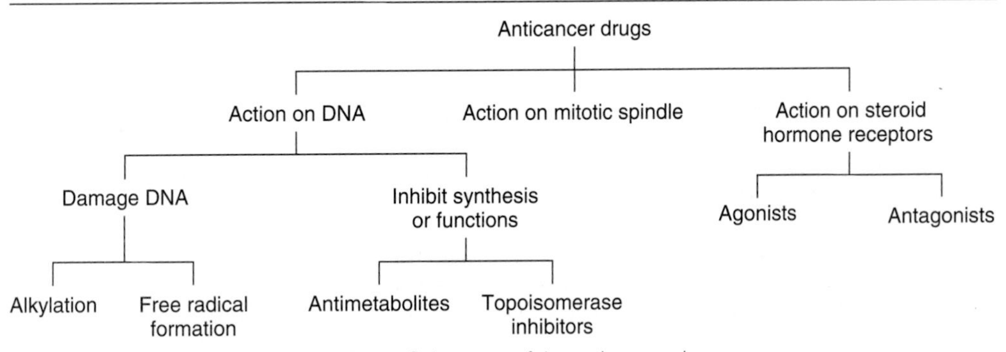

Figure 55–1. Subgroups of the anticancer drugs.

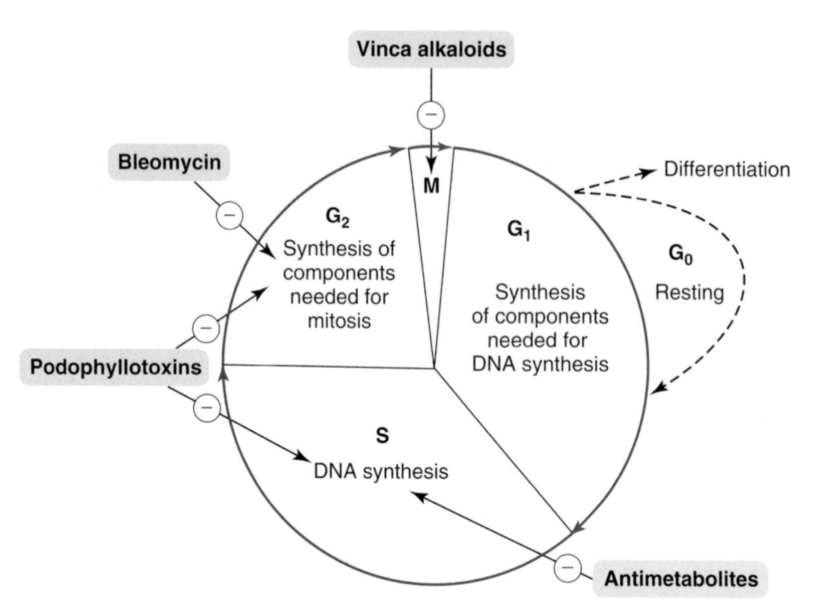

Figure 55–2. Phases of the cell cycle that are susceptible to the actions of cell cycle-specific (CCS) drugs. All cells—normal and neoplastic—must traverse these cell cycle phases before and during cell division. CCS drug actions may not be restricted to a specific phase, but tumor cells are usually most responsive to specific drugs (or drug groups) in the phases indicated. Cell cycle-nonspecific (CCNS) drugs act on tumor cells while they are actively cycling and while they are in the resting phase (G_0). (Adapted, with permission, from Katzung BG [editor]: *Basic & Clinical Pharmacology,* 7th ed. Originally published by Appleton & Lange. Copyright © 1998 by The McGraw-Hill Companies, Inc.)

1. **Increased DNA repair:** An increased rate of DNA repair in tumor cells can be responsible for resistance and is particularly important in the case of most alkylating agents and cisplatin.
2. **Formation of trapping agents:** Some tumor cells increase their production of thiol trapping agents (eg, glutathione), which interact with anticancer drugs that form reactive electrophilic species. This mechanism of resistance is seen with the alkylating agent bleomycin, cisplatin, and the anthracyclines.
3. **Changes in target enzymes:** Changes in the drug sensitivity of a target enzyme, dihydrofolate reductase, and increased synthesis of the enzyme are mechanisms of resistance of tumor cells to methotrexate.
4. **Decreased activation of prodrugs:** Resistance to the purine antimetabolites (mercaptopurine, thioguanine) and the pyrimidine antimetabolites (cytarabine, fluorouracil) can result from a decrease in the activity of the tumor cell enzymes needed to convert these prodrugs to their cytotoxic metabolites.
5. **Inactivation of anticancer drugs:** Increased activity of enzymes capable of inactivating anticancer drugs is a mechanism of tumor cell resistance to most of the purine and pyrimidine antimetabolites.
6. **Decreased drug accumulation:** This form of multidrug resistance involves the increased expression of a normal gene (the *MDR1* gene) for a cell surface glycoprotein (P-glycoprotein). This transport molecule is involved in the accelerated efflux of many anticancer drugs in resistant cells.

ALKYLATING AGENTS

The alkylating agents include nitrogen mustards **(chlorambucil, cyclophosphamide, mechlorethamine),** nitrosoureas **(carmustine [BCNU], lomustine [CCNU]),** and alkylsulfonates **(busulfan).** Other drugs that act in part as alkylating agents include **cisplatin, dacarbazine,** and **procarbazine.**

The alkylating agents are CCNS drugs. They form reactive molecular species that alkylate nucleophilic groups on DNA bases, particularly the N-7 position of guanine. This leads to cross-linking of bases, abnormal base pairing, and DNA strand breakage. Tumor cell resistance to the drugs occurs through increased DNA repair, decreased drug permeability, or the production of trapping agents such as thiols.

A. Cyclophosphamide:

1. **Pharmacokinetics:** Hepatic cytochrome P450-mediated biotransformation of cyclophosphamide is needed for antitumor activity. One of the breakdown products is acrolein.
2. **Clinical use:** Uses of cyclophosphamide include non-Hodgkin's lymphoma, breast and ovarian cancers, and neuroblastoma.
3. **Toxicity:** Gastrointestinal distress, myelosuppression, and alopecia are expected adverse effects. Hemorrhagic cystitis due to the formation of acrolein may be decreased by vigorous hydration and by use of **mercaptoethanesulfonate** (mesna). Cyclophosphamide may also cause cardiac dysfunction, pulmonary toxicity, and a syndrome of inappropriate ADH secretion.

B. Mechlorethamine:

1. **Mechanism and pharmacokinetics:** Mechlorethamine spontaneously converts in the body to a reactive cytotoxic product.
2. **Clinical use:** Mechlorethamine is best known for use in the MOPP regimen (see below) for Hodgkin's disease.
3. **Toxicity:** Gastrointestinal distress, myelosuppression, and alopecia are common. Mechlorethamine has marked vesicant actions.

C. Carmustine (BCNU) and Lomustine (CCNU):

1. **Pharmacokinetics:** BCNU and CCNU are nitrosoureas with high lipophilicity that facilitates CNS entry.
2. **Clinical use:** BCNU and CCNU are used as adjuncts in the treatment of brain tumors.
3. **Toxicity:** Adverse effects include gastrointestinal distress, myelosuppression, and CNS dysfunction.

D. Cisplatin and Carboplatin:

1. **Pharmacokinetics:** Cisplatin is used intravenously; the drug distributes to most tissues and is cleared in unchanged form by the kidney.
2. **Clinical use:** Cisplatin is commonly used as a component of regimens for testicular carcinoma and for cancers of the bladder, lung, and ovary. Carboplatin has similar uses.
3. **Toxicity:** Cisplatin causes gastrointestinal distress and mild hematotoxicity and is neurotoxic (peripheral neuritis and acoustic nerve damage) and nephrotoxic. Renal damage may be reduced by the use of mannitol with forced hydration. Carboplatin is less nephrotoxic than cisplatin and is less likely to cause tinnitus and hearing loss, but it has greater myelosuppressant actions.

E. Procarbazine:

1. **Mechanisms:** Procarbazine is a reactive agent that forms hydrogen peroxide, which generates free radicals that cause DNA strand scission.
2. **Pharmacokinetics:** Procarbazine is orally active and penetrates into most tissues, including the cerebrospinal fluid. It is eliminated via hepatic metabolism.
3. **Clinical use:** The primary use of the drug is as a component of the MOPP regimen for Hodgkin's disease.
4. **Toxicity:** Procarbazine is myelosuppressant and causes gastrointestinal irritation, CNS dysfunction, peripheral neuropathy, and skin reactions. Procarbazine inhibits many enzymes, including MAO and those involved in hepatic drug metabolism. Disulfiram-like reactions have occurred with ethanol. The drug is leukemogenic.

F. Other Alkylating Agents: Busulfan is sometimes used in chronic myelogenous leukemia. It causes adrenal insufficiency, pulmonary fibrosis, and skin pigmentation. Dacarbazine is used in Hodgkin's disease as part of the ABVD regimen. It causes alopecia, skin rash, gastrointestinal distress, myelosuppression, phototoxicity and a flu-like syndrome.

ANTIMETABOLITES

The antimetabolites are structurally similar to endogenous compounds and are antagonists of folic acid **(methotrexate),** purines **(mercaptopurine, thioguanine),** or pyrimidines **(fluorouracil, cytarabine).** Antimetabolites are CCS drugs acting primarily in the S phase of the cell cycle. Their sites of action on DNA synthetic pathways are shown in Figure 55–3. In addition to their cytotoxic effects on neoplastic cells, the antimetabolites also have immunosuppressant actions. Some of the uses of the antimetabolites in neoplastic disease are listed in Table 55–2.

A. Methotrexate:

1. **Mechanisms of action and resistance:** Methotrexate is a substrate for and inhibitor of dihydrofolate reductase. This action leads to a decrease in the synthesis of thymidylate, purine nucleotides, and amino acids and thus interferes with nucleic acid and protein metabolism. The formation of polyglutamate derivatives of methotrexate appears to be important for cytotoxic actions. Tumor cell resistance mechanisms include decreased drug accumulation, changes in the drug sensitivity or activity of dihydrofolate reductase, and decreased formation of polyglutamates.
2. **Pharmacokinetics:** Oral and intravenous administration of methotrexate affords good tissue distribution except to the CNS. Methotrexate is not metabolized, and its clearance is dependent on renal function. Adequate hydration is needed to prevent crystallization in renal tubules.
3. **Clinical use:** Methotrexate is effective in choriocarcinoma, acute leukemias, non-Hodgkin's and cutaneous T cell lymphomas, and breast cancer. Methotrexate is used also in rheumatoid arthritis and psoriasis and is an abortifacient.
4. **Toxicity:** Common adverse effects include bone marrow suppression and toxic effects on the skin and gastrointestinal mucosa (mucositis). The toxic effects of methotrexate on normal cells may be reduced by administration of folinic acid (leucovorin); this strategy is called **"leucovorin rescue."** Long-term use of methotrexate has led to hepatotoxicity and to pulmonary infiltrates and fibrosis. Salicylates, NSAIDs, sulfonamides, and sulfonylureas enhance the toxicity of methotrexate.

B. Mercaptopurine (6-MP) and Thioguanine (6-TG):

1. **Mechanisms of action and resistance:** Mercaptopurine and thioguanine are purine antimetabolites. Both drugs are activated by hypoxanthine-guanine phosphoribosyltransferases (HGPRTases) to toxic nucleotides that inhibit several enzymes involved in purine

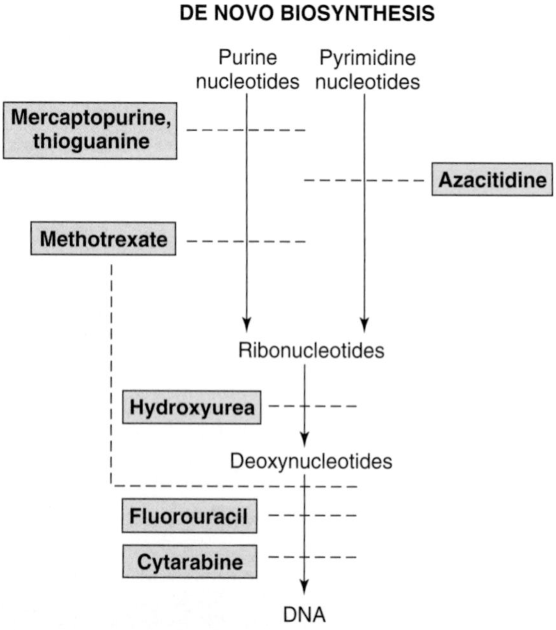

DE NOVO BIOSYNTHESIS
Purine nucleotides
Pyrimidine nucleotides
Mercaptopurine, thioguanine
Azacitidine
Methotrexate
Ribonucleotides
Hydroxyurea
Deoxynucleotides
Fluorouracil
Cytarabine
DNA

Figure 55–3. Sites of action of antimetabolites on DNA synthetic pathways.

Table 55–2. Selected examples of effective cancer chemotherapy.*

Diagnosis[1]	Current Drug Therapy of Choice
Acute lymphocytic leukemia	Induction: vincristine plus prednisone plus asparaginase plus doxorubicin with or without cyclophosphamide. Maintenance: mercaptopurine plus methotrexate
Acute myelogenous leukemia	Induction: Cytarabine plus daunorubicin with or without etoposide. Postinduction: Cytarabine plus other drugs
Breast carcinoma (stages I and II)	CMF regimen: Cyclophosphamide plus methotrexate and fluorouracil, or doxorubicin for methotrexate (CAF regimen); tamoxifen if hormone receptor-positive
Breast carcinoma (stages III and IV)	As above, plus paclitaxel, plus trastuzumab (if HER2 protein) with or without aromatase inhibitors
Ewing's sarcoma	Cyclophosphamide plus doxorubicin and vincristine
Hodgkin's lymphoma	ABVD regimen: doxorubicin (Adriamycin) plus bleomycin plus vincristine plus dacarbazine
Non-Hodgkin's lymphoma, Burkitt's, lymphoblastic, or diffuse	Cyclophosphamide plus doxorubicin plus methotrexate and vincristine with or without prednisone
Small cell lung carcinoma	Multiple combinations that include cyclophosphamide, cisplatin, doxorubicin, etoposide, and vincristine
Prostate carcinoma	Leuprolide with or without flutamide; additonal drugs include estrogens and ketoconazole
Testicular carcinoma	PEB regimen: Cisplatin (Platinol) plus etoposide plus bleomycin
Wilms' tumor	Dactinomycin plus vincristine with or without doxorubicin with or without cyclophosphamide

*Modified and reproduced, with permission, from Katzung BG (editor): *Basic & Clinical Pharmacology,* 8th ed. McGraw-Hill, 2001.
[1]Cancers that respond to chemotherapy with prolonged patient survival and some cures.

metabolism. Resistant tumor cells have a decreased activity of HGPRTase, or they may increase their production of alkaline phosphatases that inactivate the toxic nucleotides.

2. **Pharmacokinetics:** Mercaptopurine and thioguanine have low oral bioavailability due to first-pass metabolism by hepatic enzymes. The metabolism of 6-MP by xanthine oxidase is inhibited by allopurinol.
3. **Clinical use:** Purine antimetabolites are used mainly in the acute leukemias and chronic myelocytic leukemia.
4. **Toxicity:** Bone marrow suppression is dose-limiting, but hepatic dysfunction (cholestasis, jaundice, necrosis) also occurs.

C. Cytarabine (Ara-C):

1. **Mechanisms of action and resistance:** Cytarabine (cytosine arabinoside) is a pyrimidine antimetabolite. The drug is activated by kinases to AraCTP, an inhibitor of DNA polymerases. Of all the antimetabolites, cytarabine is the most specific for the S phase of the tumor cell cycle. Resistance to cytarabine can occur as a result of its decreased uptake or its decreased conversion to AraCTP.
2. **Pharmacokinetics:** The drug is used parenterally and with slow intravenous infusion may reach appreciable levels in the cerebrospinal fluid. Ara-C is eliminated via hepatic metabolism.
3. **Clinical use:** Cytarabine is an important component in regimens for the treatment of acute leukemias.
4. **Toxicity:** Ara-C causes gastrointestinal irritation and myelosuppression. High doses have led to neurotoxicity (cerebellar dysfunction and peripheral neuritis).

D. Fluorouracil (5-FU):

1. **Mechanisms:** Fluorouracil is biotransformed to 5-fluoro-2′-deoxyuridine-5′-monophosphate (5-FdUMP), which inhibits thymidylate synthase and leads to "thymineless death" of cells. Tumor cell resistance mechanisms include decreased activation of 5-FU, increased thymidylate synthase activity, and reduced drug sensitivity of this enzyme.
2. **Pharmacokinetics:** When given intravenously, fluorouracil is widely distributed, including into the cerebrospinal fluid. Elimination is mainly by metabolism.

3. **Clinical use:** Fluorouracil is used in bladder, breast, colon, head and neck, liver, and ovarian cancers. The drug can be used topically for keratoses and superficial basal cell carcinoma.
4. **Toxicity:** Gastrointestinal distress, myelosuppression, and alopecia are common.

PLANT ALKALOIDS

The most important of these CCS drugs are the vinca alkaloids **(vinblastine, vincristine),** the podophyllotoxins **(etoposide, teniposide),** and the taxanes **(paclitaxel, docetaxel).**

A. Vinblastine and Vincristine:

1. **Mechanisms:** Vinblastine and vincristine are **spindle poisons** which, by preventing the assembly of tubulin dimers into microtubules, block the formation of the mitotic spindle. They act primarily in the M phase of the cancer cell cycle. Resistance may occur from increased efflux of the drugs from tumor cells via the membrane drug transporter.
2. **Pharmacokinetics:** Both drugs must be given parenterally. They penetrate most tissues except the cerebrospinal fluid. Both drugs are cleared mainly via biliary excretion.
3. **Clinical use:** Vincristine is a component of the MOPP and COP combination drug regimens and is used in acute leukemias, lymphomas, Wilms' tumor, and choriocarcinoma. Vinblastine is a component of the ABVD regimen for Hodgkin's disease and is used for other lymphomas, neuroblastoma, testicular carcinoma, and Kaposi's sarcoma.
4. **Toxicity:** Vinblastine causes gastrointestinal distress, alopecia, and bone marrow suppression. Vincristine does not cause serious myelosuppression but has neurotoxic actions and may cause areflexia, peripheral neuritis, and paralytic ileus.

B. Etoposide and Teniposide:

1. **Mechanisms:** Etoposide increases degradation of DNA, possibly via interaction with topoisomerase II, and also inhibits mitochondrial electron transport. The drug is most active in the late S and early G_2 phases of the cell cycle. Teniposide is an analog with very similar pharmacologic characteristics.
2. **Pharmacokinetics:** Etoposide is well absorbed after oral administration and distributes to most body tissues. Elimination of etoposide is mainly via the kidneys, and dose reductions should be made in patients with renal impairment.
3. **Clinical use:** These agents are used in combination drug regimens for therapy of lung (small cell), prostate, and testicular carcinoma.
4. **Toxicity:** Etoposide and teniposide are gastrointestinal irritants and cause alopecia and bone marrow suppression.

C. Paclitaxel and Docetaxel:

1. **Mechanisms:** Paclitaxel and docetaxel are spindle poisons and act differently from vinca alkaloids—they prevent microtubule *disassembly* into tubulin monomers.
2. **Pharmacokinetics:** Paclitaxel and docetaxel are given intravenously.
3. **Clinical use:** The taxanes are used in advanced breast and ovarian cancers.
4. **Toxicity:** Paclitaxel causes neutropenia, thrombocytopenia, a high incidence of peripheral neuropathy, and possible hypersensitivity reactions during infusion. Docetaxel causes neurotoxicity and bone marrow depression.

ANTIBIOTICS

This category of antineoplastic drugs is made up of several structurally dissimilar agents, including **doxorubicin, daunorubicin, bleomycin, dactinomycin, mitomycin,** and **mithramycin.**

A. Doxorubicin and Daunorubicin:

1. **Mechanisms:** These anthracyclines can intercalate between base pairs, inhibit topoisomerase II, and generate free radicals. They block the synthesis of RNA and DNA and cause DNA strand scission. Membrane disruption also occurs. Anthracyclines are CCNS drugs.
2. **Pharmacokinetics:** Doxorubicin and daunorubicin must be given intravenously. They are metabolized in the liver, and the products are excreted in the bile and the urine (the red color is not hematuria).

3. **Clinical use:** Doxorubicin is a component of the ABVD regimen used in Hodgkin's disease and is used in treatment of myelomas, sarcomas, and breast, endometrial, lung, ovarian, and thyroid cancers. The main use of daunorubicin is in the treatment of acute leukemias. **Idarubicin,** a new anthracycline, is approved for use in acute myelogenous leukemia.
4. **Toxicity:** Both drugs cause bone marrow suppression, gastrointestinal distress, and severe alopecia. Their most distinctive adverse effect is cardiotoxicity, which includes initial electrocardiographic abnormalities (with the possibility of arrhythmias) and slowly developing cardiomyopathy and congestive heart failure. **Dexrazoxane,** a free radical scavenger, may protect against cardiotoxicity. Liposomal formulations of doxorubicin may be less cardiotoxic.

B. Bleomycin:

1. **Mechanisms:** Bleomycin is a mixture of glycopeptides that generates free radicals which bind to DNA, cause strand breaks, and inhibit DNA synthesis. Bleomycin is a CCS drug active in the G_2 phase of the tumor cell cycle.
2. **Pharmacokinetics:** Bleomycin must be given parenterally. It is inactivated by tissue aminopeptidases, but some renal clearance of intact drug also occurs.
3. **Clinical use:** Bleomycin is a component of drug regimens for Hodgkin's disease and testicular cancer. It is also used for treatment of lymphomas and for squamous cell carcinomas.
4. **Toxicity:** The toxicity profile of bleomycin includes pulmonary dysfunction (pneumonitis, fibrosis), which develops slowly and is dose-limiting. Hypersensitivity reactions (chills, fever, anaphylaxis) are common, as are mucocutaneous reactions (alopecia, blister-formation, hyperkeratosis).

C. Dactinomycin:

1. **Mechanisms and pharmacokinetics:** Dactinomycin is a CCNS drug that binds to double-stranded DNA and inhibits DNA-dependent RNA synthesis. Dactinomycin must be given parenterally, and both intact drug and metabolites are excreted in the bile.
2. **Clinical use:** Dactinomycin is used in melanoma and Wilms' tumor.
3. **Toxicity:** This drug causes bone marrow suppression, skin reactions, and gastrointestinal irritation.

D. Mitomycin:

1. **Mechanisms and pharmacokinetics:** Mitomycin is a CCNS drug that is metabolized by liver enzymes to form an alkylating agent which cross-links DNA. Mitomycin is given intravenously and is rapidly cleared via hepatic metabolism.
2. **Clinical use:** Mitomycin acts against hypoxic tumor cells and is used in combination regimens for adenocarcinomas of the cervix, stomach, pancreas, and lung.
3. **Toxicity:** Mitomycin causes severe myelosuppression and is toxic to the heart, liver, lung, and kidney.

Skill Keeper: Management of Anticancer Drug Hematotoxicity (see Chapter 33)

Bone marrow suppression is a characteristic toxicity of most cytotoxic anticancer drugs. What agents are now available for the treatment of anemia and neutropenia, and for platelet restoration in patients undergoing cancer chemotherapy? *The Skill Keeper Answer appears at the end of the chapter.*

HORMONAL ANTICANCER AGENTS

A. Glucocorticoids: **Prednisone** is the most commonly used glucocorticoid in cancer chemotherapy. The steroid has applications in drug regimens for acute and chronic lymphocytic leukemia, Hodgkin's disease (MOPP regimen), and other lymphomas. Toxicity is described in Chapter 39.

B. Sex Hormones: The estrogens, progestins, and androgens are used in some hormone-dependent cancers to change the hormone balance. Fluoxymesterone, an androgenic steroid, may be used in women with advanced breast cancer. Estrogenic steroids (eg, diethylstilbestrol) are sometimes used in men with prostate carcinoma.

C. **Sex Hormone Antagonists:** **Tamoxifen,** an estrogen receptor partial agonist, blocks the binding of estrogen to receptors of estrogen-sensitive cancer cells in breast tissue. The drug is used in receptor-positive breast carcinoma and may have a preventive effect in women at high risk for breast cancer. Tamoxifen has activity in progestin-resistant endometrial carcinoma but may activate estrogen receptors in endometrial cells to cause hyperplasia and neoplasia. Toxicity includes nausea and vomiting, hot flushes, vaginal bleeding, hypercalcemia, ocular dysfunction, and peripheral edema. **Toremifene** is a newer estrogen receptor antagonist used in advanced breast cancer. **Flutamide** is an androgen receptor antagonist used in prostatic carcinoma. Adverse effects include gynecomastia, hot flushes, and hepatic dysfunction.

D. **Gonadotropin-Releasing Hormone Analogs:** **Leuprolide, goserelin,** and **nafarelin** are GnRH agonists. When administered in constant doses so as to maintain stable blood levels, they *inhibit* release of pituitary LH and FSH. These agents are as effective as diethylstilbestrol in prostatic carcinoma and cause fewer adverse effects. Leuprolide may cause bone pain, gynecomastia, hematuria, impotence, and testicular atrophy.

E. **Aromatase Inhibitors:** Anastrozole and letrozole inhibit aromatase, the enzyme that catalyzes the conversion of androstenedione (an androgenic precursor) to estrone (an estrogenic hormone). Both drugs are used in advanced breast cancer. Toxicity includes nausea, diarrhea, hot flushes, bone and back pain, dyspnea, and peripheral edema.

MISCELLANEOUS ANTICANCER AGENTS

A. **Asparaginase:** Asparaginase is an enzyme that depletes serum asparagine; it is used in the treatment of T cell auxotrophic cancers (leukemia and lymphomas) that require exogenous asparagine for growth. Asparaginase is given intravenously and may cause severe hypersensitivity reactions, acute pancreatitis, and bleeding.

B. **Mitoxantrone:** This anthracene compound probably acts via the alkylation of DNA bases. Mitoxantrone is used in combination regimens for refractory acute leukemia and in breast carcinoma. Myelosuppression, gastrointestinal effects, and cardiac arrhythmias are toxic effects of the drug.

C. **Interferons:** The interferons are endogenous glycoproteins with antineoplastic, immunosuppressive, and antiviral actions. Alpha-interferons (see Chapter 56) are effective against a number of neoplasms, including hairy cell leukemia, the early stage of chronic myelogenous leukemia, and T cell lymphomas. Toxic effects of the interferons include myelosuppression and neurologic dysfunction.

D. **Monoclonal Antibodies:** **Rituximab** is a monoclonal antibody to a surface protein in non-Hodgkin's lymphoma cells. It is presently used with conventional anticancer drugs (eg, cyclophosphamide plus vincristine plus prednisone) in low grade lymphomas. **Trastuzumab** is a monoclonal antibody to a surface protein in breast cancers that overexpress the HER2 protein. Acute toxicity of these antibodies includes nausea and vomiting, chills, fevers, and headache. Rituximab use is associated with hypersensitivity reactions and myelosuppression. Trastuzumab may cause cardiac dysfunction, including congestive heart failure.

STRATEGIES IN CANCER CHEMOTHERAPY

A. **Principles of Combination Therapy:** Chemotherapy with combinations of anticancer drugs usually increases log kill markedly, and in some cases synergistic effects are achieved (see ¶B, below). Combinations are often cytotoxic to a heterogeneous population of cancer cells and may prevent development of resistant clones. Drug combinations using CCS and CCNS drugs may be cytotoxic to both dividing and resting cancer cells. The following principles are important for selecting appropriate drugs to use in combination chemotherapy:

(1) Each drug should be active when used alone against the particular cancer.
(2) The drugs should have different mechanisms of action.

(3) Cross-resistance between drugs should be minimal.
(4) The drugs should have different toxic effects (Table 55–3).

B. Examples of Combination Chemotherapy:

1. Hodgkin's disease:

a. MOPP regimen: Mechlorethamine, Oncovin (vincristine), procarbazine, and prednisone. This regimen is effective and was the mainstay of drug treatment of stages III and IV of the disease for many years. It has now been replaced—for initial therapy—by the ABVD regimen.

b. ABVD regimen: Adriamycin (doxorubicin), bleomycin, vinblastine, and dacarbazine. The ABVD regimen is equally effective and appears to be less likely than the MOPP regimen to cause sterility and secondary malignancies (leukemia). If the neoplasm becomes resistant, the MOPP regimen may be alternated with the ABVD regimen.

2. Non-Hodgkin's lymphoma: The COP regimen, which includes cyclophosphamide, Oncovin (vincristine), and prednisone, is commonly used with or without doxorubicin (COP-D).

3. Testicular carcinoma: The PVB regimen, which includes Platinol (cisplatin), vinblastine, and bleomycin, is the original treatment. A more recently introduced regimen (PEB), in which vinblastine is replaced by etoposide, is equally effective and better tolerated, so it is now considered first-line.

4. Breast carcinoma: Postoperative chemotherapy commonly involves use of the CMF regimen (cyclophosphamide, methotrexate, and fluorouracil) with or without tamoxifen, or the CAF regimen in which doxorubicin (Adriamycin) replaces methotrexate. Tamoxifen (or toremifene) is added to such regimens for receptor-positive cancers, and trastuzumab may be included if tumors overexpress HER2 protein.

C. Additional Strategies for Cancer Chemotherapy:

1. Pulse therapy: Pulse therapy involves intermittent treatment with very high doses of an anticancer drug—doses that are too toxic to be used continuously. Intensive drug treatment every 3–4 weeks allows for maximum effects on neoplastic cells, with hematologic and immunologic recovery between courses. This type of regimen is used successfully in therapy of acute leukemias, testicular carcinomas, and Wilms' tumor.

2. Recruitment and synchrony: The strategy of **recruitment** involves initial use of a CCNS drug to achieve a significant log kill, which results in the recruitment into cell division of previously resting cells in the G_0 phase of the cell cycle. With subsequent administration of a CCS drug that is active against dividing cells, maximal cell kill may be achieved. A similar approach involves **synchrony,** one example being the use of vinca alkaloids to hold cancer cells in the M phase. Subsequent treatment with another CCS drug,

Table 55–3. Selected examples of anticancer drug toxicity.

Drug	Toxicity
Bleomycin	Pneumonitis, pulmonary fibrosis, hyperpigmentation, alopecia, "marrow-sparing"
Cisplatin	Nephrotoxicity, ototoxicity, bone marrow suppression
Cyclophosphamide	Bone marrow suppression, hemorrhagic cystitis (consider mesna), alopecia, pulmonary infiltrates
Doxorubicin	Bone marrow suppression, cardiotoxicity (often delayed, consider dexrazoxane or liposomal formulations)
Etoposide	Bone marrow suppression, alopecia
Fluorouracil	Bone marrow suppression, oral and gastrointestinal ulcers, diarrhea, cardiac dysfunction
Mercaptopurine	Bone marrow suppression, cholestasis, oral and gastrointestinal ulcers, pancreatitis
Methotrexate	Bone marrow suppression, oral and gastrointestinal ulcers, hepatoxicity, pulmonary dysfunction. Note that use of folinic acid ("leucovorin rescue") is standard.
Paclitaxel	Bone marrow suppression, peripheral neuropathy, alopecia
Rituximab	Bone marrow suppression, fever, chills, hypersensitivity reactions
Trastuzumab	Fever, chills, rash, cardiac dysfunction
Vinblastine	Bone marrow suppression, alopecia, jaw and muscle pain
Vincristine	Peripheral neuropathy, paralytic ileus, jaw pain, "marrow-sparing"

such as the S phase-specific agent cytarabine, may result in a greater killing effect on the neoplastic cell population.

3. **Rescue therapy:** Toxic effects of anticancer drugs can sometimes be alleviated by rescue strategy. For example, high doses of methotrexate may be given for 36–48 hours and terminated before severe toxicity occurs to cells of the gastrointestinal tract and bone marrow. **Leucovorin** (formyl tetrahydrofolate), which is accumulated more readily by normal than by neoplastic cells, is then administered. This results in rescue of the normal cells, since leucovorin bypasses the dihydrofolate reductase step in folic acid synthesis. Mercaptoethanesulfonate (mesna) "traps" acrolein released from cyclophosphamide and thus reduces the incidence of hemorrhagic cystitis. Dexrazoxane is a free radical "trapper" that affords protection against the cardiac toxicity of anthracyclines (eg, doxorubicin).

DRUG LIST

The following drugs are important members of the group discussed in this chapter. Prototypes should be learned in detail; features of the major variants should be known well enough to distinguish the variants from the prototypes and from each other; the other significant agents should be recognized as belonging to a specific subclass.

Subclass	Prototype	Major Variants	Other Significant Agents
Alkylating agents			
Nitrogen mustards	Mechlorethamine		Cyclophosphamide, chlorambucil
Nitrosoureas	Carmustine	Lomustine	
Alkylsulfonates	Busulfan		
Platinum complex	Cisplatin	Carboplatin	
Triazenes	Dacarbazine		
Hydrazines	Procarbazine		
Antimetabolites			
Folate analogs	Methotrexate		
Purine analogs	Mercaptopurine		Thioguanine
Pyrimidine analogs	Fluorouracil		Cytarabine
Plant alkaloids			
Vinca alkaloids	Vinblastine	Vincristine	
Podophyllotoxins	Etoposide	Teniposide	
Other	Paclitaxel		Docetaxel
Antibiotics			
Anthracyclines	Doxorubicin	Daunorubicin	
Bleomycins	Bleomycin		
Actinomycins	Dactinomycin		
Mitomycins	Mitomycin		
Hormones			
Adrenocorticoids	Prednisone	Hydrocortisone	
Androgens	Testosterone	Fluoxymesterone	
Estrogens	Diethylstilbestrol	Ethinyl estradiol	
Progestins	Hydroxyprogesterone	Medroxyprogesterone	
Antiestrogens			
Receptor blockers	Tamoxifen	Toremifene	
Aromatase inhibitors	Anastrozole	Letrozole	
Antiandrogens	Flutamide		
Gonadotropin-releasing hormone agonists	Leuprolide	Goserelin, naferelin	
Monoclonal antibodies	Rituximab trastuzumab		

QUESTIONS

DIRECTIONS: Each of the numbered items or incomplete statements in this section is followed by answers or by completions of the statement. Select the ONE lettered answer or completion that is BEST in each case.

Items 1–3: A 32-year-old woman underwent segmental mastectomy for a breast tumor of 3 cm diameter. Lymph node sampling revealed two involved nodes. Since chemotherapy is of established value in her situation, she underwent postoperative treatment with antineoplastic drugs. The FAC-V regimen was employed, consisting of fluorouracil, doxorubicin (Adriamycin), and cyclophosphamide, plus vincristine. Six cycles 1 month apart of this chemotherapy regimen were planned. Adjunctive drugs included tamoxifen, since the tumor cells were hormone receptor-positive.

1. Regarding the mechanisms of action and resistance of the antineoplastic drugs used in this case, which one of the following statements is most accurate?
(A) Resistance to fluorouracil occurs via decreased activity of hypoxanthine-guanine phosphoribosyl transferase (HGPRTase)
(B) Cyclophosphamide is an irreversible inhibitor of dihydrofolic acid reductase
(C) Resistance to doxorubicin occurs through the formation of enzymes that can degrade the drug
(D) Vincristine causes DNA strand scission through effects on topoisomerase II
(E) A metabolite of fluorouracil is cytotoxic because it causes "thymineless death" of cells

2. The chemotherapy undertaken by this patient caused considerable gastrointestinal and hematologic toxicity. Which one of the following statements concerning these and other adverse effects of the drugs she was taking is LEAST accurate?
(A) The administration of doxorubicin probably caused local tissue necrosis
(B) The patient should have been advised to maintain a high fluid intake to decrease the risk of dysuria and hematuria
(C) The nausea and vomiting that she experienced was mainly due to tamoxifen
(D) Granulocyte and platelet counts should be determined immediately prior to each cycle of drug treatment
(E) Of the cytotoxic drugs used, vincristine was the least likely to contribute to myelosuppression

3. Between drug cycles 3 and 4, the patient was found to have a high resting pulse rate. A noninvasive radionuclide scan revealed evidence of cardiotoxicity, and a change in the drug regimen was suggested for the next cycle of treatment. Which one of the following changes is most likely to have been made?
(A) The dosage of doxorubicin was reduced by 20%
(B) Mercaptoethanesulfonate (mesna) was added to the drug regimen
(C) Mitoxantrone was added and doxorubicin discontinued
(D) Methotrexate replaced doxorubicin
(E) Vincristine was discontinued

4. In a patient with diffuse lymphoma, the oncologist suggests a treatment strategy that involves the initial administration of doxorubicin to obtain a significant log-kill, followed by the cell cycle-specific drugs cytarabine and vincristine. This therapeutic strategy is called
(A) Pulse therapy
(B) Recruitment
(C) Rescue therapy
(D) Sequential blockade
(E) Synchrony

5. Which one of the following statements about the mechanisms of action of drugs used in cancer chemotherapy is LEAST accurate?
(A) Alkylating agents commonly attack the nucleophilic N-7 position in guanine
(B) Anthracyclines intercalate with base pairs to block nucleic acid synthesis
(C) In steady doses, leuprolide inhibits the release of pituitary gonadotropins
(D) Mercaptopurine is an irreversible inhibitor of HGPRTase
(E) Paclitaxel acts mainly in the M phase of the cell cycle

Items 6–7: A patient with metastatic choriocarcinoma is to be treated with methotrexate (MTX) in a pulse dosage regimen, with the first drug course to continue for no more than 72 hours. Serum creatinine levels will be monitored, and rescue treatment with leucovorin is planned. Prior to drug treatment, glucose and bicarbonate will be given over 8–12 hours. Urine pH will be maintained above pH 6.5.

6. It is important to monitor serum MTX levels during the initial course of drug treatment because
- **(A)** High MTX levels in the blood require additional leucovorin rescue
- **(B)** Levels of MTX in the blood are predictive of gastrointestinal mucositis
- **(C)** MTX readily penetrates into the cerebrospinal fluid
- **(D)** Renal toxicity due to MTX is likely to occur
- **(E)** Resistance to MTX occurs within a few days

7. Maintenance of a high urinary pH is important during methotrexate treatment in this patient because
- **(A)** Bladder irritation is reduced
- **(B)** It decreases renal tubular secretion of methotrexate
- **(C)** Leucovorin toxicity is increased in a dehydrated patient
- **(D)** Methotrexate is a weak acid
- **(E)** Reabsorption of purine metabolites occurs at high urinary pH

8. An adult patient is being treated for acute leukemia with a combination of anticancer drugs that includes cyclophosphamide, mercaptopurine, methotrexate, vincristine, and prednisone. He is also using dronabinol for emesis, a chlorhexidine mouthwash to reduce mucositis, and laxatives. The patient complains of "pins and needles" sensations in the extremities and muscle weakness. He is not able to execute a deep knee bend or get up out of a chair without using his arm muscles. He is also very constipated. If these problems are related to the chemotherapy, the most likely causative agent is
- **(A)** Cyclophosphamide
- **(B)** Dronabinol
- **(C)** Mercaptopurine
- **(D)** Prednisone
- **(E)** Vincristine

9. Which of the following agents used in drug combination regimens to treat testicular carcinoma is most likely to cause nephrotoxicity?
- **(A)** Bleomycin
- **(B)** Cisplatin
- **(C)** Etoposide
- **(D)** Leuprolide
- **(E)** Vinblastine

10. Which one of the following is LEAST likely to be a mechanism of cancer cell resistance to antineoplastic drugs?
- **(A)** Change in properties of a target enzyme
- **(B)** Decreased activity of activating enzymes
- **(C)** Increase in drug-metabolizing cytochrome P450
- **(D)** Increase in DNA repair
- **(E)** Increase in production of drug-trapping molecules

Items 11–12: A 23-year-old man with Hodgkin's disease was treated unsuccessfully with the MOPP regimen. He subsequently underwent a successful course of therapy with the ABVD regimen.

11. Which one of the following classes of anticancer drugs used in the treatment of this patient is cell cycle-specific (CCS) and is used in both the MOPP and ABVD regimens?
- **(A)** Alkylating agents
- **(B)** Antibiotics
- **(C)** Antimetabolites
- **(D)** Glucocorticoids
- **(E)** Plant alkaloids

12. During the second course of drug treatment (ABVD regimen), this patient developed dyspnea, a nonproductive cough, and intermittent fever. Chest x-ray revealed pulmonary infiltration. If these problems are due to the anticancer drugs that he has been exposed to, the most likely causative agent is
- **(A)** Bleomycin
- **(B)** Dacarbazine
- **(C)** Doxorubicin
- **(D)** Prednisone
- **(E)** Vinblastine

13. All of the following agents have been used in drug regimens for the treatment of breast carcinoma. Which one has specific activity in a subset of female breast cancers?
 (A) Anastrozole
 (B) Doxorubicin
 (C) Fluoxymesterone
 (D) Methotrexate
 (E) Trastuzumab

DIRECTIONS: The matching questions in this section consist of a list of lettered options followed by several numbered items. For each numbered item, select the ONE lettered option that is most closely associated with it. Each lettered option may be selected once, more than once, or not at all.
 (A) Bleomycin
 (B) Cytarabine
 (C) Dacarbazine
 (D) Diethylstilbestrol
 (E) Doxorubicin
 (F) Etoposide
 (G) Flutamide
 (H) Leuprolide
 (I) Mechlorethamine
 (J) Mercaptopurine
 (K) Methotrexate
 (L) Paclitaxel
 (M) Procarbazine
 (N) Tamoxifen
 (O) Vincristine

14. If allopurinol is used adjunctively in cancer chemotherapy to offset hyperuricemia, the dosage of this drug should be reduced to 25% of normal.
15. This drug is used in combination therapy for testicular carcinoma. It is a CCS drug that acts in the late S and early G_0 phases of the tumor cell cycle via interactions with topoisomerase II.
16. This antimetabolite inhibits DNA polymerase and is one of the most active drugs in leukemias. Although myelosuppression is dose-limiting, the drug may also cause cerebellar dysfunction, including ataxia and dysarthria.

ANSWERS

1. Fluorouracil (5-FU) undergoes metabolism to form 5-fluoro-2′-deoxyuridine 5′-phosphate (5-dUMP). This metabolite forms a covalently bound ternary complex with thymidylate synthase and its coenzyme *N*-methylenetetrahydrofolate. The synthesis of thymine nucleotides is blocked, and a "thymineless death" of cells results. The answer is **(E).**
2. Cytotoxic anticancer drugs are much more likely to be the cause of nausea and vomiting than the estrogen receptor antagonist tamoxifen. Metoclopramide, ondansetron, dronabinol, dexamethasone, and phenothiazines are effective antiemetics used in cancer chemotherapy. The vesicant properties of doxorubicin may cause local tissue necrosis at injection sites; adequate hydration reduces the risk of hemorrhagic cystitis due to cyclophosphamide; vincristine is relatively sparing of the bone marrow. Blood counts are essential immediately before each cycle of pulse therapy since the drug dosages to be used depend on the extent of hematologic recovery. The answer is **(C).**
3. A high resting pulse rate is one of the first signs of cardiotoxicity due to anthracyclines, which can include arrhythmias, cardiomyopathies, and congestive heart failure. The risk of cardiotoxicity depends on cumulative dosage, so doxorubicin should be discontinued and replaced by another agent with activity against breast tumors. The most logical drug for replacement is methotrexate, since the CMF regimen (cyclophosphamide, methotrexate, fluorouracil) has been commonly used in the postoperative chemotherapy of breast cancers. Dexrazoxane may have protected this patient against the toxicity of doxorubicin. The answer is **(D).**
4. Recruitment strategy in cancer chemotherapy involves the initial use of a CCNS drug (eg, doxorubicin) to achieve a significant log kill. This results in the recruitment into cell division of resting

cells in the G_0 phase of the cell cycle. Subsequently, the administration of CCS drugs (eg, cytarabine, vincristine) active against dividing cells will achieve maximal cell kill. The answer is **(B).**

5. To exert anticancer activity, mercaptopurine (and thioguanine) must first be activated to nucleotides by HGPRTase. If mercaptopurine were an irreversible inhibitor of this enzyme, this bioactivation process could not occur. The answer is **(D).**
6. Resistance to methotrexate does not occur within a few days—a longer time period is required. Serum methotrexate levels are not predictive of mucositis but are related to potential myelosuppressive toxicity of the drug. Renal toxicity is unlikely to occur in this patient with the proposed protocol. Intrathecal administration of methotrexate is required for central nervous system leukemia. The answer is **(A).**
7. Nephrotoxicity can be a problem with high doses of methotrexate, but it is less likely to occur than myelosuppression, especially if the patient is well hydrated and the urine is alkalinized. MTX is a weak acid and is more water-soluble at alkaline pH; it is thus eliminated more rapidly in alkaline urine. The answer is **(D).**
8. Neuropathy is a toxic side effect of vincristine. In its mildest form paresthesias occur, but it progresses to significant muscle weakness—initially in the quadriceps muscle group. Constipation is the most common symptom of autonomic neuropathy. The answer is **(E).**
9. The characteristic nephrotoxicity of cisplatin may be reduced by slow intravenous infusion, the maintenance of good hydration, and the administration of mannitol (to maximize urine flow). Bear in mind that cisplatin also has dose-dependent neurotoxic effects. The answer is **(B).**
10. Increases in the activity of cytochrome P450 have not been reported as a mechanism of resistance to anticancer drugs. In fact, one might predict *enhanced* cytotoxic effects of drugs that are activated by this enzyme system, eg, cyclophosphamide. Increased drug inactivation through increased production of alkaline phosphatases is a mechanism of resistance to purine antimetabolites. The answer is **(C).**
11. The cell cycle-specific drugs used in standard treatment protocols for Hodgkin's disease are bleomycin and the vinca alkaloids. Vinblastine is used in the ABVD regimen, and vincristine (Oncovin) is used in the MOPP regimen. The answer is **(E).**
12. The anticancer drug most commonly associated with pulmonary toxicity is bleomycin. If pulmonary dysfunction with infiltration developed, the drug would be discontinued. High-dose steroids and empiric antibiotic therapy would also be indicated. Note that procarbazine (not listed), used in the MOPP regimen for Hodgkin's lymphoma, may also cause cough and pleural effusions. The answer is **(A).**
13. Each of the drugs listed has been used in drug regimens for breast cancer, but only trastuzumab has specificity in its actions. The drug is a monoclonal antibody to a surface protein in breast cancer cells that overexpress the HER2 protein. Consequently, trastuzumab has value in a specific subset of breast cancers. The answer is **(E).**
14. Allopurinol, a xanthine oxidase inhibitor, is given to control the hyperuricemia that occurs as a result of large cell kills in the successful drug therapy of malignant diseases. The antimetabolite mercaptopurine is metabolized by xanthine oxidase and, in the presence of an inhibitor of this enzyme (eg, allopurinol), toxic levels of the drug may be reached rapidly. The answer is **(J).**
15. Bleomycin, etoposide, and vinblastine are all CCS drugs used for the treatment of testicular carcinoma. Bleomycin is an antibiotic, not a plant alkaloid. Vinblastine is a spindle poison acting in the M phase of the cell cycle. The answer is **(F).**
16. The pyrimidine antimetabolite cytarabine (Ara-C) is commonly used in drug regimens for the acute leukemias. Cytarabine is dose-limited by hematotoxicity. Cerebellar dysfunction may also occur with Ara-C, especially if the drug is used at high doses. The answer is **(B).**

Skill Keeper Answer: Management of Anticancer Drug Hematotoxicity (see Chapter 33)

Recombinant DNA technology has provided several agents that have value in the management of hematotoxicity caused by anticancer drugs. Erythropoietin stimulates red cell formation by interaction with receptors on erythroid progenitors in bone marrow. Myeloid growth factors filgrastim (G-CSF) and sargramostim (GM-CSF) stimulate the production and function of neutrophils. Megakaryocyte growth factors oprelvekin (IL-11) and thrombopoietin stimulate the growth of platelet progenitors.

Immunopharmacology

56

OBJECTIVES

You should be able to:

- Describe the primary features of cell-mediated and humoral immunity.
- Name seven immunosuppressants and, for each, describe the mechanism of action, clinical uses, and toxicities.
- Describe the mechanisms of action, clinical uses, and toxicities of antibodies used as immunosuppressants.
- Identify the major cytokines and other immunomodulating agents and know their clinical applications.
- Describe the different types of allergic reactions to drugs.

Learn the definitions that follow.

Table 56–1. Definitions.

Term	Definition
B cells	Lymphoid cells derived from the bone marrow that mediate humoral (serologic) immunity through the formation of antibodies
T cells	Lymphoid cells derived from the thymus that mediate cellular immunity and can modify serologic immunity. The main subclasses of T cells are CD4 (helper) cells and CD8 (suppressor) cells
Antigen-presenting cells (APCs)	Dendritic and Langerhans cells, macrophages, and B lymphocytes involved in the processing of antigens into cell-surface forms recognizable by lymphoid cells
Clusters of differentiation (CDs)	Specific cell surface constituents (characterized by monoclonal antibodies) identified by number (CD1, CD2, etc)
Major histocompatibility complex (MHC)	Cell surface molecules that bind antigen fragments and, when bound to antigen fragments, are recognized by helper T cells. MHC class I molecules are expressed by all cells, whereas MHC class II molecules are expressed by antigen-presenting cells.
Cytokines	Polypeptide modulators of cellular functions include interferons, interleukins, and growth stimulating factors
Lymphokine	A cytokine that is capable of modulating lymphoid cell functions
Immunophillins	Members of a highly conserved family of cytoplasmic proteins that bind to the immunosuppressants cyclosporine, tacrolimus, and sirolimus and assist these drugs in inhibiting T and B cell function. Cyclophilin binds cyclosporine, whereas FK-binding protein (FKBP) binds tacrolimus and sirolimus

CONCEPTS

Immunopharmacology includes drugs that can suppress, modulate, or stimulate immune functions. It also includes antibodies that have been developed for use in immune disorders. The drugs available comprise a wide variety of chemical and pharmacologic types (Figure 56–1). This chapter also discusses the ways in which drugs activate the immune system and cause unwanted immunologic reactions.

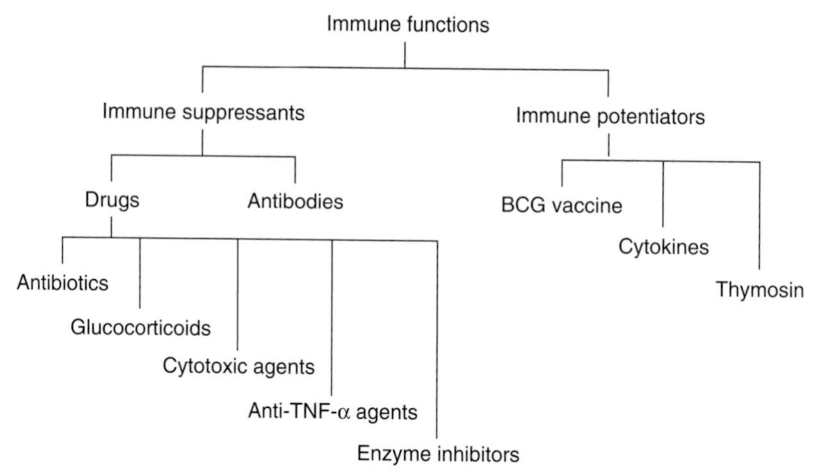

Figure 56–1. Drugs that alter immune function.

IMMUNE MECHANISMS

A. Overview: The *innate* immune system initiates the defense against pathogens and antigenic insult. It involves the concerted actions of complement components, lysozyme, macrophages, and neutrophils. If the innate response is inadequate, the *adaptive* immune response is mobilized. This culminates in the activation of T lymphocytes, the effectors of **cell-mediated immunity;** and the production of antibodies, by activated B lymphocytes, the effectors of **humoral immunity.** The cell types involved in immune responses can be identified by specific cell surface components or **clusters of differentiation (CDs).** For example, T helper cells bear the CD4 protein complex, whereas cytotoxic T lymphocytes express the CD8 protein complex. Clusters of differentiation also can be used to characterize other types of hematopoietic cells, including precursors of granulocytes, megakaryocytes, and erythrocytes (Chapter 33).

B. Antigen Recognition and Processing: This critical inaugural step in the adaptive immune response involves **antigen-presenting cells (APCs).** These cells process antigens into small peptides that can be recognized by T cell receptors (TCRs) on T helper (TH) cells. The most important antigen-presenting cell surface molecules are the **major histocompatibility complex (MHC)** class I and II antigens. The activation of TH cells involves class II MHC molecules and requires the participation of specific costimulatory and adhesion molecules in addition to activation of TCRs.

C. Cell-Mediated Immunity: Activated TH cells secrete interleukin-2 (IL-2), a cytokine that causes proliferation and activation of two subsets of T helper cells, TH1 and TH2 (Figure 56–2). TH1 cells play a major role in cell-mediated immunity and delayed hypersensitivity reactions. They produce interferon-gamma (IFN-γ), interleukin-2 (IL-2), and tumor necrosis factor-beta (TNF-β). These cytokines activate macrophages, cytotoxic T lymphocytes (CTLs), and **natural killer (NK)** cells. Activated CTLs recognize processed peptides that are bound to class I MHC molecules on the surface of virus-infected or tumor cells. The CTLs induce target cell death via lytic enzyme and nitric oxide production and by stimulation of apoptosis pathways in the target cells. CTLs also play a role in autoimmune diseases by reacting against normal tissues, such as the synovium in rheumatoid arthritis and myelin in multiple sclerosis. NK cells kill both virus-infected and neoplastic cells. They are also the main precursors of lymphokine-activated killer (LAK) cells, which are toxic to cells that do not express MHC.

D. Humoral Immunity: The **B lymphoid cells,** which are capable of differentiating into antibody-forming cells, are responsible for humoral immunity. The humoral response is triggered when B lymphocytes bind antigen via their surface immunoglobulins. The antigens are internal-

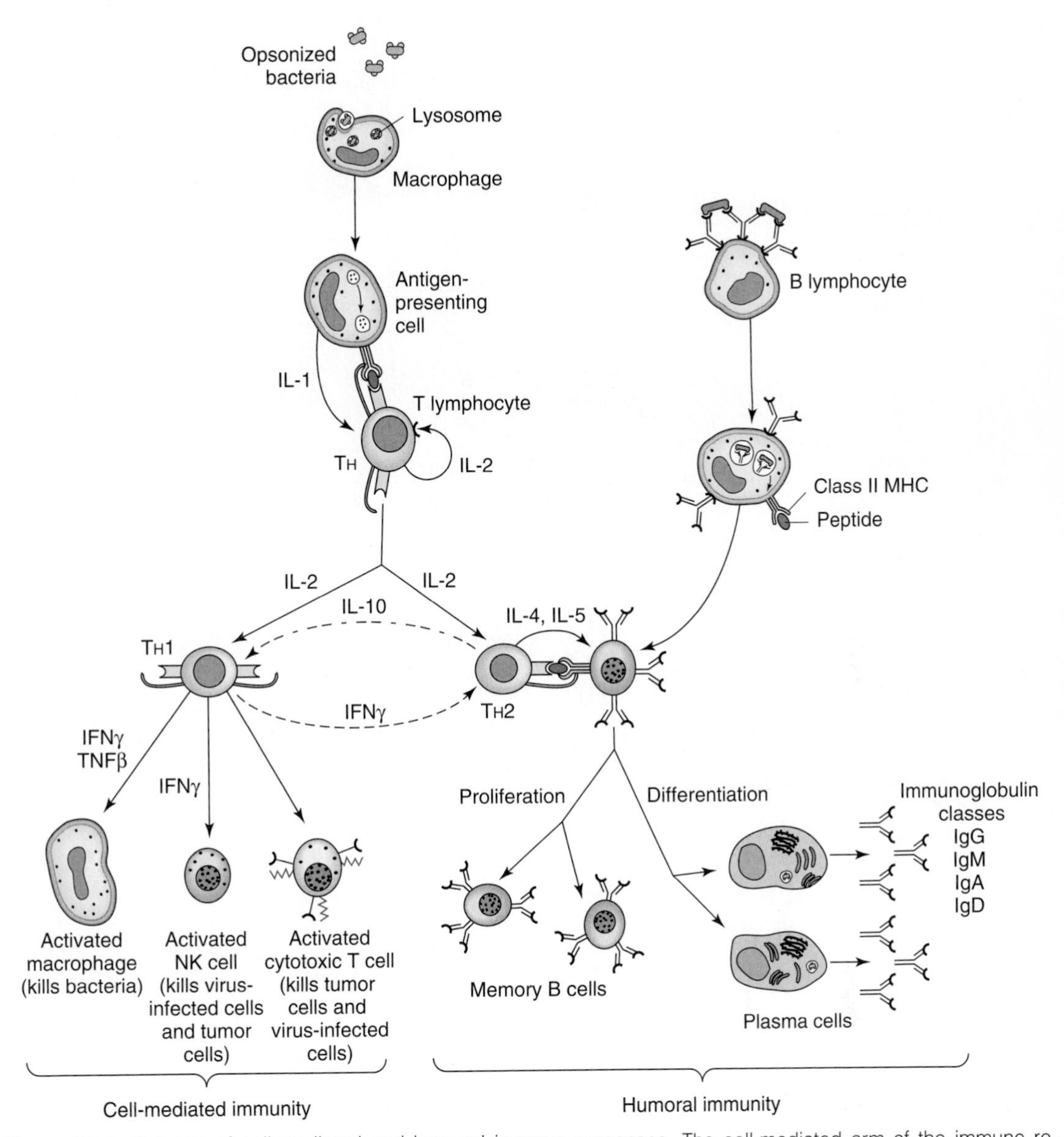

Figure 56–2. Scheme of cell-mediated and humoral immune responses. The cell-mediated arm of the immune response involves internalization and processing of antigen by APCs. The processed peptides bound to class II MHC surface proteins are recognized by the TCR on T helper cells, resulting in T cell activation. Activated TH cells secrete cytokines such as IL-2 which cause proliferation and activation of CTLs, and TH1 and TH2 cell subsets. TH1 cells also produce IFN-γ and TNF-β, which can directly activate macrophages and NK cells. The humoral response is triggered when B lymphocytes bind antigen via their surface immunoglobulins. They are then induced by TH2-derived cytokines (eg, IL-4, IL-5) to proliferate and differentiate into memory cells and antibody-secreting plasma cells. (Modified and reproduced, with permission, from Katzung BG [editor]: *Basic & Clinical Pharmacology,* 8th ed. McGraw-Hill, 2001.)

ized, processed into peptides, and presented on the cell surface bound to MHC class II molecules. When T cell receptors on TH2 cells are activated by the complexes of MHC class II molecules bound to peptides, they release interleukins (IL-4, IL-5, IL-6). These cytokines promote B lymphocyte proliferation and differentiation into memory B cells and antibody-secreting plasma cells (Figure 56–2). Antibody-antigen interactions lead to precipitation of viruses, and destruction of bacteria by phagocytic cells or lysis by the complement system.

The proliferation and differentiation of both B and T lymphocytes is under the control of a complex interplay between the cytokines (Table 56–2) and other endogenous molecules, in-

Table 56–2. Cytokines modulating immune responses.*

Cytokine	Characteristic Properties
Interferon-α (IFN-α)	Activates NK cells, antiviral, oncostatic
Interferon-β (IFN-β)	Activates NK cells, antiviral, oncostatic
Interferon-γ (IFN-γ)	Activates TH1, NK, cytotoxic T cells, and macrophages; antiviral, oncostatic
Interleukin-1 (IL-1)	T cell activation, B cell proliferation
Interleukin-2 (IL-2)	T cell proliferation, activation of TH1, NK and LAK cells
Interleukin-4 (IL-4)	TH2 and CTL activation, B cell proliferation
Interleukin-5 (IL-5)	B cell proliferation and differentiation, eosinophil proliferation
Interleukin-6 (IL-6)	Proliferation of TH2 cells, cytotoxic T cells, and B cells
Interleukin-7 (IL-7)	Proliferation of NK, cytotoxic T cells, LAK, and B cells
Interleukin-8 (IL-8)	Neutrophil chemotaxis, proinflammatory
Interleukin-9 (IL-9)	T cell proliferation
Interleukin-10 (IL-10)	TH1 suppression; cytotoxic T cell activation, B cell proliferation
Interleukin-11 (IL-11)	B cell differentiation (megakaryocyte proliferation, see Chapter 33)
Interleukin-12 (IL-12)	Proliferation and activation of TH1 and cytotoxic T cells
Interleukin-13 (IL-13)	B cell proliferation
Interleukin-14 (IL-14)	B cell proliferation and differentiation
Interleukin-15 (IL-15)	Activation of TH1, NK, and cytotoxic T cells
Interleukin-16 (IL-16)	T cell chemotaxis; HIV suppression
Interleukin-17 (IL-17)	Stromal cell cytokine production
Tumor necrosis factor-α (TNF-α)	Proinflammatory, macrophage activation, oncostatic
Tumor necrosis factor-β (TNF-β)	Proinflammatory, chemotactic, oncostatic
Granulocyte colony-stimulating factor (G-CSF)	Granulocyte production (see Chapter 33)
Granulocyte-macrophage colony-stimulating factor (GM-CSF)	Granulocyte, monocyte, eosinophil production (see Chapter 33)
Macrophage colony-stimulating factor (M-CSF)	Monocyte production, macrophage activation

*Modified and reproduced, with permission, from Katzung BG (editor): *Basic & Clinical Pharmacology,* 8th ed. McGraw-Hill, 2001.

cluding amines, leukotrienes, and prostaglandins. For example, IL-10 and IFN-γ down-regulate TH1 and TH2 responses, respectively.

E. Abnormal Immune Responses: Abnormal immune responses include hypersensitivity, autoimmunity, and immunodeficiency states. Immediate hypersensitivity is usually antibody-mediated and includes anaphylaxis and hemolytic disease of the newborn; delayed hypersensitivity, associated with extensive tissue damage, is cell-mediated. Autoimmunity arises from self-reactive lymphocytes that react to one's own molecules, or self-antigens. Examples of autoimmune diseases that are amenable to drug treatment include rheumatoid arthritis and systemic lupus erythematosus. Immunodeficiency states may be genetically acquired (eg, Di George's syndrome) or result from extrinsic factors (eg, AIDS).

F. Sites of Action of Immunosuppressant Agents: Sites of action of immunosuppressive agents are shown in Figure 56–3. Agents that act at the step of antigen recognition are antibodies and include Rh_0(D) immune globulin, antilymphocyte globulin, and muromonab-CD3. Inhibition of the lymphoid proliferation stage of immune responses occurs with most immunosuppressants, including peptide antibiotics, anti-TNF-α agents, cytotoxic drugs, enzyme inhibitors, and glucocorticoids. Lymphoid differentiation is partly inhibited by peptide antibiotics, dactinomycin, and antilymphocyte globulin. Glucocorticoids also modify tissue injury from immune responses via their anti-inflammatory properties.

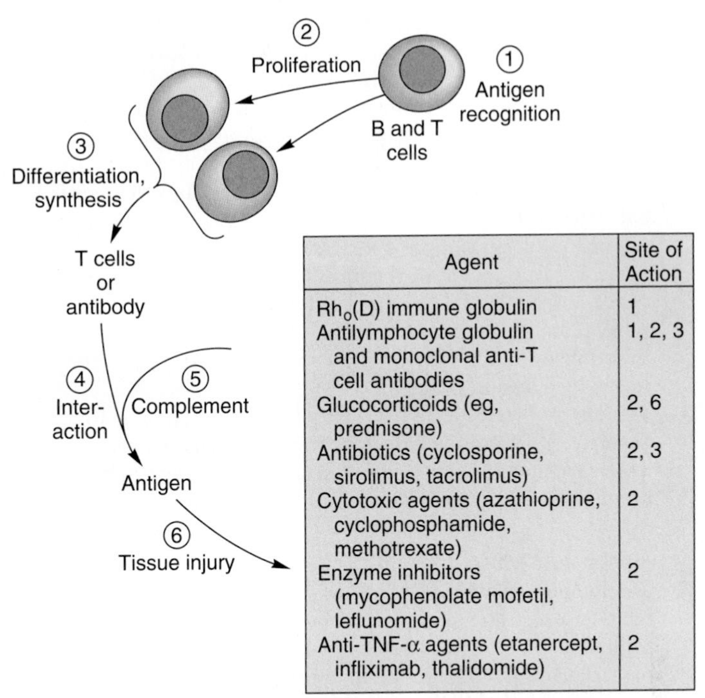

Agent	Site of Action
Rh_0(D) immune globulin	1
Antilymphocyte globulin and monoclonal anti-T cell antibodies	1, 2, 3
Glucocorticoids (eg, prednisone)	2, 6
Antibiotics (cyclosporine, sirolimus, tacrolimus)	2, 3
Cytotoxic agents (azathioprine, cyclophosphamide, methotrexate)	2
Enzyme inhibitors (mycophenolate mofetil, leflunomide)	2
Anti-TNF-α agents (etanercept, infliximab, thalidomide)	2

Figure 56–3. The sites of action of immunosuppressive agents. (Reproduced, with permission, from Katzung BG [editor]: *Basic & Clinical Pharmacology,* 8th ed. McGraw-Hill, 2001.)

IMMUNOSUPPRESSIVE AGENTS

A. Corticosteroids:

1. **Mechanism of action:** Glucocorticoids act at multiple cellular sites, leading to broad effects on inflammatory and immune processes (see Chapter 39). At the biochemical level, their actions on gene expression lead to decreases in the synthesis of prostaglandins, leukotrienes, cytokines, and other signaling molecules that participate in immune responses (eg, platelet activating factor). At the cellular level, the glucocorticoids inhibit the proliferation of T lymphocytes (suppressing cellular immunity) and, to a lesser degree, dampen humoral immunity. At doses used for immunosuppression, the glucocorticoids are cytotoxic to certain subsets of T cells. Continuous therapy lowers IgG levels by increasing catabolism of this class of immunoglobulins.
2. **Clinical use:** Glucocorticoids are used alone or in combination with other agents in a wide variety of medical conditions involving an undesirable immunologic reaction (see Chapter 39). Their ability to induce apoptosis in immune cells makes them useful for treatment of several types of cancer (see Chapter 55). Corticosteroids are also used to suppress immunologic reactions in patients who undergo organ transplantation.
3. **Toxicity:** Predictable adverse effects include adrenal suppression, growth inhibition, muscle wasting, osteoporosis, salt retention, diabetogenesis, and possible psychoses (Chapter 39).

B. Cyclosporine, Tacrolimus, and Sirolimus:

1. **Mechanism of action:** These peptide antibiotics interfere with T cell function by binding to **immunophyllins,** small cytoplasmic proteins that play critical roles in T cell responses to TCR activation and to cytokines. **Cyclosporine** binds to cyclophilin and **tacrolimus** binds to FK-binding protein (FKBP), both complexes inhibiting **calcineurin,** a cytoplasmic phosphatase. Calcineurin regulates the ability of the nuclear factor of activated T cells (NF-AT) to translocate to the nucleus and increase the production of cytokines. Cyclophilin and tacrolimus both inhibit the production of cytokines that normally occurs in response to TCR activation. **Sirolimus** also binds to FKBP, inhibiting the re-

sponse of T cells to cytokines without affecting cytokine production. Sirolimus is also a potent inhibitor of B cell proliferation, antibody production, and mononuclear cell responses to colony-stimulating factors.

2. **Clinical uses and pharmacokinetics:** Use of these immunosuppressants is a major factor in the success of solid organ transplantation. Cyclosporine is used in solid organ transplantation and in graft-versus-host syndrome in bone marrow transplants. Tacrolimus is used in liver and kidney transplant recipients and may be effective as rescue therapy in patients who fail standard therapy. Sirolimus is used alone or in combination with cyclosporine in kidney and heart transplantation. The agents, particularly cyclosporine, may also be effective in immune diseases, including rheumatoid arthritis, uveitis, psoriasis, asthma, and type 1 diabetes.

   All three agents can be used orally. However, since cyclosporine exhibits erratic bioavailability, serum levels should be monitored. The drug undergoes slow hepatic metabolism by the cytochrome P450 system and has a long half-life. Its metabolism is affected by a host of drugs.

3. **Toxicity:** Cyclosporine and tacrolimus have similar toxicity profiles. The most frequent adverse effects are renal dysfunction, hypertension, and neurotoxicity. They may also cause hyperglycemia, hyperlipidemia, and cholelithiasis. Sirolimus is more likely than the other agents to cause hyperlipidemia and hematopoietic cell toxicity.

C. Mycophenolate Mofetil:

1. **Mechanism of action:** This drug is rapidly converted into mycophenolic acid, which inhibits inosine monophosphate dehydrogenase, an enzyme in the de novo pathway of purine synthesis. This action suppresses both B and T lymphocyte activation. Lymphocytes are particularly susceptible to inhibitors of the de novo pathway because they lack the enzymes necessary for the alternative salvage pathway for purine synthesis.
2. **Clinical use:** The drug has been used successfully as a sole agent in kidney, liver, and heart transplants. In renal transplants, its use with low-dose cyclosporine has reduced cyclosporine-induced nephrotoxicity.
3. **Toxicity:** Apart from its gastrointestinal side effects, the drug appears to be quite safe.

D. Azathioprine:

1. **Mechanism of action:** This prodrug is transformed to the antimetabolite mercaptopurine, which upon further metabolic conversion inhibits enzymes involved in purine metabolism. Azathioprine is cytotoxic in the early phase of lymphoid cell proliferation and has a greater effect on the activity of T cells than B cells.
2. **Clinical use:** Azathioprine is used in autoimmune diseases (eg, systemic lupus erythematosus, rheumatoid arthritis) and for immunosuppression in renal homografts. The drug has minimal effects on established graft rejections.
3. **Toxicity:** The major toxic effect is bone marrow suppression, but gastrointestinal irritation, skin rashes, and liver dysfunction also occur. The use of azathioprine is associated with an increased incidence of cancer. The active metabolite of azathioprine, mercaptopurine, is metabolized by xanthine oxidase, and toxic effects may be increased by allopurinol given for hyperuricemia.

E. Cyclophosphamide:

1. **Mechanism of action:** This orally active prodrug is transformed by liver enzymes to an alkylating agent that is cytotoxic to proliferating lymphoid cells. The drug has a greater effect on B cells than T lymphocytes and will inhibit an established immune response. Other cytotoxic drugs that similarly suppress proliferating lymphoid cells—and are sometimes used as immunosuppressants—include **cytarabine, dactinomycin, methotrexate,** and **vincristine** (see Chapter 55).
2. **Clinical use:** Cyclophosphamide is effective in autoimmune diseases (including hemolytic anemia), antibody-induced red cell aplasia, bone marrow transplants, and possibly other organ transplant procedures. Cyclophosphamide does not prevent the graft-versus-host reaction in bone marrow transplantation.
3. **Toxicity:** Large doses of the drug (usually needed for immunosuppression) cause pancytopenia, gastrointestinal distress, hemorrhagic cystitis, and alopecia. Cyclophosphamide (and other alkylating agents) may cause sterility.

F. New Immunosuppressants:

1. **Etanercept:** This chimeric protein is a recombinant form of the human TNF receptor. The agent binds TNF-α, a proinflammatory cytokine, and thereby decrease formation of interleukins and adhesion molecules involved in leukocyte activation. Etanercept is used in rheumatoid arthritis and is being investigated in other inflammatory diseases. Injection site reactions and hypersensitivity may occur.
2. **Leflunomide:** This drug inhibits dihydroorotic acid dehydrogenase, an enzyme involved in ribonucleotide synthesis. Leflunomide arrests lymphocytes in the G_1 phase of the cell cycle. Leflunomide is used in rheumatoid arthritis. The drug causes alopecia, rash, and diarrhea.
3. **Thalidomide:** This sedative drug, notorious for its teratogenic effects, has immunosuppressant actions that appear to be due to suppression of TNF production. Thalidomide is used for some forms of leprosy reactions, for immunologic diseases (eg, systemic lupus), and as an anticancer drug. It is also effective in treating aphthous ulcers and the wasting syndrome in AIDS patients.

ANTIBODIES AS IMMUNOSUPPRESSANTS

A. Lymphocyte Immune Globulin:

1. **Mechanism of action:** Lymphocyte immune globulin (LIG), also known as antithymocyte globulin (ATG), is usually produced in horses by immunization against human thymus cells. Lymphocyte immune globulin binds to T cells involved in antigen recognition and initiates their destruction by serum complement. Lymphocyte immune globulin selectively blocks cellular immunity rather than antibody formation, which accounts for its ability to suppress organ graft rejection, a cell-mediated process.
2. **Clinical use:** Lymphocyte immune globulin is used prior to bone marrow transplantation to prevent the graft-versus-host (GVH) reaction. It is also used in combination with cyclosporine or cytotoxic drugs (or both) for maintenance following bone marrow, heart, and renal transplantations. Lymphocyte immune globulin has induced remissions in patients with aplastic anemia.
3. **Toxicity:** Since serologic immunity may remain intact, injection of lymphocyte immune globulin may cause hypersensitivity reactions, including serum sickness and anaphylaxis. Pain and erythema occur at injection sites, and lymphoma has been noted as a late complication.

B. Rh_o(D) Immune Globulin:

1. **Mechanism of action:** Rh_oGAM is a human IgG preparation that contains antibodies against red cell Rh_o(D) antigens. Administration of this antibody to Rh_o(D)-negative, D^u-negative mothers at time of antigen exposure (ie, birth of an Rh_o(D)-positive, D^u-positive child) blocks the primary immune response to the foreign cells. The mechanism probably involves feedback immunosuppression.
2. **Clinical use:** Rh_o(D) immune globulin is used for prevention of Rh hemolytic disease of the newborn. In women treated with Rh_o(D) immune globulin, maternal antibodies to Rh-positive cells are not produced in subsequent pregnancies, and hemolytic disease of the neonate is averted.

C. Monoclonal Antibodies: Monoclonal antibodies (MAbs) have the potential advantage of high specificity, since they can be developed for interaction with a single molecule. "Humanization" of murine monoclonal antibodies has reduced the likelihood of formation of neutralizing antibodies and of immune reactions. Characteristics of some currently available MAbs are shown in Table 56–3.

1. **Muromonab-CD3:** This MAb binds to the CD3 antigen on the surface of human thymocytes and mature T cells. It blocks the killing action of cytotoxic T cells and probably interferes with other T cell functions. Muromonab-CD3 is used to manage a renal homograft rejection crisis. First-dose effects include fever, chills, dyspnea, and pulmonary edema. Hypersensitivity reactions may also occur.
2. **Daclizumab:** Daclizumab is a highly specific MAb that binds to the alpha subunit of the IL-2 receptor expressed on T cells and prevents activation by IL-2. While it facilitates the

Table 56–3. Characteristics of monoclonal antibodies (MAbs).

MAb	Characteristics and Clinical Uses
Abciximab	Antagonist of glycoprotein IIb/IIIa receptor, preventing cross-linking reaction in platelet aggregation. Used post-angioplasty and in acute coronary syndromes
Daclizumab	Binds to the alpha subunit of the IL-2 receptor, preventing lymphocyte activation. Used in renal transplants
Infliximab	Antibody targeted against TNF-α. Used in Crohn's disease and rheumatoid arthritis
Muromonab	Antibody to the T3 (CD3) antigen on thymocytes. Used in acute renal allograft rejection
Palivizumab	Antibody to surface protein of RSV. Used for prophylaxis and treatment of respiratory syncytial viral infection
Rituximab	Binds to the CD20 antigen on B-lymphocytes and recruits immune effector functions to mediate lysis. Used in B cell non-Hodgkin's lymphoma
Trastuzumab	Binds to the HER2 protein on the surface of tumor cells. Cytotoxic for breast tumors that overexpress HER2 protein

actions of other immunosuppressants in renal transplants, daclizumab is not used for acute rejection episodes. In contrast to cyclosporine, tacrolimus, or cytotoxic immunosuppressants, the adverse effects of daclizumab are equivalent to those of placebo.

3. **Infliximab:** This humanized MAb has a mechanism similar to that of etanercept since it is targeted against TNF-α. Infliximab induces remissions in treatment-resistant Crohn's disease, but long-term efficacy has not been established. In combination with methotrexate, infliximab improves symptoms in patients with rheumatoid arthritis. It also is effective in the treatment of inflammatory bowel disease. Infusion reactions and an increased rate of infection may occur.

IMMUNOMODULATING AGENTS

Agents that act as stimulators of immune responses represent a new area in immunopharmacology with the potential for important therapeutic uses, including the treatment of immune deficiency diseases, chronic infectious diseases, and cancer.

A. **Aldesleukin:** Aldesleukin is recombinant interleukin-2 (IL-2), an endogenous lymphokine that promotes the production of cytotoxic T cells and activates natural killer cells (Table 56–2). Aldesleukin is indicated for the adjunctive treatment of renal cell carcinoma. It is investigational for possible efficacy in restoring immune function in AIDS and other immune deficiency disorders.

B. **Interferons:** **Interferon-α-2a** inhibits cell proliferation and is used in hairy cell leukemia, chronic myelogenous leukemia, malignant melanoma, Kaposi's sarcoma, and hepatitis B and C. **Interferon-β-1b** has some beneficial effects in relapsing multiple sclerosis. **Interferon-γ-1b** has greater immune-enhancing actions than the other interferons and appears to act by increasing the synthesis of TNF. The recombinant form is used to decrease the incidence and severity of infections in patients with chronic granulomatous disease.

C. **BCG (Bacille Calmette-Guérin):** BCG is used in some countries for immunization against tuberculosis and also as an immunostimulant in the treatment of superficial bladder cancer. Its efficacy may be due to its activation of macrophages and the resulting enhancement of immune responses.

D. **Thymosin:** Thymosin is a protein hormone from the thymus gland that stimulates the maturation of pre-T cells and promotes the formation of T cells from ordinary lymphoid stem cells. Thymosin-containing preparations have been used in DiGeorge's syndrome (thymic aplasia), but their efficacy in other immune deficiency states has not been established.

MECHANISMS OF DRUG ALLERGY

Immunologic reactions to drugs can fall into any of the four categories of hypersensitivity reactions.

A. Type I (Immediate) Drug Allergy: This form of drug allergy involves **IgE**-mediated reactions to animal and plant stings and pollens as well as drugs. Such reactions include anaphylaxis, urticaria, and angioedema. When linked to carrier proteins, small drug molecules can act as haptens and initiate B cell proliferation and formation of IgE antibodies. These antibodies bind to Fc receptors on tissue mast cells and blood basophils. On subsequent exposure, the antigenic drug crosslinks the IgE antibodies on the surface of mast cells and basophils and triggers release of mediators of vascular responses and tissue injury, including histamine, kinins, prostaglandins, and leukotrienes. Drugs that commonly cause type I reactions include penicillins and sulfonamides.

Skill Keeper: Anaphylaxis & Sympathomimetic Drugs (see Chapters 6 and 9)

In severe anaphylactic reactions, the life-threatening events commonly involve airway obstruction, laryngeal edema, and vascular collapse due to peripheral vasodilation and reduction in blood volume. Hypoxemia can contribute to cardiac events, including arrhythmias and myocardial infarction. Drugs used to treat anaphylaxis mainly target the receptors used by neurotransmitters of the sympathetic nervous system.

1. Why is epinephrine used in anaphylaxis instead of norepinephrine?
2. What other sympathomimetic drugs might be useful in the treatment of anaphylaxis?

The Skill Keeper Answers appear at the end of the chapter.

B. Type II Drug Allergy: Type II allergy involves IgG or IgM antibodies that are bound to circulating blood cells. On reexposure to the antigen, complement-dependent cell lysis occurs. Type II reactions include autoimmune syndromes such as hemolytic anemia from methyldopa, systemic lupus erythematosus from hydralazine or procainamide, thrombocytopenic purpura from quinidine, and agranulocytosis from exposure to many drugs.

C. Type III Drug Allergy: Type III hypersensitivity is a complex type of drug allergy reaction that involves complement-fixing IgM or IgG antibodies and—possibly—IgE antibodies. Drug-induced serum sickness and vasculitis are examples of type III reactions; Stevens-Johnson syndrome (associated with sulfonamide therapy) may also result from type III mechanisms.

D. Type IV Drug Allergy: Type IV allergy is a cell-mediated reaction that can occur from topical application of drugs. It results in contact dermatitis.

E. Modification of Drug Allergies: Drugs that modify allergic responses to other drugs or toxins may act at several steps of the immune mechanism. For example, corticosteroids inhibit lymphoid cell proliferation and reduce tissue injury and edema. However, most drugs that are useful in type I reactions (eg, epinephrine, theophylline, dopamine) block mediator release or act as physiologic antagonists of the mediators.

DRUG LIST

The following drugs are important members of the group discussed in this chapter. Prototypes should be learned in detail; features of the major variants should be known well enough to distinguish the variants from prototypes and from each other; the other significant agents should be recognized as belonging to a specific subclass.

Subclass	Prototype	Major Variants	Other Significant Agents
Glucocorticoids	Prednisone		
Antibiotics	Cyclosporine	Tacrolimus	Sirolimus
Cytotoxic drugs	Azathioprine, cyclophosphamide	Mercaptopurine	Cytarabine, dactinomycin, methotrexate
Enzyme inhibitors	Mycophenolate mofetil, leflunomide		
Anti-TNF-α agents	Etanercept	Infliximab, thalidomide	
Antibodies	Lymphocytic immune globulin, muromonab-CD3, Rh_o(D) immune globulin, daclizumab		
Immunostimulants	Aldesleukin, interferon-α, -β, and -γ		BCG, thymosin

QUESTIONS

DIRECTIONS: Each of the numbered items or incomplete statements in this section is followed by answers or by completions of the statement. Select the ONE lettered answer or completion that is BEST in each case.

1. Which cell involved in immune function recognizes foreign peptides bound to MHC class II molecules on the surface of APC cells, secretes interleukin-2, and initiates the cell-mediated immunity reaction responsible for host-versus-graft reactions?
- **(A)** B lymphocyte
- **(B)** Cytotoxic T lymphocyte
- **(C)** Dendritic cell
- **(D)** Macrophage
- **(E)** TH lymphocyte

2. Cyclosporine is effective in organ transplantation. The immunosuppressant action of the drug appears to be due to
- **(A)** Activation of natural killer (NK) cells
- **(B)** Blockade of tissue responses to inflammatory mediators
- **(C)** Increased catabolism of IgG antibodies
- **(D)** Inhibition of the gene transcription of interleukins
- **(E)** Interference with antigen recognition

3. Azathioprine
- **(A)** Binds avidly to a cytoplasmic immunophillin
- **(B)** Blocks formation of tetrahydrofolic acid
- **(C)** Is a precursor of cytarabine
- **(D)** Is markedly hematotoxic and has caused neoplasms
- **(E)** Is a metabolite of mercaptopurine

Items 4–5: A renal transplant recipient is given a combination of immunosuppressive agents to prevent allograft rejection. During the course of therapy, drug toxicity occurs.

4. If the toxicity includes fever, vomiting, cutaneous lesions, and lymphadenopathy, the most likely causative agent is
- **(A)** Cyclophosphamide
- **(B)** Cyclosporine
- **(C)** Lymphocytic immune globulin
- **(D)** Mycophenolate mofetil
- **(E)** Rh_o(D) immune globulin

5. If the toxicity includes upper extremity tremor, limb paresthesias, and hallucinations, the most likely causative agent is
- **(A)** Azathioprine

(B) Cyclosporine
(C) Lymphocytic immune globulin
(D) Methotrexate
(E) Prednisone

6. Which of the following drugs is a widely used agent that suppresses cellular immunity, inhibits prostaglandin and leukotriene synthesis, and increases the catabolism of IgG antibodies?
(A) Cyclophosphamide
(B) Cyclosporine
(C) Infliximab
(D) Mercaptopurine
(E) Prednisone

7. Which of the following agents activates leukocyte-activated killer cells (LAKs) that are cytotoxic across MHC barriers and can even kill cells that do not express MHC?
(A) Aldesleukin
(B) Cyclosporine
(C) Etanercept
(D) Leflunomide
(E) Thalidomide

8. Which one of the following agents acts at the step of antigen recognition?
(A) Cyclosporine
(B) Cyclophosphamide
(C) Methotrexate
(D) Rh_0(D) immune globulin
(E) Tacrolimus

9. Tumor necrosis factor-α appears to play an important role in autoimmunity and inflammatory diseases. Which of the following is a humanized monoclonal antibody that binds to TNF-α and inhibits its action?
(A) Etanercept
(B) Infliximab
(C) Muromonab-CD3
(D) Sirolimus
(E) Thalidomide

Items 10–11: An immunosuppressed patient was treated for a bacterial infection with a parenteral penicillin. Within a few minutes of the penicillin injection, he developed severe bronchoconstriction, laryngeal edema, and hypotension. Due to the rapid administration of epinephrine, the patient survived. Unfortunately, a year later he was treated with an antipsychotic drug and developed agranulocytosis.

10. The type of drug reaction that was caused by the penicillin is
(A) An autoimmune syndrome
(B) A cell-mediated reaction
(C) A type II drug allergy
(D) Mediated by IgE
(E) Serum sickness

11. The type of drug reaction that was caused by the antipsychotic drug is
(A) A type III drug reaction
(B) A type IV drug reaction
(C) Delayed-type hypersensitivity
(D) Mediated by IgG or IgM antibodies
(E) The Stevens-Johnson syndrome

12. Which one of the following agents is able to suppress both B and T lymphocytes via its inhibition of de novo synthesis of purines?
(A) Cyclophosphamide
(B) Methotrexate
(C) Mycophenolate mofetil
(D) Prednisone
(E) Tacrolimus

13. Which one of the following statements is false?
(A) Daclizumab is an MAb that binds to the CD3 antigen on the surface of human thymocytes and mature T cells.

(B) Etanercept is a recombinant form of the TNF receptor which binds TNF-α, a proinflammatory cytokine.
(C) Leflunomide inhibits ribonucleotide synthesis and arrests lymphocytes in the G_1 phase of the cell cycle.
(D) Thalidomide is used in AIDS patients to treat aphthous ulcers.
(E) Thymosin has been used in thymic aplasia to increase T cell production.

14. Which one of the following statements about sirolimus is false?
(A) Binds to FK binding protein (FKBP)
(B) Inhibits cytokine production by activated T cells
(C) Decreases B cell proliferation
(D) Inhibits the actions of colony stimulating factors
(E) Slows antibody production

15. Which one of the following agents increases phagocytosis by macrophages in patients with chronic granulomatous disease?
(A) Aldesleukin
(B) Interferon-γ
(C) Lymphocyte immune globulin
(D) Prednisone
(E) Trastuzumab

ANSWERS

1. TH lymphocytes recognize foreign antigens presented by APC cells and, once activated, secrete cytokines that drive cell-mediated immunity (see Figure 56–2). The answer is **(E).**

2. Cyclosporine inhibits calcineurin, a serine phosphatase that is needed for activation of T cell-specific transcription factors. Gene transcription of IL-2, IL-3, and interferon-γ is inhibited. The answer is **(D).**

3. Azathioprine blocks both cellular and serologic immunity. For azathioprine to exert its cytotoxic actions it must first be metabolized to mercaptopurine, an inhibitor of purine synthesis. As is true for most purine antimetabolites, hematotoxicity is dose-limiting; the use of these agents as immunosuppressants is associated with an increase in cancer risk. The answer is **(D).**

4. Lymphocytic immune globulin is produced mainly through the immunization of large animals. As a mixture of foreign proteins, the agent may cause a wide range of hypersensitivity reactions, including skin reactions, serum sickness, and even anaphylaxis. The symptoms described are typical of serum sickness. The answer is **(C).**

5. Neurotoxic effects associated with the use of cyclosporine include limb paresthesias (incidence 50%), distal tremor (incidence 25%), hallucinations, and seizures. The answer is **(B).**

6. The corticosteroid prednisone is used extensively as an immunosuppressant in autoimmune diseases and organ transplantation. Glucocorticoids have multiple actions, including those described. The answer is **(E).**

7. Aldesleukin (IL-2) and several other interleukins activate natural killer cells (NK cells) and lymphokine-activated killer cells (LAK cells; "promiscuous killers"). The investigational use of aldesleukin in AIDS patients is partly based on the fact that lymphocytes from such individuals produce significantly less IL-2 than lymphocytes from healthy controls. The answer is **(A).**

8. $Rh_0(D)$ immune globulin contains antibodies against $Rh_0(D)$ antigens. Administration to an Rh-negative mother within 72 hours after the birth of an Rh-positive baby prevents Rh hemolytic disease of the newborn (erythroblastosis fetalis) in subsequent pregnancies. The answer is **(D).**

9. Infliximab is a humanized monoclonal antibody that binds to TNF-α. Etanercept also binds to TNF-α, but it is a chimeric protein containing a portion of the human TNF-α receptor linked to the Fc region of a human IgG. Thalidomide is a small molecule that appears to inhibit production of TNF-α. The answer is **(B).**

10. The patient experienced an anaphylactic response to the penicillin. This is a type I (immediate) drug reaction, mediated by IgE antibodies. The answer is **(D).**

11. Agranulocytosis (and systemic lupus erythematosus) are autoimmune syndromes that can be drug-induced. They are type II reactions involving IgM and IgG antibodies that bind to circulating blood cells. The patient was probably treated with clozapine for his psychosis (see clozapine toxicity, Chapter 29). The answer is **(D).**

12. Mycophenolic acid, formed from mycophenolate mofetil, inhibits inosine monophosphate dehydrogenase in the de novo pathway of purine synthesis. This action suppresses both B and T lymphocyte activation. Mycophenolate mofetil is used both individually and in combination with cyclosporine in organ transplants. The answer is **(C).**
13. Daclizumab is a monoclonal antibody that binds to the alpha subunit of the IL-2 receptor expressed on T cells and prevents activation by IL-2. Daclizumab is used in renal transplants and is much less toxic than muromonab-CD3. The answer is **(A).**
14. Like tacrolimus, sirolimus binds to FKBP. However, unlike both tacrolimus and cyclosporine, sirolimus inhibits the response of T cells to cytokines without affecting cytokine production. Sirolimus has all of the other actions described. The answer is **(B).**
15. Interferon-γ is approved for use in chronic granulomatous disease, a condition that results from phagocyte deficiency. The agent markedly reduces the frequency of recurrent infections. The answer is **(B).**

Skill Keeper Answers: Anaphylaxis & Sympathomimetic Drugs (see Chapters 6 and 9)

1. Epinephrine activates all adrenoceptors, whereas norepinephrine has minimal agonist activity at β_2-adrenoceptors. This difference is important in anaphylaxis because β_2-adrenoceptor activation is needed to provide a bronchodilatory effect that will oppose the anaphylaxis-induced airway obstruction. The α_1-adrenoceptor agonist effect of epinephrine opposes the anaphylaxis-induced vasodilation and, to some extent, the vascular leak (administration of fluid is also a cornerstone of the treatment of anaphylaxis), while the β_1-adrenoceptor agonist effect helps maintain cardiac output.
2. If bronchospasm is predominant, then administration by inhalation of a β_2-selective agonist like albuterol—or intravenous administration of theophylline—may be useful. If cardiovascular collapse is predominant, then vasopressor drugs may be helpful; these include α-adrenoceptor agonists such as phenylephrine and β_1-adrenoceptor agonists such as dobutamine or dopamine.

Part IX. Toxicology

57 Introduction to Toxicology

OBJECTIVES

You should be able to:

- List the major air pollutants and their clinical effects.
- Identify the major toxicities of common solvents and insecticides, including chlorinated hydrocarbons, inhibitors of cholinesterases, and botanicals.
- List two important herbicides and their major toxicities.
- Describe the toxicologic significance of environmental pollution due to dioxins and polychlorinated biphenyls (PCBs).

Learn the definitions that follow.

Table 57–1. Definitions.

Term	Definition
Toxicology	The area of pharmacology that deals with the adverse effects of chemicals on biologic systems
Occupational toxicology	The area that deals with the toxic effects of chemicals found in the workplace; regulated by the Occupational Safety & Health Agency (OSHA) in the USA
Environmental toxicology	The area that deals with the effects of agents found in the environment (air, water, etc); regulated by the Environmental Protection Agency (EPA) in the USA
Ecotoxicology	The area that deals with the untoward effects of agents found in the environment on whole populations as opposed to single individuals
Risk	The expected frequency of occurrence of a particular toxic effect in response to a particular agent
Threshold limit values (TLV)	The amount of exposure to a given agent that is deemed safe for a stated time period. It is higher for shorter periods than for longer periods
Generally recognized as safe (GRAS)	An official list of substances that through testing or experience do not appear to have significant toxicity
Bioaccumulation	The increasing concentration of a substance in the environment as the result of environmental persistence and physical properties (eg, lipid solubility) that permits it to accumulate in the tissues of organisms
Biomagnification	The further concentration of chemicals within organisms that feed on other organisms and thereby concentrate the chemicals found in the tissues of the prey species
Acceptable daily intake (ADI)	Maximum daily intake of a chemical which—during an entire lifetime—is without appreciable risk

CONCEPTS

Chemicals in the environment—home, workplace, atmosphere, etc—may constitute important health hazards. Some of these chemical groups are indicated in Figure 57–1.

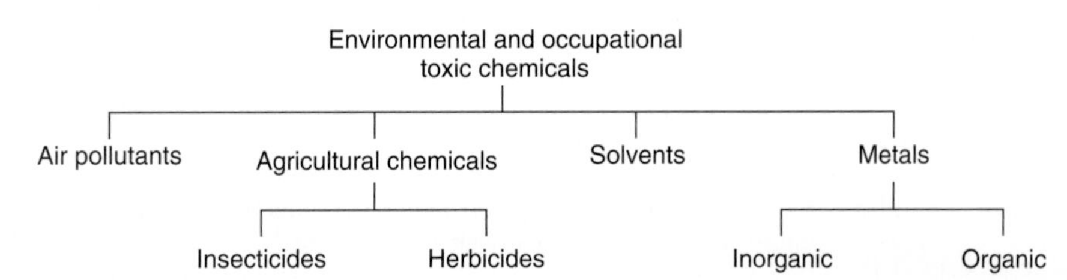

Figure 57–1. Chemical hazards in the environment. The toxicology of metals is discussed in Chapter 58.

AIR POLLUTANTS

A. Classification and Prototypes: The major air pollutants in industrialized countries include carbon monoxide (which accounts for about 50% of the total amount of air pollutants), sulfur oxides (18%), hydrocarbons (12%), particulate matter (eg, smoke particles, 10%), and nitrogen oxides (6%). Ambient air pollution appears to be a contributing factor in bronchitis, obstructive pulmonary disease, and lung cancer.

B. Carbon Monoxide: CO is an odorless, colorless gas that competes avidly with oxygen for hemoglobin. The affinity of CO for hemoglobin is more than 200-fold greater than that of oxygen. The threshold limit value (TLV) of CO for an 8-hour work day is 25 parts per million (ppm); in heavy traffic, the concentration of CO may exceed 100 ppm.

1. **Effects:** Carbon monoxide causes tissue hypoxia. Headache is one of the first symptoms, followed by confusion, decreased visual acuity, tachycardia, syncope, coma, convulsions, and death. Collapse and syncope occur when approximately 40% of hemoglobin has been converted to carboxyhemoglobin. These adverse effects may be aggravated by high ambient temperature and high altitude.
2. **Treatment:** Removal of the source of carbon monoxide and breathing pure oxygen are the major features of treatment. Hyperbaric oxygen accelerates the clearance of carbon monoxide.

C. Sulfur Dioxide: SO_2 is a colorless irritating gas formed from the combustion of fossil fuels.

1. **Effects:** SO_2 forms sulfurous acid on contact with moist mucous membranes; this acid is responsible for most of the pathologic effects. Conjunctival and bronchial irritation (especially in asthmatics) are the primary signs of exposure. Five to 10 ppm in the air is enough to cause severe bronchospasm. Heavy exposure may lead to delayed pulmonary edema. Chronic low-level exposure may aggravate cardiopulmonary disease.
2. **Treatment:** Removal from exposure and relief of irritation and inflammation comprise the major treatment.

D. Nitrogen Oxides: Nitrogen dioxide (NO_2), a brownish irritant gas, is the principal member of this group. It is formed in fires and in silage on farms.

1. **Effects:** NO_2 causes deep lung irritation and pulmonary edema. Farm workers exposed to high concentrations of the gas within enclosed silos may die rapidly of acute pulmonary edema. Irritation of the eyes, nose, and throat is common.
2. **Treatment:** No specific treatment is available. Measures to reduce inflammation and pulmonary edema are important.

E. Ozone: O_3 is a bluish irritant gas produced in air and water purification devices and in electrical fields.

1. **Effects:** Exposure to 0.01–0.1 ppm may cause irritation and dryness of the mucous membranes. Pulmonary function may be impaired at higher concentrations. Chronic exposure leads to bronchitis, bronchiolitis, pulmonary fibrosis, and emphysema.
2. **Treatment:** No specific treatment is available. Measures that reduce inflammation and pulmonary edema are emphasized.

SOLVENTS

Solvents used in industry and to clean clothing are a major source of direct exposure to hydrocarbons and also contribute to air pollution.

A. Aliphatic Hydrocarbons: This group includes halogenated solvents such as carbon tetrachloride, chloroform, and trichloroethylene.

1. **Effects:** Solvents are potent CNS depressants. The acute effects of excessive exposure are nausea, vertigo, locomotor disturbances, headache, and coma. Chronic exposure to halogenated hydrocarbons leads to both hepatic dysfunction and nephrotoxicity. Long-term exposure to tetrachloroethylene—or to trichloroethane—has caused peripheral neuropathy.
2. **Treatment:** Removal from exposure is the only specific treatment available. Serious CNS depression must be treated with support of vital signs (Chapter 60).

B. Aromatic Hydrocarbons: The aromatic hydrocarbons include benzene and toluene.

1. **Effects:** Acute exposure leads to CNS depression with ataxia and coma. Long-term exposure to benzene is associated with hematotoxicity (thrombocytopenia, leukopenia, aplastic anemia), and the compound may be leukemogenic. Toluene is not a myelosuppressant.
2. **Treatment:** Removal from exposure is the only specific way to reduce toxicity. CNS depression is managed by support of vital signs.

INSECTICIDES

A. Classification and Prototypes: The three major classes of insecticides are the chlorinated hydrocarbons (DDT and its analogs), acetylcholinesterase inhibitors (carbamates, organophosphates), and the botanical agents (nicotine, rotenone, pyrethrum alkaloids).

B. Chlorinated Hydrocarbons: These agents are persistent—very poorly metabolized—lipophilic chemicals that accumulate in body fat and thus are subject to both bioaccumulation and biomagnification (see Table 57–1).

1. **Effects:** Chlorinated hydrocarbons block physiologic inactivation in the sodium channels of nerve membranes and cause uncontrolled firing of action potentials. Tremor is usually the first sign of acute toxicity and may progress to seizures. Chronic exposure of animals to these insecticides causes increased tumorigenesis. The toxicologic impact of long-term exposure in humans is unclear. No relationship has been shown in humans between risk of breast cancer and serum levels of DDT metabolites.
2. **Treatment:** No specific treatment is available for the acute toxicity caused by chlorinated hydrocarbons. Because of their extremely long half-lives in organisms and in the environment (years), their use in North America and Europe has been curtailed.

C. Cholinesterase Inhibitors: The carbamates (eg, aldicarb, carbaryl) and organophosphates (eg, dichlorvos, malathion, parathion) are effective insecticides with short environmental half-lives. The cholinesterase inhibitors are inexpensive and are heavily used in agriculture.

1. **Effects:** As described in Chapter 7, these agents produce increased muscarinic and nicotinic stimulation. The effects include pinpoint pupils, sweating, salivation, bronchoconstriction, vomiting and diarrhea, CNS stimulation followed by depression, and muscle fasciculations, weakness, and paralysis. The most common cause of death is respiratory failure. Chronic exposure to some organophosphates (not carbamates) has resulted in a delayed neurotoxicity with axonal degeneration. The toxic mechanism appears to involve phosphorylation of a neuropathy target esterase (NTE).
2. **Treatment:** Atropine is used in large doses to control muscarinic excess; pralidoxime (2-PAM) is used to regenerate cholinesterase. Mechanical ventilation may be necessary.

D. Botanical Insecticides:

1. **Nicotine:** Nicotine has the same effects on nicotinic cholinoceptors in insects as in mammals and probably kills by the same mechanism, ie, excitation followed by paralysis of ganglionic, CNS, and neuromuscular transmission. Treatment is supportive.
2. **Rotenone:** This plant alkaloid insecticide causes gastrointestinal distress when ingested

and conjunctivitis and dermatitis following direct contact with exposed body surfaces. Treatment is symptomatic.

3. **Pyrethrum:** The most common toxic effect of this mixture of plant alkaloids is contact dermatitis. Ingestion or inhalation of large quantities may cause CNS excitation (including seizures) and peripheral neurotoxicity. Treatment is symptomatic, with anticonvulsants if necessary.

HERBICIDES

A. Paraquat: Paraquat is used extensively to kill weeds on farms and for highway maintenance.

1. **Effects:** The compound is relatively nontoxic unless ingested. After ingestion, the initial effect is gastrointestinal irritation with hematemesis and bloody stools. Within a few days, signs of pulmonary impairment occur and are usually progressive, resulting in severe pulmonary fibrosis and, often, death.
2. **Treatment:** No antidote is available; the best supportive treatment, including gastric lavage and dialysis, still results in less than 50% survival after ingestion of as little as 5 mL.

B. Phenoxyacetic Acids: 2,4-Dichlorophenoxyacetic acid (2,4-D) and 2,4,5-trichlorophenoxyacetic acid (2,4,5-T) are the two most important members of this group. During the manufacturing process, dioxin contaminants are produced. (See below for dioxin toxicology.)

1. **Effects:** Large doses of 2,4-D or 2,4,5-T cause muscle hypotonia and coma. Long-term exposure has been associated with an increased risk of non-Hodgkin's lymphoma.

ENVIRONMENTAL POLLUTANTS

The chemical compounds that contribute to environmental pollution include the chlorinated hydrocarbons (see above), the dioxins, and the polychlorinated biphenyls.

A. Dioxins:

1. **Source:** The polychlorinated dibenzo-*p*-dioxins (PCDDs) are a large group of related compounds of which the most important is 2,3,7,8-tetrachlorodibenzo-*p*-dioxin (TCDD). The dioxins have no commercial uses. They have appeared in the environment as unwanted by-products of the chemical industry. PCDDs are chemically stable and highly resistant to environmental degradation.
2. **Toxicology:** In laboratory animals, exposure to TCDD has caused multiple effects, including a wasting syndrome, hepatotoxicity, immune dysfunction, teratogenicity, and cancer. In humans, the most common signs of toxicity are dermatitis and chloracne. However, epidemiologic evidence suggests that the dioxins may have carcinogenic effects in humans, perhaps increasing the risk of non-Hodgkin's lymphoma.

B. Polychlorinated Biphenyls (PCBs):

1. **Source:** The polychlorinated biphenyls were used extensively in manufacturing electrical equipment until their potential for environmental damage was recognized. PCBs are among the most stable organic compounds known. They are poorly metabolized and lipophilic. They are therefore highly persistent in the environment and accumulate in the food chain.
2. **Toxicology:** In workers exposed to PCBs, the most common effect is dermatotoxicity (acne, erythema, folliculitis, hyperkeratosis). Less frequently, mild increases in plasma triglycerides and elevated liver enzymes have been observed. Possible teratogenicity has been suggested following several months of ingestion of cooking oils containing PCBs.

Skill Keeper: Safety of New Drugs (see Chapter 5)

The FDA requires evidence of relative safety of a new drug prior to its clinical evaluation. If a new drug is destined for chronic systemic administration, what animal toxicity testing is required? *The Skill Keeper Answer appears at the end of the chapter.*

QUESTIONS

DIRECTIONS: Each of the numbered items or incomplete statements in this section is followed by answers or by completions of the statement. Select the ONE lettered answer or completion that is BEST in each case.

1. The light brownish color of smog often apparent in the Los Angeles area on a hot summer day is mainly due to
- **(A)** Carbon monoxide
- **(B)** Hydrocarbons
- **(C)** Ozone
- **(D)** Nitrogen dioxide
- **(E)** Sulfur dioxide

2. You are stuck in traffic in New York City in summer for 3 or 4 hours and you begin to get a headache, a feeling of tightness in the temporal region, and an increased pulse rate. The most likely cause of these effects is inhalation of
- **(A)** Carbon monoxide
- **(B)** Nicotine
- **(C)** Nitrogen dioxide
- **(D)** Ozone
- **(E)** Sulfur dioxide

3. A man works all day in a storage facility that contains agricultural chemicals and solvents. Which one of the following statements about possible exposure to toxic substances in the workplace is LEAST accurate?
- **(A)** Ambient air concentrations of such chemicals should be regularly monitored
- **(B)** He may experience fatigue and possibly become ataxic if he is exposed to halogenated hydrocarbon vapors
- **(C)** He may develop a delayed neuropathy if he is working in areas where organophosphates are stored
- **(D)** The worker may develop acne from exposure to chlorophenoxy herbicides
- **(E)** He may develop a delayed pulmonary edema if he is exposed to chlorinated hydrocarbon insecticides

4. Correct pairings of toxic agent with the best method of treatment include all of the following EXCEPT
- **(A)** Carbon monoxide: 100% or hyperbaric oxygen
- **(B)** Carbon tetrachloride: Support of vital signs
- **(C)** Nitrogen dioxide: Nonspecific treatment of non-cardiogenic pulmonary edema
- **(D)** Paraquat: Hemodialysis
- **(E)** Parathion: Atropine and pralidoxime

5. Which one of the following chemicals does not undergo bioaccumulation and biomagnification and is LEAST likely to be an environmental hazard?
- **(A)** DDT
- **(B)** Dichlorvos
- **(C)** Polychlorinated biphenyls
- **(D)** TCDD
- **(E)** Toxaphene

6. An employee of a company engaged in clearing vegetation from county roadsides accidentally ingested a small quantity of a herbicidal solution that contained paraquat. Within 2 hours, he was admitted to the emergency room of a nearby hospital. Which of the following best describes his probable signs and symptoms in the emergency room?
- **(A)** Diarrhea, vomiting, sweating, and profound skeletal muscle weakness
- **(B)** Dizziness, nausea, agitation, and hyperreflexia
- **(C)** Dyspnea, pulmonary dysfunction, and elevated body temperature
- **(D)** Gastrointestinal irritation with hematemesis and bloody stools
- **(E)** Hypotension, tachycardia, and respiratory impairment

7. Chemical warfare agents that had been manufactured in the 1950s were being stored at a military installation. Several civilian workers at the facility began to feel unwell, with symptoms that included dyspnea, abdominal cramps, and diarrhea. They also had copious nasal and tracheobronchial secretions. Which type of toxic compound is most likely to be the cause of these effects?

(A) Aliphatic hydrocarbons
(B) Botulinum toxins
(C) Nitrogen mustards
(D) Organophosphates
(E) Rotenones

DIRECTIONS (Items 8–12): The matching questions in this section consist of a list of lettered options followed by several numbered items. For each numbered item, select the ONE lettered option that is most closely associated with it. Each lettered option may be selected once, more than once, or not at all.

(A) Aldicarb
(B) Benzene
(C) Carbon monoxide
(D) Carbon dioxide
(E) DDT
(F) Dioxin
(G) Malathion
(H) Nitrogen dioxide
(I) Paraquat
(J) Pyrethrum
(K) Rotenone
(L) Sulfur dioxide
(M) Tetrachloroethylene
(N) Toluene

8. Asthma is often exacerbated in patients exposed to this reducing agent when concentrations in the air are as low as 1–2 ppm. It is formed mainly from combustion of fossil fuels.
9. Acute exposure to this *aliphatic* hydrocarbon solvent causes CNS depression; chronic exposure has led to impairment of memory and peripheral neuropathy.
10. This compound is a potential environmental hazard that is formed as a contaminating by-product in the manufacture of herbicides.
11. Bone marrow cells in early stages of their development appear to be most sensitive to this agent, which has caused pancytopenia and aplastic anemia.
12. This agent is derived from a botanical source. The most frequent adverse effect reported is contact dermatitis. Accidental oral ingestion causes CNS stimulation, including seizures.

ANSWERS

1. Smog color is derived in part from suspended particulate matter. When smog is light brown, the color derives from nitrogen oxides. All of the other air pollutants listed are colorless. The answer is **(D)**.
2. The symptoms described are those of carbon monoxide inhalation. The answer is **(A)**.
3. Although DDT and related compounds are no longer used as insecticides in North America, they continue to be manufactured here for foreign markets. Exposure to such compounds causes CNS excitation, not pulmonary dysfunction. The answer is **(E)**.
4. Hemodialysis is of no value in paraquat poisoning. The answer is **(D)**.
5. Dichlorvos, an organophosphate inhibitor of acetylcholinesterase, is rapidly biotransformed and subject to inactivation by hydrolysis. Carbamates and organophosphates do not accumulate in the environment. The chlorinated hydrocarbons (DDT, toxaphene), polychlorinated biphenyls (PCBs), and the dioxins (TCDDs) are persistent chemicals. The answer is **(B)**.
6. Paraquat is highly corrosive to the gastrointestinal tract. Oral ingestion of the herbicide leads to marked gastrointestinal irritation, hematemesis, and usually blood in the stools. Gastric lavage with activated charcoal should be performed repeatedly to remove unabsorbed paraquat from the stomach. Signs of pulmonary impairment do not appear for several days and are usually progressive, resulting in severe pulmonary fibrosis and, often, death. The answer is **(D)**. (See also the answer to question 4.)
7. Too easy? Highly potent organophosphate inhibitors of acetylcholinesterase (eg, sarin, tabun) have been developed for chemical warfare purposes. Their storage represents a potential toxi-

cologic hazard. It is important to recognize the signs and symptoms of excess acetylcholine (DUMBELS; see Chapter 7), which include those described. The answer is **(D).**

8. Sulfur dioxide is a reducing agent that forms sulfurous acid on contact with moist surfaces. This is responsible for irritant effects on mucous membranes of the eye, the oropharyngeal cavity, and the respiratory tract. Asthmatics, patients with cardiac disease, and the elderly are especially sensitive to sulfur dioxide. Nitrogen dioxide causes similar problems, but it is an oxidizing agent formed from fires and in silage on farms. The answer is **(L).**

9. Three hydrocarbon solvents are listed: benzene, tetrachloroethylene, and toluene. Each of them may cause CNS effects such as headache, fatigue, and loss of appetite. Benzene and toluene are *aromatic* hydrocarbons. The answer is **(M).**

10. Dioxin is a contaminant formed in the manufacture of herbicides, including 2,4-D and 2,4,5-T ("agent orange"). The answer is **(F).**

11. Chronic exposure to benzene is markedly hematotoxic. Injury to bone marrow cells is characteristic of this aromatic hydrocarbon. Benzene has also been identified as a possible leukemogenic agent. The answer is **(B).**

12. Rotenone and pyrethrum alkaloids are both derived from plants. Both agents may cause dermatitis through skin contact. Accidental oral ingestion of rotenone causes gastrointestinal irritation but no neurotoxic effects. The answer is **(J).**

Skill Keeper Answer: Safety of New Drugs (see Chapter 5)

Acute toxicity studies in two animal species are required by the FDA for all new drugs prior to their use in humans. Subacute and chronic toxicity studies are required for drugs that are intended for chronic systemic use. Toxicity testing in animals usually involves the determination of lethal dose, monitoring of blood, hepatic, renal, and respiratory functions, gross and histopathologic examination of tissues, and tests of reproductive effects and potential carcinogenicity.

58 Heavy Metals

OBJECTIVES

You should be able to:

- Describe the general mechanism of metal chelation.
- Identify the clinically useful chelators and know their indications and their adverse effects.
- Describe the major clinical features and treatment of acute and chronic lead poisoning.
- Describe the major clinical features and treatment of arsenic poisoning.
- Describe the major clinical features and treatment of inorganic and organic mercury poisoning.
- Describe the major clinical features and treatment of iron poisoning.

Learn the definitions that follow.

Table 58–1. Definitions.

Term	Definition
Chelating agent	A molecule with two or more electronegative groups that can form stable coordinate complexes with multivalent cationic metal atoms
Erethism	Syndrome resulting from mercury poisoning characterized by insomnia, memory loss, excitability, and delirium
Pica	The ingestion of nonfood substances; in the present context, pica refers to ingestion of lead-based paint fragments by small children
Plumbism	A range of toxic syndromes due to chronic lead poisoning that may vary as a function of blood or tissue levels and patient age

CONCEPTS

The metals discussed in this chapter—lead, arsenic, mercury, and iron—frequently cause significant toxicity in humans. The toxicity profiles of metals differ, but most of their effects appear to result from interaction with sulfhydryl groups of enzymes and regulatory proteins. Chelators are organic compounds with two or more electronegative groups that can form stable covalent-coordinate bonds with cationic metal atoms. As emphasized in this chapter, these stable complexes can often be excreted readily, thus reducing the toxicity of the metal.

CHELATORS

The most useful chelators for clinical purposes are dimercaprol (BAL), succimer, penicillamine, edetate (EDTA), and deferoxamine. Variations among these agents in their affinities for specific metals govern their clinical applications. Some of these applications are outlined in Table 58–2.

A. Dimercaprol: Dimercaprol (2,3-dimercaptopropanol; BAL [British antilewisite]) is a *bidentate* chelator, ie, it forms two bonds with the metal ion, preventing the metal's binding to tissue proteins and permitting its rapid excretion.

1. **Clinical use:** Dimercaprol is used in acute arsenic and mercury poisoning—and for lead poisoning when administered with edetate. It is an oily liquid that must be given parenterally.

Table 58–2. Important characteristics of the toxicology of arsenic, iron, lead, and mercury.

Metal	Form Entering Body	Route of Absorption	Target Organs for Toxicity	Treatment[1]
Lead	Inorganic lead oxides and salts	Gastrointestinal, respiratory, skin (minor)	Hematopoietic system, CNS, kidneys	Dimercaprol, edetate, penicillamine, succimer
	Tetraethyl lead	Skin (major), gastrointestinal	CNS	Seizure control, supportive
Arsenic	Inorganic arsenic salts	All mucous surfaces	Capillaries, gastrointestinal tract, hematopoietic system	Dimercaprol, succimer, penicillamine
	Arsine gas	Inhalation	Erythrocytes	Supportive
Mercury	Elemental	Inhalation	CNS, kidneys	Dimercaprol
	Inorganic salts	Gastrointestinal	Kidneys, gastrointestinal tract	Penicillamine, dimercaprol
	Organic mercurials	Gastrointestinal	CNS	Supportive
Iron	Ferrous sulfate	Gastrointestinal	Gastrointestinal, CNS, blood	Deferoxamine

[1]In all cases, removal of the individual from the source of toxicity is the first requirement of management.

2. **Toxicity:** Dimercaprol causes a high incidence of adverse effects, possibly because it is very lipophilic and readily enters cells. Its toxicity includes transient hypertension, tachycardia, headache, nausea and vomiting, paresthesias, and fever (especially in children). It may cause pain and hematomas at the injection site. Long-term use is associated with thrombocytopenia and increased prothrombin time.

B. **Succimer:** Succimer (2,3-dimercaptosuccinic acid; DMSA) is a water-soluble bidentate congener of dimercaprol with oral bioavailability.
   1. **Clinical use:** Succimer is used for the oral treatment of lead toxicity in children and adults, and it is as effective as parenteral EDTA in reducing blood lead concentration. Succimer is effective in arsenic and mercury poisoning, if given within a few hours of exposure.
   2. **Toxicity:** While succimer appears to be less toxic than dimercaprol, gastrointestinal distress, CNS effects, skin rash, and elevation of liver enzymes may occur.

C. **Penicillamine:** Penicillamine, a derivative of penicillin, is another bidentate chelator, forming two bonds with the metal ion.
   1. **Clinical use:** The major uses of penicillamine are in the treatment of copper poisoning and of Wilson's disease. It is sometimes used as adjunctive therapy in gold, arsenic, and lead intoxication and in rheumatoid arthritis. The agent is water-soluble, well absorbed from the gastrointestinal tract, and excreted unchanged.
   2. **Toxicity:** Adverse effects are common and may be severe. They include nephrotoxicity with proteinuria, pancytopenia, and autoimmune dysfunction, including lupus erythematosus and hemolytic anemia.

D. **Edetate:** Edetate (EDTA) is a very efficient *polydentate* chelator of many divalent and trivalent cations (including calcium).
   1. **Clinical use:** The primary use of EDTA is in the treatment of lead poisoning. Because the agent is very polar, it is given parenterally and it does not enter cells. To prevent dangerous hypocalcemia, EDTA is usually given as the calcium disodium salt.
   2. **Toxicity:** The most important adverse effect of the agent is nephrotoxicity, including renal tubular necrosis. This risk can be reduced by adequate hydration and restricting treatment with EDTA to 5 days or less. Electrocardiographic changes may occur at high doses.

E. **Deferoxamine:** Deferoxamine is a polydentate bacterial product that has an extremely high and selective affinity for iron and a much lower affinity for aluminum. Fortunately, the drug competes poorly for heme iron in hemoglobin and cytochromes.
   1. **Clinical use:** Deferoxamine is used parenterally in the treatment of acute iron intoxication.
   2. **Toxicity:** Skin reactions (blushing, erythema, urticaria) may occur. With long-term use, neurotoxicity (eg, retinal degeneration), hepatic and renal dysfunction, and severe coagulopathies have been reported. Rapid intravenous administration may cause histamine release and hypotensive shock.

TOXICOLOGY OF HEAVY METALS

A. **Lead:** Lead serves no useful purpose in the body and may damage the hematopoietic tissues, liver, nervous system, kidneys, gastrointestinal tract, and reproductive system (Table 58–2). Lead represents a major environmental hazard since it is present in the air and water throughout the world.
   1. **Acute lead poisoning:** Acute inorganic lead poisoning is no longer common in the USA but may occur from industrial exposures (usually via the inhalation of dust) and in children who have ingested large quantities of chips or flakes from surfaces covered with lead-containing paint. The primary signs of this syndrome are acute abdominal colic and CNS changes. In children, the latter may take the form of acute encephalopathy. The mortality rate is high in lead encephalopathy, and prompt chelation therapy is mandatory.
   2. **Chronic lead poisoning:** Chronic inorganic lead poisoning (plumbism) is much more common than the acute form. Signs include peripheral neuropathy (wrist drop is character-

istic), anorexia, anemia, tremor, weight loss, and gastrointestinal symptoms. Treatment includes removal from the source of exposure, and chelation therapy, usually with edetate (severe cases), dimercaprol, or penicillamine. Chronic lead poisoning in children presents as growth retardation, neurocognitive deficits, and developmental delay. Succimer is generally used in such children. In workers exposed to lead, prophylaxis by means of oral chelating agents is contraindicated, since some evidence suggests that lead absorption may be enhanced by the presence of chelators. In contrast, high dietary calcium is indicated, since lead retention is reduced.

3. **Organic lead poisoning:** Poisoning by organic lead is usually due to tetraethyl lead or tetramethyl lead antiknock gasoline additives (no longer used in the USA). This form of lead is readily absorbed through the skin and lungs. The primary signs of intoxication occur in the CNS and may include hallucinations, headache, irritability, convulsions, and coma. Treatment consists of decontamination and seizure control.

B. Arsenic: This element is widely used in industrial processes and is also an environmental pollutant released during the burning of coal. Although it exists in both trivalent and pentavalent forms, its toxicity is entirely due to the trivalent form.

1. **Acute arsenic poisoning:** Acute arsenic poisoning results in severe gastrointestinal discomfort, vomiting, "ricewater" stools, and capillary damage with dehydration and shock. A sweet, garlicky odor may be detected in the breath and the stools. Treatment consists of supportive therapy to replace water and electrolytes, and chelation therapy with dimercaprol.
2. **Chronic arsenic poisoning:** Chronic arsenic intoxication is manifested by skin changes, hair loss, bone marrow depression and anemia, and chronic nausea and gastrointestinal disturbances. Dimercaprol therapy appears to be of value. Arsenic is a known human carcinogen.
3. **Arsine gas:** Arsine gas (AsH_3) is formed during the refinement and processing of certain metals and is used in the semiconductor industry; it is an occupational hazard. Arsine causes a unique form of toxicity characterized by massive hemolysis. Pigment overload from red cell breakdown may cause renal failure. Treatment is supportive.

C. Mercury: The main source of inorganic mercury as a toxic hazard is through the use of materials in dental laboratories and in the manufacture of wood preservatives, insecticides, and batteries. Organic mercury compounds are used as seed dressings and fungicides.

1. **Acute mercury poisoning:** Acute mercury poisoning usually occurs through inhalation of inorganic elemental mercury. It causes chest pain, shortness of breath, nausea and vomiting, kidney damage, gastroenteritis, and CNS damage. Chelation is effective with dimercaprol. Acute ingestion of mercuric chloride causes a severe, life-threatening hemorrhagic gastroenteritis followed by renal failure.
2. **Chronic mercury poisoning:** Chronic mercury poisoning may occur with inorganic or organic mercury. Inorganic mercury poisoning in the chronic form usually presents as a diffuse set of symptoms involving the gums and teeth, gastrointestinal disturbances, and neurologic and behavioral changes. When mercury was used in the hat-making industry, the behavioral effects (erethism) were so common that they gave rise to the epithet "mad as a hatter." Chronic inorganic mercury intoxication has been treated with penicillamine and dimercaprol.
3. **Organic mercury poisoning:** Intoxication with organic mercury compounds was first recognized in connection with an epidemic of neurologic and psychiatric disease in the village of Minamata in Japan. The outbreak was found to be the result of consumption of fish containing a high content of methylmercury, which was produced by bacteria in sea water from mercury in the effluent of a nearby vinyl plastics manufacturing plant. Similar epidemics have resulted from the consumption of grain intended for use as seed and treated with fungicidal organic mercury compounds. Treatment with chelators has been tried, but the benefits are uncertain.

D. Iron: Acute poisoning from the ingestion of ferrous sulfate tablets occurs quite frequently in small children. The initial symptoms of iron poisoning include vomiting, gastrointestinal bleeding, lethargy, and gray cyanosis. This may be followed by signs of severe gastrointestinal necrosis, pneumonitis, jaundice, seizures, and coma. Deferoxamine is the chelating agent of choice. Chronic excessive intake of iron may lead to hemosiderosis or hemochromatosis.

Skill Keeper: Iron Deficiency
(see Chapter 33)

Iron is the essential metallic element of heme, the molecule responsible for the bulk of oxygen transport in the blood.

1. How is the iron content of the body regulated?
2. How is iron deficiency diagnosed and treated?

The Skill Keeper Answers appear at the end of the chapter.

QUESTIONS

DIRECTIONS: Each numbered item or incomplete statement in this section is followed by answers or by completions of the statement. Select the ONE lettered answer or completion that is BEST in each case.

Items 1–2: A small child is brought to a hospital emergency room suffering from severe gastrointestinal distress and abdominal colic.

1. The differential diagnosis will not include
(A) Acute inorganic lead poisoning
(B) Appendicitis
(C) Exposure to arsine gas
(D) Pancreatitis
(E) Peptic ulcer

2. If this patient has severe acute lead poisoning presenting as signs and symptoms of encephalopathy, treatment should be instituted immediately with
(A) Acetylcysteine
(B) Deferoxamine
(C) EDTA
(D) Penicillamine
(E) Succimer

3. A young woman employed as a dental laboratory technician complains of conjunctivitis, skin irritation, and hair loss. On examination, she has perforation of the nasal septum and a "milk and roses" complexion. These signs and symptoms are most likely to be due to
(A) Acute mercury poisoning
(B) Chronic inorganic arsenic poisoning
(C) Chronic mercury poisoning
(D) Excessive use of supplementary iron tablets
(E) Lead poisoning

4. A patient complains of chronic headache, fatigue, loss of appetite, and constipation. He has slight weakness of the extensor muscles in the upper limbs. The following data are obtained.

Test	Result in Patient	Normal
Hemoglobin	< 13 g/dL	> 14 g/dL
Urinary coproporphyrin	> 80 μg/100 mg creatinine	< 10 μg/100 mg creatinine
Urinary aminolevulinic acid	> 2 mg/100 mg creatinine	< 0.5 mg/100 mg creatinine

The most reasonable diagnosis is that this patient is suffering from chronic poisoning due to
(A) Arsenic
(B) Hexane
(C) Inorganic lead
(D) Iron
(E) Mercuric chloride

5. In the treatment of acute inorganic arsenic poisoning, the most likely drug to be used is

(A) Deferoxamine
(B) Dimercaprol
(C) EDTA
(D) Penicillamine
(E) Succimer

6. As a general rule, chelators used in lead poisoning are more effective if administered 48 *hours* after ingestion than if administered to a patient 48 *days* after a person has ingested the same quantity of lead. The main reason for this is that
(A) Elimination of lead is 90% in the urine
(B) The half-life of lead in the blood and soft tissues is only 24 days
(C) Forty-eight days after ingestion, much of the absorbed lead is in the bone matrix
(D) Only 5% of absorbed lead is retained in the body
(E) Lead binding to erythrocytes is time-dependent

7. A 24-year-old man was employed in the supplies department of a company that manufactures semiconductors. Following an accident at the plant he presented with nausea and vomiting, headache, hypotension, and shivering. Laboratory analyses showed hemoglobinuria and a plasma free hemoglobin level greater than 1.4 g/dL. This young man was probably exposed to
(A) Arsine
(B) Inorganic arsenic
(C) Mercury vapor
(D) Methylmercury
(E) Tetraethyl lead

8. A 2-year-old child was brought to the emergency room 1 hour after ingestion of tablets he had managed to obtain from a bottle on top of the refrigerator. His symptoms included marked gastrointestinal distress, vomiting (with hematemesis), and epigastric pain. Metabolic acidosis and leukocytosis were also present. This patient is most likely to have ingested tablets containing
(A) Acetaminophen
(B) Aspirin
(C) Diphenhydramine
(D) Iron
(E) Vitamin C

DIRECTIONS: The matching questions in this section consist of a list of lettered options followed by several numbered items. For each numbered item, select the ONE lettered option that is most closely associated with it. Each lettered option may be selected once, more than once, or not at all.

(A) Arsine
(B) Deferoxamine
(C) Dimercaprol
(D) Edetate calcium disodium
(E) Inorganic mercury
(F) Iron
(G) Methylmercury
(H) Mercury vapor
(I) Penicillamine
(J) Succimer
(K) Tetraethyl lead
(L) Trivalent arsenic

9. Gingivitis, discolored gums, and loose teeth are common symptoms of chronic exposure to this agent.
10. This compound may be produced in seawater by the action of bacteria and algae. It is also synthesized chemically for commercial use as a fungicide.
11. This agent has been reported to cause lupus erythematosus and hemolytic anemia.
12. High doses of this agent may cause histamine release and extreme vasodilation.

ANSWERS

1. The diagnosis of acute lead poisoning may be difficult, since the symptoms often simulate a number of disorders of the gastrointestinal system, including acute appendicitis. In children

with recent ingestion of lead-containing materials, radiopacities may be visible on abdominal x-ray. Exposure to arsine, an industrial gas, is highly unlikely in a small child, and the symptoms are those of acute hemolysis. The answer is **(C).**

2. Encephalopathy in severe lead poisoning is a medical emergency. Of the drugs listed, intravenous EDTA is the most effective chelating agent. Dimercaprol (not listed) may also be used parenterally. Oral succimer is used in children with mild to moderate lead poisoning and may be initiated 4–5 days after the use of EDTA or dimercaprol in severe poisoning. The answer is **(C).**
3. The "milk and roses" complexion, which results from vasodilation and anemia, is one characteristic of chronic inorganic arsenic poisoning, while patients with lead poisoning often have a gray pallor. Other signs and symptoms include gastrointestinal distress, hyperpigmentation, and white lines on the nails. We hope you were not led astray by her employment. The answer is **(B).**
4. Of the agents listed, lead is most likely to cause a decrease in heme biosynthesis. Exposure to inorganic arsenic may also cause anemia. The urinary concentrations of lead before and after EDTA treatment may confirm the diagnosis. The answer is **(C).**
5. The treatment of choice in acute arsenic poisoning is intramuscular dimercaprol. While succimer is less toxic than dimercaprol, it is available only in an oral formulation and its absorption may be impaired due to the severe gastroenteritis that occurs in acute poisoning with arsenic. The answer is **(B).**
6. Depending on patient age, 10–40% of inorganic lead absorbed from the gastrointestinal tract is retained in the body, the balance being mostly eliminated in the urine. Of the fraction retained, over 90% is incorporated into the skeleton. By 2 months, a significant amount of the body burden of lead is present in the bone matrix. Chelating agents are much less able to penetrate into the bone than into more vascular tissues and thus are less effective if they are not administered soon after lead exposure. The answer is **(C).**
7. From the signs and symptoms alone, a diagnosis could not be made of arsine poisoning. However, clues to the etiology of poisoning can often be provided by knowing a patient's occupation. The laboratory reports suggest marked hemolysis. Arsine binds to hemoglobin and decreases erythrocyte glutathione levels, causing membrane fragility and resulting hemolysis. The answer is **(A).**
8. This question emphasizes that the ingestion of iron tablets is a relatively common cause of accidental poisoning in young children. The signs and symptoms described usually occur in the first 6 hours following ingestion. In a child of body weight 22 lb, the ingestion of 600 mg can cause severe, perhaps lethal, toxicity. The answer is **(D).**
9. Oral and gastrointestinal complaints are common in chronic mercury poisoning, and tremor involving the fingers and arms is often present. The answer is **(E).**
10. Methylmercury continues to be used as a fungicide to prevent mold growth in seed grain. The answer is **(G).**
11. Autoimmune diseases have occurred during the treatment of Wilson's disease with penicillamine. The answer is **(I).**
12. Deferoxamine may cause shock if given by rapid intravenous infusion. The answer is **(B).**

Skill Keeper Answers: Iron Deficiency (see Chapter 33)

1. Regulation of body iron occurs through modulation of its intestinal absorption. Ferrous ions are absorbed and oxidized in mucosal cells to the ferric form. Ferric iron can be stored in mucosal cells bound to ferritin or may be distributed throughout the body bound to transferritin. Most of the iron in the body is present in hemoglobin. Small quantities of iron are eliminated in sweat, saliva, and the exfoliation of skin and mucosal cells.
2. Iron deficiency can be diagnosed from red blood cell changes, including microcytic size and decreased hemoglobin content, and from measurement of serum and bone marrow iron stores. Iron deficiency anemia is treated by dietary ferrous iron supplements or, in severe cases, parenteral use of iron dextran.

Management of the Poisoned Patient 59

OBJECTIVES

You should be able to list or describe:

- Steps involved in the management of the poisoned patient, including the emergency treatment of a comatose patient.
- Common toxic syndromes associated with major drug groups and individual agents frequently involved in poisoning.
- Methods for identification of toxic compounds, including physical symptoms and laboratory methods.
- Methods available for decontamination of poisoned patients and for increasing the elimination of toxic compounds.
- Specific antidotes available for management of poisoning.

CONCEPTS

Toxic substances include drugs usually used for therapeutic purposes as well as agricultural and industrial chemicals that have no medical applications. Most chemicals are capable of causing toxic effects when given in excessive dosage; even for therapeutic drugs, the difference between obtaining a therapeutic action and a toxic one is a matter of dose. Many toxic effects of therapeutic agents have been discussed in previous chapters. Common toxic syndromes associated with major drug groups are summarized below. Other chemicals commonly involved in poisonings are those readily accessible in the environment: solvents, corrosives, insecticides, heavy metals, and drugs of abuse. This unit reviews the principles of management of the poisoned patient.

TOXICOKINETICS, TOXICODYNAMICS, & CAUSE OF DEATH

A. **Toxicokinetics:** This term is used to denote the disposition of poisons in the body, ie, their pharmacokinetics. Knowledge of the absorption, distribution, and elimination permits assessment of the value of procedures designed to remove particular toxins from the skin or gastrointestinal tract. For example, drugs with large apparent volumes of distribution, such as antidepressants and antimalarials, are not amenable to dialysis procedures for drug removal. Drugs with low volumes of distribution, including lithium, phenytoin, and salicylates, are more readily removed by dialysis and diuresis procedures. In some cases, it is possible to accelerate renal elimination of weak acids by urinary alkalinization and weak bases by urinary acidification. The clearance of drugs may be different at toxic concentrations than at therapeutic concentrations. For example, in overdoses of phenytoin or salicylates, the capacity of the liver to metabolize the drugs may be exceeded and elimination will change from first-order (constant half-life) to zero-order (variable half-life) kinetics.

B. **Toxicodynamics:** Toxicodynamics is a term used to denote the injurious effects of toxins, ie, their pharmacodynamics. A knowledge of toxicodynamics can be useful in the diagnosis and management of poisoning. For example, hypertension and tachycardia are typically seen in overdoses with amphetamines, cocaine, and antimuscarinic drugs. Hypotension with bradycardia occurs with overdoses of calcium channel blockers, beta-blockers, and sedative-hypnotics. Hypotension with tachycardia occurs with tricyclic antidepressants, phenothiazines, and theophylline. Hyperthermia is most frequently a result of overdose of drugs with antimuscarinic actions, the salicylates, or sympathomimetics. Hypothermia is more likely to occur with toxic doses of ethanol and other CNS depressants. Increased respiratory rate is often a feature of overdose with carbon monoxide, salicylates, and other drugs that cause metabolic acidosis or cellular asphyxia. Overdoses of agents that depress the heart are likely to affect the functions of all organ systems that are critically dependent on blood flow, including brain, liver, and kidney. Note that restoration of blood pressure after a period of hypotension may increase the tissue distribution of a toxin, which can result in waxing and waning of signs and symptoms.

C. **Cause of Death in Intoxicated Patients:** The most common causes of death from drug overdose in the USA reflect the drug groups most often selected for abuse or for suicide. Sedative-hypnotics and narcotics cause respiratory depression, coma, aspiration of gastric contents, and other respiratory malfunctions. Drugs such as cocaine, PCP, tricyclic antidepressants, and theophylline cause seizures, which may lead to vomiting and aspiration of gastric contents, and to postictal respiratory depression. Tricyclic antidepressants and cardiac glycosides cause dangerous and frequently lethal arrhythmias. Severe hypotension may occur with any of these drugs. A few intoxicants cause direct liver and kidney damage. These include acetaminophen, mushroom poisons of the *Amanita phalloides* type, certain inhalants, and some heavy metals. The metals are discussed in Chapter 58.

MANAGEMENT OF THE POISONED PATIENT

Management of the poisoned patient consists of maintenance of vital functions, identification of the toxic substance, decontamination procedures, enhancement of elimination, and, in a few instances, the use of a specific antidote.

A. **Vital Functions:** The most important aspect of treatment of a poisoned patient is maintenance of vital functions, as indicated by the mnemonic **"ABCDs."** The most commonly endangered or impaired vital function is respiration. Therefore, an open and protected airway (the "A" of the mnemonic) must be established first and effective ventilation ("B" for breathing) must be ensured. The circulation ("C") should be evaluated and supported as needed. The cardiac rhythm should be determined, and if ventricular fibrillation is present, it must be corrected at once. The blood pressure should be measured but rarely needs immediate treatment except in cases of traumatic hemorrhage. Because of the danger of brain damage from hypoglycemia, intravenous 50% dextrose ("D" of the mnemonic) should be given to comatose patients immediately after blood has been drawn for laboratory tests and before laboratory results have been obtained. Similarly, thiamine should be given to prevent Wernicke's syndrome in the suspected alcoholic or malnourished patient. In patients with signs of respiratory or CNS depression, intravenous naloxone may be administered to offset possible toxic effects of opioid analgesic overdose.

B. **Identification of Poisons:** Many intoxicants cause a characteristic syndrome of clinical and laboratory changes. Table 59–1 summarizes toxic syndromes associated with major drug groups and the key interventions called for. The toxic features of selected individual agents are listed in Table 59–2. When the toxic agent responsible for a case of poisoning cannot be directly examined and identified, the clinician must rely on indirect means to identify the type of intoxication and the progress of therapy. In addition to the history and physical examination, certain laboratory examinations may be useful. A few intoxicants can be directly identified in the blood or urine, especially when information in the history helps to narrow the search. In the more common situation (a comatose patient unable to provide a history), general tests for replacement of anions or osmotic equivalents in the blood (anion gap, osmolar gap) may be useful. A few intoxicants can be identified or strongly suspected on the basis of electrocardiographic or radiologic findings.

1. **Osmolar gap:** The osmolar gap is the difference between the measured osmolarity (measured by the freezing point depression method) and the predicted osmolarity:

$$\textbf{Gap} = \textbf{Osm (measured)} - [(2 \times \textbf{Na}^+ [\textbf{meq/L}]) + (\textbf{Glucose} [\textbf{mg/dL}] \div 18) + (\textbf{BUN} [\textbf{mg/dL}] \div 3)]$$

This gap is normally zero. A significant gap is produced by high serum concentrations of intoxicants of low molecular weight such as ethanol, methanol, and ethylene glycol.

Table 59–1. Toxic syndromes caused by major drug groups.*

Drug Group	Clinical Features	Key Interventions
Antimuscarinic drugs (atropine, some antidepressants and antihistaminics, jimsonweed, etc)	Delirium, hallucinations, seizures, coma, tachycardia, hypertension, hyperthermia, mydriasis, decreased bowel sounds, urinary retention	Control hyperthermia; physostigmine may be helpful, but not for tricyclic overdose
Cholinomimetic drugs (carbamate, organophosphate inhibitors of acetyl-cholinesterase)	Anxiety, agitation, seizures, coma, bradycardia or tachycardia, pinpoint pupils, salivation, sweating, hyperactive bowel, muscle fasciculations, then paralysis	Support respiration. Treat with atropine and pralidoxime. Decontaminate
Opioids (heroin, morphine, methadone, etc)	Lethargy, sedation, coma, bradycardia, hypotension, hypoventilation, pinpoint pupils, cool skin, decreased bowel sounds, flaccid muscles	Provide airway and respiratory support. Give naloxone as required
Salicylates	Confusion, lethargy, coma, seizures, hyperventilation, hyperthermia, dehydration, hypokalemia, anion gap metabolic acidosis	Correct acidosis and fluid and electrolyte imbalance. Provide alkaline diuresis or hemodialysis to aid elimination
Sedative-hypnotics (barbiturates, benzodiazepines, ethanol)	Disinhibition initially, later lethargy, stupor, coma. Nystagmus is common. Decreased muscle tone, hypothermia. Small pupils, hypotension, and decreased bowel sounds in severe overdose	Provide airway and respiratory support. Avoid fluid overload. Use flumazenil for benzodiazepine overdose
Stimulants (amphetamines, cocaine, phencyclidine)	Agitation, anxiety, seizures. Hypertension, tachycardia, arrhythmias. Mydriasis, vertical and horizontal nystagmus with PCP. Skin warm and sweaty, hyperthermia, increased muscle tone, possible rhabdomyolysis	Control seizures, hypertension, and hyperthermia
Tricyclic antidepressants	Antimuscarinic effects (see above). The "three C's" of coma, convulsions, cardiac toxicity (QRS prolongation, arrhythmias, hypotension)	Control seizures. Correct acidosis and cardiotoxicity with ventilation and bicarbonate. Control hyperthermia

*Modified and reproduced, with permission, from Katzung BG (editor): *Basic & Clinical Pharmacology,* 7th ed. Originally published by Appleton & Lange. Copyright © 1998 by The McGraw-Hill Companies, Inc.

2. **Anion gap:** The anion gap is the difference between the sum of the two primary cations, sodium and potassium, and the sum of the two primary anions, chloride and bicarbonate:

$$\text{Gap} = (\text{Na}^+ + \text{K}^+) - (\text{HCO}_3^- + \text{Cl}^-)$$

This gap is normally 12–16 meq/L. A significant increase may be produced by diabetic ketoacidosis, renal failure, or drug-induced metabolic acidosis. Drugs that may cause metabolic acidosis include ethanol, ethylene glycol, isoniazid, iron, methanol, phenelzine, salicylates, tranylcypromine, and verapamil.

3. **Serum potassium:** Myocardial function is critically dependent on serum potassium level. Drugs that cause hyperkalemia include beta-adrenoceptor blockers, digitalis (in suicidal overdose), fluoride, and lithium. Drugs associated with hypokalemia include barium, beta-adrenoceptor agonists, methylxanthines, most diuretics, and toluene.

C. **Decontamination:** Decontamination consists of removing any unabsorbed poison from the patient's body. In the case of ingested noncorrosive toxins, this may involve inducing vomiting (emesis) by means of **syrup of ipecac** if the patient is conscious. (*Fluid extract* of ipecac should not be used since it contains cardiotoxic alkaloids.) In unconscious patients, emesis will lead to aspiration into the respiratory tree and must be avoided. **Gastric lavage** with a large-bore tube may be used to remove noncorrosive drugs from the stomach of a comatose patient if the airway has been protected with a cuffed endotracheal tube. Corrosives (strong acids and

Table 59–2. Toxic features of specific agents.

Agent	Toxic Features
Acetaminophen	Mild anorexia, nausea, vomiting, delayed jaundice, hepatic and renal failure
Antifreeze (ethylene glycol)	Renal failure, crystals in urine, anion and osmolar gap, initial CNS excitation; eye examination normal
Botulism	Dysphagia, dysarthria, ptosis, ophthalmoplegia, muscle weakness; incubation period 12–36 hours
Carbon monoxide	Coma, metabolic acidosis, retinal hemorrhages
Cyanide	Bitter almond odor, seizures, coma, abnormal ECG
Gasoline	Distinctive odor, coughing, pulmonary infiltrates
Iron	Bloody diarrhea, coma, radiopaque material in gut (seen on x-ray), high leukocyte count, hyperglycemia
Lead	Abdominal pain, hypertension, seizures, muscle weakness, metallic taste, anorexia, encephalopathy, delayed motor neuropathy, changes in renal and reproductive function
LSD	Hallucinations, dilated pupils, hypertension
Mercury	Acute renal failure, tremor, salivation, gingivitis, colitis, erethism (fits of crying, irrational behavior), nephrotic syndrome
Methanol	Rapid respiration, visual symptoms, osmolar gap, severe metabolic acidosis
Mushrooms (*Amanita phalloides* type)	Severe nausea and vomiting 8 hours after ingestion; delayed hepatic and renal failure
Paraquat	Oropharyngeal burning, headache, vomiting, delayed pulmonary fibrosis and death
Phencyclidine (PCP)	Coma with eyes open, horizontal and vertical nystagmus, hyperacusis
Plants	
Nightshade family, jimsonweed	Hallucinations, mydriasis, seizures (these plants contain atropine-like alkaloids)
Oleander and foxglove	Digitalis poisoning
Predatory bean (rosary pea)	Delayed severe gastrointestinal distress, seizures, hemolytic anemia, death

bases) may cause severe esophageal damage during emesis and should be diluted (not neutralized) in the stomach. **Activated charcoal,** given orally or by stomach tube, may be very effective in adsorbing any remaining drug. Toxins removed by multiple treatments with activated charcoal include amitriptyline, barbiturates, carbamazepine, digitalis glycosides, phencyclidine, propoxyphene, theophylline, tricyclic antidepressants, and valproic acid. In the case of topical exposure (insecticides, solvents), the clothing should be removed and the patient washed to remove any chemical still present on the skin. Medical personnel must be careful not to contaminate themselves during this procedure.

D. Enhancement of Elimination: Enhancement of elimination is possible for a number of toxins, including manipulation of urine pH to accelerate renal excretion of weak acids and bases. For example, alkaline diuresis is effective in toxicity due to fluoride, isoniazid, fluoroquinolones, phenobarbital, and salicylates. Urinary acidification may be useful in toxicity due to weak bases, including amphetamines, nicotine, and phencyclidine, but care must be taken to avoid acidosis and renal failure in rhabdomyolysis. Hemodialysis or hemoperfusion enhances the elimination of many toxic compounds, including acetaminophen, ethylene glycol, formaldehyde, lithium, methanol, procainamide, quinidine, salicylates, and theophylline. Cathartics such as sorbitol (70%) may decrease absorption and hasten removal of toxins from the gastrointestinal tract.

E. Antidotes: Specific antidotes exist for only a few poisons (Table 59–3). Consideration must be given to the fact that the duration of action of most antidotes is shorter than that of the intoxicant, and the antidotes may need to be given repeatedly. The use of chelating agents for metal poisoning is discussed in Chapter 58.

Table 59–3. Specific antidotes.*

Antidote	Poisons
Acetylcysteine	Acetaminophen; best given within 8–10 hours after overdose
Atropine	Cholinesterase inhibitors
Bicarbonate, sodium	Membrane-depressant cardiotoxic drugs, eg, quinidine, tricyclic antidepressants
Deferoxamine (Desferal)	Iron salts
Digoxin-specific Fab antibodies (Digibind)	Digoxin and related cardiac glycosides
Esmolol	Caffeine, theophylline, metaproterenol
Ethanol	Methanol, ethylene glycol (fomepizole is now approved for ethylene glycol poisoning)
Flumazenil	Benzodiazepines, zolpidem
Glucagon	Beta-adrenoceptor blockers
Edetate (EDTA)	Lead
Dimercaprol	Lead, gold, arsenic
Penicillamine	Copper, lead, arsenic, gold
Naloxone (Narcan)	Opioid analgesics
Oxygen	Carbon monoxide
Physostigmine	Suggested for muscarinic receptor blockers, *not* for tricyclics
Pralidoxime (2-PAM)	Organophosphate cholinesterase inhibitors

*Modified and reproduced, with permission, from Katzung BG (editor): *Basic & Clinical Pharmacology,* 8th ed. McGraw-Hill, 2001.

Skill Keeper: Cyanide Poisoning (see Chapters 11 and 12)

Cyanide forms a stable complex with the ferric ion of cytochrome oxidase enzymes, inhibiting cellular respiration. What is the connection between the management of cyanide poisoning and the drugs amyl nitrite and nitroprusside? *The Skill Keeper Answer appears at the end of the chapter.*

F. Snakebite: The most common dangerous snake in the USA is the rattlesnake. Although snakebites are common (several thousand per year in the USA), severe envenomation is infrequent.

1. **Effects:** Snake venom contains a large number of enzymes and tissue toxins. The most common effects of envenomation include local tissue necrosis, vascular damage, thrombosis, hemorrhage, and neural injury.
2. **Treatment:** It is now well documented that once-popular remedies such as incision and suction, ice packs, and tourniquets are usually more dangerous than helpful. The most important prehospital therapy is to minimize movement of the bitten part to limit the spread of the venom in the tissues. Effective therapy consists of adequate dosage with antivenin. Since antivenins are prepared in horses, serum sickness frequently follows and may also require therapy.

QUESTIONS

DIRECTIONS: Each of the numbered items or incomplete statements in this section is followed by answers or by completions of the statement. Select the ONE lettered answer or completion that is BEST in each case.

Items 1–2: A patient has taken an overdose of aspirin that has caused metabolic acidosis. Serum electrolyte concentrations are Na^+, 147 meq/L; K^+, 6 meq/L; Cl^-, 100 meq/L; HCO_3^-, 15 meq/L.

1. The anion gap in this patient
  (A) Cannot be calculated from the data given
  (B) Is unchanged from normal
  (C) Is increased above normal
  (D) Is decreased below normal
  (E) Is reversed

2. Which of the following agents may cause an increase in anion gap?
  (A) Antifreeze solution
  (B) Iron tablets
  (C) Phenelzine
  (D) Verapamil
  (E) All of the above

3. Which one of the following drugs or toxins is LEAST likely to cause hyperthermia in overdosage?
  (A) Amphetamine
  (B) Aspirin
  (C) Heroin
  (D) Jimsonweed
  (E) Phencyclidine

4. A patient is brought to the emergency room suffering from nausea, vomiting, and abdominal pain. He has muscle weakness, which seems to be progressing downward from the head and neck. The patient has difficulty talking clearly and has ptosis and ophthalmoplegia. The most likely cause of these symptoms is
  (A) Accidental ingestion of paraquat
  (B) An overdose of phenobarbital
  (C) Excessive consumption of ethanol
  (D) Food poisoning
  (E) Organophosphate poisoning

5. Which one of the following is LEAST likely to cause an osmolar gap when taken in overdose?
  (A) Digoxin
  (B) Ethanol
  (C) Ethylene glycol
  (D) Isopropanol
  (E) Methanol

6. A patient with congestive heart failure has accidentally taken an overdose of digoxin. The blood concentration of the drug is eight times the threshold for toxicity. Pharmacokinetic parameters for digoxin include a clearance of 7 L/h and an elimination half-life of 56 hours. If no procedures are instituted to decontaminate this patient, the time taken to reach a safe level of digoxin will be approximately
  (A) 3.5 days
  (B) 7 days
  (C) 14 days
  (D) 28 days
  (E) 56 days

7. Regarding snakebite,
  (A) A rattlesnake bite is almost always associated with significant tissue injury
  (B) A snakebite should be treated in the field with incision, suction, and a tourniquet before the victim is moved
  (C) The most common manifestation of serious envenomation is convulsions
  (D) When a victim of a serious envenomation reaches the hospital, the most effective therapy is prompt administration of snake antivenin
  (E) All of the above are correct

Items 8–9: A patient is brought to the emergency room having taken an overdose (unknown quantity) of a sustained-release preparation of theophylline by oral administration 2 hours previously. He has marked gastrointestinal distress with vomiting, is agitated and hyperreflexic, and is hypotensive.

8. Regarding the management of this patient, which one of the following interventions is LEAST likely to be employed?

(A) Activated charcoal orally
(B) Hemoperfusion
(C) Intravenous normal saline
(D) Ipecac fluid extract
(E) Whole bowel irrigation

9. The plasma level of theophylline measured immediately upon hospitalization was 80 mg/L. If the oral bioavailability of theophylline is 98%, the clearance is 50 mL/min, volume of distribution is 35 L, and the elimination half-life is 7.5 hours, the amount ingested must have been at least
(A) 0.3 g
(B) 0.6 g
(C) 1.6 g
(D) 2.8 g
(E) 8.0 g

10. Intoxicants correctly associated with their effects include
(A) All of the following
(B) Carbon monoxide: Carboxyhemoglobinemia
(C) Cyanide: Cytochrome oxidase inactivation
(D) Paraquat: Pulmonary fibrosis
(E) Sodium nitrite: Methemoglobinemia

DIRECTIONS (Items 11–16): The matching questions in this section consist of a list of lettered options followed by several numbered items. For each numbered item, select the ONE lettered option that is most closely associated with it. Each lettered option may be selected once, more than once, or not at all.

(A) Acetaminophen
(B) Acetylsalicylic acid
(C) Benzene
(D) Carbon monoxide
(E) Heroin
(F) Hydrogen sulfide
(G) Iron
(H) Lead
(I) Methanol
(J) Physostigmine
(K) Sodium cyanide
(L) Theophylline
(M) Triazolam

11. The best antidote for overdose of this substance is atropine

12. The most likely drug to be needed in an overdose due to this substance is an anticonvulsant, but beta-blockers are appropriate when cardiac arrhythmias are present

13. Acetylcysteine should be administered to a patient who overdoses on this drug

14. The ingestion of this chemical is best managed by intravenous ethanol

15. This agent should not be used in overdose of a tricyclic antidepressant, though it would reverse many of the anticholinergic symptoms that occur

16. Intravenous flumazenil will reverse the effects of this drug in overdose

ANSWERS

1. Anion gap is calculated by subtracting measured serum anions (bicarbonate plus chloride) from cations (potassium plus sodium). Increases in anion gap above normal are due to the presence of unmeasured anions that accompany acidosis. The gap in this case (38 meq/L) is well in excess of the normal gap (12–16 meq/L). The answer is **(C).**

2. The ingestion of ethylene glycol (antifreeze), iron tablets, monoamine oxidase inhibitors used for depressive disorders (eg, phenelzine), or verapamil can result in metabolic acidosis, with an increase in anion gap. The answer is **(E).**

3. Aspirin, sympathomimetics, agents with muscarinic blocking actions, and drugs that cause muscle rigidity or seizures are all likely to cause hyperthermia at toxic doses. Hypothermia is more typical of overdoses with opioids or sedative-hypnotics. The answer is **(C).**

4. Food-borne botulism (due to *C botulinum*) may lead to a symmetric descending paralysis that results in respiratory failure. Patients are initially alert but may suffer from dysarthria and dysphagia. Ptosis and ophthalmoplegia are also characteristic symptoms. The answer is **(D)**.
5. Digoxin is lethal at levels much too low to be detected by the osmolar gap method. This method is useful only for poisonings with low-potency substances of low molecular weight, eg, methanol and ethylene glycol. The answer is **(A)**.
6. Estimations of the time period required for drug or toxin elimination may be of value in the management of the poisoned patient. If no procedures were used to hasten the elimination of digoxin in this patient, the time taken to reach a safe plasma level of the drug (12.5% of the measured level) is three half-lives, or approximately 7 days. The answer is **(B)**.
7. Only about 20% of rattlesnake bites involve significant envenomation. Incision, suction, and tourniquets are usually more damaging than helpful. Ice packs are contraindicated. Serious envenomation causes primarily local tissue damage. Antivenin is by far the most effective therapy for serious envenomation. The answer is **(D)**.
8. Activated charcoal is effective in decreasing theophylline absorption from the gastrointestinal tract, and whole bowel irrigation is especially useful for decontamination of orally administered sustained-release formulations of the drug. Hypotension is often managed by saline infusion, though vasopressors may be required. The blood levels of theophylline are decreased by charcoal hemoperfusion or by hemodialysis. Ipecac *fluid extract* contains cardiotoxic alkaloids and should never be used as an emetic. The answer is **(D)**.
9. Estimations of the quantity of a drug or toxin ingested may be of value in management of the poisoned patient. Applying toxicokinetic principles, a rough estimate of ingested dose of theophylline could be made by multiplying the peak plasma level of the drug (80 mg/L) by its volume of distribution (35 L) to give a value of 2800 mg, or 2.8 g. Because only about one-fourth of a half-life has passed since ingestion, the amount eliminated since that time will be rather small. The answer is **(D)**.
10. All are correct. The answer is **(A)**.
11. Atropine is the primary antidote for poisoning due to inhibitors of acetylcholinesterase, including carbamate (eg, physostigmine) and organophosphate insecticides (eg, malathion). Pralidoxime may be administered to regenerate inactivated enzyme in poisoning due to insecticides. The answer is **(J)**.
12. The most dangerous toxic effect of theophylline is convulsions. The cardiovascular toxicity of theophylline (eg, arrhythmias) often responds to beta-blockers. The answer is **(L)**.
13. Hepatotoxicity due to overdose of acetaminophen (more likely in alcoholic patients) is due to the formation of a toxic metabolite. Early administration of acetylcysteine can be protective. The answer is **(A)**.
14. Ethanol competes with methanol for alcohol dehydrogenase, preventing its conversion to the toxic compounds formaldehyde and formic acid. The answer is **(I)**.
15. Tricyclic antidepressant overdose includes cardiotoxicity, convulsions, and symptoms of muscarinic receptor blockade. The antidote for the quinidine-like cardiotoxicity of tricyclic antidepressants is sodium bicarbonate. Although physostigmine does effectively reverse anticholinergic symptoms, it can aggravate depression of cardiac conduction and can cause seizures. The answer is **(J)**.
16. Flumazenil displaces benzodiazepines from their binding sites on the GABA receptor-chloride ion channel macromolecular complex in neural membranes. The answer is **(M)**.

Skill Keeper Answer: Cyanide Poisoning (see Chapters 11 and 12)

The cyanide antidote kit contains amyl nitrite, sodium nitrite, and sodium thiosulfate. The nitrites convert hemoglobin to methemoglobin, which has a higher affinity for the cyanide ion (forming cyanmethemoglobin) than cytochrome oxidase. Subsequent treatment with sodium thiosulfate results in the formation of methemoglobin and thiocyanate ions.

Nitroprusside is often considered the drug of choice in severe hypertension. Prolonged use of nitroprusside may result in toxicity due to the release of cyanide and subsequent conversion to thiocyanate ions.

Part X. Special Topics

Drugs Used in Gastrointestinal Disorders

60

OBJECTIVES

You should be able to:

- List five different drug groups used in the treatment of peptic ulcer and describe their mechanisms.
- List four drugs used in the prevention of chemotherapy-induced vomiting.
- List three laxative drugs and describe their mechanisms.
- List the two most important antidiarrheal drugs.
- List two drugs used to prevent or diminish the formation of gallstones.

CONCEPTS

The gastrointestinal tract serves several functions: digestive, excretory, endocrine, exocrine, etc. These functions provide numerous important drug targets, and many of the drugs used in gastrointestinal disease have been discussed in earlier chapters of this book. However, several important drugs used in common gastrointestinal diseases do not fall into the drug groups discussed earlier; these agents are described in this chapter.

A. **Drugs Used in Acid-Peptic Disease:** Ulceration and erosion of the lining of the gastrointestinal tract are common problems, and several drug groups used in these diseases have been discussed previously (H_2 blockers [Chapter 16], antimuscarinic drugs [Chapter 8], and misoprostol [Chapter 18]). Other drugs used in peptic disease include the antacids, sucralfate, proton pump inhibitors, and antibiotics. Figure 60–1 summarizes the actions of these drugs.

1. **Antacids:** Antacids are simple physical agents that react with protons in the lumen of the gut. Some antacids (aluminum-containing antacids) may also stimulate the protective functions of the gastric mucosa. The antacids effectively reduce the recurrence rate of peptic ulcers when used regularly in the large doses needed to significantly raise the stomach pH.

   The antacids differ mainly in their absorption and effects on stool consistency. The most popular antacids in use in the USA are **magnesium hydroxide** ($Mg[OH]_2$) and **aluminum hydroxide** ($Al[OH]_3$). Neither of these weak bases is significantly absorbed from the bowel. Magnesium hydroxide has a strong laxative effect, while aluminum hydroxide has a constipating action. These drugs are available as single-ingredient products and as combined preparations. Calcium carbonate and sodium bicarbonate are also weak bases, but they differ from aluminum and magnesium hydroxides in being absorbed from the gut. Because of their systemic effects, calcium and bicarbonate salts are less popular as antacids than the magnesium and aluminum compounds listed.

2. **Sucralfate:** Sucralfate is aluminum sucrose sulfate, a small, poorly soluble molecule that polymerizes in the acid environment of the stomach. This polymer binds to injured tissue and forms a protective coating over ulcer beds. The drug has been shown to accelerate the healing of peptic ulcers and to reduce the recurrence rate. Unfortunately, sucralfate must be

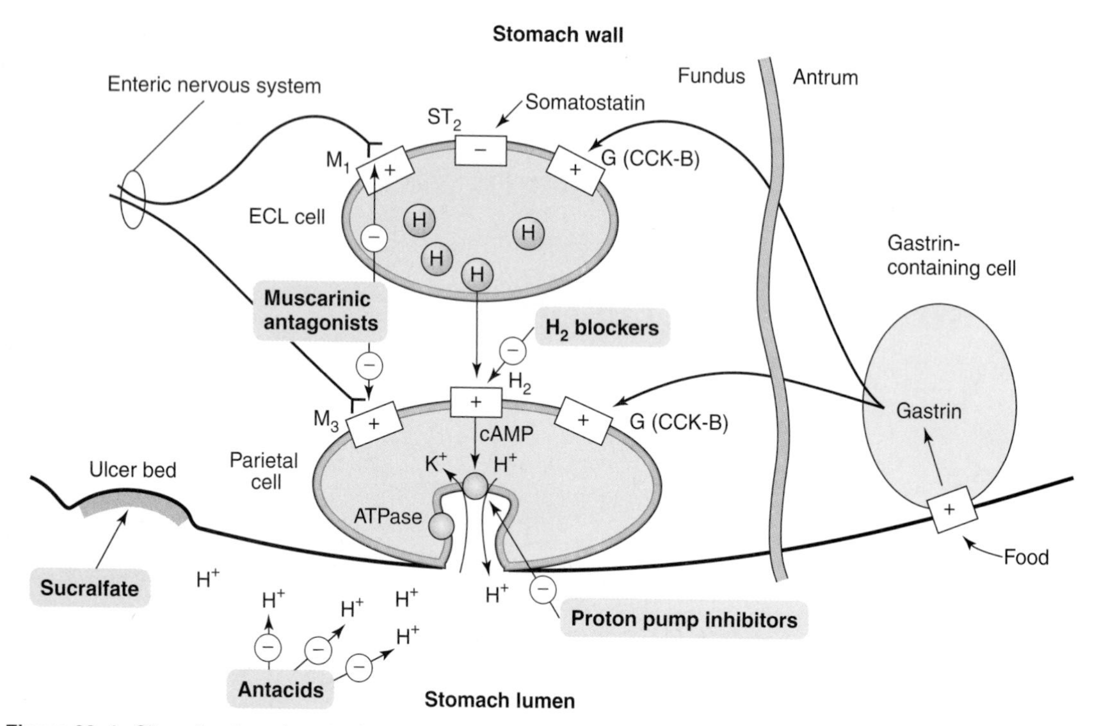

Figure 60–1. Sites of action of some drugs used in peptic ulcer disease. The site of action of misoprostol is not shown; it is thought to reduce acid secretion and increase protective factors such as mucus and bicarbonate. (Modified and reproduced, with permission, from Katzung BG [editor]: *Basic & Clinical Pharmacology,* 7th ed. Originally published by Appleton & Lange. Copyright © 1998 by The McGraw-Hill Companies, Inc.)

taken four times daily. Sucralfate is too insoluble to have significant systemic effects when taken by the oral route; toxicity is very low.

3. **Proton pump inhibitors: Omeprazole** is the prototype of the class of inhibitors of the proton pump of gastric parietal cells. This pump, an H^+/K^+ ATPase located in the luminal membrane of parietal cells, binds proton pump inhibitors irreversibly. Proton pump inhibitors are particularly useful in the treatment of Zollinger-Ellison syndrome (usually associated with a gastrin-secreting tumor), and gastroesophageal reflux disorder (GERD), conditions in which the H_2 blockers are not completely satisfactory. Other agents in the group include lansoprazole and rabeprazole. Chronic treatment with proton pump inhibitors results in hypergastrinemia. In rats, large doses have caused carcinoid tumors, but in humans no tumors have been reported and toxicity appears to be very low.
4. **Antibiotics:** Chronic infection with *Helicobacter pylori* is present in the great majority of patients with recurrent non-NSAID-induced peptic ulcers, and eradication of this organism greatly reduces the rate of recurrence of ulcer in these patients. The regimens of choice consist of a proton pump inhibitor plus a course of bismuth (Pepto-Bismol), tetracycline, and metronidazole or a course of amoxicillin plus clarithromycin.

B. **Drugs That Promote Upper Gastrointestinal Motility:** Diabetes and other diseases that damage nerves to the viscera frequently cause a marked loss of motility in the esophagus and stomach, resulting in gastric paralysis (gastroparesis). Gastroparesis is associated with delayed stomach emptying, nausea, and severe bloating. **Metoclopramide** and **cisapride** are able to stimulate motility in gastroparesis. Metoclopramide probably acts as an acetylcholine facilitator and dopamine receptor antagonist in the enteric nervous system (ENS). Cisapride appears to act as a 5-HT_4 agonist in the ENS. The "prokinetic" action of metoclopramide is also of some value in preventing emesis following surgical anesthesia and emesis induced by cancer chemotherapeutic drugs. Adverse effects of metoclopramide include induction of parkinsonism and other extrapyramidal effects. Cisapride in high concentrations is associated with long-

QT syndrome and has caused fatal arrhythmias. For this reason, cisapride is now available only on a limited basis.

C. Drugs With Antiemetic Actions: A variety of drugs have been found to be of some value in the prevention and treatment of vomiting, especially cancer chemotherapy-induced vomiting. In addition to **metoclopramide**, useful antiemetic drugs include **dexamethasone;** some **H_1 antihistamines;** several **phenothiazines;** the **5-HT_3 inhibitors;** and **dronabinol,** the active ingredient in marijuana. The 5-HT_3 inhibitors, **ondansetron, granisetron,** and **dolasetron,** are extremely useful in preventing nausea and vomiting after general anesthesia and in patients receiving cancer chemotherapy.

Skill Keeper: 5-HT Agonists & Antagonists (see Chapters 16 and 30)

List the various 5-HT receptor agonists and antagonists in current use. Describe their clinical applications. *The Skill Keeper Answer appears at the end of the chapter.*

D. Pancreatic Enzyme Replacements: Steatorrhea, a condition of decreased fat absorption coupled with an increase in stool fat excretion, results from inadequate pancreatic secretion of lipase. The abnormality of fat absorption can be significantly relieved by oral administration of pancreatic lipase **(pancrelipase)** obtained from pigs. Pancreatic lipase is inactivated at a pH below 4.0; thus, up to 90% of an administered dose will be destroyed in the stomach, unless the pH is raised with antacids or drugs that reduce acid secretion.

E. Laxatives: Laxatives increase the probability of a bowel movement by several mechanisms: an irritant or stimulant action on the bowel wall; a bulk-forming action on the stool that evokes reflex contraction of the bowel; a softening action on hard or impacted stool; and a lubricating action that eases passage of stool through the rectum. Examples of drugs that act by these mechanisms are set forth in Table 60–1.

F. Antidiarrheal Agents: The most effective antidiarrheal drugs are the opioids and derivatives of opioids that have been selected for maximal antidiarrheal and minimal CNS effect. Of the latter group, the most important are **diphenoxylate** and **loperamide,** meperidine analogs with very weak analgesic effects. **Difenoxin,** the active metabolite of diphenoxylate, is also available as a prescription medication. Diphenoxylate is formulated with antimuscarinic alkaloids to reduce the already minimal likelihood of abuse; loperamide is formulated alone and sold over the counter as such.

G. Drugs That Inhibit the Formation of Gallstones: The formation of cholesterol gallstones can be inhibited by several drugs, though none are dramatically effective. Such drugs include the bile acid derivatives **chenodiol** and **ursodiol.** Chenodiol appears to reduce the secretion of bile acids by the liver, while the mechanism of action of ursodiol is unknown.

Table 60–1. The major laxative mechanisms and some representative laxative drugs.

Mechanism	Examples
Irritant	Castor oil, cascara, senna
Bulk-forming	Saline cathartics (eg, $Mg[OH]_2$), psyllium
Stool-softening	Dioctyl sodium sulfosuccinate (docusate)
Lubricating	Mineral oil, glycerin

QUESTIONS

DIRECTIONS: Each numbered item or incomplete statement in this section is followed by answers or by completions of the statement. Select the ONE lettered answer or completion that is BEST in each case.

1. A 55-year-old woman with insulin-dependent diabetes of 40 years' duration complains of severe bloating and abdominal distress, especially after meals. Evaluation is consistent with diabetic gastroparesis. The drug you would be most likely to recommend is
(A) Docusate
(B) Dopamine
(C) Loperamide
(D) Metoclopramide
(E) Sucralfate

2. A patient who must take verapamil for hypertension and angina has become severely constipated. Which of the following drugs would be most suitable as a cathartic?
(A) Aluminum hydroxide
(B) Diphenoxylate
(C) Magnesium hydroxide
(D) Metoclopramide
(E) Mineral oil

3. Your cousin is planning a three-week trip overseas and asks your advice regarding medications for traveler's diarrhea. A drug suitable for noninfectious diarrhea is
(A) Aluminum hydroxide
(B) Diphenoxylate
(C) Magnesium hydroxide
(D) Metoclopramide
(E) Mineral oil

4. Which of the following drugs or drug groups is not useful in the prevention of nausea and vomiting induced by cancer chemotherapy:
(A) Dexamethasone
(B) Dronabinol
(C) Ketanserin
(D) Ondansetron
(E) Phenothiazines

5. A patient presents with Zollinger-Ellison syndrome due to a gastrinoma. He has two bleeding ulcers and diarrhea. A drug that irreversibly inhibits the H^+/K^+ ATPase in gastric parietal cells is
(A) Cimetidine
(B) Cisapride
(C) Glycopyrrollate
(D) Omeprazole
(E) Ondansetron

6. A drug associated with the long QT syndrome and cardiac arrhythmias is:
(A) Aluminum hydroxide
(B) Cisapride
(C) Granisetron
(D) Loperamide
(E) Metronidazole

7. On your way to an examination you experience that vulnerable feeling that an attack of diarrhea is imminent. If you stopped at a drugstore, you could buy this antidiarrheal drug without a prescription even though it is related chemically to the strong opioid-analgesic meperidine:
(A) Aluminum hydroxide
(B) Diphenoxylate
(C) Loperamide
(D) Magnesium hydroxide
(E) Metoclopramide

8. This antibiotic is not appropriate for use as an oral agent in the treatment of recurrent peptic ulcer associated with *Helicobacter pylori*
(A) Amoxicillin
(B) Clarithromycin

(C) Metronidazole
(D) Tetracycline
(E) Vancomycin

9. A patient is receiving chemotherapy for metastatic carcinoma. She threatens to stop her treatment because of severe nausea and vomiting. Which one of the following drugs is not likely to prevent such chemotherapy-induced nausea and vomiting?
(A) Dexamethasone
(B) Dronabinol
(C) Levodopa
(D) Ondansetron
(E) Prochlorperazine

DIRECTIONS: The following matching questions consist of a list of lettered options followed by several numbered items. For each numbered item, select the ONE option that is most closely associated with it. Each answer may be selected once, more than once, or not at all.

(A) Aluminum hydroxide
(B) Castor oil
(C) Cimetidine
(D) Diphenoxylate
(E) Loperamide
(F) Magnesium hydroxide
(G) Metoclopramide
(H) Mineral oil
(I) Omeprazole
(J) Pancrelipase
(K) Ondansetron
(L) Sucralfate

10. A lubricating laxative; not very effective if bowel tone is absent or severely reduced
11. Management of steatorrhea is best accomplished by the use of
12. A small molecule that polymerizes in stomach acid and coats the ulcer bed, resulting in accelerated healing and reduction of symptoms

ANSWERS

1. Of the drugs listed, only metoclopramide is considered a prokinetic agent, ie, one that increases propulsive motility in the gut. The answer is **(D)**.
2. A cathartic that mildly stimulates the gut would be most suitable in a patient taking a smooth muscle relaxant drug such as verapamil. Magnesium hydroxide, by holding water in the intestine, provides additional bulk and stimulates increased contractions. The answer is **(C)**.
3. Diphenoxylate and loperamide are the traditional traveler's antidiarrheal drugs. Diphenoxylate requires a prescription in the USA but is less expensive than loperamide. The answer is **(B)**.
4. Ketanserin is an inhibitor of 5-HT_2 receptors (Chapter 16) and has no antiemetic action. All of the other drugs listed are useful in preventing chemotherapy-induced nausea and vomiting. The answer is **(C)**.
5. Omeprazole and other members of the "prazole" family irreversibly inhibit the proton pump. The answer is **(D)**.
6. Cisapride can cause marked prolongation of the cardiac action potential and the long QT syndrome if given with another drug that inhibits cisapride's metabolism (eg, erythromycin, ketoconazole). The answer is **(B)**.
7. Aluminum hydroxide is constipating but is not related chemically to meperidine; magnesium hydroxide is a strong laxative. The two antidiarrheal drugs that are structurally related to opioids are diphenoxylate and loperamide. Loperamide is available over-the-counter; diphenoxylate is mixed with atropine alkaloids, and the product (Lomotil, others) requires a prescription. The answer is **(C)**.
8. Metronidazole (in combination with tetracycline and bismuth) is one of the antibiotic regimens sometimes used to eradicate *H pylori*. The antibiotics are combined with a proton pump inhibitor or H_2 blocker. Amoxicillin and clarithromycin are also commonly used for this pur-

pose. Vancomycin is not used and should be reserved for management of MRSA infections, for which it is the drug of choice. The answer is **(E).**

9. Antihistamines, dronabinol, glucocorticoids, and metoclopramide have antiemetic actions that are useful in the management of vomiting caused by anticancer drugs. Levodopa causes nausea because it is converted to dopamine, which activates dopamine receptors in the emetic center. The answer is **(C).**

10. Mineral oil is a lubricant. It has no irritant or bulk-forming properties. Mineral oil and other laxatives may be "abused" by persons with eating disorders. The answer is **(H).**

11. Steatorrhea is due to decreased fat absorption as a result of inadequate pancreatic secretion of lipase. The answer is **(J).**

12. Sucralfate is a small molecule that polymerizes in stomach acid and forms a protective coat over the ulcer bed. The answer is **(L).**

Skill Keeper Answer: 5-HT Agonists & Antagonists (see Chapters 16 and 30)

The only serotonin agonists in common use are the 5-HT_{1D}-selective agonists such as sumatriptan and its congeners (Chapter 16). These drugs are used in migraine. Ergot alkaloids are *partial* agonists at several 5-HT receptors and are also used in migraine and other conditions. Several valuable antidepressants are inhibitors of the serotonin reuptake pump in neurons (Chapter 30). Serotonin antagonists include 5-HT_2-blockers such as ketanserin (also an α-blocker), cyproheptadine (also an H_1 blocker), and phenoxybenzamine (also an α-blocker). Ketanserin is not available in the USA but is used for hypertension in some countries. Cyproheptadine is used for pruritus and sometimes for carcinoid tumor. Phenoxybenzamine is used for carcinoid tumor as well as for pheochromocytoma. 5-HT_3 receptors are blocked by ondansetron and its congeners. These drugs are extremely useful in preventing postoperative and cancer-chemotherapy-induced nausea and vomiting.

61 Drug Interactions

OBJECTIVES

You should be able to:

- Describe the primary pharmacokinetic mechanisms that underlie drug interactions.
- Describe how the pharmacodynamic characteristics of different drugs administered concomitantly may lead to additive, synergistic, or antagonistic effects.
- Identify specific drug interactions that occur commonly in clinical practice.

Learn the definitions that follow.

Table 61–1. Definitions.

Term	Definition
Pharmacokinetic interaction	A change in the pharmacokinetics of one drug caused by the interacting drug, eg, an inducer of hepatic enzymes
Pharmacodynamic interaction	A change in the pharmacodynamics of one drug caused by the interacting drug, eg, additive action of two drugs having similar effects
Addition	The effect of two drugs given together is equal to the sum of the responses to the same doses given separately
Antagonism	The effect of two drugs given together is less than the sum of the responses to the same doses given separately
Synergism	The effect of two drugs given together is greater than the sum of the two responses when they are given separately

CONCEPTS

Drug interactions occur when one drug modifies the actions of another drug in the body. Usually such actions are quantitative—ie, an increase or a decrease in the size of an expected response. Drug interactions may be the result of pharmacokinetic alterations, pharmacodynamic changes, or a combination of both. Interactions between drugs in vitro (eg, precipitation when mixed in solutions for intravenous administration) are usually classified as *drug incompatibilities,* not drug interactions.

Although hundreds of drug interactions have been documented, relatively few are of clinical significance and constitute a contraindication to simultaneous use or require a change in dosage. Some of these are listed in Table 61–2. In patients taking many drugs, however, the likelihood of significant drug interactions is increased. Elderly patients have a high incidence of drug interactions because they often have age-related changes in drug clearance and commonly take multiple medications.

PHARMACOKINETIC INTERACTIONS

A. Interactions Based on Absorption: Absorption from the gastrointestinal tract may be influenced by agents that bind drugs (eg, resins, antacids, calcium-containing foods), by agents that increase or decrease gastrointestinal motility (eg, metoclopramide or antimuscarinics, respectively), and by drugs that alter the P-glycoprotein transporter in the wall of the intestine. Problems caused by slowed gastric emptying may be unexpected because the antimuscarinic action of a particular agent is often not a desired but an unwanted side effect. Concomitant use of antacids has resulted in decreased gut absorption of digoxin, ketoconazole, quinolone antibiotics, and tetracyclines. On the other hand, erythromycin appears to increase oral bioavailability of digoxin in some patients, probably by reducing gut flora that degrade digoxin. Compounds in grapefruit juice and some drugs inhibit the P-glycoprotein drug transporter in the intestinal epithelium and increase the net absorption of drugs that are normally expelled by the transporter. These agents may also induce CYP3A4 in the intestinal wall. Absorption from subcutaneous sites may be slowed predictably by vasoconstrictors given simultaneously (eg, local anesthetics and epinephrine) and by cardiac depressants that decrease tissue perfusion (eg, beta-blockers).

B. Interactions Based on Distribution and Binding: Distribution of a drug may be altered by other drugs that compete for binding sites on plasma proteins. For example, antibacterial sulfonamides can displace methotrexate, phenytoin, sulfonylureas, and warfarin from binding sites on albumin. However, it is difficult to document many clinically significant interactions of this type, and they seem to be the exception rather than the rule. The ability of quinidine to raise the blood levels of digoxin was originally attributed to displacement from tissue binding sites but probably involves a reduction in the clearance of digoxin. Changes in drug distribution can occur if one agent alters the size of the physical compartment in which another drug distributes. For example, diuretics, by reducing total body water, can increase plasma levels of aminoglycosides and of lithium, possibly enhancing drug toxicities.

Table 61–2. Some important drug interactions.

Drug or Drug Group	Drugs Involved	Comment
Alcohol	Sedative-hypnotics, opioid analgesics, tricyclic antidepressants, antihistamines	Additive CNS depression, sedation, ataxia, increased risk of accidents
Aminoglycosides	Loop diuretics	Enhanced ototoxicity
Antacids	Iron supplements, fluoroquinolones, ketoconazole, tetracyclines	Decreased gut absorption, due either to reaction with the drug affected or to reduced gut acidity
Antibiotics	Estrogens, including oral contraceptives	Many antibiotics lower estrogen levels and reduce contraceptive effectiveness
Antihistamines (H_1-blockers)	Antimuscarinics, sedatives	Additive effects with the drugs involved
Antimuscarinic drugs	Drugs absorbed from the small intestine	Slowed onset of effect because stomach emptying is delayed
Barbiturates, especially phenobarbital	Azoles, calcium channel blockers, propranolol, quinidine, steroids, warfarin, and many other drugs metabolized in the liver	Increased clearance of the affected drugs due to enzyme induction, possibly leading to decreases in drug effectiveness
Beta-blockers	Insulin	Masking of symptoms of hypoglycemia
	Prazosin	Increased "first-dose" syncope
Bile acid-binding resins	Acetaminophen, digitalis, thiazides, thyroxine	Reduced absorption of the affected drug
Carbamazepine	Doxycycline, estrogen, haloperidol, theophylline, warfarin	Reduced effect because of induction of metabolism
Cimetidine	Benzodiazepines, lidocaine, phenytoin, quinidine, theophylline, warfarin	Increased effect due to inhibition of hepatic metabolism
Disulfiram, metronidazole, certain cephalosporins	Ethanol	Increased hangover effect of ethanol because aldehyde dehydrogenase is blocked
Erythromycin	Cisapride, quinidine, sildenafil, theophylline	Risk of toxicity due to inhibition of metabolism of these drugs
Ketoconazole and other azoles	Benzodiazepines, cisapride, cyclosporine, fluoxetine, lovastatin, omeprazole, quinidine, tolbutamide, warfarin	Risk of toxicity due to inhibition of metabolism of these drugs
MAO inhibitors	Catecholamine releasers (amphetamine, ephedrine)	Increased NE in sympathetic nerve endings released by the interacting drugs
	Tyramine-containing foods and beverages	Hypertensive crisis
Nonsteroidal anti-inflammatory drugs	Anticoagulants	Increased bleeding tendency because of reduced platelet aggregation
	ACE inhibitors	Decreased antihypertensive efficacy of ACE inhibitor
	Loop diuretics, thiazides	Reduced diuretic efficacy
Phenytoin	Doxycycline, methadone, quinidine, steroids, verapamil	Increased metabolism due to enzyme induction; decreased efficacy
Quinidine	Digoxin	Increased digoxin levels due to decreased clearance; displacement may play a role
Rifampin	Azole antifungal drugs, corticosteroids, methadone, theophylline, tolbutamide	Decreased efficacy of these drugs due to induction of hepatic P450 isozymes
Salicylates	Corticosteroids	Additive toxicity to gastric mucosa
	Heparin, warfarin	Increased bleeding tendency
	Methotrexate	Decreased clearance causing greater methotrexate toxicity
	Sulfinpyrazone	Decreased uricosuric effect

(continued)

Table 61–2. Some important drug interactions. (continued)

Drug or Drug Group	Drugs Involved	Comment
Selective serotonin reuptake inhibitors	MAO inhibitors, meperidine, tricyclic antidepressants	Serotonin syndrome: hypertension, tachycardia, muscle rigidity, hyperthermia, seizures
Thiazides	Digitalis	Increased risk of digitalis toxicity because thiazides diminish potassium stores
	Lithium	Increased plasma levels of lithium due to decreased total body water
Warfarin	Cimetidine, erythromycin, lovastatin, metronidazole	Increased anticoagulant effect via inhibition of warfarin metabolism
	Anabolic steroids, aspirin, NSAIDs, quinidine, thyroxine	Increased anticoagulant effects via pharmacodynamic mechanisms
	Barbiturates, carbamazepine, phenytoin, rifampin	Decreased anticoagulant effects due to increased clearance of warfarin via induction of hepatic P450 isozymes

C. Interactions Based on Metabolic Clearance: Many interactions of this type are well-documented and have considerable clinical significance. The metabolism of many drugs can be increased by other agents that cause the induction of hepatic drug-metabolizing enzymes, especially cytochrome P450 isozymes. Induction of drug-metabolizing enzymes occurs predictably with the chronic administration of **barbiturates, carbamazepine, ethanol, phenytoin,** or **rifampin.** Conversely, the metabolism of some drugs may be decreased by other drugs that inhibit drug-metabolizing enzymes. Such inhibitors of drug-metabolizing enzymes include **cimetidine, disulfiram, erythromycin, ketoconazole, propoxyphene, quinidine,** and **sulfonamides.** The CYP3A4 isozyme of cytochrome P450, the dominant form in the human liver, is particularly sensitive to such inhibitory actions.

Drugs that reduce hepatic blood flow, eg, **propranolol,** may also reduce the clearance of other drugs metabolized in the liver, especially those subject to flow-limited hepatic clearance such as morphine and verapamil.

A modified form of an interaction based on metabolic clearance results from the ability of some drugs to increase the stores of endogenous substances by blocking their metabolism. These endogenous drugs may subsequently be released by other exogenous drugs, resulting in an unexpected action. The best-documented reaction of this type is the sensitization of patients taking **MAO inhibitors** to indirectly acting sympathomimetics (amphetamine, phenylpropanolamine, etc). Such patients may suffer a severe hypertensive reaction in response to ordinary doses of cold remedies, decongestants, and appetite suppressants.

D. Interactions Based on Renal Function: Excretion of drugs by the kidney may be changed by drugs that reduce renal blood flow (eg, beta-blockers) or inhibit specific renal transport mechanisms (eg, the action of aspirin on uric acid secretion in the S_2 segment of the proximal tubule). Drugs that alter urinary pH may change the ionization state of drugs that are weak acids or weak bases, leading to changes in renal tubular reabsorption.

PHARMACODYNAMIC INTERACTIONS

A. Interactions Based on Opposing Actions or Effects: Antagonism, the simplest type of drug interaction, is often predictable. For example, antagonism of the bronchodilating effects of β_2-adrenoceptor activators used in asthma is to be anticipated if a beta-blocker is given for another condition. Likewise, the action of a catecholamine on heart rate (via β-adrenoceptor activation) is antagonized by an inhibitor of acetylcholinesterase that acts through ACh (via muscarinic receptors). Antagonism by mixed agonist-antagonist drugs (eg, pentazocine) or by partial agonists (eg, pindolol) is not as easily predicted but should be expected when such drugs are used with pure agonists. Some drug antagonisms do not appear to be based on receptor interactions. For example, NSAIDs may decrease the antihypertensive action of ACE inhibitors by reducing renal elimination of sodium.

Table 61–3. Selected interactions of herbal medications with other drugs.

Herbal Medication	Other Drug	Interaction
Dong quai	Warfarin	Increased anticoagulant effect of warfarin; bleeding
Garlic, ginkgo	Anticoagulants, antiplatelet agents	Increased risk of bleeding
Ginseng	Antidepressants	Increased antidepressant effect, mania
Kava	Sedative-hypnotics	Additive sedation
Licorice root	Aldosterone, antihypertensive drugs	Licorice root extract (not candy) increases salt retention; hypertension
Ma-huang, other ephedra preparations	Sympathomimetics	Ephedrine in Ma-huang is additive with other sympathomimetics; hypertension, stroke
St. John's wort	Oral contraceptives, digoxin	Increased metabolism of drug, decreased efficacy
	Antidepressants	Increased antidepressant effect

B. Interactions Based on Additive Effects: Additive interaction describes the algebraic summing of the effects of two drugs. The two drugs may or may not act on the same receptor to produce such effects. The combined use of tricyclic antidepressants with diphenhydramine or promethazine predictably causes excessive atropine-like effects since all of these drugs have significant muscarinic receptor-blocking actions. Tricyclic antidepressants may increase the pressor responses to sympathomimetics by interference with amine transporter systems.

One of the most common and important drug interactions is the additive depression of CNS function caused by concomitant administration of sedatives, hypnotics, and opioids with each other or associated with the consumption of ethanol. In such cases, multiple receptor systems in the brain are presumed to be involved. Similarly, the patient with moderate to severe hypertension maintained on one drug is at risk of excessive lowering of blood pressure if another drug with a different site of action is added at high dosage. This interaction is the basis for the use of "stepped care" therapy in hypertension because it permits the use of lower, less toxic doses. Additive effects of anticoagulant drugs can lead to bleeding complications. In the case of warfarin, the potential for such adverse effects is enhanced by aspirin (via an antiplatelet action), quinidine (additive hypoprothrombinemia), thrombolytics (via plasminogen activation), and the thyroid hormones (via enhanced clotting factor catabolism).

Supra-additive interactions and potentiation appear to be much less common than antagonism and the simple additive interactions described above. Supra-additive (synergistic) interaction is said to occur if the result of interaction is greater than the sum of the drugs used alone; the best example is the therapeutic synergism of certain antibiotic combinations such as sulfonamides and dihydrofolic acid reductase inhibitors such as trimethoprim. Potentiation is said to occur when a drug's effect is increased by another agent that has no such effect. The best example of this type of interaction is the therapeutic interaction of beta-lactamase inhibitors such as clavulanic acid with lactamase-susceptible penicillins.

INTERACTIONS OF HERBAL MEDICATIONS WITH OTHER DRUGS

Because of the marked increase in use of herbal medications, more interactions of these agents with purified drugs are being reported. Some of the reported or suspected interactions are listed in Table 61–3.

QUESTIONS

DIRECTIONS: Each of the numbered items or incomplete statements in this section is followed by answers or by completions of the statement. Select the ONE lettered answer or completion that is BEST in each case.

1. Which one of the following drugs increases digoxin plasma concentration by a pharmacokinetic mechanism?

(A) Captopril
(B) Hydrochorothiazide
(C) Lidocaine
(D) Quinidine
(E) Sulfasalazine

2. A 55-year-old patient currently receiving other drugs for another condition is to be started on diuretic therapy for mild heart failure. Thiazides are known to reduce the excretion of
(A) Diazepam
(B) Fluoxetine
(C) Imipramine
(D) Lithium
(E) Potassium

3. A hypertensive patient has been using nifedipine for some time without untoward effects. If he experiences a rapidly developing enhancement of the antihypertensive effect of the drug, it is probably due to
(A) Concomitant use of antacids
(B) Foods containing tyramine
(C) Grapefruit juice
(D) Induction of drug metabolism
(E) Over-the-counter decongestants

4. Which one of the following agents is LEAST likely to enhance the anticoagulant effects of warfarin?
(A) Aspirin
(B) Cholestyramine
(C) Cimetidine
(D) Quinidine
(E) Thyroxine

5. Patients should be cautioned not to consume alcoholic beverages when given a prescription for any of the following drugs EXCEPT
(A) Cefixime
(B) Chloral hydrate
(C) Chlorpropamide
(D) Glipizide
(E) Metronidazole

6. A patient suffering from a depressive disorder is being treated with imipramine. If he uses diphenhydramine for allergic rhinitis, a drug interaction is likely to occur because
(A) Diphenhydramine inhibits imipramine metabolism
(B) Both drugs block reuptake of norepinephrine released from sympathetic nerve endings
(C) Imipramine inhibits the metabolism of diphenhydramine
(D) Both drugs block muscarinic receptors
(E) The drugs compete with each other for renal elimination

7. If phenelzine is administered to a patient taking fluoxetine, the most likely result is
(A) Antagonism of the antidepressant action of fluoxetine
(B) A decrease in the plasma levels of fluoxetine
(C) Hypertensive crisis
(D) Priapism
(E) Agitation, muscle rigidity, hyperthermia, seizures

8. Following organ transplantation, a patient is being maintained on cyclosporine. Which one of the following drugs is LEAST likely to enhance the nephrotoxicity of cyclosporine?
(A) Carbamazepine
(B) Diltiazem
(C) Gentamicin
(D) Ketoconazole
(E) Verapamil

9. Which one of the following antibiotics is a potent inducer of hepatic drug-metabolizing enzymes?
(A) Ciprofloxacin
(B) Cyclosporine
(C) Erythromycin

(D) Rifampin
(E) Tetracycline

10. The antihypertensive effects of captopril can be antagonized (reduced) by
(A) Angiotensin II receptor blockers
(B) Loop diuretics
(C) NSAIDs
(D) Sulfonylurea hypoglycemics
(E) Thiazides

11. Which one of the following drugs has no effect on prothrombin but increases the likelihood of bleeding in patients who are also taking warfarin?
(A) Carbamazepine
(B) Cholestyramine
(C) Naproxen
(D) Rifampin
(E) Vitamin K

12. Which one of the following drugs has resulted in severe hematotoxicity when administered to a patient being treated with azathioprine?
(A) Allopurinol
(B) Cholestyramine
(C) Digoxin
(D) Lithium
(E) Theophylline

DIRECTIONS (Items 13–15): The following section consists of a list of lettered options followed by several numbered items. For each numbered item, select the ONE option that is most closely associated with it. Each answer may be selected once, more than once, or not at all.
(A) Allopurinol
(B) Carbamazepine
(C) Cholestyramine
(D) Cimetidine
(E) Cisapride
(F) Cyclosporine
(G) Digoxin
(H) Erythromycin
(I) Ethinyl estradiol
(J) Ibuprofen
(K) Lithium
(L) Phenelzine
(M) Rifampin
(N) Tetracycline
(O) Theophylline

13. A meal with a high content of fermented foods would be dangerous in a person taking this drug.

14. This drug is capable of blocking potassium channels in cardiac cell membranes; inhibition of its metabolism has led to cardiac arrhythmias.

15. This drug enhances the toxicity of methotrexate by decreasing its renal clearance.

ANSWERS

1. Quinidine and thiazide diuretics can both enhance the toxicity of digitalis. The action of quinidine is attributed to pharmacokinetic mechanisms, especially inhibition of its clearance. The plasma concentration of digoxin predictably increases when quinidine is added. The enhancement of digitalis toxicity by thiazides is due to a pharmacodynamic mechanism, namely, the action of these diuretics to reduce extracellular potassium. Sulfasalazine decreases plasma levels of digitalis by interfering with gut absorption of the drug. The answer is **(D).**

2. Thiazides reduce the clearance of lithium by about 25%. They do not alter the clearance of the other agents mentioned except for potassium, the clearance of which is increased. The answer is **(D).**

3. Compounds in grapefruit juice such as naringenin and 6′,7′-dihydroxybergamottin can increase the rate and extent of bioavailability of several dihydropyridine calcium channel blockers, including felodipine and nifedipine. This interaction may be due to inhibition of the metabolism of the dihydropyridines by intestinal wall CYP3A4 or inhibition of the P-glycoprotein transporter in the same location. The answer is **(C).**
4. Cholestyramine interferes with the oral absorption of many drugs (including warfarin), resulting in decreased effectiveness. Aspirin and thyroid hormones enhance the action of warfarin via pharmacodynamic mechanisms. Increased anticoagulant effects with cimetidine or quinidine result from the inhibition of metabolism of warfarin. The answer is **(B).**
5. Only a few cephalosporins (eg, cefoperazone, cefotetan, moxalactam) cause disulfiram-like reactions with ethanol. Sulfonylureas used in type 2 diabetes may cause such reactions, and ethanol may enhance their hypoglycemic actions, especially in fasting patients. The answer is **(A).**
6. This is a good example of an additive drug interaction resulting from two drugs acting on the same type of receptor. Most tricyclic antidepressants, phenothiazines, and older antihistaminic drugs (those available without prescription) are blockers of muscarinic receptors. Used concomitantly, any pair of these agents will demonstrate a predictable increase in atropine-like adverse effects. The answer is **(D).**
7. The drug interaction between the inhibitors of monoamine oxidase used for depression and the drugs which selectively block serotonin reuptake (SSRIs) is called the serotonin syndrome. In the case of phenelzine and fluoxetine, the interaction has resulted in a fatal outcome. Key interventions include control of hyperthermia and seizures. The answer is **(E).**
8. Concomitant use of nephrotoxic drugs (eg, aminoglycosides, amphotericin B, vancomycin) with cyclosporine leads to enhanced nephrotoxicity. Diltiazem, ketoconazole, and verapamil inhibit the metabolism of cyclosporine, enhancing its toxic effects unless dosage is reduced. Carbamazepine induces cytochrome P450 and reduces both the therapeutic and the toxic effects of the immunosuppressant drug. The answer is **(A).**
9. Rifampin is an effective inducer of hepatic P450 isozymes. Cyclosporine and tetracycline have no effects on drug metabolism. Ciprofloxacin and erythromycin are inhibitors of drug metabolism. The answer is **(D).**
10. NSAIDs interfere with the antihypertensive action of angiotensin-converting enzyme inhibitors; the other drugs listed enhance the blood pressure-lowering effects of captopril and other members of the "pril" drug family. The answer is **(C).**
11. Warfarin reduces the synthesis of prothrombin and several other clotting factors. Carbamazepine and rifampin interfere with this action by increasing the metabolism of warfarin. Cholestyramine decreases the oral absorption of warfarin and other acidic drugs. Vitamin K is the antidote to excessive effects of warfarin. Antiplatelet drugs such as naproxen enhance the anticoagulant effects of warfarin. The answer is **(C).**
12. Azathioprine is converted to mercaptopurine, which is responsible for both its immunosuppressant action and its hematotoxicity. Allopurinol inhibits xanthine oxidase, the enzyme that metabolizes mercaptopurine. The answer is **(A).**
13. Monoamine oxidase inhibitors used in depressive disorders (phenelzine, tranylcypromine) increase the stores of norepinephrine in sympathetic nerve endings. They also inhibit the metabolism of tyramine, which at high levels in the blood can act as an indirect sympathomimetic to release norepinephrine. The answer is **(L).**
14. Cisapride is metabolized by a cytochrome P450 isozyme that is inhibited by erythromycin and by ketoconazole. Decreased clearance of the antihistaminic drugs astemizole and terfenadine (now withdrawn) may also result in cardiotoxicity. The answer is **(E).**
15. Several NSAIDs, including aspirin, ibuprofen, and piroxicam, increase serum levels of methotrexate by interfering with its renal clearance. The adverse effects of methotrexate, including its hematotoxicity are predictably increased. The answer is **(J).**

62 Vaccines, Immune Globulins, & Other Complex Biologic Products

OBJECTIVES

You should be able to:

- Describe the principles of active and passive immunization, and know the differences between them.
- List the types of materials available for passive immunization and the special uses of immune globulin.
- List the types of materials available for active immunization, and describe the relative merits and disadvantages of live versus dead immunogens.
- List the vaccines recommended for the active immunization of children.

CONCEPTS

A. **Passive Immunization:** In passive immunization, **preformed antibodies** of human or animal origin are used to transfer immunity to the host. Such materials, usually **immunoglobulins,** may contain high titers of specific or relatively nonspecific antibodies (eg, **immune globulin**). Their clinical uses include prevention or amelioration of diseases after exposure (eg, hepatitis, measles, poliomyelitis), treatment of certain snake and insect bites, and management of hypogammaglobulinemia. The most commonly used preparation is **immune globulin**, a 25-fold concentration of gamma globulins from human plasma, available in formulations for intramuscular and intravenous use. The biologic half-life of immune globulin is about 23 days, and hypersensitivity reactions are rare. Immune globulin is used for passive immunization to hepatitis A, measles, poliomyelitis, and rubella and for hypogammaglobulinemia and idiopathic thrombocytopenic purpura (ITP). More specific products include diphtheria antitoxin, snake and spider antivenins, Rh_0(D) immune globulin, and immune globulins for cytomegalovirus (CMV), hepatitis B, pertussis, rabies, respiratory syncytial virus (RSV), tetanus, vaccinia, and varicella. Such antibodies usually have a half-life of only 5–7 days. Because animal antibodies can act as antigens in humans, allergic reactions to antibodies from nonhuman sources are more common and severe than those from human sources. Examples of materials used in passive immunization are shown in Table 62–1.

B. **Active Immunization:** In active immunization, **antigens** are used to stimulate antibody formation and host cell-mediated immunity, giving protection against disease vectors. The major advantage of active over passive immunization is that it confers stronger host resistance by stimulating higher antibody levels. Immunization can be produced by live (attenuated) or dead (inactivated) immunogens. Live attenuated products stimulate natural resistance and confer longer-lasting immunity than dead immunogens; however, the risk of disease is greater. Examples of the use of live attenuated immunogens include the vaccines for measles, mumps, poliovirus, rubella, and varicella. Materials utilizing dead immunogens include diphtheria and tetanus toxoids, rabies vaccine, and both hepatitis A and B viruses. *Haemophilus influenzae* type b conjugate (Hib-conjugate), derived from a bacterial polysaccharide, is used in children and in selected high-risk persons. Similar polysaccharide vaccines are also available for active immunization of individuals at high risk of infection from meningococci and pneumococci. Selected examples of products used in active immunization are shown in Table 62–2.

C. **Active Immunization of Children:** Recommended schedules for active immunization of children are shown in Table 62–3. They include hepatitis B vaccine, DTP (toxoids of diphtheria

Table 62–1. Materials used for passive immunization.*

Indication	Product	Comments
Black widow spider bite	Black widow spider antivenin (equine)	Treatment; use in hypertensive cardiovascular disease or age < 16 or > 60 years
Botulism	ABE polyvalent antitoxin (equine)	Treatment and prophylaxis
Cytomegalovirus	CMV immune globulin	Prophylaxis in organ or tissue transplantation
Hepatitis A	Immune globulin	Prophylaxis; postexposure and chronic exposure
Hepatitis B	Hepatitis B immune globulin (HBIG)	Prophylaxis; postexposure
Hypogammaglobulinemia	Immune globulin	Treatment
Organ or tissue transplantation	Immune globulin	Adjunctive immunosuppression
Rabies	Rabies immune globulin	Also need rabies vaccine
Rh isoimmunization	Rh_o(D) immune globulin	To suppress formation of anti-Rh_o(D) in Rh_o(D)-negative, Du-negative women exposed to Rh-positive blood during delivery
Respiratory syncytial virus	RSV immune globulin	Palivizumab usually preferred
Snakebite	Coral snake antivenin (equine); crotalid antivenin (equine)	Treatment; also need antitetanus therapy
Tetanus	Tetanus immune globulin	Only for major or contaminated wounds
Vaccinia	Vaccinia immune globulin	Treatment; generalized, ocular, skin infections
Varicella	Varicella-zoster immune globulin	Immunosuppressed children in contact with the index case

*Adapted, with permission, from Katzung BG (editor): *Basic & Clinical Pharmacology,* 8th ed. McGraw-Hill, 2001.

Table 62–2. Materials for active immunization.*

Pathogen or Disease	Product	Comments
Haemophilus influenzae type b conjugate	Bacterial polysaccharide conjugate	For all children, asplenics, and others at risk
Hepatitis A	Inactivated virus	Give 2–4 weeks prior to travel to endemic areas, household contacts, intravenous drug users
Hepatitis B	Inactivated viral antigen, recombinant	Give (before exposure) to infants and high risk individuals (> 90% effective). Duration: years
Influenza	Inactivated virus or viral components	Annually for the elderly, those with chronic disease, and other high risk individuals
Lyme disease	Bacterial protein, recombinant	Persons who live in or have frequent exposure to tick-infested habitats
Measles	Live virus	Prophylaxis
Meningococci	Bacterial polysaccharides	Epidemic situations
Pneumococci	Bacterial polysaccharides	High-risk individuals (asplenia, hemoglobinopathies, cardiovascular disease)
Rabies	Inactivated virus	Prophylaxis for individuals at risk; postexposure after bites (plus rabies immune globulin)
Rubella	Live virus	Avoid during pregnancy
Tetanus-diphtheria (Td)	Toxoids	Recommended every 10 years
Varicella	Live virus	All children, high risk persons, postexposure

*Adapted, with permission, from Katzung BG (editor): *Basic & Clinical Pharmacology,* 8th ed. McGraw-Hill, 2001.

Table 62–3. Recommended schedule for active immunization of children.*

Age	Product Administered
Birth	HBV (hepatitis B vaccine)
2 months	DTaP (toxoids of diphtheria and tetanus, acellular pertussis vaccine); inactivated poliovirus (IPV); *Haemophilus influenzae* type b conjugate (Hib); HBV (second dose)
4 months	DTaP; IPV; Hib
6 months	DTaP; Hib
6–18 months	IPV; HBV (third dose)
12–18 months	DTaP; Hib; measles, mumps, rubella vaccines (MMR); varicella vaccine
4–6 years	DTaP; IPV; MMR
11–12 years	Td (tetanus and diphtheria toxoids)

*Adapted, with permission, from Katzung BG (editor): *Basic & Clinical Pharmacology,* 8th ed. McGraw-Hill, 2001.

and tetanus with pertussis antigen), Hib-conjugate vaccine, MMR (measles, mumps, and rubella) vaccines, poliovirus vaccine, and varicella vaccine.

QUESTIONS

DIRECTIONS: Each of the numbered items or incomplete statements in this section is followed by answers or by completions of the statement. Select the ONE lettered answer or completion that is BEST in each case.

1. Which one of the following antibodies has the longest half-life?
(A) Black widow spider antivenin
(B) Botulinum antitoxin
(C) Diphtheria antitoxin
(D) Hepatitis B immune globulin
(E) Snake bite antivenin

2. Passive immunization involves
(A) Live immunogens
(B) Polysaccharide vaccines
(C) Stimulation of antibody formation
(D) Use of antigens
(E) Use of preformed antibodies

3. A businessman intends to travel abroad in a geographical region where several diseases are endemic. He would not be able to be vaccinated against
(A) Cholera
(B) Malaria
(C) Meningococcal infections
(D) Typhoid fever
(E) Yellow fever

4. Which one of the following statements about passive immunization is LEAST accurate?
(A) Rabies immune globulin is recommended only in patients who demonstrate an antibody response from preexposure prophylaxis
(B) Patients with IgA deficiency may develop hypersensitivity reactions to immune globulin
(C) Equine-derived antivenins are used in the treatment of snake bite
(D) Passive immunization is useful in the treatment of certain diseases that are normally prevented by active immunization (eg, tetanus)
(E) Cytomegalovirus immune globulin is useful in bone marrow transplantation

5. Which one of the following statements about active immunization is LEAST accurate?
(A) Immunization against hepatitis B involves the use of a purified and inactivated virus coat protein
(B) Poliovirus vaccine containing live virus can be administered orally
(C) The vaccine against *Haemophilus influenzae* type b is a polysaccharide conjugate

(D) Some protective factors may not be stimulated with the use of inactivated (killed) products
(E) Active immunization results in permanent protection

6. Which of the following is used in active immunization of children and combines bacterial toxoids with a bacterial antigen?
   (A) BCG
   (B) BSA
   (C) DTP
   (D) ISG
   (E) Rh_o(D)
7. Which of the following is a polysaccharide used for active immunization in patients with chronic cardiorespiratory ailments?
   (A) Antilymphocyte immune serum
   (B) BCG vaccine
   (C) Mumps virus vaccine
   (D) Pertussis immune globulin
   (E) Pneumococcal vaccine
8. Which one of the following statements about the administration of Rh_o(D) immune globulin is LEAST accurate?
   (A) It provides Rh isoimmunization from fetal-maternal transfusion
   (B) Its administration more than 48 hours after exposure is not effective
   (C) It is used for nonimmune females only
   (D) Its use is a form of passive immunization
   (E) It has been used for transfusion of Rh-positive blood to a Rh-negative woman
9. A needlestick injury is sustained by a health care worker, and the blood is known to contain HBV surface antigens. The health care worker should be given
   (A) Nothing
   (B) Immune globulin
   (C) Hepatitis B immune globulin
   (D) Hepatitis B vaccine
   (E) Hepatitis B vaccine and hepatitis B immune globulin
10. Hepatitis B vaccine is LEAST likely to be recommended for prophylactic use in
    (A) Dialysis patients
    (B) Intravenous drug abusers
    (C) Newborns
    (D) Raw oyster eaters
    (E) Surgeons

ANSWERS

1. Antibodies derived from human serum not only diminish the risk of hypersensitivity but also have much longer half-lives than those from animal sources. For example, human IgG antibodies have a half-life of more than 20 days compared with 5–7 days for the antibodies derived from animals. Smaller doses of human antibodies can be administered to provide therapeutic levels for several weeks. The answer is **(D).**
2. Passive immunization utilizes preformed immunologic products (immunoglobulins) of human or animal origin to transfer immunity to the host. Other products of the cellular immune system, including interferons, have clinical uses in hematologic, infectious, and neoplastic diseases. The answer is **(E).**
3. Vaccines are available for active immunization against all of the diseases listed except malaria. Drug prophylaxis against malaria is described in Chapter 53. A vaccine is also available for travelers to hepatitis A-endemic geographical regions. The answer is **(B).**
4. Rabies immune globulin should be given as soon as possible after exposure and must be combined with immunization using human diploid cell-derived rabies vaccine. Passive immunization is not recommended for individuals with demonstrated antibody response to preexposure prophylaxis with rabies vaccine. The answer is **(A).**
5. Active immunization does not always result in permanent protection. Primary immunization against measles, mumps, poliomyelitis, and rubella appears to be permanent, and in each case

live viruses are used. However, the duration of effect of active immunization with killed virus products is about 6 months for cholera, 1–3 years for influenza, and more than 3 years for tetanus. The answer is **(E).**

6. DTP contains diphtheria and tetanus toxoids and pertussis antigen. The answer is **(C).**

7. The pertussis and antilymphocyte preparations are used in passive immunization. Both the mumps vaccine and BCG (used for tuberculosis) are used in active immunization, but they are live organisms. Pneumococcal vaccine is a polysaccharide recommended for individuals at high risk for pneumococcal disease. The *Haemophilus* and meningococcal vaccines (not listed) are also polysaccharides. The answer is **(E).**

8. Ideally, $Rh_0(D)$ should be administered to an Rh(D)-negative woman within 72 hours after abortion, amniocentesis, obstetric delivery of an Rh-positive child, or transfusion of Rh-positive blood. However, the product may be effective at much greater postexposure intervals and should be given even if more than 72 hours have elapsed. The answer is **(B).**

9. The HBV needlestick situation is best handled by a combination passive-active immunization approach. Immediate and long-term protection is afforded by the administration of hepatitis B vaccine and hepatitis B immune globulin at different intramuscular sites. The answer is **(E).**

10. Too easy? Hepatitis A commonly arises from fecally contaminated water or from foods grown in such water and consumed raw. The administration of hepatitis B vaccine is prophylactic in all of the other situations. The answer is **(D).**

63 Botanical Medications & Nutritional Supplements

OBJECTIVES

You should be able to:

- Appreciate that these substances are marketed without governmental review of efficacy and safety.
- Recognize that in many cases the medical value of these substances has not been demonstrated in controlled clinical studies.
- Identify the most widely used botanical products and describe their purported medical uses, adverse effects, and potential for drug interactions.
- Describe the proposed medical uses and adverse effects of dehydroepiandrosterone and melatonin.

CONCEPTS

The use of botanical or "herbal" medications has increased markedly in the past decade. Popular botanical products in the USA include echinacea, garlic, ginseng, gingko, Ma-huang, psyllium, St. John's wort, and saw palmetto. These "natural" medicinals are available without prescription and, unlike over-the-counter medications, are considered to be nutritional supplements rather than drugs. As such, these substances are marketed without FDA review of efficacy or safety and there are no mandated requirements governing purity, variations in potency, or the chemical identities of all constituents in a herbal product. Purified nonherbal nutritional supplements such as dehydroepiandrosterone (DHEA) and melatonin are also used widely by the general public in pursuit of "alternative medicine."

In the case of many herbal products and nutritional supplements, evidence for their medical effectiveness based on controlled clinical studies is incomplete or nonexistent. Clinical trials of herbal products have been characterized by multiple variables, including their formulation, their chemical constitution, the dosages used, and the duration of treatment. Thus it has often been difficult to make recommendations regarding possible therapeutic benefits.

A summary of those herbal products whose clinical efficacy has been tested is presented in Table 63–1. Some botanicals are known to cause severe adverse effects and should be used cautiously or not at all (Table 63–2). In addition, interactions between herbal medications and conventional drugs are increasingly reported.

BOTANICAL SUBSTANCES

A. Echinacea:

1. **Nature:** Leaves and roots of echinacea species (eg, *E purpurea*) contain flavonoids, polyacetylenes, and caffeoyl conjugates.
2. **Pharmacology:** In vitro studies have shown that echinacea has cytokine activation (increased interleukins and tumor necrosis factor) and anti-inflammatory properties. At the clinical level, two reasonably well-controlled studies have documented a reduction in duration of cold symptoms with the use of freshly pressed juice of the aerial parts of *E purpurea.*
3. **Toxicity and drug interactions:** Unpleasant taste and gastrointestinal effects may occur, sometimes with dizziness or headache. Some preparations have a high alcohol content, but no drug interactions have been reported.

B. Feverfew:

1. **Nature:** Feverfew *(Tanacetum parthenium)* contains flavonoid glycosides, monoterpenes, and parthenolide, a lactone that forms covalent bonds with thiol groups on proteins.
2. **Pharmacology:** In vitro studies have shown decreased histamine release from mast cells, inhibition of prostaglandin and leukotriene formation, and decreased TNF expression. The fresh leaves of feverfew are thought to have prophylactic value in migraine. Three of five randomized, double-blind, placebo-controlled trials in migraine showed reductions in headache frequency and severity and in nausea. The only well-controlled study of feverfew in rheumatoid arthritis failed to show clinical benefit.
3. **Toxicity and drug interactions:** Mouth ulcers and gastrointestinal effects occur commonly. Possible antiplatelet action warrants caution in patients taking anticoagulants or conventional antiplatelet drugs.

Table 63–1. Clinical effectiveness of botanicals and nutritional supplements.

Botanical or Nutritional Supplement	Established or Possible Effectiveness
Echinacea	Decreases duration and intensity of cold symptoms
Feverfew	Decreases headache frequency and severity in migraine
Ginkgo	Some value in intermittent claudication; mild, temporary effects in Alzheimer's disease
Ginseng	Therapeutic value remains to be proved
Kava	Effective in chronic anxiety states
Ma-huang	Established uses as for ephedrine and pseudoephedrine
Milk thistle	Improves liver function in viral hepatitis; antidote to *Amanita* mushroom poisoning
Saw palmetto	Improvement in symptoms of benign prostatic hyperplasia
St. John's wort	Possibly effective in moderate to severe depressive disorder
Dehydroepiandrosterone	Possible value in AIDS and SLE in women
Melatonin	Decreases jet lag symptoms and useful as a sleep aid

Table 63–2. Potential toxicity of selected botanicals.

Name	Intended Use	Potential Toxicity
Aconite (monkshood, wolfsbane)	Analgesic (topical and oral)	Cardiac and CNS toxicity with oral use
Borage (beebread, burrage)	Anti-inflammatory, diuretic	Oral use causes gastrointestinal distress and possible hepatotoxicity
Chaparral (creosote bush, greasewood)	Anti-infective, antioxidant	Hepatotoxicity and renal dysfunction
Coltsfoot (coughwort)	Respiratory tract and oral infections	Allergic reactions, phototoxicity, liver dysfunction
Ephedra (Ma-huang, sea grape, yellow horse)	Bronchodilator, diet aid, CNS stimulant	Hypertension, cardiac arrhythmias, stroke, seizures
Germander	Diet aid, digestive aid, gastrointestinal dysfunction	Multiple cases of hepatitis and death. (Still used as flavoring agent in USA)
Jimsonweed (*Datura*, devil's apple, stinkweed)	Respiratory tract diseases, hallucinogen	Marked adverse effects due to atropine and related M-blockers
Pennyroyal	Abortifacient, digestive aid, induction of menstrual flow	Gastrointestinal distress (hematemesis), CNS dysfunction, hepatotoxicity, renal dysfunction, disseminated intravascular coagulation
Pokeweed berries and root (American nightshade)	Berries used as food coloring; root extracts for emesis, rheumatism	Oral use highly toxic: bloody diarrhea, hypotension, coma, blindness, respiratory failure
Royal jelly	Tonic, immune potentiation, hyperlipidemia	Allergic reactions including anaphylaxis and death
Sassafras	Blood thinner, urinary tract disorders; oil used topically as antiseptic	Diaphoresis, hot flushes with oral use of bark; ingestion of sassafas oil may be lethal (coma, cardiovascular collapse and respiratory paralysis)

C. Garlic:

1. **Nature:** Garlic *(Allium sativum)* contains organic thiosulfinates that can form allicin (responsible for the characteristic odor) via enzymes that are activated by disruption of the garlic bulb.
2. **Pharmacology:** In vitro studies show that allicin inhibits HMG-CoA reductase and ACE, blocks platelet aggregation, increases NO, has antimicrobial activity, and reduces carcinogen activation. Claims for clinical efficacy are based largely on epidemiologic evidence. For example, high dietary garlic consumption is associated with a decrease in aortic stiffness and possible decreases in the incidence of stomach cancer. A few controlled studies have shown small reductions in total cholesterol and in blood pressure.
3. **Toxicity and drug interactions:** Nausea, hypotension, and allergic reactions may occur. Possible antiplatelet action warrants caution in patients receiving anticoagulants or conventional antiplatelet drugs.

D. Ginkgo:

1. **Nature:** Prepared from the leaves of *Ginkgo biloba,* ginkgo contains flavone glycosides and terpenoids.
2. **Pharmacology:** In vitro studies have documented antioxidant and radical-scavenging effects and increased formation of NO. Animal studies have revealed reduced blood viscosity and changes in CNS neurotransmitters. At the clinical level, ginkgo appears to have value in intermittent claudication, and it reduces markers of oxidative stress in coronary artery bypass surgery. Several studies show a mild benefit of ginkgo in Alzheimer's dementia.
3. **Toxicity and drug interactions:** Gastrointestinal effects, anxiety, insomnia, and headache occur. Possible antiplatelet action suggests caution in patients receiving anticoagulants or antiplatelet drugs.

E. Ginseng:

1. **Nature:** Most ginseng products are derived from plants of the genus *Panax* that contain multiple triterpenoid saponin glycosides (ginsenosides). Siberian or Brazilian ginseng does not contain these chemicals.

2. **Pharmacology:** Ginseng is purported to improve mental and physical performance, but the clinical evidence for such effects is limited. A small clinical trial suggested a possibility of some value in type 2 diabetes.
3. **Toxicity and drug interactions:** Estrogenic effects include mastalgia and vaginal bleeding. Insomnia, nervousness, and hypertension have been reported. Ginseng should be used cautiously in patients receiving antihypertensive, hypoglycemic, or psychiatric medications.

F. Kava:

1. **Nature:** Kava is derived from the root of *Piper methysticum*, which contains kawain, methysticin, and yangonin.
2. **Pharmacology:** In vitro studies have led to suggestions that kava facilitates the actions of GABA in the CNS. Use of large quantities of kava extract causes drowsiness, sedation, and possibly a state of intoxication ("drunken" feeling). Controlled clinical trials have shown effectiveness in anxiety states but only after several weeks of use. In one study, kava was compared favorably with oxazepam and caused fewer side effects.
3. **Toxicity and drug interactions:** Tingling in the mouth and gastrointestinal effects occur. Ataxia, muscle weakness, paresthesias, and dystonias have also been reported. A reversible syndrome characterized by skin exfoliation, photosensitivity, and facial swelling may occur with high doses of kava. Potentiation of conventional CNS depressants and alcohol is predictable. Kava use should be avoided in patients taking dopamine agonist or antagonist drugs and in those with liver dysfunction.

G. Ma-huang:

1. **Nature:** Ma-huang is one of many names given to extracts from various plants of the genus *Ephedra,* the major chemical constituents of which are ephedrine and pseudoephedrine. Ephedrine is a prescription drug in the USA; pseudoephedrine is available in over-the-counter decongestants.
2. **Pharmacology:** The actions of ephedra products are those of ephedrine and pseudoephedrine, which release norepinephrine from sympathetic nerve endings. In addition to nasal decongestion, the established clinical use of ephedrine is as a pressor agent. Ephedra herbal products are commonly used for treatment of respiratory dysfunction (including bronchitis and asthma) and as mild CNS stimulants. In Chinese medicine, ephedra products are also used for relief of cold and flu symptoms, for diuresis, and for bone or joint pain.
3. **Toxicity and drug interactions:** Toxic effects are those of ephedrine including dizziness, insomnia, anorexia, flushing, palpitations, tachycardia, and urinary retention. In high doses, ephedra can cause a marked increase in blood pressure, cardiac arrhythmias, and a toxic psychosis. Contraindications are those for ephedrine and include anxiety states, bulimia, cardiac arrhythmias, diabetes, heart failure, hypertension, glaucoma, hyperthyroidism, and pregnancy. As a weak base, renal elimination of ephedrine overdose can be facilitated by urinary acidification.

H. Milk Thistle:

1. **Nature:** Milk thistle is derived from the fruit and seeds of *Silybum marianum,* which contain flavonolignans such as silymarin.
2. **Pharmacology:** In vitro studies show that milk thistle reduces lipid peroxidation, scavenges free radicals, enhances superoxide dismutase, inhibits formation of leukotrienes, and increases hepatocyte RNA polymerase activity. In animal models, milk thistle protects against liver injury caused by alcohol, acetaminophen, and amanita mushrooms. The outcomes of clinical trials in patients with liver disease caused by alcohol have been mixed. In viral hepatitis and liver injury caused by amanita mushrooms, results of clinical trials have been mainly favorable. A commercial preparation of silybin (an isomer of silymarin) is available in some countries as an antidote to *Amanita phalloides* mushroom poisoning.
3. **Toxicity and drug interactions:** Other than loose stools, milk thistle does not cause significant toxicity and there are no reports of drug interactions.

I. St. John's Wort:

1. **Nature:** St. John's wort is made from dried flowers of *Hypericum perforatum,* the active constituents of which include hypericin and hyperforin.
2. **Pharmacology:** In vitro studies with hyperforin have shown decreased activity of serotonergic reuptake systems. In animals, chronic treatment with commercial extracts led to

down-regulation of adrenoceptors and up-regulation of 5-HT receptors. Some (but not all) clinical trials of the extract in patients with mild to moderate depression have shown efficacy similar to that of tricyclic drugs, with fewer adverse effects. Hypericin, when photoactivated, may have antiviral and anticancer effects.

3. **Toxicity and drug interactions:** Mild gastrointestinal side effects occur and photosensitization has been reported. St. John's wort should be avoided in patients using SSRIs or MAO inhibitors and in those with a history of bipolar or psychotic disorder.

J. Saw Palmetto:

1. **Nature:** Saw palmetto is derived from the berries of *Serenoa repens* or *Sabal serrulata* and contains phytosterols, aliphatic alcohols, polyprenes, and flavonoids.
2. **Pharmacology:** In vitro studies have shown inhibition of 5α-reductase and antagonistic effects at androgen receptors. Clinical trials of saw palmetto in benign prostatic hyperplasia (BPH) have shown improvement in urologic function and in urinary flow. When compared with finasteride in BPH, saw palmetto did not lower prostate-specific antigen or dihydrotestosterone levels. However, sexual dysfunction was less with saw palmetto than with finasteride. Clinical improvement of BPH with saw palmetto appears to be less than that with alpha-blockers.
3. **Toxicity and drug interactions:** Abdominal pain with gastrointestinal distress, decreased libido, headache, and hypertension occur with an overall incidence of less than 3%.

Skill Keeper: Drugs from Plant Sources

Many conventional drugs, strictly regulated by governmental agencies such as the FDA, originated from plant sources. How many of these compounds can you identify? *The Skill Keeper Answer appears at the end of the chapter.*

PURIFIED NUTRITIONAL SUBSTANCES

A. Dehydroepiandrosterone:

1. **Nature:** Dehydroepiandrosterone (DHEA), derived mainly from the adrenal cortex, is an androgen precursor and in peripheral tissues is converted by aromatase to estradiol. In the plasma, DHEA is converted to DHEA sulfate (DHEAS). No specific physiologic function has been defined for DHEA or DHEAS. However, DHEA levels decrease during aging and possibly in some disease states, including advanced AIDS, diabetes, and systemic lupus erythematosus (in women).
2. **Pharmacology:** DHEA supplementation has been advocated for a variety of indications, including Alzheimer's disease, cardiovascular disease, hypercholesterolemia, diabetes and insulin resistance, slowing or reversing the aging process, treatment of viral infections and cancers, and weight loss. For most of these indications, there is incomplete evidence for the efficacy of DHEA supplementation. For example, in elderly men DHEA increases free testosterone by 5–10%, but this effect has not been correlated with improvement of sexual function.

   In AIDS, DHEA supplementation has been shown to increase body weight and CD4 cell count in women but not in men. All patients reported improvement in "well being," but no reductions in viral load were detectable. Women with SLE had fewer symptoms or flare-ups of the disease while using DHEA, but problems with androgenic side effects led to a 60% discontinuance rate before a 1-year study could be completed.
3. **Toxicity:** Endocrine side effects depend on gender. In premenopausal women, androgenization occurs because DHEA is converted to testosterone. In young men, feminization occurs because DHEA is converted mainly to estradiol. Elevation of testosterone levels in elderly men has caused concern regarding possible BPH and cancer, though clinical studies are lacking. Similarly, in postmenopausal women, the risk of breast cancer and the risk of cardiovascular morbidity is reported to be greater with elevated DHEA and DHEAS levels.

B. Melatonin:

1. **Nature:** Melatonin is a serotonin derivative produced mainly in the pineal gland. It is thought to regulate sleep-wake cycles, and its release coincides with darkness (9 PM to

4 AM). Other purported activities include contraception, prevention of aging, protection against oxidative stress, and the treatment of cancer, major depression, and HIV infection.

2. **Pharmacology:** Melatonin has been used extensively for jet lag and as an alternative to prescription drugs for insomnia. In jet lag, clinical studies have shown subjective improvements in mood, more rapid recovery times, and reductions in daytime fatigue.

   Exposure to daylight in the new time zone also facilitates regulation of the sleep-wake cycle. Melatonin improves sleep onset, duration, and quality when given to patients with sleep disorders.

3. **Toxicity and drug interactions:** Sedation and next-day drowsiness and headache have been reported. Melatonin may suppress the midcycle surge of LH and should not be used in pregnancy or in women attempting to conceive. Since it may decrease prolactin levels, melatonin should not be used by nursing mothers.

QUESTIONS

DIRECTIONS: Each of the numbered items or incomplete statements in this section is followed by answers or by completions of the statement. Select the ONE lettered answer or completion that is BEST in each case.

1. Which one of the following statements concerning the use of herbal products in the USA is accurate?
- **(A)** Classified as dietary supplements
- **(B)** Herbal products do not have to be pure
- **(C)** Labeling of such products is under the purview of the FDA
- **(D)** Safety does not have to demonstrated
- **(E)** All of these statements are accurate

2. You have accidentally ingested mushrooms identified as *Amanita phalloides.* Which of the following herbals is most likely to protect against hepatic dysfunction?
- **(A)** Echinacea
- **(B)** Ginkgo
- **(C)** Pennyroyal
- **(D)** Milk thistle
- **(E)** Saw palmetto

3. Which one of the following statements about ephedra is false?
- **(A)** Chemical constituents release norepinephrine from sympathetic nerve endings
- **(B)** Effective as a nasal decongestant
- **(C)** High doses may cause sudden death due to a cardiac arrhythmia
- **(D)** Ma-huang is one name for extracts from plants of the genus *Ephedra*
- **(E)** Useful as a sleep aid

4. You suffer from migraine and your botanist friend points out a plant she calls *Tanacetum parthenium,* saying that the fresh leaves of the plant may help you. One conventional name for this botanical is
- **(A)** Echinacea
- **(B)** Feverfew
- **(C)** Kava
- **(D)** St. John's wort
- **(E)** Sassafras

5. Which one of the following statements about kava is false?
- **(A)** Comes from the root of a pepper plant
- **(B)** Effective in management of acute anxiety states
- **(C)** Exfoliation on the palms of the hands and soles of the feet may occur
- **(D)** Potentiates the effects of ethanol and other CNS depressants
- **(E)** Used as a ceremonial drink in Polynesia

6. Which one of the following drugs most resembles the psychoactive constituent(s) of St. John's wort in terms of proposed mechanism of action?
- **(A)** Alprazolam
- **(B)** Fluoxetine
- **(C)** Levodopa
- **(D)** Methylphenidate
- **(E)** Selegiline

7. Dietary supplementation with DHEA is best documented to have therapeutic value in the treatment of
   (A) Acne
   (B) Diabetes insipidus
   (C) Hirsutism in female patients
   (D) Postmenopausal osteoporosis
   (E) Systemic lupus erythematosus
8. Which one of the following compounds has been shown to have value in managing symptoms of jet lag?
   (A) DHEA
   (B) Garlic
   (C) Ginseng
   (D) Melatonin
   (E) Sassafras
9. Many plant products that have traditionally been used as medications are known to cause adverse effects. Which one of the following pairs of botanical:toxicity is false?
   (A) Chaparral: hepatotoxicity
   (B) Germander: hepatitis
   (C) Milk thistle: leukemia
   (D) Pennyroyal: disseminated intravascular coagulation
   (E) Royal jelly: anaphylaxis
10. Which one of the following compounds enhances immune function in vitro and in clinical trials decreases the symptoms of the common cold?
    (A) Echinacea
    (B) Feverfew
    (C) Garlic
    (D) Melatonin
    (E) Milk Thistle

ANSWERS

1. Although regulations concerning dietary supplements are administered by the FDA, there are no provisions for establishing the potency or purity of herbal products. Such products do not have to be proved safe for the consumer. The answer is **(E).**
2. Milk thistle contains compounds that may have cytoprotective actions against liver toxins including those present in amanita mushrooms. The answer is **(D).**
3. Extracts of ephedra contain ephedrine, a CNS stimulant contraindicated in persons who suffer from insomnia. The peripheral effects of ephedrine in overdose can be lethal. The answer is **(E).**
4. Several clinical trials have shown that the air-dried or freeze-dried leaves of feverfew reduce headache and nausea in patients who suffer from migraine. The answer is **(B).**
5. Regarding the use of kava in anxiety states, the crucial word in statement (B) is "acute." Kava is effective as an anxiolytic—perhaps equivalent to benzodiazepines—but it has a *slow* onset of action. Most patients respond only after 4–8 weeks of treatment. The answer is **(B).**
6. Extracts of the flowers of St. John's wort contain chemicals with possible antidepressant activity. In vitro studies have shown that these chemicals interfere with the neuronal reuptake of amine neurotransmitters in a fashion similar to the proposed mechanism of antidepressant actions of tricyclics and SSRIs. The answer is **(B).**
7. DHEA has some therapeutic value in women with SLE, at least temporarily. Androgenic side effects due to the formation of testosterone, including acne and hirsutism, are predictable when DHEA is used in premenopausal female patients. DHEA may prove to have some value in diabetes mellitus, not diabetes insipidus. It is not known if DHEA has value in postmenopausal osteoporosis. However, postmenopausal women with high levels of DHEA are at greater risk for both cancer and cardiovascular morbidity. The answer is **(E).**
8. Garlic might get you a row of seats to yourself, but the compound that will help in jet lag is melatonin. The answer is **(D).**
9. Milk thistle is remarkably nontoxic. In murine models of skin cancer the herbal product reduced tumor initiation and promotion. The answer is **(C).**

10. The freshly pressed juice of the aerial parts of *Echinacea purpurea* have been shown to significantly reduce the symptoms of the common cold and the time of recovery. The answer is **(A).**

Skill Keeper Answer: Drugs from Plant Sources

The clinical application of drugs that originated from plant sources has contributed greatly to conventional medicine. Such compounds include aspirin, atropine, cocaine, codeine, colchicine, digoxin, ephedrine, ergonovine, ergotamine, etoposide, methysergide, morphine, nicotine, physostigmine, pilocarpine, quinidine, quinine, reserpine, scopolamine, taxanes (eg, paclitaxel), tubocurarine, vinblastine, and vincristine.

Appendix I

Key Words for Key Drugs

The following list is a compilation of the drugs that are most likely to appear on examinations. Some of them are old, some are quite new. The brief descriptions should serve as a rapid review. The list can be used in two ways. First, cover the column of properties and test your ability to recall descriptive information about drugs picked at random from the left column; second, cover the left column and try to name a drug that fits the properties described.

Common abbreviations and acronyms: ANS, autonomic nervous system; AV, atrioventricular; BP, blood pressure; CHF, congestive heart failure; CNS, central nervous system; CV, cardiovascular system; DMARD, disease-modifying antirheumatic drug; ECG, electrocardiogram; ENS, enteric nervous system; EPS, extrapyramidal system; GI, gastrointestinal; HR, heart rate; HTN, hypertension; MI, myocardial infarct; NSAID, nonsteroidal anti-inflammatory drug; PANS, parasympathetic nervous system; RA, rheumatoid arthritis; SANS, sympathetic nervous system; TNF, tumor necrosis factor; *Tox,* toxicity; TCA, tricyclic antidepressant.

Drug	Properties
Abciximab	Monoclonal antibody (MAb) to fibrin receptor (glycoprotein IIb/IIIa) on platelets. Used to prevent clotting after coronary angioplasty and in acute coronary syndrome. Eptifibatide and tirofiban have a similar action on this receptor to inhibit platelet cross-linking.
Acetaminophen	Antipyretic analgesic: very weak cyclooxygenase inhibitor; not anti-inflammatory. Less GI distress than aspirin but dangerous in overdose. *Tox:* hepatic necrosis. *Antidote:* acetylcysteine.
Acetazolamide	Carbonic anhydrase-inhibiting diuretic acting in the proximal convoluted tubule (PCT): produces a $NaHCO_3$ diuresis, results in bicarbonate depletion, and therefore has self-limited action. Used in glaucoma and mountain sickness. *Tox:* paresthesias, hepatic encephalopathy. Dorzolamide and brinzolamide are topical analogs for glaucoma.
Acetylcholine	Cholinomimetic prototype: transmitter in CNS, ENS, all ANS ganglia, parasympathetic postganglionic synapses, sympathetic postganglionic fibers to sweat glands, and skeletal muscle end plate synapses.
Acyclovir	Antiviral: inhibits DNA synthesis in herpes simplex (HSV) and varicella-zoster (VZV). Requires activation by viral thymidine kinase (TK^- strains are resistant). *Tox:* behavioral effects and nephrotoxicity (crystalluria) but not myelosuppression. Famciclovir, penciclovir, and valacyclovir are similar but with longer half-lives.
Adenosine	Antiarrhythmic: unclassified ("group V"); parenteral only. Hyperpolarizes AV nodal tissue, blocks conduction for 10–15 seconds. Used for nodal reentry arrhythmias. *Tox:* hypotension, flushing.
Albuterol	Typical β_2 agonist; important use in asthma. *Tox:* tachycardia, arrhythmias, tremor. Other drugs with similar action: metoproterenol, salmeterol, terbutaline.
Alendronate	Bisphosphonate stabilizer of bone structure and increases bone mineral density. Used in postmenopausal and steroid-induced osteoporosis. *Tox:* esophageal

ulceration. Other bisphosphonates (eg, etidronate, pamidronate) are used in Paget's disease.

Allopurinol Antigout: suicide inhibitor of xanthine oxidase; reduces production of uric acid. Used in gout and adjunctively in cancer chemotherapy.

Alprazolam Benzodiazepine sedative-hypnotic: widely used in anxiety states, selectivity for panic attacks and phobias; possible antidepressant actions. *Tox:* psychologic and physiologic dependence, additive effects with other CNS depressants.

Alprostadil PGE_1 analog: used in male erectile dysfunction.

Alteplase (rt-PA) Thrombolytic: human recombinant tissue plasminogen activator. Used in acute MI (to recanalize the occluded coronary), pulmonary embolism, stroke. *Tox:* bleeding.

Amiloride K^+-sparing diuretic: blocks Na^+ channels in cortical collecting tubules (CCT). *Tox:* hyperkalemia.

Amiodarone Class IA and class III antiarrhythmic: broad spectrum; blocks sodium, potassium, calcium channels, beta receptors. High efficacy and very long half-life (weeks to months). *Tox:* deposits in tissues; hypo- or hyperthyroidism; pulmonary fibrosis.

Amitriptyline Tricyclic antidepressant (TCA): blocks reuptake of norepinephrine and serotonin. *Tox:* atropine-like, postural hypotension, sedation, cardiac arrhythmias in overdose, additive effects with other CNS depressants. Other TCAs: imipramine, clomipramine, doxepin.

Amoxicillin Penicillin: wider spectrum than penicillin G with activity similar to ampicillin but greater oral bioavailability; less adverse effects on GI tract than ampicillin. Susceptible to penicillinases unless used with clavulanic acid. *Tox:* penicillin allergy.

Amphetamine Indirectly acting sympathomimetic: displaces stored catecholamines in nerve endings. Marked CNS stimulant actions; high abuse liability. Used in attention deficit hyperactivity disorder, for short-term weight loss, and for narcolepsy. *Tox:* psychosis, HTN, MI, seizures.

Amphotericin B Antifungal: polyene drug of choice for some systemic mycoses; binds to ergosterol to disrupt fungal cell membrane permeability. *Tox:* chills and fever, hypotension, nephrotoxicity (dose-limiting; less with liposomal forms).

Ampicillin Penicillin: wider spectrum than penicillin G, susceptible to penicillinases unless used with sulbactam. Activity similar to that of penicillin G, plus *E coli, H influenzae, P mirabilis,* shigella. Synergy with aminoglycosides versus enterococci and listeria. *Tox:* penicillin allergy; more adverse effects on GI tract than other penicillins; maculopapular skin rash.

Anastrozole Prototype aromatase inhibitor used in estrogen-dependent cancers. Letrozole is similar.

Aspirin NSAID prototype: inhibits cyclooxygenase (COX)-1 and -2 irreversibly. Potent antiplatelet agent as well as antipyretic analgesic and anti-inflammatory drug. *Tox:* GI ulcers, allergy, bronchoconstriction, salicylism.

Atenolol $Beta_1$-selective blocker: low lipid solubility, less CNS effect; used for HTN. (Names of β_1-selective blockers start with A through M except for carteolol, carvedilol, and labetalol.) *Tox:* bradycardia, AV block, congestive heart failure.

Atropine Muscarinic cholinoceptor blocker prototype: lipid-soluble, CNS effects. *Tox:* "red as a beet, dry as a bone, blind as a bat, mad as a hatter," urinary retention, mydriasis. Cyclopentolate, tropicamide: antimuscarinics for ophthalmology; shorter duration than atropine (a few hours or less); cause cycloplegia and mydriasis.

Azithromycin — Macrolide antibiotic: similar to erythromycin but greater activity against *H influenzae*, chlamydiae, and streptococci; long half-life due to tissue accumulation; renal elimination. *Tox:* GI distress, but no inhibition of drug metabolism.

Baclofen — GABA analog, orally active: spasmolytic; activates $GABA_B$ receptors in the spinal cord.

Benztropine — Centrally acting antimuscarinic prototype for parkinsonism. *Tox:* excess antimuscarinic effects.

Bethanechol — Muscarinic agonist: choline ester with good resistance to cholinesterase; used for atonic bowel or bladder. *Tox:* excess muscarinic effects. Another ester, carbachol, is a nonselective muscarinic and nicotinic agonist, used for glaucoma.

Botulinum — Toxins: produced by *Clostridium botulinum;* interacts with synaptobrevin to block release of acetylcholine vesicles. *Tox:* neuromuscular paralysis.

Bromocriptine — Ergot derivative: prototype dopamine agonist in CNS; inhibits prolactin release. Alternative drug in parkinsonism and hyperprolactinemia. *Tox:* CNS, dyskinesias, hypotension.

Bupivacaine — Long-acting amide local anesthetic prototype: *Tox:* greater cardiovascular toxicity than most local anesthetics.

Buspirone — Anxiolytic: atypical drug that interacts with $5\text{-}HT_{1A}$ receptors; slow onset (1–2 weeks). Minimal potentiation of CNS depressants, including ethanol; negligible abuse liability.

Captopril — Angiotensin-converting enzyme inhibitor prototype: used in HTN, diabetic nephropathy, and CHF. *Tox:* hyperkalemia, fetal renal damage, cough ("sore throat"). Other "prils": benzepril, enalapril, lisinopril, quinapril.

Carbamazepine — Anticonvulsant: used for tonic-clonic and partial seizures; blocks Na^+ channels in neuronal membranes. Drug of choice for trigeminal neuralgia; backup drug in bipolar disorder. *Tox:* CNS depression, hematotoxic, induces liver drug-metabolizing enzymes, teratogenicity.

Carvedilol — Adrenoceptor blocker: combines two isomers, one a nonselective beta-blocker and the other an α_1-blocker. Possible antioxidant actions. Prolongs survival in CHF.

Cefazolin — First-generation cephalosporin prototype: bactericidal beta-lactam inhibitor of cell wall synthesis. Active against gram-positive cocci, *E coli, K pneumoniae,* but does not enter CSF. *Tox:* potential allergy; partial cross-reactivity with penicillins.

Cefoxitin — Second-generation cephalosporin: active against a wide spectrum of gram-negative bacteria, including anaerobes *(B fragilis).* Does not enter the CNS. Cefotetan is similar.

Ceftriaxone — Third-generation cephalosporin: active against many bacteria, including pneumococci, gonococci (a drug of choice), and gram-negative rods. Enters the CNS and is used in bacterial meningitis. Cefotaxime and ceftazidime are other third-generation cephalosporins.

Celecoxib — Selective COX-2 inhibitor: acts mainly on enzymes of cells involved in inflammation. Used in rheumatoid arthritis and other inflammatory disorders. *Tox:* GI toxicity, but less than that of aspirin and other NSAIDs. Rofecoxib is similar.

Chloramphenicol — Antibiotic: broad-spectrum agent; inhibits protein synthesis (50S); uses restricted to backup drug for bacterial meningitis, infections due to anaerobes, salmonella. *Tox:* reversible myelosuppression, aplastic anemia, gray baby syndrome.

Chloroquine — Antimalarial: blood schizonticide used for treatment and as a chemosuppressant where *P falciparum* is susceptible. Binds to hemin, causing dysfunctional cell membranes; resistance due to efflux via P-glycoprotein pump. *Tox:*

GI distress and skin rash at low doses; peripheral neuropathy, skin lesions, auditory and visual impairment, quinidine-like cardiotoxicity at high doses.

Chlorpheniramine
Antihistamine first generation H_1 blocker prototype: *Tox:* mild sedation, little antimuscarinic action.

Chlorpromazine
Phenothiazine antipsychotic drug prototype: blocks most dopamine receptors in the CNS. *Tox:* atropine-like, EPS dysfunction, hyperprolactinemia, postural hypotension, sedation, seizures (in overdose), additive effects with other CNS depressants.

Cholestyramine
Bile acid-binding resin: sequesters bile acids in gut and diverts more cholesterol from the liver to bile acids instead of circulating lipoproteins. *Tox:* constipation, bloating; interferes with absorption of some drugs. Colestipol is similar.

Cimetidine
H_2 blocker prototype: used in acid-peptic disease. *Tox:* inhibits hepatic drug metabolism; antiandrogen effects. Less toxic analogs: ranitidine, famotidine, nizatidine.

Ciprofloxacin
Fluoroquinolone antibiotic: bactericidal inhibitor of topoisomerases; active against *E coli, H influenzae,* campylobacter, enterobacter, pseudomonas, shigella. *Tox:* CNS dysfunction, GI distress, superinfection, collagen dysfunction (avoid in children and pregnant women). *Interactions:* inhibits metabolism of caffeine, theophylline, warfarin.

Cisplatin
Platinum-containing alkylating anticancer drug. Used for solid tumors (eg, testes, lung). *Tox:* Neurotoxic and nephrotoxic. Carboplatin is similar.

Clindamycin
Lincosamide antibiotic: bacteriostatic inhibitor of protein synthesis (50S); active against gram-positive cocci, *B fragilis. Tox:* GI distress, pseudomembranous colitis.

Clomiphene
Estrogen partial agonist: synthetic used in infertility to induce ovulation. May result in multiple births.

Clonidine
$Alpha_2$ agonist: acts centrally to reduce SANS outflow, lowers BP. Used in HTN and in drug dependency states. *Tox:* mild sedation, rebound HTN if stopped suddenly.

Clozapine
Atypical antipsychotic: low affinity for dopamine D_2 receptors, higher for D_4 and $5\text{-}HT_{2A}$ receptors; less EPS adverse effects than other antipsychotic drugs. *Tox:* ANS effects, agranulocytosis (infrequent but significant).

Cocaine
Indirectly acting sympathomimetic: blocks amine reuptake into nerve endings. Local anesthetic (ester type). Marked CNS stimulation, euphoria; high abuse and dependence liability. *Tox:* psychosis, cardiac arrhythmias, seizures.

Colchicine
Microtubule assembly inhibitor: reduces mobility and phagocytosis by WBCs in gout-inflamed joints; useful in acute gout. *Tox:* GI (often severe), hepatic, renal damage.

Cyclophosphamide
Antineoplastic, immunosuppressive: cell cycle-nonspecific alkylating agent. *Tox:* alopecia, gastrointestinal distress, hemorrhagic cystitis (use mesna), myelosuppression

Cyclosporine
Immunosuppressant: antibiotic; inhibits synthesis of interleukins and interferon gamma, suppressing T cell activation. *Tox:* nephrotoxicity (dose-limiting), hirsutism, hypertension, seizures (in overdose). Not a myelosuppressant.

Cytokines
Recombinant DNA technology products: aldesleukin (IL-2, used in renal cancer); erythropoietin (epoetin alfa, used in anemias); filgrastim (G-CSF, used in neutropenia); interferon alpha (used in hepatitis B and C and in cancer), interferon beta (used in multiple sclerosis); interferon gamma (used in chronic granulomatous disease); oprelvekin (IL-11, used in thrombocytopenia); thrombopoietin (used in thrombocytopenia); and sargramostim (GM-CSF, used in neutropenia).

Dantrolene	Muscle relaxant: blocks Ca^{2+} release from sarcoplasmic reticulum of skeletal muscle. Used in muscle spasm (cerebral palsy, multiple sclerosis, cord injury) and in emergency treatment of malignant hyperthermia.
Desmopressin	ADH analog, selective for V_2 receptors: used for pituitary diabetes insipidus and to increase factor VIII in bleeding disorders.
Dexamethasone	Glucocorticoid: very potent, long-acting; no mineralocorticoid activity. Betamethasone is similar; triamcinolone has shorter half-life.
Diazepam	Benzodiazepine prototype: binds to BZ receptors of the $GABA_A$ receptor-chloride ion channel complex; facilitates the inhibitory actions of GABA by increasing the *frequency* of channel opening. Uses: anxiety states, ethanol detoxification, muscle spasticity, status epilepticus. *Tox:* dependence, additive effects with other CNS depressants.
Didanosine (ddI)	Antiviral: nucleoside inhibitor of HIV reverse transcriptase (NRTI). Used in combination regimens. *Tox:* peripheral neuropathy, pancreatitis. Other NRTIs: lamivudine (3TC), stavudine (d4T), zalcitabine (ddC), and the prototype, zidovudine (see below).
Digoxin	Cardiac glycoside prototype: positive inotropic drug for CHF, half-life 40 hours; renal excretion; inhibits Na^+/K^+ ATPase, also a cardiac parasympathomimetic. *Tox:* calcium overload arrhythmias, GI upset. Digitoxin: half-life 168 hours, excreted in the bile (partially as digoxin).
Diloxanide	Antiprotozoal: used as sole drug in asymptomatic intestinal amebiasis and with metronidazole in mild to severe intestinal forms of the disease.
Diphenhydramine	Antihistamine H_1 blocker prototype: used in hay fever, motion sickness, dystonias. *Tox:* antimuscarinic, α-adrenoceptor blocker, sedative.
Dopamine	Neurotransmitter and agonist drug at dopamine receptors: used in shock to increase renal blood flow (low dose) and positive inotropic effects (moderate dose).
Doxorubicin	Antineoplastic: anthracycline drug (cell cycle-nonspecific); intercalates between base pairs to disrupt DNA functions, inhibits topoisomerases, and forms cytotoxic free radicals. *Tox:* cardiotoxicity (consider dexrazoxane), myelosuppression. Daunorubicin is similar.
Doxycycline	Tetracycline antibiotic: protein synthesis inhibitor (30S), more effective than other tetracyclines against chlamydia and in Lyme disease. Unlike other tetracyclines, it is eliminated mainly in the feces. *Tox:* see tetracycline.
Echothiophate	Organophosphate cholinesterase inhibitor: less lipid-soluble than most organophosphates; used topically in glaucoma.
Edrophonium	Cholinesterase inhibitor: very short duration of action (15 minutes). Used in diagnosis of myasthenia gravis and to distinguish myasthenic crisis from cholinergic crisis.
Efavirenz	Nonnucleoside reverse transcriptase inhibitor (NNRTI): used in combination regimens for HIV. *Tox:* skin rash, CNS effects. Other NNRTIs: delavirdine, nevirapine.
Enoxaparin	Low-molecular-weight (LMW) heparin. Primary effect is on anti-factor X. The aPTT test is unreliable. Other LMW heparin-like products: dalteparin, danaparoid. *Tox:* bleeding.
Entacapone	COMT inhibitor: enhances levodopa access to CNS neurons; adjunctive use in Parkinson's disease. *Tox:* exacerbates levodopa effects. Tolcapone is similar in action and use but may be hepatotoxic.
Ephedrine	Indirectly acting sympathomimetic: like amphetamine but less CNS stimulation, more smooth muscle effects. In botanicals (eg, Ma-huang). *Tox:* hypertension, stroke, MI.

Epinephrine	Adrenoceptor agonist prototype: product of adrenal medulla, some CNS neurons. Affinity for all alpha and all beta receptors. Used in asthma; as hemostatic and as adjunct with local anesthetics; drug of choice in anaphylaxis. *Tox:* tachycardia, hypertension, MI, pulmonary edema and hemorrhage.
Ergot alkaloids	Ergonovine: causes prolonged uterine contraction. Used in postpartum bleeding and in migraine. Ergotamine: causes prolonged vasoconstriction, uterine contraction. Used in migraine, obstetrics. *Tox:* vasospasm (including coronaries).
Erythromycin	Macrolide antibiotic: bacteriostatic inhibitor of protein synthesis (50S); activity includes gram-positive cocci and bacilli, *M pneumoniae, Legionella pneumophila, C trachomatis. Tox:* cholestatic jaundice (avoid estolate in pregnancy), inhibits liver drug-metabolizing enzymes, interactions with cisapride, theophylline, warfarin.
Etanercept	DMARD: recombinant fusion protein that binds TNF. Infliximab (see under Mabs) has a similar mechanism of action. Effective (by injection) in RA and possibly other severe inflammatory diseases. *Tox:* injection site reactions include erythema, itching and swelling; possible increased infection rate.
Ethanol	A sedative-hypnotic. Acute actions include impaired judgment, ataxia, loss of consciousness, vasodilation and cardiovascular and respiratory depression. Chronic use leads to dependence and dysfunction of multiple organ systems. *Note:* zero-order elimination kinetics.
Ethosuximide	Anticonvulsant: used in absence seizures; may block T-type Ca^{2+} channels in thalamic neurons. *Tox:* GI distress; safe in pregnancy.
Fenoldopam:	Dopamine receptor agonist: D_1-selective; used in hypertensive emergencies to lower BP.
Finasteride	Steroid inhibitor of 5α-reductase: inhibits synthesis of dihydrotestosterone. Used in benign prostatic hyperplasia and male pattern baldness.
Flecainide	Class IC antiarrhythmic prototype: used in ventricular tachycardia and rapid atrial arrhythmias with Wolff-Parkinson-White syndrome. *Tox:* arrhythmogenic, CNS excitation.
Fluconazole	Imidazole antifungal: inhibits ergosterol synthesis. Used in esophageal and vaginal candidiasis, in coccidioidomycosis, and in the prophylaxis and treatment of fungal meningitis. Adverse effects similar to those of ketoconazole (see below), but less severe.
Fludrocortisone	Synthetic corticosteroid: high mineralocorticoid and moderate glucocorticoid activity; long duration of action.
Flumazenil	Benzodiazepine receptor antagonist: used to reverse CNS depressant effects of benzodiazepines.
Fluorouracil	Antineoplastic: pyrimidine antimetabolite (cell cycle-specific), causes "thymine-less" cell death; used mainly for solid or superficial tumors. *Tox:* GI distress, myelosuppression.
Fluoxetine	Antidepressant: serotonin selective reuptake inhibitor (SSRI) prototype. Less ANS adverse effects and cardiotoxic potential than tricyclics. *Tox:* CNS stimulation, sexual dysfunction, seizures in overdose, serotonin syndrome. Other SSRIs: citalopram, paroxetine, sertraline.
Flutamide	Androgen receptor antagonist: used in prostatic carcinoma.
Foscarnet	Antiviral: effective against herpes viruses (CMV and HSV including TK^- strains). Not an antimetabolite, not bioactivated. *Tox:* electrolyte imbalance, nephrotoxicity, seizures at high dose.
Furosemide	Loop diuretic prototype: blocks $Na^+/K^+/2Cl^-$ transporter in thick ascending limb (TAL); high efficacy; used in acute pulmonary edema, refractory edematous states, hypercalcemia, and HTN. *Tox:* ototoxicity, K^+ wasting, hypo-

volemia, increased serum uric acid. Ethacrynic acid is similar but has less effect on uric acid.

Gabapentin — Anticonvulsant: structural analog of GABA facilitating its CNS inhibitory actions; used for partial seizures, neuropathic pain and in bipolar disorder. *Tox:* sedation, movement disorders. For other novel antiseizure drugs see Chapter 24.

Ganciclovir — Antiviral: effective against herpes viruses (CMV and HSV); for CMV requires bioactivation via viral phosphotransferase. *Tox:* myelosuppression, nephrotoxicity, neurotoxicity.

Gemfibrozil — Antilipemic: stimulates lipoprotein lipase in endothelial cells and peripheral tissues. Used in hypertriglyceridemias and mixed triglyceridemia/hypercholesterolemia. *Tox:* GI distress, cholelithiasis, skin rashes.

Gentamicin — Aminoglycoside prototype: bactericidal inhibitor of protein synthesis (30S); active against many aerobic gram-negative bacteria. Narrow therapeutic window; dose reduction required in renal impairment. *Tox:* renal dysfunction, ototoxicity; once-daily dosing is effective (postantibiotic effect) and less toxic. Amikacin and tobramycin are similar.

Glipizide — Oral hypoglycemic: second-generation sulfonylurea, very potent. Blocks K^+ channels in pancreatic B cells, causing depolarization and release of insulin. *Tox:* hypoglycemia, weight gain. Related drugs: glyburide and older sulfonylureas (see Tolbutamide).

Glucagon — Hormone from pancreatic A cells. Increases blood sugar via increased cAMP. Used in hypoglycemia and as an antidote in beta-blocker overdose.

Guanethidine — Postganglionic sympathetic neuron blocker: enters nerve ending via uptake-1 and effects reversed by TCAs, cocaine. *Tox:* severe orthostatic hypotension, sexual dysfunction.

Haloperidol — Antipsychotic butyrophenone: blocks brain dopamine D_2 receptors. *Tox:* marked EPS dysfunction, hyperprolactinemia; fewer ANS adverse effects than phenothiazines.

Halothane — General anesthetic prototype: inhaled halogenated hydrocarbon. *Tox:* cardiovascular and respiratory depression and relaxation of skeletal and smooth muscle. Use is declining because of sensitization of heart to catecholamines and occurrence (rare) of hepatitis.

Heparin — Anticoagulant: large polymeric molecule with antithrombin and anti-factor X activity. Rapid onset, in vitro and in vivo anticoagulation. *Antidote:* protamine. See also Enoxaparin.

Hydralazine — Antihypertensive: arteriolar vasodilator, orally active; used in severe HTN, CHF. *Tox:* tachycardia, salt and water retention, lupus-like syndrome.

Hydrochlorothiazide — Thiazide diuretic prototype: acts in distal convoluted tubule (DCT) to block Na^+/Cl^- transporter; used in HTN, CHF, nephrolithiasis. *Tox:* a sulfonamide; increased serum lipids, uric acid, glucose; K^+ wasting.

Hydroxychloroquine — DMARD: decreases leukocyte chemotaxis, stabilizes lysosomes, and traps free radicals. *Tox:* GI distress, ototoxicity, myopathy, neuropathy. Other older DMARDs: methotrexate, prednisone, sulfasalazine, gold salts, penicillamine.

Imipenem — Antibiotic: carbapenem active against many aerobic and anaerobic bacteria, including penicillinase-producing organisms; a bactericidal inhibitor of cell wall synthesis. Used with cilastatin (which inhibits metabolism by renal dehydropeptidases). *Tox:* allergy (partial cross-reactivity with penicillins), seizures (overdose). Meropenem is similar but does not require cilastatin.

Indinavir — Antiviral; HIV protease inhibitor (PI) used as a component of combination regimens in AIDS. *Tox:* anemia, nephrolithiasis, metabolic disorders, inhibits P450 drug metabolism. Other PIs: amprenavir, nelfinavir, ritonavir (major P450 inhibitor), and saquinavir.

Indomethacin — NSAID prototype: highly potent. Usually reserved for acute inflammation (eg, acute gout), not chronic; neonatal patent ductus arteriosus. *Tox:* GI (bleeding), renal damage. Other NSAIDs: aspirin, ibuprofen, ketorolac, naproxen, and piroxicam.

Ipratropium — Antimuscarinic agent: aerosol for asthma, chronic obstructive pulmonary disease. Good bronchodilator in 20–30% of patients. Not as efficacious as β_2 agonists. *Tox:* dry mouth.

Isoniazid — Antimycobacterial: primary drug in combination regimens for tuberculosis; used as sole agent in prophylaxis. Metabolic clearance via N-acetyltransferases (genetic variability). *Tox:* hepatotoxicity (age-dependent), peripheral neuropathy (reversed by pyridoxine), hemolysis (in G6PD deficiency).

Isoproterenol — $Beta_1$ and β_2 agonist catecholamine prototype: bronchodilator, cardiac stimulant. Always causes tachycardia because both direct and reflex actions increase HR. *Tox:* arrhythmias, tremor, angina.

Ivermectin — Anthelmintic: drug of choice for onchocerciasis and for threadworm infections. Intensifies GABA-mediated neurotransmission in nematodes, but no access to CNS in humans. *Tox:* in onchocerciasis causes headache, fever, hypotension, joint pain.

Ketoconazole — Antifungal azole prototype: active systemically; inhibits the synthesis of ergosterol. Used for *C albicans,* dermatophytosis, and non-life-threatening systemic mycoses. *Tox:* hepatic dysfunction, inhibits steroid synthesis and P450-dependent drug metabolism.

Labetalol — $Alpha_1$- and nonselective β-blocker: used in HTN and CHF. *Tox:* AV block, hypotension.

Leflunomide — DMARD: dihydroorotate dehydrogenase inhibitor that arrests T cell proliferation. Used orally in RA. *Tox:* diarrhea, increased liver enzymes.

Leuprolide — GnRH analog: synthetic peptide used in pulse therapy to stimulate gonadal steroid synthesis (infertility); used in continuous or depot therapy to shut off steroid synthesis, especially in prostatic carcinoma and endometriosis.

Levodopa — Dopamine precursor: used in parkinsonism, usually combined with carbidopa (a peripheral inhibitor of dopamine metabolism). *Tox:* dyskinesias, hypotension, on-off phenomena, behavioral changes.

Lidocaine — Local anesthetic, medium duration amide prototype: highly selective use-dependent class IB antiarrhythmic; used for nerve block and post-MI ischemic ventricular arrhythmias. *Tox:* CNS excitation. Mexiletine: like lidocaine, but orally active.

Linezolid — Antibiotic (prototype oxazoladinone): binds to 50S ribosomal subunit to inhibit bacterial protein synthesis. Used for drug-resistant gram-positive organisms, including MRSA and VRE strains.

Lithium — Antimanic prototype: drug of choice in mania and bipolar affective disorders; blocks recycling of the phosphatidylinositol second messenger system. *Tox:* tremor, diabetes insipidus, goiter, seizures (in overdose), teratogenic potential (Ebstein's malformations).

Loratadine — Second-generation H_1 antihistamine: used in hay fever. *Tox:* Much less sedation than first generation antihistamines; no ANS effects. Others: cetirizine, fexofenadine.

Losartan — Angiotensin AT_1 receptor blocker prototype: used in HTN. Effects and toxicity similar to those of ACE inhibitors but causes less cough. Other AT_1 blockers: candesartan, valsartan.

Lovastatin — Antilipemic HMG-CoA reductase inhibitor prototype: acts in liver to reduce synthesis of cholesterol. Other "statins": atorvastatin, fluvastatin, pravastatin, simvastatin. *Tox:* liver damage (elevated enzymes), muscle damage.

MAbs	Monoclonal antibodies include: abciximab (see above), daclizumab (blocks IL-2 receptors—used in renal transplants), infliximab (binds TNF—used in RA and Crohn's disease), palivizumab (used in RSV), rituximab (used in non-Hodgkin's lymphoma), and trastuzumab (used in breast cancers with HER2/neu receptors).
Malathion	Organophosphate insecticide cholinesterase inhibitor: prodrug converted to malaoxon. Less toxic in mammals and birds because metabolized to inactive products.
Mebendazole	Anthelmintic: important drug for pinworm and whipworm infections. Inhibits microtubule synthesis and glucose uptake in nematodes. *Tox:* GI distress, caution in pregnancy. Albendazole and thiabendazole are related anthelmintics.
Mefloquine	Antimalarial: unknown mechanism of action. Used for prophylaxis against and treatment of chloroquine-resistant malaria. *Tox:* GI distress, dizziness, seizures in overdose.
Meperidine	Opioid analgesic: synthetic, equivalent to morphine in efficacy but orally bioavailable. Strong agonist at mu opioid receptors; blocks muscarinic receptors. *Tox:* see morphine; normeperidine accumulation may cause seizures.
Mestranol	Synthetic estrogen: used in many oral contraceptives.
Metformin	Oral biguanide hypoglycemic: is euglycemic and does not release insulin from pancreatic B cells; proposed mechanisms include decreased hepatic gluconeogenesis and stimulation of glycolysis. Minimal hypoglycemia or weight gain. *Tox:* GI distress, potential lactic acidosis, but rare.
Methadone	Opioid analgesic: synthetic mu agonist, equivalent to morphine in efficacy but orally bioavailable and with a longer half-life. Used as analgesic, to suppress withdrawal symptoms, and in maintenance programs. *Tox:* see morphine.
Methotrexate	Antineoplastic, immunosuppressant: cell cycle-specific drug that inhibits dihydrofolate reductase. Major dose reduction required in renal impairment. *Tox:* GI distress, myelosuppression, crystalluria. Leucovorin rescue used to reduce toxicity.
Methyldopa	Antihypertensive: prodrug of methylnorepinephrine, a CNS-active α_2 agonist. Reduces SANS outflow from vasomotor center. *Tox:* sedation, positive Coombs test, hemolysis.
Methysergide	Semisynthetic ergot alkaloid: used as prophylactic in migraine. *Tox:* retroperitoneal and subendocardial fibroplasia.
Metronidazole	Antiprotozoal antibiotic: drug of choice in extraluminal amebiasis and trichomoniasis; effective against bacterial anaerobes, including *B fragilis* and in antibiotic-induced colitis due to *C difficile*. *Tox:* peripheral neuropathy, gastrointestinal distress, ethanol intolerance, mutagenic potential.
Mifepristone	Progestin and glucocorticoid receptor antagonist: abortifacient, antineoplastic.
Minoxidil	Antihypertensive: prodrug of minoxidil sulfate, a high-efficacy arteriolar vasodilator. Used in HTN; topically for baldness. *Tox:* tachycardia, salt and water retention, pericardial effusion.
Misoprostol	PGE_1 derivative: orally active prostaglandin used for GI ulcers caused by NSAIDs. *Tox:* diarrhea.
Morphine	Opioid analgesic prototype: strong mu receptor agonist. Poor oral bioavailability. *Tox:* constipation, emesis, sedation, respiratory depression, miosis, and urinary retention. Tolerance may be marked; high potential for psychologic and physiologic dependence. Additive effects with other CNS depressants.

Nafcillin	Penicillinase-resistant penicillin prototype: used for suspected or known staphylococcal infections; not active against MRSA. *Tox:* penicillin allergy. Others in group include oxacillin, cloxacillin, and dicloxacillin.
Nalbuphine	Opioid: mixed agonist-antagonist analgesic that activates kappa and weakly blocks mu receptors. Effective analgesic, but with lower abuse liability and less respiratory depressant effects than most strong opioid analgesics. Pentazocine is similar but with less analgesic efficacy.
Naloxone	Opioid mu receptor antagonist: used to reverse CNS depressant effects of opioid analgesics (overdose or when used in anesthesia). Naltrexone (orally active), a related compound, is used in ethanol dependency states.
Neostigmine	Cholinesterase inhibitor prototype: quaternary nitrogen carbamate with little CNS effect. *Tox:* excess cholinomimetic effects. Pyridostigmine is similar.
Niacin	Antilipemic: reduces release of VLDL from liver into circulation. *Tox:* flushing, pruritus, liver dysfunction.
Nifedipine	Dihydropyridine calcium channel blocker prototype: vasoselective (less cardiac depression than verapamil, diltiazem); used in angina, HTN. *Tox:* constipation, headache, gingival overgrowths, tachycardia, arrhythmias (avoid rapid-onset forms). Others in group include amlodipine (used in CHF), nimodipine (used in subarachnoid hemorrhage), and nicardipine.
Nitric oxide	Endogenous vasodilator released from vascular endothelium; neurotransmitter. Mediates vasodilating effect of acetylcholine, histamine, and hydralazine. Active metabolite of nitroprusside and of nitrates used in angina. Used as pulmonary dilator in neonatal hypoxia. *Tox:* excessive vasodilation, hypotension.
Nitroglycerin	Antianginal vasodilator prototype: releases nitric oxide (NO) in smooth muscle of veins, less in arteries, and causes relaxation. Standard of therapy in angina (both atherosclerotic and variant). *Tox:* tachycardia, orthostatic hypotension, headache.
Norepinephrine	Adrenoceptor agonist prototype: acts at β_1- and all α-adrenoceptors; used as vasoconstrictor. Causes reflex bradycardia. *Tox:* ischemia, arrhythmias, HTN.
Norgestrel	Progestin: used in many oral contraceptives and Norplant implantable contraceptive.
Olanzapine	Atypical antipsychotic; high-affinity antagonist at 5-HT_2 receptors, with minimal extrapyramidal side effects; improves both positive and negative symptoms of schizophrenia. Other atypicals: quetiapine (short half-life), risperidone (possible EPS dysfunction), sertindole (QT prolongation).
Omeprazole	Proton pump inhibitor prototype: irreversible blocker of H^+/K^+ ATPase proton pump in parietal cells of stomach. Used in GI ulcers, Zollinger-Ellison syndrome, gastroesophageal reflux disease (GERD). Other "prazoles": lansoprazole, rabeprazole. *Tox:* hypergastrinemia.
Ondansetron	5-HT_3 receptor blocker prototype: very important antiemetic for cancer chemotherapy; also used postoperatively to reduce vomiting. *Tox:* extrapyramidal effects. Other "setrons": granisetron, dolasetron.
Oseltamivir	Neuraminidase inhibitor: facilitates clumping of mature virions of influenza A and B and decreases their infectivity. Shortens duration of flu symptoms. Zanamivir is similar in action and use.
Oxybutynin	Muscarinic cholinoceptor blocker: used to relieve bladder spasm and incontinence. Tolterodine, more selective for M_3 receptors, has similar uses.
Parathion	Organophosphate acetylcholinesterase inhibitor prototype: used as insecticide. Prodrug: converted in body to paraoxon. Other organophosphates: DFP, soman, tabun, echothiophate. *Tox:* "DUMBELS" mnemonic (Chapter 7).

Penicillamine — Chelator, immunomodulator: copper and sometimes lead, mercury, arsenic. Used in Wilson's disease and rheumatoid arthritis.

Penicillin G — Penicillin prototype: active against common streptococci, gram-positive bacilli, gram-negative cocci, spirochetes (drug of choice in syphilis), and enterococci (if used with an aminoglycoside); penicillinase-susceptible. *Tox:* penicillin allergy.

Phenobarbital — Long-acting barbiturate: used as a sedative and for tonic-clonic seizures. Facilitates GABA-mediated neuronal inhibition (by increasing *duration* of channel opening) and may block excitatory neurotransmitters. Partial renal clearance that can be increased by urinary alkalinization. Chronic use leads to induction of liver drug-metabolizing enzymes and ALA synthase. *Tox:* psychologic and physiologic dependence; additive effects with other CNS depressants.

Phenoxybenzamine — Alpha-blocker prototype: irreversible action. Phentolamine: reversible action. Used in pheochromocytoma. *Tox:* excess hypotension; GI distress.

Phenytoin — Anticonvulsant: used for tonic-clonic and partial seizures; blocks Na^+ channels in neuronal membranes. Serum levels variable due to first-pass metabolism and nonlinear elimination kinetics. *Tox:* sedation, diplopia, gingival hyperplasia, hirsutism, teratogenic potential. Drug interactions via effects on plasma protein binding or induction of hepatic metabolism.

Physostigmine — Acetylcholinesterase inhibitor prototype: alkaloid tertiary amine carbamate, enters eye and CNS readily. Used in glaucoma. *Tox:* excess cholinomimetic effects.

Pilocarpine — Muscarinic agonist prototype: tertiary amine alkaloid. May cause paradoxic hypertension by activating muscarinic excitatory postsynaptic potential receptors in postganglionic sympathetic neurons. Used in glaucoma. *Tox:* muscarinic excess.

Pioglitazone — Thiazolidinedione stimulator of peroxisome proliferator-activator receptors (PPARs) enhances target tissue sensitivity to insulin. Used in type 2 diabetes as monotherapy, or with other oral hypoglycemics. Less hypoglycemia and weight gain than sulfonylureas. Other "glitazones": rosiglitazone, troglitazone (the latter drug discontinued in USA due to hepatotoxicity).

Piperacillin — Extended-spectrum penicillin active against selected gram-negative bacteria, including *Pseudomonas aeruginosa* (synergistic with aminoglycosides). Susceptible to penicillinases unless used with tazobactam. *Tox:* penicillin allergy.

Pralidoxime — Acetylcholinesterase regenerator (antidote for organophosphate poisoning): very high affinity for phosphorus in organophosphates. *Tox:* neuromuscular weakness.

Praziquantel — Anthelmintic: important drug for trematode (fluke) and cestode (tapeworm) infections. Increases membrane permeability to Ca^{2+} causing muscle contraction followed by paralysis. *Tox:* headache, dizziness, GI distress, fever; potential abortifacient.

Prazosin — $Alpha_1$-selective blocker prototype: used in HTN and benign prostatic hyperplasia. *Tox:* first-dose orthostatic hypotension. Other "osins": terazosin, doxazosin.

Prednisone — Glucocorticoid prototype: potent, short-acting; much less mineralocorticoid activity than cortisol but more than dexamethasone or triamcinolone.

Probenecid — Uricosuric: inhibitor of renal weak acid secretion and reabsorption in S_2 segment of proximal tubule; prolongs half-life of penicillin, accelerates clearance of uric acid. Used in gout. Sulfinpyrazole is similar.

Procainamide — Class IA antiarrhythmic drug: short half-life, metabolized by *N*-acetyltransferase. Similar to quinidine but more cardiodepressant and may cause lupus erythematosus.

Propranolol	Nonselective beta-blocker prototype: local anesthetic action but no partial agonist effect. Used in HTN, angina, arrhythmias, migraine, hyperthyroidism, tremor. *Tox:* asthma, AV block, CHF.
Propylthiouracil	Antithyroid drug prototype: inhibits tyrosine iodination and coupling reactions; orally active. *Tox:* rash, agranulocytosis (rare). Methimazole is similar but more lipid-soluble.
Prostacyclin	PGI_2 prostaglandin vasodilator and inhibitor of platelet aggregation. An analog, epoprostenol, is used in primary pulmonary HTN.
Pyrantel pamoate	Anthelmintic: important drug for nematode infections, especially hookworm and roundworm. Activates muscle endplate nicotinic receptors causing contraction, then paralysis. *Tox:* GI distress, headache, lassitude.
Pyrimethamine	Antiprotozoal: antifol inhibiting DHF reductase and synergistic, via sequential blockade, with sulfadiazine against *Toxoplasma gondii.* Folinic acid is needed to offset hematologic toxicity.
Quinidine	Class IA antiarrhythmic prototype: used in atrial and ventricular arrhythmias. *Tox:* cinchonism, GI upset, thrombocytopenic purpura, arrhythmogenic (torsade de pointes).
Quinine	Antimalarial: blood schizonticide; no effect on liver stages. Interferes with nucleic acid metabolism in plasmodium. Isomer of quinidine, same toxicity.
Raloxifene	Selective estrogen receptor modulator (SERM): agonist at bone receptors (used in osteoporosis), antagonist at breast receptors (used in cancer) but does not stimulate endometrial receptors.
Repaglinide	Oral hypoglycemic (prototype meglitinide): blocks K^+ channels in pancreatic B cells, causing depolarization and release of insulin. Used in type 1 diabetes alone, or in combinations; rapid onset and short duration. *Tox:* hypoglycemia, increases liver enzymes.
Reserpine	Antihypertensive (rarely used): selective inhibitor of vesicle catecholamine-H^+ antiporter; used in HTN, causes depletion of catecholamines and 5-HT from their stores. *Tox:* severe depression, suicide, ulcers.
Rifampin	Antimicrobial: inhibitor of DNA-dependent RNA polymerase used in drug regimens for tuberculosis and the meningococcal carrier state. *Tox:* hepatic dysfunction, induction of liver drug-metabolizing enzymes (drug interactions), flu-like syndrome with intermittent dosing. Rifabutin similar but associated with fewer drug interactions.
Ropinirole	Dopamine receptor agonist: used in Parkinson's disease; less toxicity than bromocriptine. *Tox:* dyskinesias, sedation. Pramipexole is similar.
Selegiline	MAO-B inhibitor: selective inhibitor of the enzyme that metabolizes dopamine (no tyramine interactions). Used in Parkinson's disease.
Spironolactone	Aldosterone receptor antagonist: K^+-sparing diuretic action in the collecting tubules; used in aldosteronism, HTN, and female hirsutism. *Tox:* hyperkalemia, gynecomastia.
Sotalol	Class III antiarrhythmic prototype: blocks I_{Kr} channels. Used for atrial and ventricular arrhythmias. *Tox:* torsade de pointes arrhythmias. Others in group: ibutilide, dofetilide.
Streptogramins	Antibiotics: Synercid is the combination of quinupristin and dalfopristin; bactericidal inhibitors of protein synthesis. Intravenous use for drug-resistant gram-positive cocci including MRSA, VRE, and pneumococci. *Tox:* infusion-related pain, arthralgia, myalgia.
Streptokinase	Thrombolytic: protein from streptococci that accelerates plasminogen-to-plasmin conversion. *Tox:* bleeding, allergy. Anistreplase combines streptokinase with human plasminogen.

Succinylcholine	Depolarizing neuromuscular relaxant prototype: short duration (5 minutes) if patient has normal plasma cholinesterase (genetically determined). No antidote (compare with tubocurarine). Implicated in malignant hyperthermia.
Sumatriptan	5-HT_{1D} receptor agonist: used to abort migraine attacks. *Tox:* coronary vasospasm, chest pain or pressure. Other "triptans": naratriptan, rizatriptan, zolmitriptan.
Tamoxifen	Selective estrogen receptor modulator (SERM): blocks estrogen (E) receptors in breast tissue; activates endometrial E receptors. Used in E receptor-positive cancers, possibly prophylactic in high-risk patients. Toremifene is similar.
Tetracaine	Local anesthetic: long-acting ester prototype. *Tox:* CNS excitation.
Tetracycline	Antibiotic: tetracycline prototype; bacteriostatic inhibitor of protein synthesis (30S). Broad spectrum, but many resistant organisms. Used for mycoplasmal, chlamydial, rickettsial infections, chronic bronchitis, acne, cholera; a backup drug in syphilis. *Tox:* GI upset and superinfections, antianabolic actions, Fanconi's syndrome, photosensitivity, dental enamel dysplasia.
Tetrodotoxin	Toxin: potent sodium channel blocker; blocks action potential propagation in nerve, heart, and skeletal muscle. From puffer fish, California newt. *Tox:* paresthesias, paralysis. Saxitoxin (paralytic shellfish poison) is similar.
Thioridazine	Antipsychotic phenothiazine: blocks most dopamine receptors in the CNS. *Tox:* atropine-like effects (marked), electrocardiographic abnormalities, postural hypotension, retinal pigmentation, sedation, additive effects with other CNS depressants (but less EPS dysfunction than with other phenothiazines).
Ticlopidine	Antiplatelet agent that blocks ADP receptors; irreversible inhibitor of fibrin binding to platelets. Used in transient ischemic attacks and to prevent strokes. Clopidogrel has a similar mechanism and use. *Tox:* bleeding, diarrhea, leukopenia.
Tolbutamide	Oral hypoglycemic: older sulfonylurea group prototype. See Glipizide. Blocks K^+ channels in pancreatic B cells, causing depolarization and release of insulin. *Tox:* hypoglycemia, weight gain. Others: acetohexamide, tolazamide, and chlorpropamide (longest duration of action).
Trimethoprim-sulfamethoxazole	Antimicrobial drug combination: causes synergistic sequential blockade of folic acid synthesis. Active against many gram-negative bacteria, including aeromonas, enterobacter, *H influenzae,* klebsiella, moraxella, salmonella, serratia, and shigella. *Tox:* mainly due to sulfonamide; includes hypersensitivity, hematotoxicity, kernicterus, and drug interactions due to competition for plasma protein binding.
Tubocurarine	Nondepolarizing neuromuscular blocking agent prototype: competitive nicotinic blocker. Releases histamine and may cause hypotension. Analogs: pancuronium, atracurium, vecuronium, and other "-curiums" and "-curoniums." *Antidote:* cholinesterase inhibitor, eg, neostigmine.
Tyramine	Indirectly acting sympathomimetic prototype: releases or displaces norepinephrine from stores in nerve endings. Presence in certain foods may cause potentially lethal hypertensive responses in patients taking MAO inhibitors.
Valproic acid	Anticonvulsant: primary drug in absence, clonic-tonic, and myoclonic seizure states. *Tox:* GI distress, hepatic necrosis (rare), teratogenic (spina bifida); inhibits drug metabolism.
Vancomycin	Glycopeptide bactericidal antibiotic: inhibits synthesis of cell wall precursor molecules. Drug of choice for methicillin-resistant staphylococci and effective in antibiotic-induced colitis. Dose reduction required in renal impairment (or hemodialysis). *Tox:* ototoxicity, hypersensitivity, renal dysfunction (rare).
Verapamil	Calcium channel blocker prototype: blocks "L-type" channels; cardiac depressant and vasodilator; used in HTN, angina, and arrhythmias. *Tox:* AV block, CHF, constipation. Diltiazem: like verapamil, has more depressant effect on heart than dihydropyridines (eg, nifedipine).

Vincristine	Antineoplastic plant alkaloid: cell cycle (M phase)-specific agent; inhibits mitotic spindle formation. *Tox:* peripheral neuropathy. Vinblastine, a congener, causes myelosuppression.
Warfarin	Oral anticoagulant prototype: causes synthesis of nonfunctional versions of the vitamin K-dependent clotting factors (II, VII, IX, X). *Tox:* bleeding, teratogenic. *Antidote:* vitamin K, fresh plasma.
Zidovudine (ZDV)	Antiviral: prototype NRTI used in combinations for HIV infections and sometimes as individual agent in prophylaxis for needlesticks and vertical transmission. *Tox:* severe myelosuppression.
Zolpidem	Nonbenzodiazepine hypnotic, acts via the BZ_1 receptor subtype and is reversed by flumazenil; less amnesia and muscle relaxation; lower dependence liability. Zaleplon similar, but shorter-acting.

Appendix II

Examination 1

The following examination consists of 120 questions, mostly in the format ("single best answer") used in USMLE examinations. As in an actual examination, clinical descriptions, tables, or graphs are provided in many of the question stems.

It is suggested that you time yourself in taking this examination—in current USMLE examinations the time allotted is approximately 1 minute per question; thus, 2 hours would be appropriate for this examination.

DIRECTIONS: Each numbered item or incomplete statement in this section is followed by answers or by completions of the statement. Select the ONE lettered answer or completion that is BEST in each case.

1. Phase II clinical trials typically involve
- **(A)** Measurement of the pharmacokinetics of the new drug in normal volunteers
- **(B)** Double-blind evaluation of the new drug in thousands of patients with the target disease
- **(C)** Postmarketing surveillance of drug toxicities
- **(D)** Evaluation of the new drug in 50 to several hundred patients with the target disease
- **(E)** Collection of data regarding late-appearing toxicities from patients previously studied in phase I trials

2. A patient is admitted to the emergency department for treatment of a drug overdose. The identity of the drug is unknown, but it is observed that when the urine pH is acidic, the renal clearance of the drug is less than the glomerular filtration rate and that when the urine pH is alkaline, the clearance is greater than the glomerular filtration rate. The drug is probably a
- **(A)** Strong acid
- **(B)** Weak acid
- **(C)** Nonelectrolyte
- **(D)** Weak base
- **(E)** Strong base

3. A 45-year-old patient is to have reconstructive surgery on a hand that was recently injured in an accident. The anesthesiologist plans to use regional anesthesia of the arm for a fairly long procedure. The amide-type local anesthetic with the longest duration of action is
- **(A)** Cocaine
- **(B)** Bupivacaine
- **(C)** Lidocaine
- **(D)** Procaine
- **(E)** Tetracaine

4. A 60-year-old woman is in the coronary care unit following an acute myocardial infarction. She has developed signs of pulmonary edema of rapidly increasing severity. Aminophylline, dobutamine, and digoxin can each
- **(A)** Increase the amount of cAMP in cardiac muscle cells
- **(B)** Increase cardiac contractile force
- **(C)** Decrease conduction velocity in the atrioventricular node
- **(D)** Increase peripheral vascular resistance
- **(E)** Decrease venous return

5. Regarding peptide agents, which one of the following statements is false?
- **(A)** Angiotensin I is an endogenous vasodilator
- **(B)** Bradykinin is inactivated by angiotensin-converting enzyme
- **(C)** Most of the actions of angiotensin II are mediated by the AT_1 receptor subtype, a G protein-coupled receptor

(D) Patients with heart failure usually have high plasma levels of atrial natriuretic peptide (ANP)
(E) The endothelium is the source of peptides (endothelins) that cause vasoconstriction in most vascular beds

6. A patient with Zollinger-Ellison syndrome has been receiving high doses of cimetidine for 7 weeks. A frequent adverse effect of cimetidine is
(A) Agranulocytosis
(B) Systemic lupus erythematosus
(C) Inhibition of hepatic metabolism of other drugs
(D) Antiestrogenic effects
(E) Hypertension

7. A 67-year-old patient has recovered from the acute phase of a myocardial infarction but requires an antiarrhythmic drug for ventricular tachycardia. One property of quinidine that is not associated with procainamide is its
(A) Ability to control atrial as well as ventricular arrhythmias
(B) Activity by the oral route
(C) Prolongation of the PR interval
(D) Prolongation of the QRS interval
(E) Tendency to produce cinchonism

8. A patient discharged from the hospital after a myocardial infarction had been receiving small doses of quinidine to suppress a ventricular tachycardia. One month later, his local physician prescribed high-dose hydrochlorothiazide therapy for ankle edema, which was ascribed to congestive heart failure. Three weeks after beginning thiazide therapy, the patient was readmitted to the hospital with a rapid multifocal ventricular tachycardia. The most probable cause of this arrhythmia is
(A) Quinidine toxicity caused by inhibition of quinidine metabolism by the thiazide
(B) Direct effects of hydrochlorothiazide on the pacemaker of the heart
(C) Thiazide toxicity caused by the effects of quinidine on the kidneys
(D) Block of calcium current by the combination of quinidine plus thiazide
(E) Reduction of serum potassium caused by the diuretic action of hydrochlorothiazide

9. An important therapeutic or toxic effect of loop diuretics is
(A) Decreased blood volume
(B) Decreased heart rate
(C) Increased serum sodium
(D) Increased total body potassium
(E) Metabolic acidosis

10. The most appropriate drug for reversing myasthenic crisis in a patient who is experiencing diplopia, dysarthria, and difficulty swallowing is
(A) Neostigmine
(B) Pilocarpine
(C) Pralidoxime
(D) Succinylcholine
(E) Tubocurarine

11. Soon after being put to bed for a nap, a 4-year-old child is found convulsing. Diarrhea, sweating, and urination are apparent. The heart rate is 70/min, and the pupils are markedly constricted. Drug intoxication is suspected. The most probable cause is
(A) Acetaminophen overdose
(B) Amphetamine-containing diet pills
(C) Exposure to an organophosphate-containing insecticide
(D) Ingestion of a cold medication containing atropine
(E) Ingestion of phenylephrine-containing eye drops

12. A patient is admitted to the emergency room 2 hours after taking an overdose of phenobarbital. The plasma level of the drug at time of admission is 100 mg/L, and the apparent volume of distribution, half-life, and clearance of phenobarbital are 35 L, 4 days, and 6.1 L/d, respectively. The ingested dose was approximately
(A) 1 g
(B) 3.5 g
(C) 6.1 g
(D) 40 g
(E) 70 g

13. Most weak acid drugs as well as weak base drugs are absorbed primarily from the small intestine after oral administration because
(A) Both types are more ionized in the small intestine
(B) Both types are less ionized in the small intestine
(C) The blood flow is greater in the small intestine than that of other parts of the gut
(D) The surface area of the small intestine is greater than other parts of the gut
(E) The small intestine has nonspecific carriers for most drugs

14. The primary site of action of tyramine is
(A) Ganglionic receptors
(B) Gut and liver catechol-*O*-methyltransferase
(C) Postganglionic sympathetic nerve terminals
(D) Preganglionic sympathetic nerve terminals
(E) Vascular smooth muscle cell receptors

15. A semiconscious patient in the intensive care unit is being artificially ventilated. Random spontaneous respiratory movements are rendering the mechanical ventilation ineffective. A useful drug to reduce the patient's ineffective spontaneous respiratory activity is
(A) Baclofen
(B) Dantrolene
(C) Pancuronium
(D) Pyridostigmine
(E) Succinylcholine

16. Which one of the following drugs has been used in ophthalmology, but causes mydriasis and cycloplegia lasting more than 24 hours?
(A) Atropine
(B) Echothiophate
(C) Edrophonium
(D) Ephedrine
(E) Tropicamide

17. A 45-year-old surgeon has developed symmetric early morning stiffness in her hands. She wishes to take a nonsteroidal anti-inflammatory drug to relieve these symptoms and wants to avoid gastrointestinal side effects. Which one of the following drugs is most appropriate?
(A) Aspirin
(B) Celecoxib
(C) Ibuprofen
(D) Indomethacin
(E) Piroxicam

18. A 59-year-old woman with a 60 pack-year smoking history was diagnosed with lung cancer 2 months ago. She now enters the hospital in coma. Her serum calcium is 16 mg/dL. Which of the following (given with IV fluids) would be most useful to reduce serum calcium in this patient rapidly?
(A) Acetazolamide
(B) Furosemide
(C) Hydrochlorothiazide
(D) Mannitol
(E) Spironolactone

19. A 50-year-old man has a macrocytic anemia and early signs of neurologic abnormality. The drug that will probably be required in this case is
(A) Erythropoietin
(B) Filgrastim
(C) Folic acid
(D) Iron dextran
(E) Vitamin B_{12}

20. A patient in the coronary care unit has been receiving warfarin for 2 weeks. As a result of this therapy, the patient will probably have
(A) Reduced plasma factor II activity
(B) Reduced plasma factor VIII activity
(C) Reduced plasma plasminogen activity
(D) Increased tissue plasminogen activator
(E) Increased platelet adenosine stores

Items 21–22: A 55-year-old man with a strong family history of cardiovascular disease has moderate hypertension and angina pectoris. Blood pressure is 160/109 mm Hg and the ECG shows left ventricular hypertrophy. The rest of his physical examination and laboratory results are normal. His angina is precipitated by exercise. You have been asked to recommend a drug regimen for both conditions.

21. The antihypertensive drug most likely to aggravate angina pectoris is
- **(A)** Clonidine
- **(B)** Guanethidine
- **(C)** Hydralazine
- **(D)** Methyldopa
- **(E)** Propranolol

22. A drug lacking vasodilator properties that is useful in angina is
- **(A)** Isosorbide dinitrate
- **(B)** Metoprolol
- **(C)** Nifedipine
- **(D)** Nitroglycerin
- **(E)** Verapamil

23. Which one of the following statements regarding eicosanoids is false?
- **(A)** Leukotriene B_4 has potent chemotactic effects
- **(B)** Prostacyclin stimulates platelet aggregation
- **(C)** Prostaglandin E_2 increases uterine tone
- **(D)** Prostaglandin F_2 endometrial levels increase in primary dysmenorrhea
- **(E)** Thromboxane A_2 formation is inhibited by NSAIDs

24. Which one of the following drugs is used in the treatment of male impotence and activates prostaglandin E_1 receptors?
- **(A)** Alprostadil
- **(B)** Fluoxetine
- **(C)** Mifepristone
- **(D)** Sildenafil
- **(E)** Zafirlukast

25. A drug useful in the treatment of asthma but lacking bronchodilator action, is
- **(A)** Cromolyn
- **(B)** Ephedrine
- **(C)** Isoproterenol
- **(D)** Metaproterenol
- **(E)** Metoprolol

26. The toxicity spectrum of aspirin does not include
- **(A)** Increased risk of encephalopathy in children with viral infections
- **(B)** Increased risk of peptic ulcers
- **(C)** Hyperprothrombinemia
- **(D)** Metabolic acidosis
- **(E)** Respiratory alkalosis

27. Although it does not act at any histamine receptor, epinephrine reverses many effects of histamine. Epinephrine is a
- **(A)** Competitive inhibitor of histamine
- **(B)** Noncompetitive antagonist of histamine
- **(C)** Physiologic antagonist of histamine
- **(D)** Chemical antagonist of histamine
- **(E)** Metabolic inhibitor of histamine

28. Most drug receptors are
- **(A)** Small molecules with a molecular weight between 100 and 1000
- **(B)** Lipids arranged in a bilayer configuration
- **(C)** Proteins located on cell membranes or in the cytosol
- **(D)** DNA molecules
- **(E)** RNA molecules

29. After an intravenous bolus injection of lidocaine, the major factors determining the initial plasma concentration are
- **(A)** Dose and clearance
- **(B)** Dose and apparent volume of distribution
- **(C)** Apparent volume of distribution and clearance

(D) Clearance and half-life
(E) Half-life and dose

30. The graph shows the serum insulin level resulting from a two-injection regimen given to a child with type 1 diabetes. Assume that both injections (indicated by arrows along the time line) contain the same medication(s). Which one of the following is MOST likely to generate the levels of insulin depicted in the figure?
(A) 100% Regular insulin
(B) 100% Lispro insulin
(C) 70% NPH insulin plus 30% regular insulin
(D) 100% NPH insulin
(E) 100% Ultralente insulin

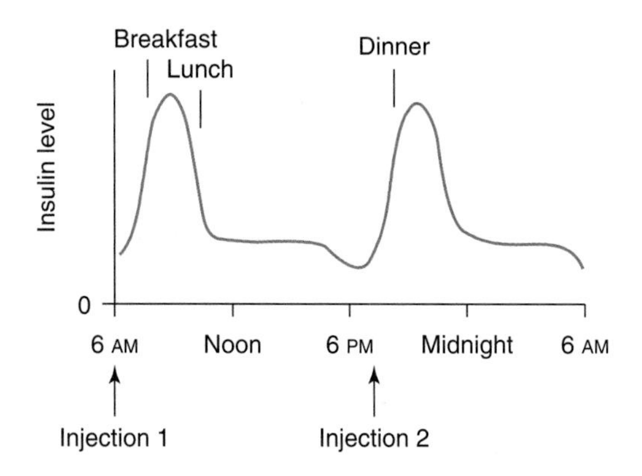

31. Intravenous administration of norepinephrine in a patient already taking an effective dose of atropine will often
(A) Increase heart rate
(B) Decrease total peripheral resistance
(C) Decrease blood sugar
(D) Increase skin temperature
(E) Reduce pupil size

32. A 26-year-old woman comes to the outpatient clinic with a complaint of rapid heart rate and easy fatigability. Laboratory work up reveals low hemoglobin and microcytic red cell size. The most suitable therapy will be
(A) Ferrous sulfate
(B) Folic acid
(C) Iron dextran
(D) Pyridoxine
(E) Vitamin B_{12}

33. Which of the following statements is most correct?
(A) Maximum efficacy of a drug is directly correlated with its potency
(B) The therapeutic index is the LD_{50} (or TD_{50}) divided by the ED_{50}
(C) A partial agonist has no effect on its receptors unless another drug is present
(D) Graded dose-response data provide information about the standard deviation of sensitivity to the drug in the population studied
(E) Quantal dose-response curves provide information about the efficacy of a drug

34. The heart rate response to the infusion of a moderate dose of phenylephrine in conscious patients is not blocked by
(A) Atropine
(B) Hexamethonium
(C) Phenoxybenzamine
(D) Reserpine
(E) Scopolamine

35. Which one of the following statements about scopolamine is false ?
(A) It has depressant actions on the CNS
(B) It may cause hallucinations
(C) It is poorly distributed across the placenta to the fetus

(D) It may prevent motion sickness and vertigo when applied as a patch to the skin
(E) It is similar to atropine in reducing gastrointestinal motility

36. Which of the following statements about antiplatelet drugs is false ?
(A) Abciximab is a monoclonal antibody that binds to the glycoprotein IIb/IIIa receptor
(B) Decreased formation of thromboxane underlies the antiplatelet action of aspirin
(C) Ibuprofen reversibly inhibits cyclooxygenase in platelets
(D) Ticlopidine is an inhibitor of the platelet thrombin receptor
(E) Dipyridamole is occasionally used with warfarin in patients with artificial heart valves

37. A 70-year-old man has severe urinary hesitancy associated with benign prostatic hyperplasia. He has tried alpha blockers with little relief. His physician recommends a drug that blocks 5α-reductase in the prostate and writes a prescription for
(A) Cyproterone
(B) Finasteride
(C) Flutamide
(D) Ketoconazole
(E) Leuprolide

38. The increase in heart rate and the force of cardiac contraction normally induced by electrical stimulation of sympathetic nerves can be blocked by which of the following?
(A) Atropine
(B) Clonidine
(C) Hydralazine
(D) Neostigmine
(E) Propranolol

39. A treatment of angina that consistently decreases the heart rate and can prevent vasospastic angina attacks is
(A) Isosorbide dinitrate
(B) Nifedipine
(C) Nitroglycerin
(D) Propranolol
(E) Verapamil

40. Verapamil and diltiazem diminish the symptoms of angina pectoris by causing all of the following EXCEPT
(A) Increase in diastolic interval
(B) Reduction in blood pressure
(C) Reduction in cardiac contractile force
(D) Reduction in heart rate
(E) Reduction in heart size

41. In a study of new diuretics, a new drug was given twice daily for eight days. The following data were obtained.

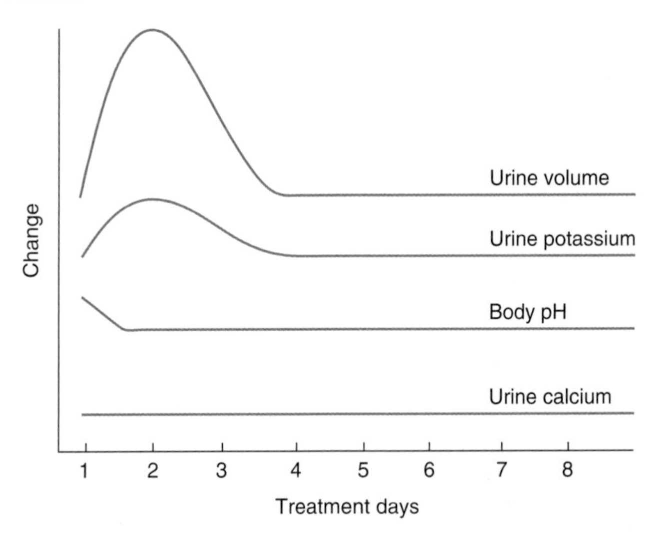

Which of the following mechanisms best explains the effects shown on the graph?

(A) Carbonic anhydrase inhibition
(B) Blockade of a $Na^+/K^+/2Cl^-$ transporter in the ascending limb of the loop of Henle
(C) Blockade of a NaCl transporter in the distal convoluted tubule
(D) Osmotic diuresis
(E) Block of aldosterone in the cortical collecting tubule

42. Diuretics that increase the delivery of poorly absorbed solute to the thick ascending limb of the nephron include
(A) Furosemide
(B) Indapamide
(C) Mannitol
(D) Spironolactone
(E) All of the above

Items 43–44. A 65-year-old man with cardiomyopathy has recurrent congestive heart failure. Addition of digitalis to his regimen is being considered.

43. In a patient receiving digoxin for congestive heart failure, conditions that may facilitate the appearance of toxicity include
(A) Hyperkalemia
(B) Hypernatremia
(C) Hypocalcemia
(D) Hypomagnesemia
(E) All of the above

44. The primary cause of digitalis toxicity is
(A) Intracellular calcium overload
(B) Intracellular potassium overload
(C) Increased parasympathetic activity
(D) Increased adrenocorticosteroid levels
(E) All of the above

45. Methylxanthine drugs such as aminophylline cause which one of the following?
(A) Vasoconstriction in many vascular beds
(B) Decrease in the amount of cAMP in mast cells
(C) Bronchodilation
(D) Activation of the enzyme phosphodiesterase
(E) Sedation

46. Drugs used in asthma that often cause tachycardia and tremor include
(A) Beclomethasone
(B) Cromolyn sodium
(C) Ipratropium
(D) Metaproterenol
(E) All of the above

47. The drug with the most useful effects in the treatment of inoperable metastatic pheochromocytoma secreting mostly norepinephrine is:
(A) Clonidine
(B) Minoxidil
(C) Phenoxybenzamine
(D) Propranolol
(E) Reserpine

48. Agents that can readily cause edema if released or injected near capillaries include
(A) Angiotensin II
(B) Epinephrine
(C) Histamine
(D) Norepinephrine
(D) Serotonin

49. Typical results of beta-receptor activation include which one of the following?
(A) Hypoglycemia
(B) Lipolysis
(C) Glycogen synthesis
(D) Decreased skeletal muscle tremor
(E) Decreased renin secretion

50. A patient has been taking aspirin for rheumatoid arthritis for 8 years. Exacerbations are becoming worse and she asks the physician about drugs that might stop the progression of the disease. Which one of the following is not a disease-modifying (slow-acting) antirheumatic drug?

(A) Auranofin
(B) Hydroxychloroquine
(C) Methotrexate
(D) Penicillamine
(E) Rofecoxib

51. A neuronal cell body is located in the raphe nuclei with fine axonal projections to most brain levels. The neurotransmitter that it releases, which can be either excitatory or inhibitory, is most likely to be

(A) Acetylcholine
(B) Dopamine
(C) Glutamic acid
(D) Norepinephrine
(E) Serotonin

Items 52–53. A 40-year-old man had been consuming alcoholic beverages at lunch and in the evenings all his adult life. During the last 2 years, his alcohol consumption had steadily increased, continuing throughout the day. In response to family pressures, he abruptly stopped drinking alcohol, and within a few hours he became increasingly anxious and agitated and showed symptoms of autonomic hyperexcitability. He developed a hand tremor and the following day had delusions and visual hallucinations. At this point he was brought to the hospital.

52. Which of the following statements about the chronic consumption of alcohol in this patient is MOST accurate?

(A) Because of his gender, he is more susceptible to hepatotoxicity than a female in the same situation
(B) Intravenous thiamine will reverse the symptoms he is experiencing
(C) The rate of his metabolism of ethanol is dependent on its blood level
(D) He is probably tolerant to ethanol as a result of an increase in the activity of liver alcohol dehydrogenase
(E) Delirium tremens would be an appropriate preliminary diagnosis of his present condition

53. In the emergency room, the symptoms increased in severity, with hyperreflexia progressing to seizures. He was given an intravenous injection of a drug which controlled the seizure activity and was then hospitalized. During the recovery period, the same agent was used in oral form with gradual dose-tapering. The drug most likely to have been used is

(A) Clonidine
(B) Diazepam
(C) Haloperidol
(D) Naltrexone
(E) Phenytoin

54. The pharmacokinetic characteristics of several hydantoin derivatives, each with anticonvulsant activity equivalent to that of phenytoin, were examined in phase I clinical trials. The rationale was to identify a drug with more desirable kinetic properties than those of phenytoin.

Drug	Oral Bioavailability (%)	Plasma Protein Binding (%)	Elimination Kinetics	Cytochrome P450 Induction
ABC	10	90	First order	++
DEF	90	50	First order	++
GHI	50	98	Zero order	None
JKL	85	10	First order	None
MNO	95	10	First order	++

Based on the data shown in the table above, which drug has the optimum pharmacokinetic properties for oral use in the management of patients with seizure disorders?

(A) ABC
(B) DEF
(C) GHI
(D) JKL
(E) MNO

55. Which of the following statements concerning anesthetic agents is most accurate?
(A) Anesthetic potency is quantitated by the minimum alveolar concentration (MAC) that causes 50% of subjects to fail to respond to a standardized painful stimulus
(B) General anesthesia is associated with increased blood pressure and total peripheral resistance
(C) If an anesthetic agent is very soluble in the blood, it will have a relatively fast onset of action
(D) Inhalational agents are used for long procedures because intravenous anesthetics are too toxic to use for more than a few minutes
(E) The state of surgical anesthesia is associated with complete muscle paralysis

56. A patient is to undergo day surgery for a short procedure, and intravenous anesthesia will be used. Which of the following statements about the intravenous anesthetic agents is MOST accurate?
(A) Emesis is more likely to occur with propofol than with other agents
(B) Hypotension is the major limitation to the use of ketamine
(C) Postoperative respiratory depression due to midazolam may be attenuated by flumazenil
(D) The main value of fentanyl is its ability to cause muscle relaxation
(E) Thiopental is likely to increase cerebral blood flow

57. A patient with terminal cancer is suffering from pain that is gradually increasing in intensity. In the management of pain in such a patient
(A) Physical dependency occurs universally in the later stages of the disease
(B) To delay the development of dependency, opioid analgesics should never be given for initial management of chronic pain
(C) Meperidine is more effective than morphine in cancer pain states
(D) Nonsteroidal anti-inflammatory drugs may control symptoms during a significant portion of the course of the disease
(E) The placebo effect is absent

58. Which one of the following effects of the opioid analgesics is most likely to be mediated via activation of mu receptors?
(A) Cough suppression
(B) Elevation of arterial P_{CO_2}
(C) Emesis
(D) Sedation
(E) Vasodilation

59. Recreational use of drugs sometimes leads to dependence. Which of the following is LEAST likely to cause physical dependence?
(A) Amphetamine
(B) Cocaine
(C) Heroin
(D) Mescaline
(E) Secobarbital

60. This agent is currently a first-choice drug in the management of absence seizures as well as partial, primary generalized, and tonic-clonic seizures.
(A) Carbamazepine
(B) Clonazepam
(C) Ethosuximide
(D) Phenytoin
(E) Valproic acid

61. If one patient is taking amitriptyline and another patient is taking chlorpromazine, they are both likely to experience
(A) Excessive salivation
(B) Extrapyramidal dysfunction
(C) Gynecomastia

(D) Increased gastrointestinal motility
(E) Postural hypotension

62. The following data concern the relative activities of hypothetical investigational drugs as blockers of the membrane transporters (reuptake systems) for three CNS neurotransmitters.

	Blocking Actions on CNS Transporters for		
Drug	**Dopamine**	**Serotonin**	**Norepinephrine**
UCSF 1	+++	None	None
UCSF 2	+++	++++	++
UCSF 3	None	++	++
UCSF 4	None	+++	++
UCSF 5	+	+	None

Key: Number of + signs denotes intensity of blocking actions.

Which one of the drugs is likely to be effective in the treatment of major depressive disorders, but may also cause marked adverse effects including thought disorders, delusions, hallucinations, and paranoia?
(A) UCSF 1
(B) UCSF 2
(C) UCSF 3
(D) UCSF 4
(E) UCSF 5

63. A 38-year-old divorced woman who lived alone visited a psychiatrist because she was depressed. Her symptoms included low self-esteem, with frequent ruminations on her worthlessness, and hypersomnia. She was hyperphagic and complained that her limbs felt heavy. An initial diagnosis was made of a major depressive disorder with atypical symptoms. Treatment was initiated with amitriptyline, but after 2 months the patient had not improved significantly. Which one of the following drugs is MOST likely to have therapeutic value in this depressed patient?
(A) Buprenorphine
(B) Diazepam
(C) Paroxetine
(D) Methylphenidate
(E) Risperidone

64. Psychiatric evaluation of a patient after 6 weeks of treatment with a monoamine oxidase inhibitor (MAOI) shows no improvement. The psychiatrist now writes a prescription for fluoxetine which the patient starts two days after her final dose of the MAOI. Since the MAOIs used as antidepressants continue to exert effects for 2 or more weeks after discontinuance, the most likely result of the administration of fluoxetine now will be to cause
(A) A rapid amelioration of her depressive symptoms
(B) Electrocardiographic abnormalities
(C) Extrapyramidal dysfunction
(D) The serotonin syndrome
(E) Weight gain

65. The phenothiazines have a variety of actions at different receptor types. However, they do NOT appear to interact with receptors for
(A) Dopamine
(B) Histamine
(C) Nicotine
(D) Norepinephrine
(E) Muscarine

66. Which of the following statements about tardive dyskinesias is most accurate?
(A) Symptoms may be temporarily alleviated by raising antipsychotic drug dosage
(B) Their severity can be reduced by muscarinic receptor blocking drugs
(C) They occur during the first few weeks of treatment with antipsychotic drugs
(D) Clozapine is likely to exacerbate the symptoms
(E) They are parkinsonism-like movement disorders

67. A psychiatric patient taking medications develops a tremor, thyroid enlargement, and leukocytosis. The drug he is taking is most likely to be
(A) Clomipramine
(B) Haloperidol
(C) Imipramine
(D) Lithium
(E) Sertraline

68. The mechanism of action of benzodiazepines is
(A) Activation of $GABA_B$ receptors
(B) Antagonism of glycine receptors in the spinal cord
(C) Blockade of the action of glutamic acid
(D) Increased GABA-mediated chloride ion conductance
(E) Inhibition of GABA aminotransferase

69. A drug that is used in the treatment of parkinsonism and will also attenuate reversible extrapyramidal side effects of neuroleptics is
(A) Amantadine
(B) Levodopa
(C) Pergolide
(D) Selegiline
(E) Trihexyphenidyl

70. Following a very large overdose of a benzodiazepine, a patient is admitted to hospital. Which one of the following is not likely to be of therapeutic value in the management of this patient?
(A) Administration of naloxone
(B) Gastric lavage if an endotracheal tube is in place
(C) Intravenous flumazenil
(D) Protection of the airway
(E) Ventilatory support

71. A 65-year-old man with bacteremia is to be treated with a combination of antibiotics. If amikacin is included in the drug regimen, it is not likely to be effective against
(A) *B fragilis*
(B) *E coli*
(C) Enterobacter species
(D) *K pneumoniae*
(E) *Serratia marcescens*

72. If an aerobic gram-negative rod causing bacteremia proves to be resistant to aminoglycosides, the mechanism of resistance is most likely due to
(A) Changed pathway of bacterial folate synthesis
(B) Decreased intracellular accumulation of the drug
(C) Drug inactivation by bacterial group transferases
(D) Induced synthesis of beta-lactamases
(E) Production of drug-trapping thiol compounds

73. The characteristics of once-daily dosing with aminoglycosides compared with conventional dosing protocols (every 6–12 hours) include
(A) Decreased drug uptake into the renal cortex
(B) Higher peak serum drug levels to MIC ratios
(C) Postantibiotic actions
(D) All of the above
(E) None of the above

74. Beta-lactamase production by strains of *Haemophilus influenzae, Moraxella catarrhalis,* and *Neisseria gonorrhoeae* confers resistance against penicillin G. Which one of the following antibiotics is most likely to be effective against all strains of each of the above organisms?
(A) Ampicillin
(B) Ceftriaxone
(C) Clindamycin
(D) Gentamicin
(E) Piperacillin

Items 75–76. A 36-year-old patient is hospitalized following injuries sustained in an automobile accident. After several days, he develops a urinary tract infection due to *Pseudomonas aeruginosa.*

Current drug treatment of the patient is limited to opioid analgesics and ibuprofen for pain. The patient's past drug history includes a severe skin rash following treatment of otitis media with cefaclor. The following data show the antimicrobial sensitivity of aerobic isolates from urine sources in the hospital.

	Percentage of Isolates from Urine Sources Susceptible to				
Organism	**Ampicillin**	**Ciprofloxacin**	**Tobramycin**	**Cefipime**	**Ticarcillin-Clavulanate**
E coli	50	99	98	100	50
K pneumoniae	5	100	99	100	50
P mirabilis	90	98	98	100	90
P aeruginosa	0	86	90	94	90
S marcescens	8	70	80	85	82
S aureus	13	67	0	0	13
S epidermidis	14	67	0	0	12

75. If a single drug is to be administered to this patient the most appropriate choice in terms of efficacy and safety is
(A) Ampicillin
(B) Cefipime
(C) Ciprofloxacin
(D) Ticarcillin-clavulanate
(E) Tobramycin

76. Since the mortality rate approaches 50% in patients who develop sepsis due to *Pseudomonas aeruginosa,* it is usually advisable to use a combination of antibiotics known to have synergistic activity against this microorganism. Which one of the following pairs of antibiotics is known to be synergistic against *Pseudomonas aeruginosa?*
(A) Ampicillin and tobramycin
(B) Cefipime and vancomycin
(C) Ciprofloxacin and ampicillin
(D) Tobramycin and ticarcillin
(E) Trimethoprim and sulfamethoxazole

77. A 24-year-old mother of a young infant is to be treated with ciprofloxacin for a urinary tract infection. In providing the patient with information about the ciprofloxacin which one of the following statements is false?
(A) Antacids taken concomitantly may interfere with oral absorption of ciprofloxacin
(B) Ciprofloxacin will also be effective against an accompanying yeast infection
(C) If she is breast-feeding, she should stop while taking ciprofloxacin
(D) Tendonitis has occurred in some patients
(E) The drug may increase stimulant effects of caffeine

78. A 19-year-old woman with recurrent sinusitis has been treated with different antibiotics on several occasions. During the course of one such treatment she developed a severe diarrhea and was hospitalized. Sigmoidoscopy revealed colitis, and pseudomembranes were confirmed histologically. Which of the following drugs, administered orally, is most likely to be effective in the treatment of colitis due to *C difficile?*
(A) Ampicillin
(B) Cefazolin
(C) Clindamycin
(D) Metronidazole
(E) Tetracycline

79. In the management of patients with AIDS, the sulfonamides are often used in combination with inhibitors of folate reductase. However, such combinations have minimal activity against
(A) *Escherichia coli*
(B) Nocardia species
(C) *Pneumocystis carinii*
(D) *Toxoplasma gondii*
(E) *Treponema pallidum*

Items 80–81. A patient with metastatic choriocarcinoma was treated first with methotrexate plus dactinomycin and subsequently with a combination of cisplatin and vincristine. In both regimens, drug dosage was maximized to a toxicity limit of a 2-log decrease in blood platelets. The effects of chemotherapy were monitored by urinary chorionic gonadotropin (UCG, U/24 h), as shown in the data below.

	Urinary Chorionic Gonadotropin (units per 24 h)	
Drug Regimen	**Initial**	**After Treatment**
Methotrexate plus dactinomycin	10^8	10^5
Cisplatin plus vincristine	10^7	10^3

80. Which one of the following statements about the data is MOST accurate?
- **(A)** The maximal effect of methotrexate plus dactinomycin was a 2-log decrease in UCG titer
- **(B)** The drug-induced changes in UCG titer are directly proportionate to decreases in platelet count
- **(C)** The maximal effect of the cisplatin plus vincristine regimen was a 4-log decrease in UCG titer
- **(D)** The effects of the anticancer drugs on UCG titer have a direct relationship to cell kill
- **(E)** The final UCG titer demonstrates that the patient was cured

81. Which one of the following statements about the drugs used in this case is false?
- **(A)** Cardiotoxicity is the dose-limiting toxicity of dactinomycin
- **(B)** Leucovorin rescue is used in patients treated with methotrexate
- **(C)** Methotrexate and vincristine are both cell cycle-specific drugs
- **(D)** Saline hydration will be employed during treatment with cisplatin to reduce its nephrotoxicity
- **(E)** The cisplatin plus vincristine regimen is likely to be neurotoxic

82. A 20-year-old foreign exchange student attending college in California is to be treated for pulmonary tuberculosis acquired while he was living in Southeast Asia. Since drug resistance is anticipated, the proposed antibiotic regimen includes ethambutol, isoniazid (with supplementary vitamin B_6), pyrazinamide, and rifampin. Provided that his disease responds well to the drug regimen and that the microbiology laboratory results show sensitivity to the drugs, it would be appropriate after 2 months to
- **(A)** Change his drug regimen to prophylaxis with isoniazid
- **(B)** Discontinue pyrazinamide
- **(C)** Establish baseline ocular function
- **(D)** Monitor amylase activity
- **(E)** Stop the supplementary vitamin B_6

83. Which one of the following statements about the pharmacodynamics of antifungal drugs is accurate?
- **(A)** Amphotericin B blocks the conversion of lanosterol to ergosterol
- **(B)** Flucytosine is currently the drug of choice for esophageal candidiasis
- **(C)** Griseofulvin inhibits hepatic cytochrome P450
- **(D)** Ketoconazole binds to ergosterol to form artificial pores in fungal cell membranes
- **(E)** Oral fluconazole is prophylactic against fungal meningitis

Items 84–85. A 20-year-old college student is brought to the emergency room after taking an overdose of a nonprescription drug. The patient is confused and lethargic. He has been hyperventilating and is now dehydrated with an elevated temperature. Serum analyses demonstrate that the patient has an anion gap metabolic acidosis.

84. The most likely cause of these signs and symptoms is overdosage of
- **(A)** Aspirin
- **(B)** Acetaminophen
- **(C)** Dextromethorphan
- **(D)** Diphenhydramine
- **(E)** Ethanol

85. In the management of this patient, which one of the following procedures is not likely to have therapeutic value ?
(A) Alkalinization of the urine
(B) Correction of metabolic acidosis and electrolyte imbalance
(C) Gastric lavage with an endotracheal tube in place
(D) Hemodialysis, if pH or CNS signs are not readily controlled
(E) Treatment with acetylcysteine

86. A young mother is breast-feeding her 2-month-old infant. Which one of the following drug situations involving the mother is MOST likely to be safe for the nursing infant?
(A) Doxycycline, for Lyme disease
(B) Metronidazole, for trichomoniasis
(C) Nystatin, for a yeast infection
(D) Phentermine, used for weight reduction
(E) Triazolam, used as a sleeping pill

87. Chemoprophylaxis for travelers to geographic regions where chloroquine-resistant *P falciparum* is endemic is best provided by
(A) Atovaquone
(B) Mefloquine
(C) Primaquine
(D) Pyrimethamine plus sulfadoxine
(E) Quinine

88. A cardiac Purkinje fiber was isolated from an animal heart and placed in a recording chamber. One of the Purkinje cells was impaled with a microelectrode, and action potentials were recorded while the preparation was stimulated at 1 stimulus per second. A representative control action potential is shown in black in the graph. After equilibration, a drug was added to the perfusate while recording continued. A representative action potential obtained at the peak of drug action is shown as the superimposed action potential (color). Identify the drug from the following list.

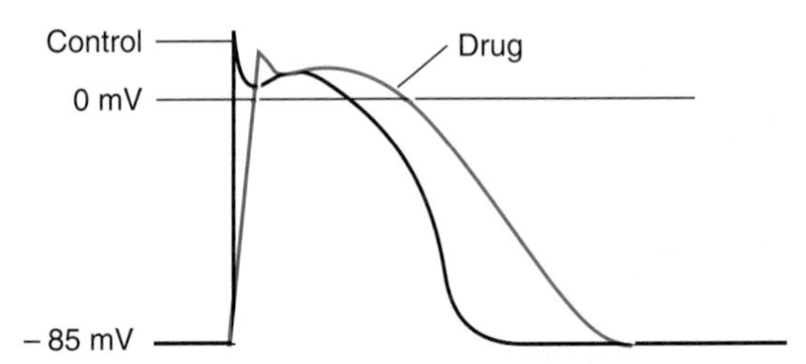

(A) Amiodarone
(B) Bretylium
(C) Diltiazem
(D) Flecainide
(E) Fluoxetine
(F) Lidocaine
(G) Nitroglycerin
(H) Propranolol
(I) Sotalol
(J) Verapamil

89. In patients with chronic granulomatous disease which of the following agents increases the synthesis of tumor necrosis factor, leading to activation of phagocytosis?
(A) Aldesleukin
(B) Cyclosporine
(C) Filgrastim
(D) Infliximab
(E) Interferon gamma

90. A 43-year-old woman was brought to a hospital emergency room by her brother. Visiting the halfway house in which she lived, he had found her to be lethargic, with slurred speech. The patient had a long history of treatment for psychiatric problems, and the brother feared that she might have overdosed on one or more of the several drugs that had been prescribed for her.

Physical examination revealed tachycardia with irregular heart rate, shallow respiration, decreased bowel sounds, dilated pupils, and hyperthermia. An ECG revealed a widened QRS complex with diffuse T wave changes. If this patient had taken a drug overdose the most likely causative agent was

(A) Clozapine
(B) Fluoxetine
(C) Lithium
(D) Thioridazine
(E) Zolpidem

91. Cocaine intoxication has become a common problem in hospital emergency rooms. Which one of the following drugs is not likely to be of any value in the management of cocaine overdose?

(A) Dantrolene
(B) Diazepam
(C) Lidocaine
(D) Naltrexone
(E) Nitroprusside

Items 92–93. A 30-year-old hospitalized AIDS patient has a CD4 cell count of 50/μL. He is being treated with a highly active antiretroviral therapy (HAART) regimen consisting of zidovudine (ZDV), lamivudine (3TC), and indinavir. Other drugs being administered to this patient include acyclovir, clarithromycin, foscarnet, rifabutin, and trimethoprim-sulfamethoxazole.

92. Which one of the following statements about the drug management of this patient is accurate?

(A) Acyclovir is highly effective in CMV infections
(B) Foscarnet has activity against TK^- strains of HSV
(C) Indinavir induces the formation of liver drug-metabolizing enzymes
(D) Pancreatitis is the dose-limiting toxicity of zidovudine
(E) Viral RNA will be undetectable in the blood of this patient

93. None of the drugs being administered to this patient are useful for prevention or treatment of opportunistic infections due to

(A) *Candida albicans*
(B) Cytomegalovirus
(C) *M avium-intracellulare*
(D) *Pneumocystis carinii*
(E) *Toxoplasma gondii*

94. After an all-night party, a 38-year-old man is brought to the emergency room at 5 AM by friends. In the early morning hours the patient had become very happy, excited, and talkative. An hour later he had become dizzy and quite pale and then vomited. Subsequently, his friends noticed that his lips and fingers were twitching and that he seemed to be hallucinating. In the hospital, the physical examination reveals a well-dressed, apparently affluent young man who is very agitated and incoherent. His blood pressure is 180/110 mm Hg, with a heart rate of 100/min and a respiratory rate of 20/min. Other signs and symptoms include pale and dry mucous membranes, mydriasis, hyperthermia, and increased deep tendon reflexes. The most reasonable preliminary diagnosis in this case is that the patient is intoxicated by

(A) Cocaine
(B) Ethanol
(C) Flunitrazepam
(D) Hashish
(E) Heroin

95. Which one of the following is LEAST characteristic of chronic lead poisoning?

(A) Acute tubular necrosis
(B) Infertility
(C) Hemorrhagic pulmonary edema
(D) Microcytic hypochromic anemia
(E) Radial nerve palsy

96. Which one of the following statements about reserpine is false?

(A) Blocks a carrier mechanism located in the membrane of synaptic transmitter storage vesicles
(B) Causes symptoms like those of a severe depressive disorder at high doses
(C) Derived from a botanical source

(D) Hypertension is an indication, but the drug is now rarely used
(E) Used in the management of pheochromocytoma

97. Which one of the following agents used in hypertension is a prodrug that is converted to its active form in the brain?
(A) Clonidine
(B) Doxazosin
(C) Methyldopa
(D) Nitroprusside
(E) Verapamil

98. Which one of the following statements about cocaine is false?
(A) Blocks sodium channels in axonal membranes
(B) Blood pressure increase is due to its ability to release norepinephrine from sympathetic nerve terminals
(C) Cardiac arrhythmias may occur at high doses
(D) Derived from a botanical source
(E) Topical application can provide local anesthesia and restrict bleeding

99. The consumption of shellfish harvested during a "red tide" (due to a large population of a dinoflagellate species) is not recommended. This is because the shellfish are likely to contain
(A) Arsenic
(B) Botulinum toxins
(C) Cyanide
(D) Saxitoxin
(E) Tetrodotoxin

100. Which one of the following statements about beta-adrenoceptor antagonists is false?
(A) One should avoid nonselective beta-blockers in asthma
(B) Both alpha- and beta-adrenoceptors are blocked by labetalol
(C) Glucagon can be useful in reversing cardiac depression caused by a beta blocker
(D) They mask the signs of developing hyperthyroidism
(E) Treatment of glaucoma commonly involves the topical use of propranolol

101. A 35-year-old female who has never been pregnant suffers each month from pain, discomfort, and mood depression at the time of menses. She may benefit from the use of this selective inhibitor of the reuptake of serotonin.
(A) Amitriptyline
(B) Bupropion
(C) Mirtazapine
(D) Paroxetine
(E) Trazodone

102. A 23-year-old heroin addict was brought to a hospital suffering from marked bradykinesia, muscle rigidity, and tremor at rest. Unfortunately, the extrapyramidal dysfunction was permanent in this patient, since he had self-administered this agent that is cytotoxic to nigrostriatal dopaminergic neurons.
(A) MDMA
(B) MPTP
(C) Ma-huang
(D) Meperidine
(E) Mescaline

103. Which one of the following statements about pentazocine is false?
(A) Analgesia is at least equivalent to that of codeine
(B) Causes sedation
(C) Classified as a mixed agonist-antagonist
(D) Full agonist at mu receptors
(E) May interfere with the analgesic effects of morphine

104. A 24-year-old schizophrenic man has been treated for several years with haloperidol but, since parkinsonism-like effects are worsening, the drug is discontinued and treatment is started with olanzapine. Which one of the following statements about the new medication is false?
(A) Antipsychotic effects may take several weeks to develop
(B) Alleviates some of the negative symptoms of schizophrenia
(C) Causes agranulocytosis

(D) Has a greater affinity for serotonin receptors than for dopamine receptors in the CNS
(E) Less effect on pituitary function than haloperidol

105. A 44-year-old patient suffering from alcoholism enters a residential treatment program that emphasizes group therapy but uses pharmacologic agents adjunctively. The patient is given a drug that decreases the craving for alcohol, possibly by interference with the neuroregulatory functions of opioid peptides. Since the drug will not cause adverse effects if the patient consumes alcoholic beverages, it can be identified as
(A) Bupropion
(B) Disulfiram
(C) Nalbuphine
(D) Naltrexone
(E) Sertraline

106. A 32-year-old woman presents with left lower quadrant abdominal pain and a purulent vaginal discharge which on Gram stain revealed gram-negative rods. A preliminary diagnosis is pelvic inflammatory disease. Which one of the following statements about the management of this patient is accurate?
(A) Aminoglycosides are active against anaerobes
(B) Cefoxitin has activity against *Bacteroides fragilis*
(C) Chlamydial infection in pelvic inflammatory disease requires the use of ampicillin
(D) A single dose of azithromycin is usually curative
(E) Patients with pelvic inflammatory disease must be hospitalized

107. This agent, which is used in the chemotherapy of Hodgkin's lymphoma, is potentially leukemogenic.
(A) Dacarbazine
(B) Doxorubicin
(C) Prednisone
(D) Procarbazine
(E) Vinblastine

108. Bleomycin is used in most effective drug combination regimens for the chemotherapy of testicular carcinoma. Which one of the following statements about the drug is accurate?
(A) Acts mainly in the M phase of the cell cycle
(B) Derived from the bark of yew trees
(C) Myelosuppression is dose-limiting
(D) Peripheral neuropathy occurs in more than 50% of patients
(E) Pulmonary infiltrates and fibrosis may occur

109. A high school student presents with headache, fever, and cough of 2 days' duration. Sputum is scant and nonpurulent and a Gram stain reveals many white cells but no organisms. Since this patient appears to have atypical pneumonia, you should initiate treatment with
(A) Cefazolin
(B) Clindamycin
(C) Erythromycin
(D) Gentamicin
(E) Trovafloxacin

110. Which one of the following statements about ciprofloxacin is false?
(A) Bactericidal against sensitive organisms
(B) Inhibits bacterial topoisomerases
(C) Resistant strains of gram-positive cocci are increasingly reported
(D) Safety in pregnancy has been established
(E) Tendonitis is a possible side effect

111. The drug of choice for the management of osteoporosis caused by high-dose use of glucocorticoids is
(A) Alendronate
(B) Calcitonin
(C) Mestranol
(D) Oxandrolone
(E) Vitamin D

112. The mechanism of action of cyclosporine involves
(A) Activation of calcineurin
(B) Binding to cyclophilin to cause inhibition of a cytoplasmic phosphatase

(C) Blockade of interleukin-2 receptors
(D) Inhibition of phospholipase A_2
(E) Suppression of bone marrow progenitors

113. Accidental poisonings are common with both aspirin and ibuprofen, two OTC drugs available in tasty chewable tablets. In cases of overdose, aspirin is more likely than ibuprofen to cause
(A) Autonomic instability
(B) Hepatic necrosis
(C) Metabolic acidosis
(D) Thrombocytopenia
(E) Ventricular arrhythmias

Items 114–115: An anesthetized subject was given an intravenous bolus dose of a drug **(Drug 1)** while the systolic and diastolic blood pressures (color) and the heart rate were recorded, as shown on the left side of the graph below. While the recorder was stopped, **Drug 2** was given (center). Drug 1 was then administered again, as shown on the right side of the graph.

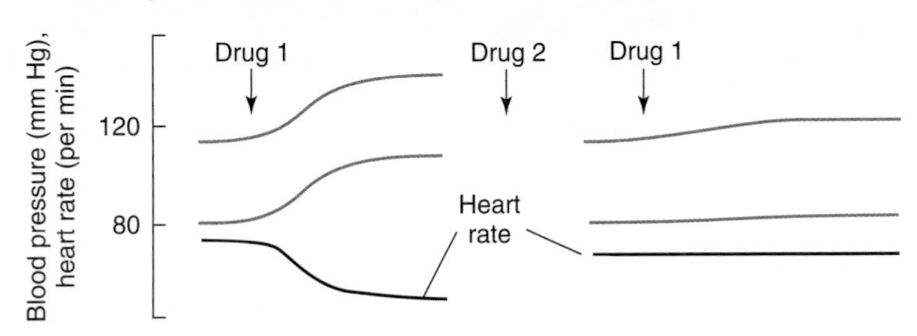

114. Identify Drug 1 from the following list
(A) Atropine
(B) Diphenhydramine
(C) Echothiophate
(D) Endothelin
(E) Epinephrine
(F) Histamine
(G) Isoproterenol
(H) Norepinephrine
(I) Phentolamine
(J) Phenylephrine
(K) Terbutaline

115. Identify Drug 2 from the following list
(A) Angiotensin II
(B) Atropine
(C) Bethanechol
(D) Diphenhydramine
(E) Endothelin
(F) Epinephrine
(G) Isoproterenol
(H) Norepinephrine
(I) Phentolamine
(J) Phenylephrine
(K) Terbutaline

116. Which one of the following statements about mebendazole is false ?
(A) It is a drug of first choice for hookworm and pinworm infections
(B) It causes the Mazzotti reaction, which is due to toxic products from dying worms
(C) It should be avoided in pregnancy
(D) It inhibits microtubule aggregation
(E) It has a high therapeutic index

117. In the treatment of hypothyroidism, thyroxine is preferred over liothyronine because thyroxine
(A) Can be made more easily by recombinant DNA technology
(B) Has a longer half-life
(C) Has higher affinity for thyroid hormone receptors

(D) Is faster-acting
(E) Is more likely to improve a patient's mood

118. Which one of the following statements about insulin secretagogues is false?
(A) Block potassium channels in pancreatic B cell membranes
(B) Chronic use leads to a decrease in glucagon
(C) Effective in both type 1 and type 2 diabetes
(D) Hypoglycemia can be severe with the more potent sulfonylureas
(E) Repaglinide has a rapid onset but a very short duration of action

119. A young woman seeks advice because she had unprotected sexual intercourse 12 hours earlier. Based on her menstrual cycle, she believes that conception is possible. Which of the following drugs should she use as a postcoital contraceptive?
(A) Clomiphene
(B) Diethylstilbestrol plus raloxifene
(C) Ethinyl estradiol combined with norethindrone
(D) Flutamide
(E) Letrozole plus finasteride

120. Regarding the thiazolidinediones used in diabetes mellitus, which one of the following statements is false?
(A) They are inducers of liver drug-metabolizing enzymes
(B) They interact with peroxisome-proliferator-activated receptors
(C) Hypoglycemia is a major problem when they are used as sole agents in type 2 diabetes
(D) They reduce both fasting and postprandial hyperglycemia
(E) Though rare, troglitazone has caused liver failure

Answer Key for Examination 1*

1. D (5)
2. B (1)
3. B (26)
4. B (9, 13, 20)
5. A (17)
6. C (16)
7. E (14)
8. E (14, 15)
9. A (11, 15)
10. A (7)
11. C (7)
12. B (3)
13. D (1)
14. C (6, 9)
15. C (27)
16. A (8)
17. B (36)
18. B (15)
19. E (33)
20. A (34)
21. C (11, 12)
22. B (12)
23. B (18)
24. A (18, 19)
25. A (20)
26. C (36)
27. C (2)
28. C (1)
29. B (3)
30. C (41)
31. A (6, 8, 9)
32. A (33)
33. B (2)
34. D (9)
35. C (8)
36. D (34)
37. B (40)
38. E (10)
39. E (12)
40. E (12)
41. A (15)
42. C (15)
43. D (13)
44. A (13)
45. C (20)
46. D (20)
47. C (10, 11)
48. C (16)
49. B (9)
50. E (36)
51. E (21)
52. E (23, 32)
53. B (22, 23, 59)
54. D (3, 24)
55. A (25)
56. C (22, 25)
57. D (31, 36)
58. B (31)
59. D (32)
60. E (24)
61. E (29, 30)
62. B (29, 30)
63. C (30)
64. D (30)
65. C (29)
66. A (29)
67. D (29)
68. D (21, 22)
69. E (28, 29)
70. A (22, 59)
71. A (45, 51)
72. C (45)
73. D (45)
74. B (43, 51)
75. E (43, 51)
76. D (43, 45)
77. B (46)
78. D (43, 50, 51)
79. E (46, 53)
80. C (55)
81. A (55)
82. B (47)
83. E (48)
84. A (36, 59)
85. E (59)
86. C (48)
87. B (53)
88. A (14)
89. E (56)
90. D (30, 59)

* Numbers in parentheses are chapters in which answers may be found.

91. D (58)
92. B (49)
93. A (48, 49)
94. A (32, 59)
95. C (58, 59)
96. E (6, 11)
97. C (11)
98. B (6, 9)
99. D (6)
100. E (10, 11, 12)
101. D (30)
102. B (28, 32)
103. D (31)
104. C (29)
105. D (23, 31, 32)
106. B (43, 51)
107. D (55)
108. E (55)
109. C (44, 51)
110. D (46)
111. A (42)
112. B (56)
113. C (36, 57)
114. J (9)
115. I (10)
116. B (54)
117. B (38)
118. C (41)
119. C (40)
120. C (41)

Appendix III

Examination 2

DIRECTIONS: Each numbered item or incomplete statement in this section is followed by answers or by completions of the statement. Select the ONE lettered answer or completion that is BEST in each case.

1. Which of the following is a common effect of muscarinic stimulant drugs?
- **(A)** Decreased peristalsis
- **(B)** Decreased secretion by salivary glands
- **(C)** Hypertension
- **(D)** Inhibition of sweat glands
- **(E)** Miosis

2. Which of the following statements about nitric oxide is false?
- **(A)** Nitric oxide is synthesized in vascular endothelium and the brain
- **(B)** Nitric oxide is released from storage vesicles by acetylcholine
- **(C)** Nitric oxide is released from exogenous molecules, eg, nitrates and nitroprusside
- **(D)** Nitric oxide synthase is stimulated by histamine
- **(E)** Nitric oxide synthase exists in both inducible and constitutive forms

3. With regard to distribution of a drug from the blood into tissues
- **(A)** Blood flow to the tissue is an important determinant
- **(B)** Solubility of the drug in the tissue is an important determinant
- **(C)** Concentration of the drug in the blood is an important determinant
- **(D)** Size (volume) of the tissue is an important determinant
- **(E)** All of the above are important determinants

4. Receptors that communicate their activation by turning on an integral intracellular tyrosine kinase are typically
- **(A)** Acetylcholine nicotinic receptors
- **(B)** G protein-coupled
- **(C)** Insulin or epidermal growth factor receptors
- **(D)** Steroid receptors
- **(E)** Vitamin D receptors

5. A patient with an arrhythmia is to receive lidocaine by constant IV infusion. The target plasma concentration is 3 mg/L. The pharmacokinetic parameters for lidocaine in the general population are V_d 70 L, CL 35 L/h, and $t_{1/2}$ 1.4 hours. An infusion is begun. The plasma concentration of lidocaine is measured 2.8 hours later and reported to be 1.5 mg/L. This indicates that the final steady state plasma concentration in this patient will be
- **(A)** 1.5 mg/L
- **(B)** 2.0 mg/L
- **(C)** 3.0 mg/L
- **(D)** 6.0 mg/L
- **(E)** Insufficient data to answer

6. A new drug is to be evaluated. Before human trials are begun, FDA regulations require that
- **(A)** The drug be studied in three mammalian species
- **(B)** All acute and chronic animal toxicity data be submitted to the FDA
- **(C)** The drug must be shown to be safe in animals with the target disease
- **(D)** The drug must be shown to be free of carcinogenic effects
- **(E)** The effect of the drug on reproduction must be studied in at least two animal species

7. A drug that blocks the heart rate effect of a slow IV infusion of phenylephrine is

(A) Atropine
(B) Haloperidol
(C) Physostigmine
(D) Pilocarpine
(E) Propranolol

8. A patient is admitted to the emergency room with orthostatic hypotension and evidence of marked GI bleeding. Which of the following most accurately describes the probable autonomic response to this bleeding?
(A) Slow heart rate, dilated pupils, damp skin
(B) Rapid heart rate, dilated pupils, damp skin
(C) Slow heart rate, dry skin, increased bowel sounds
(D) Rapid heart rate, dry skin, constricted pupils, increased bowel sounds
(E) Rapid heart rate, constricted pupils, warm skin

9. A 65-year-old man has open-angle glaucoma. The drug LEAST likely to have therapeutic value for this condition is
(A) Acetazolamide
(B) Epinephrine
(C) Isoproterenol
(D) Pilocarpine
(E) Timolol

10. A new drug was administered to a group of normal volunteers. Intravenous bolus doses produced the changes in blood pressure and heart rate shown in the graph below. The most probable receptor affinities of this new drug are
(A) α_1, α_2, and β_1
(B) α_1 and α_2 only
(C) β_1 and β_2 only
(D) Muscarinic M_3 only
(E) Nicotinic N_N only

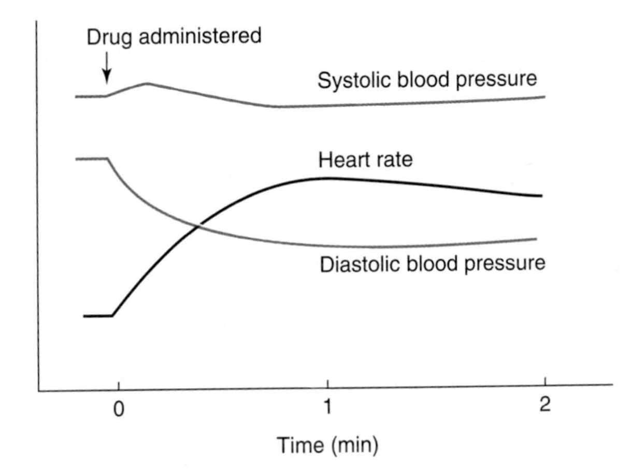

11. A 14-year-old boy is developing signs of anaphylaxis after an injection of penicillin in the doctor's office. If an intramuscular injection of epinephrine is administered, which of the following is LEAST likely?
(A) Bronchodilation
(B) Hyperkalemia
(C) Hypoglycemia
(D) Leukocytosis
(E) Tachycardia

12. Infusion of phentolamine into the cerebrospinal fluid of an experimental animal will prevent the blood pressure-lowering action of
(A) Clonidine
(B) Enalapril
(C) Guanethidine

(D) Reserpine
(E) Trimethaphan

Items 13–14: A 52-year-old plumber comes to the office with a complaint of periodic onset of chest pain, described as a sensation of heavy pressure over the sternum that comes on when he exercises and disappears within 15 minutes when he stops. After a full physical examination and further evaluation, you make the diagnosis of angina of effort.

13. In considering medical therapy for this patient, which of the following correctly describes the beneficial action of nitroglycerin in this condition?
(A) Dilation of coronary arterioles reduces resistance and increases coronary flow through ischemic tissue
(B) Dilation of peripheral arterioles increases cardiac work
(C) Dilation of systemic veins results in decreased diastolic cardiac size
(D) Increased sympathetic outflow increases coronary flow
(E) Tachycardia increases diastolic coronary flow

14. A drug that is useful in angina but causes constipation, edema, and increased cardiac size is
(A) Diltiazem
(B) Hydralazine
(C) Isosorbide dinitrate
(D) Nitroglycerin
(E) Propranolol

15. A drug suitable for producing a brief (5- to 15-minute) increase in cardiac vagal tone is
(A) Digoxin
(B) Edrophonium
(C) Ergotamine
(D) Pralidoxime
(E) Pyridostigmine

16. A patient with a 30-year history of type 1 diabetes comes to you with a complaint of bloating and sour belching after meals. On several occasions, vomiting has occurred after a meal. Evaluation reveals delayed emptying of the stomach, and you diagnose diabetic gastroparesis. Which of the following drugs would be most useful in this patient?
(A) Famotidine
(B) Metoclopramide
(C) Misoprostol
(D) Omeprazole
(E) Ondansetron

17. Drugs that block the α receptor on effector cells at adrenergic nerve endings
(A) Antagonize the effects of isoproterenol on the heart rate
(B) Antagonize some of the effects of epinephrine on the blood pressure
(C) Antagonize the effects of epinephrine on adenylyl cyclase
(D) Cause mydriasis
(E) Decrease blood glucose levels

Items 18–19: A 47-year-old sales associate has developed cardiomyopathy with severe congestive heart failure and digoxin is prescribed for his condition. In addition to the signs and symptoms of heart failure, he has become very depressed about his poor prognosis.

18. The most accurate description of the mechanism of action of digitalis in congestive heart failure is that
(A) Reduction of the inward sodium gradient results in increased calcium stores in sarcoplasmic reticulum
(B) Blockade of the sodium pump results in increased calcium entry through calcium channels
(C) Blockade of potassium transport results in increased intracellular potassium
(D) Actin-myosin filaments are sensitized to calcium
(E) Increased inward trigger calcium influx causes increased release of calcium from the sarcoplasmic reticulum

19. Six months after starting digoxin therapy, the patient attempts suicide by swallowing 75 digoxin tablets (0.25 mg each). He is discovered by his wife and brought to the emergency

room by paramedics. His blood pressure is 100/50 mm Hg, heart rate 40/min, and respirations 15/min. Toxicity caused by suicidal digoxin overdose should be treated by
(A) Administration of digoxin antibodies
(B) Administration of phenytoin intravenously
(C) Administration of sodium bicarbonate
(D) Lowering the serum magnesium
(E) Raising the serum potassium to 7 meq/L

Items 20–21: A 70-year-old woman fell 2 years ago and broke her hip. Now she is to be treated for a blood pressure of 170/100 mm Hg.

20. When treating hypertension chronically, orthostatic hypotension is greatest with
(A) Clonidine
(B) Guanethidine
(C) Hydralazine
(D) Prazosin
(E) Propranolol

21. Which of the following is associated with orthostatic hypotension for the first few doses only?
(A) Clonidine
(B) Guanethidine
(C) Hydralazine
(D) Prazosin
(E) Propranolol

22. Which one of the following agents is LEAST likely to protect the upper gastrointestinal tract from ulcer formation?
(A) Antacids
(B) Celecoxib
(C) Cimetidine
(D) Misoprostol
(E) Sucralfate

Items 23–24: A 52-year-old woman is admitted to the emergency room with a history of drug treatment for several conditions. Her serum electrolytes are found to be as follows (normal values in parentheses):

Na^+: 140 meq/L (135–145) K^+: 3 meq/L (3.5–5)
Cl^-: 100 meq/L (98–107) pH: 7.50 (7.31–7.41)

23. This patient has probably been taking
(A) Acetazolamide
(B) Amiloride
(C) Digoxin
(D) Furosemide
(E) Quinidine

24. In view of the electrolyte panel shown (and regardless of its cause), the patient will be more sensitive to the toxic actions of all of the following drugs EXCEPT
(A) Digoxin
(B) Imipramine
(C) Procainamide
(D) Quinidine
(E) Warfarin

25. A drug that decreases blood pressure and has analgesic and spasmolytic effects when given intrathecally is
(A) Atenolol
(B) Clonidine
(C) Morphine
(D) Nitroprusside
(E) Prazosin

26. Ventricular muscle from a cardiac biopsy was prepared for transmembrane potential recording in an isolated muscle chamber. Action potentials were recorded before and after application of drug X. Identify drug X from the following list.

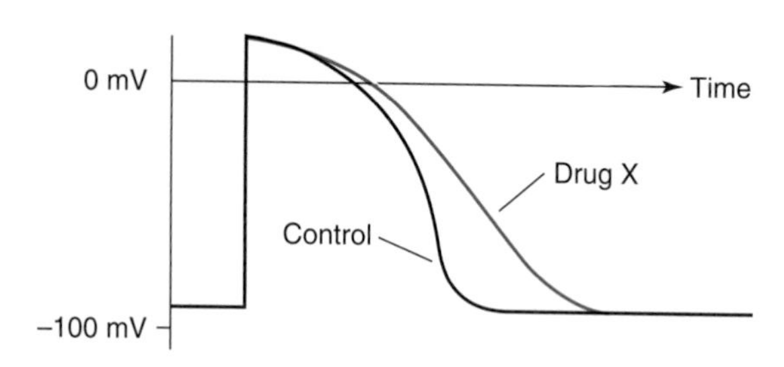

(A) Adenosine
(B) Esmolol
(C) Ibutilide
(D) Quinidine
(E) Verapamil

27. Propranolol and hydralazine have which of the following effects in common?
(A) Decreased cardiac force
(B) Decreased cardiac output
(C) Decreased mean arterial blood pressure
(D) Increased systemic vascular resistance
(E) Tachycardia

28. A 54-year-old farmer has a 5-year history of frequent, recurrent, and very painful kidney stones. Appropriate chronic therapy for this man is
(A) Furosemide
(B) Hydrochlorothiazide
(C) Morphine
(D) Spironolactone
(E) Triamterene

29. A 55-year-old executive has cardiomyopathy and congestive heart failure. He is being treated with diuretics. The mechanism of action of furosemide is best described as
(A) Interference with H^+/HCO_3^- exchange
(B) Blockade of a $Na^+/K^+/2Cl^-$ transporter
(C) Blockade of a Na^+/Cl^- cotransporter
(D) Blockade of carbonic anhydrase
(E) Inhibition of genetic expression of DNA in the kidney

30. Which one of the following peptides is not a vasodilator?
(A) Atrial natriuretic factor (ANF)
(B) Calcitonin gene-related peptide
(C) Endothelin
(D) Substance P
(E) Vasoactive intestinal peptide

31. Cyclooxygenase-1 and -2 are responsible for
(A) The synthesis of prostaglandins from arachidonate
(B) The synthesis of leukotrienes from arachidonate
(C) The conversion of ATP to cAMP
(D) The metabolic degradation of cAMP
(E) The conversion of GTP to cGMP

Items 32–33: A 16-year-old student has had asthma for 8 years. The number of episodes of severe bronchospasm has increased recently and you have been asked to review the therapeutic plan.

32. Which one of the following agents is LEAST likely to be of therapeutic value in an ordinary acute bronchospastic attack?
(A) Albuterol
(B) Ipratropium
(C) Metaproterenol
(D) Nedocromil
(E) Theophylline

33. Which of the following is a recognized toxicity of theophylline?
(A) AV blockade
(B) Bradycardia

(C) Convulsions
(D) Cycloplegia
(E) Dry mouth

34. Toxicities of local anesthetics do not include
(A) Cardiovascular arrhythmias and collapse (bupivacaine)
(B) Convulsions (lidocaine)
(C) Dizziness, sedation (lidocaine)
(D) Hypertensive emergencies, strokes (procaine)
(E) Methemoglobinemia (prilocaine)

35. Early in an anesthesia procedure which includes the use of succinylcholine and halothane a surgical patient develops severe muscle rigidity, hypertension, and hyperthermia. Management of this patient will almost certainly include the administration of
(A) Baclofen
(B) Cyclobenzaprine
(C) Dantrolene
(D) Naloxone
(D) Tubocurarine

36. A 56-year-old man is admitted to the coronary care unit with myocardial infarction. You would like to attempt dissolution of the coronary occlusion with a thrombolytic agent. Recent medical history includes a streptococcal throat infection (1 month previously) and hemorrhage from a tooth socket following a difficult extraction (6 months previously). His problem list includes renal parenchymal disease. He has been taking aspirin, one 325-mg tablet daily, for the last 6 years. Which of the following is most correct?
(A) Because of his history of bleeding, all thrombolytics are contraindicated
(B) Because of his history of strep infection, alteplase carries a high risk of anaphylaxis
(C) Because of his history of strep infection, streptokinase will be less effective than would otherwise be expected
(D) Thrombolytics would be extremely hazardous in this patient because of his recent consumption of aspirin
(E) Urokinase should not be used in a patient with a history of renal disease

37. Which of the following drugs is correctly associated with its clinical application?
(A) Erythropoietin: Macrocytic anemia
(B) Filgrastim: Thrombocytopenia due to myelocytic leukemia
(C) Iron dextran: Severe macrocytic anemia
(D) Ferrous sulfate: Microcytic anemia of pregnancy
(E) Folic acid: Hemochromatosis

38. Regarding trimethoprim-sulfamethoxazole (TMP-SMZ), which one of the following statements is false?
(A) Active against some strains of MRSA
(B) Bactericidal actions occur through sequential blockade of folic acid synthesis
(C) Folinic acid will reduce hematologic side effects
(D) Respiratory tract infections often respond since TMP-SMZ has activity against pneumococci, *H influenzae,* and *M catarrhalis*
(E) The trimethoprim component of TMP-SMZ is responsible for the enhanced hypoglycemia seen with certain sulfonylureas used in diabetes

39. Which one of the following matches of antifungal agent: characteristic feature is LEAST accurate?
(A) Amphotericin B: Dose-limiting nephrotoxicity
(B) Flucytosine: Causes "thymine-less" death of fungal cells
(C) Ketoconazole: Inhibition of cytochromes P-450
(D) Itraconazole: Binds to ergosterol to form artificial membrane "pores"
(E) Terbinafine: Effective treatment of onychomycosis

40. The CD4 count of an AIDS patient drops below 200/μL and prophylaxis is initiated to prevent pneumocystis pneumonia. Which one of the following is LEAST likely to be effective?
(A) Atovaquone
(B) Pentamidine
(C) Primaquine
(D) Pyrimethamine plus sulfadiazine
(E) Trimethoprim plus sulfamethoxazole

41. Regarding antiparasitic drugs which one of the following statements is not accurate?
(A) Common tapeworm infections are usually responsive to praziquantel
(B) Diethylcarbamazine is effective in filariasis
(C) Ivermectin has been used for the mass treatment of onchocerciasis
(D) Metrifonate is the drug of choice for intestinal nematode infections
(E) Pinworm and whipworm infections respond well to mebendazole

42. This agent is the drug of choice in severe amebic disease and for hepatic abscess. It is activated to toxic intermediates by the pyruvate-ferredoxin oxidoreductase enzyme system present in the parasite.
(A) Diloxanide furoate
(B) Emetine
(C) Iodoquinol
(D) Metronidazole
(E) Paromomycin

43. A 14-year-old girl is brought to the emergency room of a hospital by her friends after being thrown from a horse and hitting a fence. She does not appear to be seriously hurt, but she does have dirty abrasions and scratches over her arms and face. The teenager does not recall any immunizations she might have received in early childhood but states that none have been given since she was 4 or 5 years old. This patient should be treated with
(A) A broad spectrum antibiotic
(B) Tetanus-diphtheria toxin
(C) Tetanus immune globulin
(D) Tetanus-diphtheria toxin and a broad spectrum antibiotic
(E) Tetanus-diphtheria toxin and tetanus immune globulin

44. A young patient with end stage renal disease receives a kidney transplant from a living related donor who is HLA-identical and red blood cell ABO-matched. To prevent rejection, the transplant recipient is treated with cyclosporine. Which one of the following statements about this immunosuppressant drug is false?
(A) Cyclosporine decreases activation of transcription factor for interleukin-2
(B) Cyclosporine has no direct actions on B cell-mediated immune responses
(C) Myelosuppression is dose-limiting
(D) Nephrotoxicity occurs in more than 10% of patients
(E) Seizures may occur in overdosage

45. Blizzard weather conditions have forced a family living on welfare to stay in their poorly ventilated apartment for several days. During this time, all family members have developed slight nausea, headache, and dizziness. When the youngest member of the family becomes confused, starts breathing rapidly, and then faints she is brought to the emergency room of the local hospital. The condition of this patient is most likely due to
(A) Glue sniffing
(B) Ingestion of lead-based paints (pica)
(C) Inhalation of carbon monoxide
(D) Malnutrition
(E) Sulfur dioxide poisoning

46. A young female patient using an oral contraceptive is to be treated for pulmonary tuberculosis. She is advised to use an additional method of contraception since the efficacy of the oral agents is commonly decreased if her drug regimen includes
(A) Amikacin
(B) Ethambutol
(C) Isoniazid
(D) Pyrazinamide
(E) Rifampin

47. Which one of the following statements about heavy metal poisoning is false?
(A) Acute necrotizing gastroenteritis may occur with ingestion of iron tablets
(B) Chelation with succimer is the standard management of copper poisoning
(C) Ingestion of flaking paint is a major source of lead poisoning in young children
(D) An odor of garlic on the breath and "ricewater" stools are signs of poisoning due to inorganic arsenic
(E) Pneumonitis may occur following inhalation of mercury vapor

48. Inhalation of carbon monoxide remains one of the leading causes of poisoning deaths in the

United States. Which one of the following statements about such poisoning and its management is false?
(A) Administration of oxygen (100%) via a tight-fitting nonrebreather mask should be instituted immediately
(B) A preliminary diagnosis would be confirmed by determination of the carboxyhemoglobin blood level
(C) Hyperbaric oxygen (2–3 atm) is usually recommended if the patient has electrocardiographic abnormalities, is unconscious, or is pregnant
(D) Permanent neurologic deficits may occur in survivors of severe poisoning
(E) Red mucous membranes and nail bed lunulae are present in over 90% of cases

49. Which one of the following statements about the fluoroquinolone group of antibiotics is false?
(A) Antibacterial spectrum of ciprofloxacin includes common pathogens of the urogenital system and the gastrointestinal tract
(B) Fluoroquinolones may interfere with collagen metabolism
(C) Levofloxacin has good activity against pathogens causing upper respiratory tract infections
(D) Resistance mechanisms include point mutations in the gene for DNA-dependent RNA polymerase
(E) Sparfloxacin causes a high incidence of phototoxicity

50. This neurotransmitter, located in the spinal cord, is inhibitory to motor neurons via an increase in chloride ion conductance
(A) Acetylcholine
(B) Dopamine
(C) Glycine
(D) Serotonin
(E) Substance P

Items 51–52: The research division of a pharmaceutical corporation has characterized the receptor blocking actions of five new drugs, each of which may have potential therapeutic value. The relative intensities of their blocking actions are shown in the following table. Since each of these drugs is lipophilic and can cross the blood-brain barrier, they are expected to have CNS effects.

Blocking Action on CNS Receptors

Drug	Adrenergic (Beta)	Cholinergic (M)	Dopaminergic (D_2)	GABAergic (A)
A	++	+++	+++	None
B	None	None	None	++++
C	None	++++	+	None
D	+	None	+++	+
E	None	+	+	+

Key: Number of + signs denotes intensity of blocking actions.

51. Based on the data shown in the table above, which drug is most likely to exacerbate the symptoms of Parkinson's disease?
(A) Drug A
(B) Drug B
(C) Drug C
(D) Drug D
(E) Drug E

52. Based on the data shown in the table above, which drug is most likely to lower the threshold to seizures
(A) A
(B) B
(C) C
(D) D
(E) E

53. A 20-year-old male who had become physiologically dependent following illicit use of seco-

barbital ("reds") is undergoing severe withdrawal symptoms including nausea, vomiting, delirium, and periodic seizures. Which one of the following drugs will not alleviate these symptoms?
(A) Buspirone
(B) Chlordiazepoxide
(C) Diazepam
(D) Midazolam
(E) Phenobarbital

54. Benzodiazepines are LEAST effective in
(A) Alcohol withdrawal syndromes
(B) Balanced anesthesia regimens
(C) Initial management of phencyclidine overdose
(D) Obsessive-compulsive disorders
(E) Social phobias

55. An individual has ingested an antifreeze solution containing ethylene glycol and is brought to a hospital emergency room. Which one of the following statements about this poisoning case is false?
(A) Dialysis is indicated in the treatment
(B) Ethanol is likely to be administered in management
(C) Metabolic acidosis is very likely
(D) Oxalate crystals may be present in the urine
(E) Visual dysfunction will include flickering white spots ("like a snowstorm")

56. Which one of the following drugs exerts its anticonvulsant effects by blocking sodium channels in neuronal membranes?
(A) Acetazolamide
(B) Carbamazepine
(C) Diazepam
(D) Gabapentin
(E) Vigabatrin

57. A young woman suffering from myoclonic seizures was receiving effective single-drug therapy with valproic acid. Since she was planning a pregnancy, her physician switched her to an alternative medication with less potential for teratogenicity. Which one of the following drugs is effective in myoclonic seizures but often makes the patient extremely drowsy at the dose level required for effective seizure control?
(A) Carbamazepine
(B) Clonazepam
(C) Ethosuximide
(D) Lamotrigine
(E) Topiramate

58. Regarding the pharmacodynamic actions of local anesthetics, which one of the following statements is most accurate?
(A) All local anesthetics with ester bonds are vasodilators
(B) Amides cause a high incidence of hypersensitivity reactions
(C) Protonated forms of such drugs readily penetrate biomembranes
(D) The ionized forms of local anesthetics cause a use-dependent blockade of sodium ion channels
(E) Type A alpha nerve fibers are highly sensitive to blockade

59. A patient is brought to the emergency room suffering from an overdose of an illicit drug. She is agitated, has disordered thought processes, suffers from paranoia, and "hears voices." The drug most likely to be responsible for her condition is
(A) Gamma-hydroxybutyrate (GHB)
(B) Hashish
(C) Heroin
(D) Marijuana
(E) Methamphetamine

60. A patient undergoing surgery is given a drug for muscle relaxation. The anesthesiologist notes a marked drop in blood pressure and an increase in airway resistance immediately after the injection. Intravenous administration of diphenhydramine quickly restores the patient's blood pressure and airway diameter. The muscle relaxant used was probably

(A) Atracurium
(B) Baclofen
(C) Diazepam
(D) Tubocurarine
(E) Vecuronium

61. The following table contains data on two properties of different compounds under study for use as inhalational anesthetics.

Properties of Inhalational Anesthetics

Anesthetic	Blood: Gas Partition Coefficient	Minimal Alveolar Anesthetic Concentration (%)
A	0.8	9.7
B	1.4	1.46
C	9.8	0.66
D	2.3	0.86
E	1.8	1.76

The agent most likely to have the slowest rate of recovery from its anesthetic action is
(A) Anesthetic A
(B) Anesthetic B
(C) Anesthetic C
(D) Anesthetic D
(E) Anesthetic E

62. Which one of the following statements about opioid analgesics is false?
(A) Analgesic actions of methadone are reversed by naloxone
(B) Codeine has antitussive effects at subanalgesic doses
(C) Morphine has limited oral bioavailability
(D) Nalbuphine is less likely to depress respiratory function than meperidine
(E) Tolerance to ocular and gastrointestinal effects develops rapidly during chronic use

63. Mental retardation, microcephaly, and underdevelopment of the mid face region in an infant is associated with chronic maternal abuse of
(A) Amphetamine
(B) Cocaine
(C) Ethanol
(D) Mescaline
(E) Phencyclidine

64. After ingestion of a meal that included sardines, cheese, and red wine, a patient taking an antidepressant drug experiences a hypertensive crisis. The drug most likely to be responsible is
(A) Bupropion
(B) Fluoxetine
(C) Imipramine
(D) Phenelzine
(E) Trazodone

65. Following a stroke, a 54-year-old man develops marked muscle spasticity. A number of spasmolytics could be used to reduce muscle spasm without significant loss of muscle strength. Which one of the following drugs would not be effective in this patient?
(A) Baclofen
(B) Cyclobenzaprine
(C) Dantrolene
(D) Diazepam
(E) Tizanidine

66. A 48-year-old surgical patient was anesthetized with an intravenous bolus dose of propofol, then maintained on isoflurane with vecuronium as the skeletal muscle relaxant. At the end of the surgical procedure, she was given pyridostigmine and glycopyrrolate. Postoperative pain was managed by parenteral morphine. Which of the following statements about the drugs used in this case is most accurate?

(A) Continuous infusion of propofol is contraindicated because of its emetic effects
(B) Glycopyrrolate protects against potential cardiovascular effects of pyridostigmine
(C) Muscle fasciculation due to vecuronium causes postoperative pain
(D) Pyridostigmine is likely to cause CNS effects
(E) Isoflurane has less skeletal muscle-relaxing effects than other inhalation anesthetics

67. A woman taking haloperidol develops a spectrum of adverse effects that include the amenorrhea-galactorrhea syndrome and extrapyramidal dysfunction, including bradykinesia, muscle rigidity, and tremor at rest. Her psychiatrist prescribes a newer antipsychotic drug that improves both positive and negative symptoms of schizophrenia with few of the side effects that result from dopamine receptor blockade. Since weekly blood tests are not deemed necessary the drug prescribed by the psychiatrist is probably
(A) Bupropion
(B) Clozapine
(C) Nefazodone
(D) Olanzapine
(E) Sertraline

68. Naloxone will not antagonize or reverse
(A) Analgesic effects of morphine in a cancer patient
(B) Drug actions resulting from activation of mu opioid receptors
(C) Opioid-analgesic overdose in a patient on methadone maintenance
(D) Pupillary constriction caused by levorphanol
(E) Respiratory depression caused by overdose of nefazodone

69. Which one of the following statements about the drugs used in Parkinson's disease is false?
(A) Adjunctive use of entacapone is based on its ability to inhibit catechol-*O*-methyltransferase (COMT)
(B) CNS side effects are reduced when carbidopa is used in combination with levodopa
(C) Pramipexole is a non-ergot dopamine agonist
(D) Response fluctuations ("on-off" phenomena) are common in patients treated with levodopa
(E) Selective serotonin reuptake inhibitors (SSRIs) should be avoided if the patient is taking selegiline

70. Five patients are scheduled for a short surgical procedure during which succinylcholine will be used for muscle relaxation. Selected blood laboratory values for each patient are shown in the table.

	Aspartate Aminotransferase	Urea Nitrogen (BUN)	Dibucaine (% Inhibition)
Patient No.	Normal Range 8–20 units/L	Normal Range 7–18 mg/dL	Normal 80%
1	28 units/L	12 mg/dL	78%
2	6 units/L	30 mg/dL	83%
3	13 units/L	14 mg/dL	18%
4	26 units/L	25 mg/dL	90%
5	18 units/L	6 mg/dL	64%

Which patient is most likely to experience a prolonged respiratory paralysis following the administration of a bolus dose of succinylcholine?
(A) Patient 1
(B) Patient 2
(C) Patient 3
(D) Patient 4
(E) Patient 5

Items 71–72. A young man comes to a community clinic with a urogenital infection that, based on the Gram stain, appears to be due to *Neisseria gonorrhoeae*. Questioning suggests that the patient acquired the infection while vacationing abroad. The physician is concerned about drug resistance of the gonococcus. He notes that the patient experienced an anaphylactic reaction to penicillin G administered intramuscularly 6 months earlier.

71. Which one of the following drugs is most likely to be effective in the treatment of gonorrhea in this patient and safe to use?
(A) Amoxicillin-clavulanate
(B) Ceftriaxone
(C) Clarithromycin
(D) Ofloxacin
(E) Tetracycline

72. The physician is also concerned about the possibility of a nongonococcal urethritis in this patient. Such infections are usually eradicated by the administration of a single dose of
(A) Azithromycin
(B) Doxycycline
(C) Erythromycin
(D) Tetracycline
(E) Trimethoprim-sulfamethoxazole

73. Which one of the following statements about the mechanisms of action of antibiotics is false?
(A) Binding of aminoglycosides to the 30S ribosomal subunit can block initiation of bacterial protein synthesis
(B) Cephalosporins bind to PBPs and activation of autolytic enzymes is contributory to their bactericidal action
(C) Fluoroquinolones inhibit bacterial topoisomerases II and IV
(D) Streptogramins are recently introduced inhibitors of bacterial nucleic acid synthesis
(E) Vancomycin inhibits the synthesis of precursors of the linear peptidoglycan chains of the bacterial cell wall

74. A 26-year-old woman with chronic bronchitis lives in a region of the country where winter conditions are harsh. Her physician recommends prophylactic use of oral tetracycline during the winter season. Which one of the following statements about the drug is false?
(A) Absorption from the GI tract may be decreased by milk products
(B) Decreased intracellular accumulation is a mechanism of bacterial resistance
(C) Elimination is predominantly via biliary excretion
(D) The patient should discontinue the tetracycline if she becomes pregnant
(E) Vaginal candidiasis may occur during treatment

Items 75–76: A 52-year-old insurance agent receiving chemotherapy for leukemia is given intramuscular cefazolin (500 mg) for treatment of pneumococcal pneumonia. Within a few minutes, he is wheezing, develops an urticarial rash, and his systolic blood pressure falls markedly. The patient recovers following the administration of epinephrine, dexamethasone, and fluids.

75. Which one of the following statements regarding this case is most accurate?
(A) A first-generation cephalosporin should not be used in a patient who is likely to be immunosuppressed
(B) Gentamicin would be more effective against pneumococci in an immunosuppressed patient
(C) It would have been preferable to use nafcillin in this patient
(D) Penicillin G is a more appropriate drug for pneumococcal pneumonia
(E) The reaction could have been avoided with a lower dose of the drug

76. Regarding the drug reaction in this case, which one of the following statements is false?
(A) It is likely that the reaction would have been less severe if a test dose (50 mg) of cefazolin was administered initially
(B) Reactions of this type are more frequent after use of the penicillins than with the cephalosporins
(C) Skin testing with a dilute solution of cefazolin is routinely used to detect hypersensitivity
(D) The reaction was IgE-mediated
(E) This was a type I allergic reaction

77. Which one of the following statements about the macrolide group of antibiotics is false?
(A) Cholestatic hepatitis is associated with the use of erythromycin estolate
(B) Clarithromycin has activity against *M avium-intracellulare*
(C) High tissue levels, prolonged half-life, and minimal liability for drug interactions are distinctive features of azithromycin
(D) Organisms sensitive to macrolides include gram-positive cocci, mycoplasma, and chlamydia
(E) Stimulation of the activity of hepatic drug-metabolizing enzymes commonly occurs during erythromycin treatment

78. A 30-year-old male patient who is HIV-positive has a CD4 count of 450/μL and a viral RNA load of 11,000/mL. His treatment involves a three-drug antiviral regimen (HAART) consisting of zidovudine, didanosine, and ritonavir. Nystatin had been used for oral candidiasis, but for the past week the patient has been taking ketoconazole. Because of weight loss, he has just started using dronabinol. Which one of the following statements about this case is not accurate?
(A) Bitter taste and GI distress with ritonavir impedes patient compliance
(B) Ketoconazole may increase blood levels of ritonavir
(C) Ritonavir decreases the blood levels of dronabinol
(D) Serum amylase activity should be monitored
(E) The anti-HIV "cocktail" of multiple drugs should slow progression of the disease

Items 79–80: A 73-year-old patient has chronic pulmonary dysfunction requiring daily hospital visits for respiratory therapy. She is hospitalized with pneumonia, and it is not clear whether the infection is community- or hospital-acquired.

79. If she has a community-acquired pneumonia, coverage must be provided for pneumococci and atypical pathogens. In such a case, the most appropriate drug treatment in this patient is
(A) Ampicillin plus tobramycin
(B) Ceftriaxone plus erythromycin
(C) Penicillin G plus norfloxacin
(D) Ticarcillin-clavulanic acid
(E) Trimethoprim-sulfamethoxazole

80. If she has a hospital-acquired pneumonia, coverage must be provided for coliforms, pneumococci, and anaerobes. In such a case, empiric treatment is likely to involve the parenteral administration of
(A) Amoxicillin-clavulanic acid
(B) Cefazolin plus metronidazole
(C) Imipenem-cilastatin
(D) Quinupristin-dalfopristin
(E) Vancomycin plus piperacillin

81. Which one of the following statements about the mechanisms of antiviral drug resistance is false?
(A) CMV resistance to ganciclovir can involve mutations in the gene for viral phosphotransferase
(B) Famciclovir is active against TK^- strains of HSV
(C) Point mutations in the gene for reverse transcriptase lead to zidovudine resistance
(D) Resistance to cidofovir results from changes in viral DNA polymerase
(E) There is incomplete cross-resistance between saquinavir and other protease inhibitors

82. A male patient with AIDS has a CD4 count of 50/μL. He is being maintained on a multidrug regimen consisting of acyclovir, clarithromycin, dronabinol, fluconazole, lamivudine, ritonavir, trimethoprim-sulfamethoxazole, and zidovudine. The drug most likely to provide prophylaxis against cryptococcal infections of the meninges is
(A) Acyclovir
(B) Clarithromycin
(C) Fluconazole
(D) Ritonavir
(E) Trimethoprim-sulfamethoxazole

Items 83–84. A patient with diffuse non-Hodgkin's lymphoma is treated with a combination drug regimen (BACOP) that includes bleomycin, cyclophosphamide, vincristine, doxorubicin, and prednisone.

83. Concerning the adverse effects of these drugs, which one of the following is least likely to occur?
(A) Cardiotoxicity
(B) Hemorrhagic cystitis
(C) Hypoglycemia
(D) Peripheral neuropathy
(E) Pulmonary fibrosis

84. Dexrazoxane is thought to protect against the distinctive toxicity of this drug used in the BACOP regimen.

(A) Bleomycin
(B) Cyclophosphamide
(C) Doxorubicin
(D) Prednisone

85. Following delivery of a healthy baby, a young woman begins to bleed extensively because her uterus has failed to contract. Which one of the following drugs should be administered to this woman?
(A) Desmopressin
(B) Octreotide
(C) Oxytocin
(D) Prolactin
(E) Triamcinolone

86. Which one of the following statements about antiandrogens is false?
(A) Estrogens can reduce circulating levels of free androgens
(B) Exposure of a pregnant woman to finasteride can cause feminization of the external genitalia of her male fetus
(C) Flutamide is an androgen receptor antagonist
(D) Leuprolide indirectly inhibits endogenous androgen synthesis
(E) Oxandrolone selectively blocks androgen receptors in bone tissue

87. Based on the data in the table below concerning the antimicrobial drug sensitivity of bacterial isolates, which one of the drugs listed appears to be the best choice for treatment of acute otitis media?
(A) Amoxicillin
(B) Ceftriaxone
(C) Ciprofloxacin
(D) Erythromycin
(E) TMP-SMZ

Antimicrobial Sensitivity of Aerobic Isolates from Non-Urine Sources

	% of Isolates Susceptible to				
Organism	**Amoxicillin**	**Ceftriaxone**	**Ciprofloxacin**	**Erythromycin**	**TMP-SMZ**
E coli	50	99	98	20	70
H influenzae	5	95	97	23	87
K pneumoniae	90	98	98	98	90
M catarrhalis	20	86	76	91	96
L pneumophila	8	20	48	100	88
S pneumoniae	13	97	85	90	39
S aureus	14	87	65	50	50

88. Relative to fexofenadine, diphenhydramine is more likely to
(A) Be used for treatment of asthma
(B) Be used for treatment of gastroesophageal reflux disease
(C) Cause cardiac arrhythmias in overdose
(D) Have efficacy in the prevention of motion sickness
(E) Increase the serum concentration of warfarin

89. Which one of the following drugs predictably prolongs the PR interval and increases cardiac contractility?
(A) Digoxin
(B) Lidocaine
(C) Propranolol
(D) Quinidine
(E) Verapamil

90. Which one of the following drugs inhibits the synthesis of thyroid hormone by preventing coupling of iodotyrosine molecules?
(A) Dexamethasone
(B) Ipodate

(C) Lithium
(D) Methimazole
(E) Propranolol

91. A patient suffering from the pain of terminal cancer requires administration of a powerful analgesic. If meperidine is used, the drug is not likely to cause
(A) Constipation
(B) Dependence
(C) Pupillary constriction
(D) Respiratory depression
(E) Development of tolerance

92. Which of the following is the drug of choice for management of cardiac arrhythmias that occur in digitalis toxicity?
(A) Amiodarone
(B) Lidocaine
(C) Propranolol
(D) Sotalol
(E) Verapamil

93. Which one of the following statements about drugs used in coagulation disorders is false?
(A) Activated partial thromboplastin time reliably measures the anticoagulant effect of low-molecular-weight (LMW) heparins
(B) Cimetidine increases the anticoagulant activity of warfarin
(C) Coumarin anticoagulants reduce the activities of clotting factors II, VII, IX, and X
(D) Heparins are safe to use in the pregnant patient
(E) Treatment with cholestyramine decreases the anticoagulant effects of warfarin

94. This compound reduces the need for platelet transfusions in patients undergoing cancer chemotherapy.
(A) Cyanocobalamin
(B) Erythropoietin
(C) Interleukin-11
(D) Iron dextran
(E) Tranexamic acid

95. A 54-year-old woman with severe hypercholesterolemia is to be treated with a combination of niacin and atorvastatin. With this drug combination, it is important that the patient be monitored closely for signs of
(A) Agranulocytosis
(B) Gallstones
(C) Lactic acidosis
(D) Myopathy
(E) Thyrotoxicosis

96. A drug was given as an IV bolus to an anesthetized subject while the blood pressure was recorded. The result are shown in the figure below. Systolic and diastolic blood pressures in response to **Drug X** are shown. Identify Drug X from the following list.

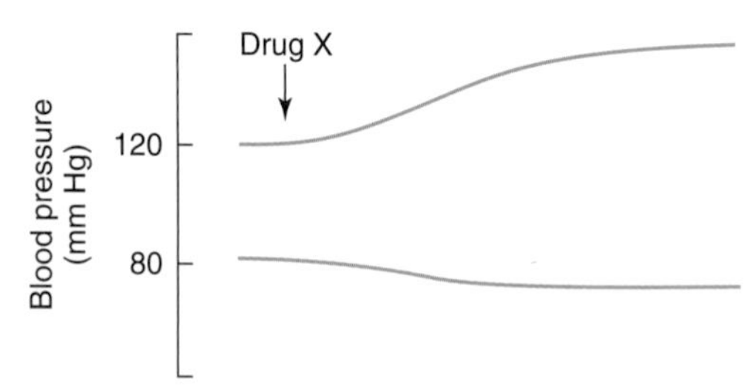

(A) Angiotensin
(B) Epinephrine
(C) Isoproterenol
(D) Norepinephrine
(E) Phenylephrine
(F) Terbutaline
(G) Tyramine

97. Which one of the following statements about hormone replacement therapy (HRT) regimens in menopause is accurate?
(A) It commonly includes a progestin to reduce the risk of endometrial cancer
(B) It has been shown in clinical trials to reduce migraine attacks
(C) It includes steroids that induce cytochrome P450
(D) It should be avoided in women with a history of diabetes
(E) It uses the same effective doses of steroids as those in combined oral contraceptives

98. Hypercoagulability and dermal vascular necrosis due to protein C deficiency is known to be an early-appearing adverse effect of treatment with
(A) Aspirin
(B) Clopidogrel
(C) Heparin
(D) Streptokinase
(E) Warfarin

99. Which one of the following drugs is most selective in preventing recurrence of peptic ulcers in patients using NSAIDs for rheumatoid arthritis?
(A) Aluminum hydroxide
(B) Metoclopramide
(C) Misoprostol
(D) Omeprazole
(E) Ranitidine

100. A 24-year-old man with a history of partial seizures has been treated with standard anticonvulsants for several years. He is currently taking valproic acid, which is not fully effective and his neurologist prescribes a new drug approved for adjunctive use in partial seizures. Unfortunately, the patient develops toxic epidermal necrolysis. The new drug prescribed was
(A) Felbamate
(B) Gabapentin
(C) Lamotrigine
(D) Tiagabine
(E) Vigabatrin

101. The introduction of this drug may represent a novel approach to the treatment of major depressive disorders since it appears to act as an antagonist at $alpha_2$-adrenoceptors in the CNS.
(A) Amoxapine
(B) Bupropion
(C) Citalopram
(D) Mirtazapine
(E) Paroxetine

102. Which one of the following statements about antiarrhythmic drugs is false?
(A) Adenosine is the drug of choice for cardioversion in patients with AV nodal arrhythmias
(B) Clearance of digoxin is increased by quinidine
(C) Procainamide causes a reversible syndrome similar to lupus erythematosus
(D) Pulmonary fibrosis and thyroid dysfunction are known adverse effects of amiodarone
(E) Torsade de pointes arrhythmias are often associated with drugs that prolong action potential duration

103. Which one of the following pairs of drug: indication is accurate?
(A) Amphetamine: Alzheimer's dementia
(B) Bupropion: Acute anxiety
(C) Fluoxetine: Insomnia
(D) Ropinirole: Parkinson's disease
(E) Trazodone: Attention deficit disorder

104. Which one of the following pairs of toxic compound: antidote is not accurate?
(A) Acetaminophen: Acetylcysteine
(B) Beta blocker: Glucagon
(C) Cyanide: Sodium nitrite
(D) Methanol: Ethanol
(E) Tricyclic antidepressants: Physostigmine

105. This cell cycle nonspecific agent is commonly used as a component of cancer chemotherapy regimens including those for non-Hodgkin's lymphoma and for breast cancers; administration of mercaptoethanesulfonate (mesna) decreases the risk of hematuria.

(A) Cyclophosphamide
(B) Cytarabine
(C) Fluorouracil
(D) Methotrexate
(E) Vinblastine

106. Regarding ritonavir, which one of the following statements is false?
(A) Blocks the enzymic cleavage of protein precursors needed for the formation of mature HIV virions
(B) Central adiposity and insulin resistance are potential adverse effects
(C) Myelosuppression is dose-limiting
(D) Potent inhibitor of the CYP 3A isoform of hepatic cytochrome P450
(E) Used with reverse transcriptase inhibitors in treatment of AIDS

107. Regarding drugs used for malaria, which one of the following statements is false?
(A) Chloroquine is the drug of choice for acute attacks of nonfalciparum malaria
(B) Cinchonism is associated with the use of quinine
(C) Hemolysis has occurred with primaquine in patients deficient in G6P dehydrogenase
(D) Mefloquine is used for prophylaxis in regions where chloroquine resistance occurs
(E) Quinine is safe to use in pregnancy

108. Which one of the following anticancer drugs acts in the M-phase of the cell cycle to prevent disassembly of the mitotic spindle?
(A) Dactinomycin
(B) Etoposide
(C) Paclitaxel
(D) Procarbazine
(E) Vinblastine

109. The dose of this immunosuppressive prodrug must be significantly reduced in patients who are also taking the xanthine oxidase inhibitor allopurinol.
(A) Azathioprine
(B) Cyclosporine
(C) Hydroxychloroquine
(D) Methotrexate
(E) Tacrolimus

110. While colchicine has been used in acute gout, the drug often causes severe gastrointestinal distress. Consequently, many authorities now consider that the drug of choice for acute gout is
(A) Acetaminophen
(B) Aspirin
(C) Indomethacin
(D) Methotrexate
(E) Sulfinpyrazone

111. The primary objective for designing drugs that selectively inhibit COX-2 is to
(A) Decrease the risk of nephrotoxicity
(B) Improve anti-inflammatory effectiveness
(C) Lower the risk of gastrointestinal toxicity
(D) Reduce the cost of treatment of rheumatoid arthritis
(E) Selectively decrease thromboxane A_2 without effects on other eicosanoids

112. A newborn was diagnosed as having a congenital abnormality that resulted in transposition of her great arteries. While preparing the infant for surgery, the medical team needed to keep the ductus arteriosus open. They did this by infusing
(A) Cortisol
(B) Indomethacin
(C) Ketorolac
(D) Misoprostol
(E) Tacrolimus

113. A 42-year-old woman requires treatment for diabetes insipidus following surgical removal of part of her pituitary gland. The advantage of treating this patient with desmopressin instead of vasopressin is that desmopressin
(A) Causes less formation of factor VIII
(B) Causes less hypernatremia
(C) Causes less hyperprolactinemia

(D) Is more selective for the V_2 receptor subtype
(E) Provides greater relief of the excessive thirst the patient is experiencing

114. Relative to Lugol's solution propylthiouracil has
(A) A faster onset of antithyroid action
(B) A greater inhibitory effect on the proteolytic release of hormones from the thyroid gland
(C) Increased likelihood of causing exophthalmos during the first week of treatment
(D) Increased risk of fetal toxicity
(E) More sustained antithyroid activity when used continuously for several months

115. Regarding verapamil, which one of the following statements is false?
(A) Angina pectoris is an important indication for the use of verapamil
(B) Contraindicated in the asthmatic patient
(C) Relaxes vascular smooth muscle
(D) Slows the depolarization phase of the action potential in AV nodal cells
(E) Used in management of supraventricular tachycardias

116. Raloxifene is a selective estrogen receptor modulator (SERM). Its characteristic properties make the drug MOST suitable for treatment of a female patient who
(A) Decides to start using an oral contraceptive
(B) Has postmenopausal osteoporosis and is at risk for breast cancer
(C) Needs postcoital contraception
(D) Suffers from hirsutism
(E) Wants a therapeutic abortion

117. Which one of the following drugs is most likely to cause hypoglycemia when used as monotherapy in the treatment of type 2 diabetes?
(A) Acarbose
(B) Glipizide
(C) Metformin
(D) Miglitol
(E) Rosiglitazone

118. Anticoagulation is needed immediately in a patient with pulmonary embolism. Since there is some concern about a possible drug-induced thrombocytopenia, the most appropriate drug for parenteral administration in this patient is
(A) Clopidogrel
(B) Enoxaparin
(C) Heparin
(D) Ticlopidine
(E) Warfarin

Items 119–120: A drug (**Drug 1**) was given as an IV bolus to a subject while blood pressure and heart rate were recorded as shown on the left side of the graph below. After recovery from the effects of Drug 1, a long-acting dose of **Drug 2** was given. After the recorder was turned back on, Drug 1 was repeated with the results shown on the right side of the graph.

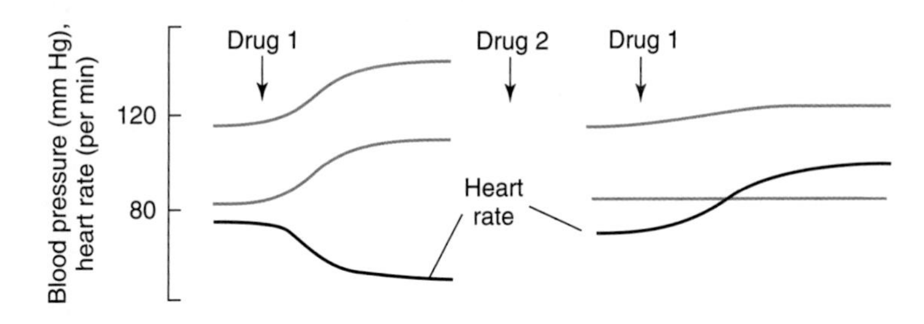

119. Identify Drug 1 from the following list.
(A) Angiotensin
(B) Endothelin
(C) Epinephrine
(D) Guanethidine
(E) Hexamethonium
(F) Isoproterenol
(G) Norepinephrine
(H) Phenylephrine
(I) Prazosin
(J) Propranolol

120. Identify Drug 2 from the following list.
(A) Angiotensin
(B) Endothelin
(C) Epinephrine
(D) Guanethidine
(E) Hexamethonium
(F) Isoproterenol
(G) Norepinephrine
(H) Phenylephrine
(I) Prazosin
(J) Propranolol

Answer Key for Examination 2

1. E (7)
2. B (19)
3. E (1)
4. C (2)
5. B (3)
6. E (5)
7. A (6, 8, 9)
8. B (6)
9. C (10)
10. C (9)
11. C (9)
12. A (11)
13. C (12)
14. A (12)
15. B (7)
16. B (60)
17. B (10)
18. A (13)
19. A (13)
20. B (11)
21. D (11)
22. B (36, 60)
23. D (15)
24. E (13, 14)
25. B (11)
26. C (14)
27. C (10, 11)
28. B (15)
29. B (15)
30. C (17)
31. A (18)
32. D (20)
33. C (20)
34. D (26)
35. C (25, 27)
36. C (34)
37. D (33)
38. E (46)
39. D (48)
40. C (53)
41. D (53, 54)
42. D (53)
43. E (62)
44. C (56)
45. C (57)
46. E (47, 61)
47. B (58)
48. E (57, 59)
49. D (46)
50. C (21)
51. D (21, 28)
52. B (21, 24)
53. A (22)
54. D (22)
55. E (23)
56. B (24)
57. B (24)
58. D (26)
59. E (32)
60. D (27)
61. C (25)
62. E (31)
63. C (23)
64. D (30, 61)
65. B (27)
66. B (7, 8, 27)
67. D (29)
68. E (30, 31)
69. B (28)
70. C (27)
71. D (45, 46)
72. A (44)
73. D (43–46)
74. C (44)
75. D (43)
76. C (43, 56)
77. E (44)
78. C (49)
79. B (43, 44, 46)
80. C (43, 44, 46)
81. B (49)
82. C (48)
83. C (55)
84. C (55)
85. C (37)
86. E (40)
87. B (43, 51)
88. D (16)
89. A (13, 14)
90. D (38)
91. C (31)
92. B (14)
93. A (34)
94. C (33)
95. D (35)
96. B (9, 10)
97. A (40)
98. E (34)
99. C (18, 36)
100. C (24)
101. D (30)
102. B (14)
103. D (28)
104. E (59)
105. A (55)
106. C (49)
107. E (53)
108. C (55)
109. A (55, 56)
110. C (36)
111. C (36)
112. D (18)
113. D (37)
114. E (38)
115. B (12, 14)
116. B (40)
117. B (41)
118. B (34)
119. G (9, 10)
120. I (10)

Appendix IV

Strategies for Improving Test Performance

There are many strategies for studying and exam taking, and decisions about which ones to use are partly a function of individual habit and preference. However, basic study rules may be applied to any learning exercise; test-taking strategies depend upon the type of examination. For those interested in test-*writing* strategies, the Case and Swanson reference is strongly recommended (see References).

FIVE BASIC STUDY RULES

1. Never read more than a few pages of dense textual material without stopping to write out the gist of it from memory. This is a universal rule for effective study. If necessary, refer to the material just read. After finishing a chapter, make up your own tables of the major drugs, receptor types, mechanisms, etc, and fill in as many of the blanks as you can. Refer to tables and figures in the book as needed to fill in your own notes. Make up and write down your own mnemonics if possible. Look up other mnemonics in books if you can't think of one yourself.* This is active learning; just reading is passive and far less effective unless you happen to have a photographic memory. Notes should be legible and saved for ready access when reviewing before exams.
2. Experiment with additional study methods until you find out what works for you. This may involve solo study or group study, flash cards, or text reading. You won't know how effective these techniques are until you have tried them.
3. Don't scorn "cramming," but don't rely on it either. Some steady, day-by-day reading and digestion of conceptual material is usually needed to avoid last-minute indigestion. Similarly, don't substitute memorization of lists (eg, the Key Words list, Appendix I) for more substantive understanding.
4. If you are preparing for a course examination, make every effort to attend all the lectures. The lecturer's view of what is important may be very different from that of the author of the textbook, and the chances are good that exam questions will be based on the instructor's own lecture notes.
5. If old test questions are legitimately available (as they are for the USMLE and courses in most medical schools) be sure to make use of these guides to study. By definition, they are a strong indicator of what the examination writers have considered core information in the recent past (also see 4 above).

STRATEGIES APPLICABLE TO ALL EXAMINATIONS

Three general rules apply to all examinations.

1. When starting the examination, scan the entire question set before answering any. If the examination has several parts, allot time to each part in proportion to its length. Within each part, answer the easy questions first, placing a mark in the margin by the questions to which you will return. Practice saving enough time for the more difficult questions by scheduling

* This book contains many mnemonics. Another good source is Bhushan V et al: *First Aid for the USMLE Step 1.* McGraw-Hill. (An annual publication.)

one minute or less for each question on practice examinations such as those in Appendices II and III in this book. (The time available in the USMLE examination is approximately 55–60 seconds per question.)

2. When answering multiple choice questions such as those on the USMLE, don't change your first guess unless you find a convincing reason for doing so.
3. Understand the method for scoring wrong answers. The USMLE does not penalize for wrong answers; it scores you only on the total number of correct answers. Therefore, even if you have no idea as to the correct answer, make a guess anyway; there is no penalty for an incorrect answer. In other words, *do not leave any blanks on a USMLE answer sheet or computer screen.* Note that this may not be true for some local examinations; some scoring algorithms do penalize for incorrect answers. Make sure you understand the rules for such local examinations.

STRATEGIES FOR SPECIFIC QUESTION FORMATS

A certain group of students—often characterized as "good test-takers"—may not know every detail about the subject matter being tested but seem to perform extremely well most of the time. The strategy used by these people is not a secret, though few instructors seem to realize how easy it is to break down their questions into much simpler ones. Lists of these strategies are widely available, eg, in the descriptive material distributed by the National Board of Medical Examiners to its candidates. A paraphrased compendium of this advice is presented below.

A. Strategies for the "Choose the One Best Answer" (of Five Choices) Type Question:

1. Many of the newer "clinical correlation" questions on the Board exam have an extremely long stem that provides a great deal of clinical data. Much of the data presented may be irrelevant. The challenge becomes one of *finding out what is being asked.* One method for rapidly narrowing the search is to scan the answer list *first* when confronted with a very long stem. The nature of the answers will provide a clue to the parts of the stem that are relevant and those that are not.
2. If two statements are contradictory (ie, only one can be correct), chances are good that one of the two is the correct answer, ie, the other three choices may be distracters. For example, consider the following:

   In treating quinidine overdose, the best strategy would be to

   (A) Alkalinize the urine
   (B) Acidify the urine
   (C) Give procainamide
   (D) Give potassium chloride
   (E) Administer a calcium chelator such as EDTA

   The correct answer is **(B)**, acidify the urine. The instructor revealed what was being tested in the first pair of choices and used the last three as "filler." Therefore, if you don't know the answer, you are better off guessing **(A)** or **(B)** (a 50% success probability) than **(A)** or **(B)** or **(C)** or **(D)** or **(E)** (a 20% success probability). Note that this strategy is only valid if you **must** guess; many instructors now introduce contradictory pairs as distracters. Another "rule" which should only be used if you must guess is the "longest choice" rule. When all the answers in a multiple choice question are relatively long, the correct answer is often the longest one. Note again that sophisticated question writers may introduce especially long **incorrect** choices to foil this strategy.
3. Statements that contain the words "always," "never," "must," etc, are usually false. For example,

   Acetylcholine always increases the heart rate when given intravenously because it lowers blood pressure and evokes a strong baroreceptor-mediated reflex tachycardia.

   The statement is false because although acetylcholine often increases the heart rate, it can also cause bradycardia. (When given as a bolus, it may reach the sinus node in high enough concentration to cause initial bradycardia.) The use of "trigger" words such as "always" and "must" suggests that the instructor had some exception in mind. However, be aware that there are a few situations in which the statement with a trigger word is correct.

4. Choices that do not fit the stem grammatically are usually wrong. For example:

   A drug that acts on a beta receptor and produces a maximal effect that is equal to one-half the effect of a large dose of isoproterenol is called a

   (A) Agonist
   (B) Partial agonist
   (C) Antagonist
   (D) Analog of isoproterenol

   The use of the article *a* at the end of the stem rather than *an* implies that the answer must start with a consonant, ie, choice **(B).** Similar use may be made of disagreements in number. Note that careful question writers will avoid this problem by placing the articles in the choice list, not in the stem.
5. A statement is not false just because changing a few words will make it somewhat more true than you think it is now. "Choose the one best answer" does not mean "Choose the only correct statement."

B. Strategies for Matching Type Questions: Matching questions usually test name recognition, and the most efficient approach consists of reading each stem item and then scanning the list of choices from the start and picking the first clear "hit." This is especially important on extended matching questions in which just reading the list can be time-consuming. (It should be noted, however, that the strategy suggested by the National Board of Medical Examiners for the USMLE differs from the above; see their *General Instructions* publication.) Occasionally, the strategies described above for the single best answer type question can be applied to the matching and extended matching type.

C. Strategies for the "Answer A if 1, 2, and 3 Are Correct" Type Question: This type of question, known as the "K type," has been dropped from the USMLE and therefore is no longer represented among the practice questions provided in this *Review.* However, it is still used in many local examinations.

For this type of question, one rarely must know the truth about all four statements to arrive at the correct answer. The instructions are to select

(A) if only (1), (2), and (3) are correct;
(B) if only (1) and (3) are correct;
(C) if only (2) and (4) are correct;
(D) if only (4) is correct;
(E) if all are correct.

Useful strategies include the following:

1. If statement (1) is correct and (2) is wrong, the answer must be **(B),** ie, (1) and (3) are correct. You don't need to know anything about (3) or (4).
2. If statement (1) is wrong, then answers **(A), (B),** and **(E)** are automatically excluded. Concentrate on statements (2) and (4).
3. The converse of 1 above: If choice (1) is wrong and (2) is correct, the answer must be (C), ie, (2) and (4) are correct.
4. If statement (2) is correct and (4) is wrong, the answer is **(A),** ie, (1) and (3) must be correct and you need not even look at them. (See example below.)
5. If statements (1), (2), and (4) are correct, the answer must be **(E).** You need not know anything about (3).
6. Similarly, if statements (2) and (3) are correct and (4) is wrong, the answer must be **(A),** and statement (1) must be correct.
7. If statements (2), (3), and (4) are correct, then the answer must be **(E),** and statement (1) must be correct.

No doubt more of these rules exist. In general, if you know whether two or three of the four statements in each question are right or wrong (ie, 50–75% the material), you should achieve a perfect score on this kind of question. The best way to learn these rules is to apply them to practice questions until the principles are firmly ingrained.

Consider the following question. Using the above rules, you should be able to answer it correctly even though there is no reason why you should know anything about the information contained in two of the four statements. The answer follows.

Which of the following statements is (are) correct?

1. The "struck bushel" is equal to 2150.42 cubic inches.
2. Medicine is one of the health sciences.
3. The fresh meat of the Atlantic salmon contains 220 IU of vitamin A per 100 g edible portion.
4. Hippocrates was the founder of modern psychoanalysis.

The answer is **(A).** Since statement (2) is clearly correct, and (4) is just as patently incorrect (let's give Freud the credit), the answer can only be **(A),** and statements (1) and (3) must be correct. (The data are from Lentner C [editor]: *Geigy Scientific Tables,* 8th ed. Vol. 1. Ciba-Geigy, 1981.)

REFERENCES

Bhushan V et al: *First Aid For The USMLE STEP 1.* McGraw-Hill, 2001.

Case SM, Swanson DB: Constructing written test questions for the basic and clinical sciences. Second Edition. National Board of Medical Examiners, 1998. Available only from the World Wide Web (www.nbme.org; Guide for Writing Test Items).

2001 Step 1 Content description and sample test materials. National Board of Medical Examiners, 2001. See also the USMLE World Wide Web page at www.usmle.org.

Index

NOTE: Page numbers in **boldface** type indicate a major discussion. A *t* following a page number indicates tabular material, an *f* following a page number indicates a figure.